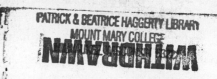

M A Y O · C L I N I C

Diet Manual

A Handbook of Nutrition Practices

MAYO · CLINIC
Diet Manual

A Handbook of Nutrition Practices

Jennifer K. Nelson, M.S., R.D., C.N.S.D.

Karen E. Moxness, M.S., R.D.

Michael D. Jensen, M.D.

Clifford F. Gastineau, Ph.D., M.D.

By the Dietetic Staffs of Mayo Clinic—Rochester MN, Jacksonville FL, Scottsdale AZ,
Rochester Methodist Hospital and Saint Marys Hospital—Rochester MN,
and St Lukes Hospital—Jacksonville FL

SEVENTH EDITION

with 33 illustrations

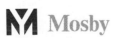
Mosby

St. Louis Baltimore Berlin Boston Carlsbad Chicago London Madrid
Naples New York Philadelphia Sydney Tokyo Toronto

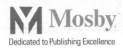

Mosby
Dedicated to Publishing Excellence

**A Times Mirror
Company**

Editor: Laura DeYoung
Project Manager: Linda Clarke
Book Design: Jeanne Wolfgeher
Cover Design: Margie Durhman, Mayo Clinic
Composition Specialist: Christine H. Poullain

SEVENTH EDITION
Copyright © 1994 Mayo Foundation
Previous editions copyrighted 1949, 1954, 1961, 1971, 1981, 1988

Printed in the United States of America

Composition by Mosby Electronic Production, Philadelphia
Printing/binding by R.R. Donnelley & Sons Company

Mosby–Year Book, Inc.
11830 Westline Industrial Drive
St. Louis, Missouri 63146

Library of Congress Cataloging-in-Publication Data

Mayo clinic diet manual: a handbook of nutrition practices / Jennifer K. Nelson . . . [et al.]. — 7th ed.
    p.   cm.
  Includes bibliographical references and index.
  ISBN 0-8151-6348-7
   1. Diet therapy—Handbooks, manuals, etc. 2. Diet in disease—Handbooks, manuals, etc.
3. Nutrition—Handbooks, manuals, etc.
I. Nelson, Jennifer K. II. Mayo Clinic.
   [DNLM: 1. Diet Therapy. 2. Nutrition. WB 400 M473 1994]
RM217.2.M38 1994
615.8'54—dc20
DNLM/DCL
for Library of Congress

93-43747
CIP

96 97 98 / 9 8 7 6 5 4 3 2

Contributors

J. Eric Ahlskog, M.D.
Parkinson's Disease

Virginia Anderson, R.D.
Cancer—Adult

Margaret R. Baker, R.D.
Cancer—Pediatrics
Diarrhea—Pediatrics
Enteral Nutrition—Pediatrics
Healthy Infants, Children, and Adolescents
Inflammatory Bowel Disease—Pediatrics
Nutrition in Transplantation
Pancreas Transplantation and Pancreas-
*   Kidney Transplantation*
Sick Infants, Children and Adolescents
Pediatric Appendix

Kathy Bates, R.D., C.N.S.D.
Enteral Nutrition—Adult
Adult Appendix

Marylin Borges, Pharm.D.
Parenteral Nutrition—Adult
Adult Appendix

Sheri Boyden, R.D., C.D.E.
Diabetes Mellitus—Adult
Food Exchange Lists for Diabetes
Adult Appendix

Jenny Buccicone, M.S., R.D.
National Cholesterol Education Program
*   Guidelines for Treatment of*
*   Hyperlipidemia*

Mary Ann Burke, Dietitian
Nutrition Screening and Assessment—Adult

Michaeleen Burroughs, M.S., R.D.
Potassium Control
Urolithiasis
Pediatric Appendix

Shawn Craig, R.D.
Congestive Heart Failure
Myocardial Infarction

Connie Davila, R.D.
Bariatric Surgery
Inflammatory Bowel Disease—Adult
Nutrition in Transplantation
Thoracic Organ Transplantation

Steve DeBoer, M.P.H., R.D.

Food Guide Pyramid
Geriatric Nutrition
Hypertension—Adult

Sara R. DiCecco, M.S., R.D.

Diarrhea—Adult
Hepatobiliary Diseases
Jewish Dietary Practices
Liver Transplantation
Low Bacteria Diet
Nutrition in Transplantation
*Pancreas Transplantation and Pancreas-
    Kidney Transplantation*

Susan Kraus Eckert, R.D.

Allergy—Pediatrics
Cystic Fibrosis
Failure to Thrive
Gluten Sensitive Enteropathy: Celiac Disease
Hyperlipidemia—Adult and Pediatric
Hypertension—Pediatric

Mary Ann Evans, M.S., R.D., C.N.S.D.

Enteral Nutrition—Adults

Kristine Fitzpatrick, R.D.

Cardiac Surgery—Adult
Low Bacteria Diet
Myocardial Infarction
Thoracic Organ Transplantation

Linda Foster, M.S., R.D.

Diabetes Mellitus
Food Exchange Lists for Diabetes Mellitus
*Hospital Diet Progressions: General Diet,
    Clear Liquid Diet, Full Liquid Diet,
    Pureed Diet, Mechanical Soft Diet, Soft
    Diet, Preoperative Diet, Postoperative
    Diet, Tonsillectomy and Adenoidectomy
    Diet, Intermaxillary Fixation Diet*
Adult Appendix

Marsha Sayre Frick, R.D.

Bariatric Surgery
Developmental Disability
Nutrition Assessment—Pediatrics
Young Athletes

Margaret Gall, R.D.

Hypertension—Adult
Obesity
Osteoporosis

Janet Gannon, R.D.

Dysphagia
Parenteral Nutrition—Adult

Joan Gartner, R.D.

Acute Renal Failure—Adult
Fat Malabsorption—Adult
*Gluten Sensitivity—Celiac Sprue and
    Dermatitis Herpetiformis*
Lactose Intolerance
Nephrotic Syndrome—Adult
100 Gram Fat Test Diet
Potassium Control

Stephanie Geinert, R.D.

Food Allergy and Intolerance—Adult

Cathy Glovka, M.S., R.D.

Pediatric Appendix

Janelle Gonyea, R.D.

Chronic Renal Failure—Adult and Pediatric
Constipation and Encopresis
Dialysis—Adult and Pediatric
*Food Exchange Lists for Protein, Sodium
    and Potassium Control*
Kidney Transplantation
Nephrotic Syndrome—Adult and Pediatric
Nutrition and Transplantation
Potassium Control
Urolithiasis
Adult Appendix

Carol Grover, R.D.

Hyperlipidemia—Adult

Heidi Gunderson, M.S., R.D., C.D.E.

Diabetes Mellitus—Adult
Dietary Guidelines for Americans
Food Exchange Lists for Diabetes
Adult Appendices

Lisa Harnack, R.D.

Diabetes Mellitus—Adult
Food Exchange Lists for Diabetes
Kidney Transplantation
Urolithiasis
Adult Appendix

Diane M. Huse, M.S., R.D.

Anorexia Nervosa and Bulimia Nervosa
Diabetes Mellitus—Pediatrics
Fat Absorption Test Diet—Pediatrics
Healthy Infants, Children and Adolescents
Hyperlipidemia—Pediatrics
Hypertension—Pediatrics
Inborn Errors of Metabolism
Ketogenic Diet
Low Birth Weight Infants
Maple Syrup Urine Disease
Phenylketonuria
Weight Control—Pediatrics

Denise Janzow, R.D.

Parenteral Nutrition—Adult

M.D. Jensen, M.D.

Obesity

Rita Jones, R.D., C.D.E.

Diabetes Mellitus—Adult
Food Exchange Lists for Diabetes
Adult Appendix

Martin E. Kochevar, R.Ph., M.S., B.C.N.S.P.

Parenteral Nutrition—Adult
Adult Appendix

Kathleen A. Krause, R.D., C.D.E.

Diabetes Mellitus—Adult
Food Exchange Lists for Diabetes
Nutritional Needs for Physical Performance
Adult Appendix

Maren Kryzer, R.D.

Cardiac Surgery—Adult

Audrey A. Lally, M.S., R.D., C.D.E.

Diabetes Mellitus—Adult
Food Exchange Lists for Diabetes
Food, Facts, Fads, and Fallacies
Irritable Bowel Syndrome
Adult Appendix

Therese Liffrig, R.D., C.N.S.D.

Nutrition Screening and Assessment—Adult
Adult Appendix

A.R. Lucas, M.D.

Anorexia Nervosa and Bulimia Nervosa

Noreen Lundberg, R.D.

Obesity

Peggy A. Menzel, R.D.

Hyperlipidemia—Adult
Food Labeling
Adult Appendix

Jean Mortenson, R.D., C.D.E.

Diabetes Mellitus—Adult
Food Exchange Lists for Diabetes
Nutritional Needs for Physical Performance
Adult Appendix

Karen E. Moxness, M.S., R.D.

Introduction to Nutritional Care
Tyramine Control
Adult Appendices

Jennifer Kay Nelson, M.S., R.D., C.N.S.D.

Diets in Preparation for Diagnostic Tests
Inflammatory Bowel Disease—Adult
Food Allergy and Intolerance—Adult
Adult Appendices

Yvette Newborn, M.S., R.D.

Vegetarian Diet—Adult

Helen Griffith-O'Connor, M.S., R.D.

Urolithiasis

Lavonne Oenning, R.D.

Copper Metabolism
Delayed Gastric Emptying
Sclerotherapy

F. Karen Olson, R.D.

Geriatric Nutrition
Tyramine Control

Diane L. Olson, R.D., C.N.S.D., C.D.E.

Glycogen Storage Diseases
Nutrition Assessment—Pediatrics
Parenteral Nutrition—Pediatrics
Vegetarian Diets—Pediatrics
Young Athletes

Kris Orton, R.D.

Cardiac Surgery—Adult and Pediatrics
Congestive Heart Failure
Nutrition Screening and Assessment—Adult

Rose Prissel, R.D.

Bariatric Surgery Diets
Obesity

Lorraine Reck, M.Ag., R.D.

Congestive Heart Failure
Myocardial Infarction

Marsha Andresen Reid, M.S., R.D.

Congestive Heart Failure
Myocardial Infarction

Sara Roberts, R.D.

Acute Renal Failure—Adult
Parenteral Nutrition—Adult

Charla Schultz, R.D.

Food Allergy and Intolerance—Adult
Geriatric Nutrition
Hypertension—Adult
Osteoporosis

Jacalyn See, M.S., R.D.

Abdominal Gas and Flatulence
Cancer—Adult
Delayed Gastric Emptying
Diet and Cancer Risk
Fiber and Residue Modification
Hyperlipidemia—Adult
Post-Gastrectomy Dumping Syndrome
Adult Appendix

Ann Skemp, R.D.

Chronic Renal Failure—Adult
*Food Exchange Lists for Protein, Sodium,
    and Potassium Control*

Susan Starkson, R.D.

American Heart Association Dietary Guidelines
Fat Substitutes
Geriatric Nutrition
Penicillin and Mold Controlled Diet
Recommended Dietary Allowances
Adult Appendix

Joan Vruwink, R.D., C.D.E.

Cancer—Adult
Bone Marrow Transplantation
Low Bacteria Diet
Nutrition in Transplantation

Constance L. Weber, M.S., R.D.

Irritable Bowel Syndrome
Parkinson's Disease

Jody Weckwerth, R.D., C.N.S.D.

Cancer—Adult
Enteral Nutrition—Adult
Adult Appendix

Rosemary White, R.D.

Cancer—Adult

Eve Marie Wiitanen, M.Ed., R.D., C.D.E.

Diabetes Mellitus—Adults
Food Exchange Lists for Diabetes
Geriatric Nutrition
Adult Appendix

Carol L. Willett, R.D., C.D.E.

Diabetes Mellitus—Adult
Food Exchange Lists for Diabetes
Adult Appendix

Stephanie V. Wood, R.D.

Chronic Renal Failure
Pregnancy and Lactation
Urolithiasis

Georgia Ziegler, R.D., C.D.E.

Diabetes Mellitus—Adult
Food Exchange Lists for Diabetes
Adult Appendix

Nickie Francisco-Ziller, R.D.

Esophageal Reflux
Peptic Ulcer Disease

REVIEWERS*

The following physicians, dietitians, nurses, pharmacists and healthcare professionals are thanked for their extensive reviews and helpful comments:

D.A. Ahlquist, M.D., Division of Gastroenterology and Internal Medicine

C.F. Anderson, M.D., Division of Nephrology and Internal Medicine

C.A.S. Arndt, Department of Pediatric and Adolescent Medicine—Hematology and Oncology

R.W. Beart, M.D., Department of Surgery, Colon and Rectal—Mayo Clinic, Scottsdale, Arizona

P.A. Burch, M.D., Department of Oncology, Medical Oncology

J.U. Burnes, R.N., M.S.N., C.N.S.N., Division of Gastroenterology and Internal Medicine

A.J. Cameron, M.D., Division of Gastroenterology and Internal Medicine

M. Camilleri, M.D., Division of Gastroenterology and Internal Medicine

*Unless otherwise specified the reviewers are staff of Mayo Medical Center, Rochester, MN

D.S. Chutka, M.D., Division of Community Internal Medicine

R.C. Colligan, Ph.D., Department of Psychiatry and Psychology

E.T. Creagan, M.D., Department of Oncology, Medical Oncology

A.J. Cunnien, M.D., Department of Psychiatry, Mayo Clinic, Scottsdale, Arizona

L.C. Dale, M.D., Division of Community Internal Medicine

K.R. DeVault, M.D., Division of Gastroenterology and Internal Medicine, Mayo Clinic, Jacksonville, Florida

D.J. Driscoll, M.D., Department of Pediatric and Adolescent Medicine—Cardiology

S.B. Erickson, M.D., Division of Nephrology and Internal Medicine

Richard Ferdinande, E.Sp., Department of Psychiatry and Psychology—Adolescent Psychiatry

P.M. Fitzpatrick, M.D., Division of Nephrology and Internal Medicine, Mayo Clinic, Jacksonville, Florida

C.R. Fleming, M.D., Division of Gastroenterology and Internal Medicine, Mayo Clinic, Jacksonville, Florida

W.N. Folger, M.D., Department of Neurology, Mayo Clinic, Jacksonville, Florida

T.P. Fox, M.D., Division of Endocrinology, Metabolism and Internal Medicine, Mayo Clinic, Jacksonville, Florida

Rabbi David Freedman, B'Nai Israel Synagogue, Rochester, Minnesota

M.A. Gertz, M.D., Division of Hematology and Internal Medicine

M.R. Gomez, M.D., Department of Pediatrics—Neurology

C.J. Gostout, M.D., Division of Gastroenterology and Internal Medicine

J.B. Gross, M.D., Division of Gastroenterology and Internal Medicine

R.I. Heigh, M.D., Division of Gastroenterology and Internal medicine, Mayo Clinic, Scottsdale, Arizona

S.F. Hodgson, M.D., Division of Endocrinology, Metabolism and Internal Medicine

R.F. House, Jr., M.D., Department of Pediatrics—Community Pediatric Service

D.L. Hurley, M.D., Division of Endocrinology, Metabolism and Internal Medicine

P.S. Kamath, M.D., Division of Gastroenterology and Internal Medicine

D.G. Kelly, M.D., Ph.D., Division of Gastroenterology and Internal Medicine

F.P. Kennedy, M.D., Division of Endocrinology, Metabolism and Internal Medicine

S. Khosla, M.D., Division of Endocrinology, Metabolism and Internal Medicine

J.E. King, M.D., Division of Gastroenterology and Internal Medicine

G.C. Kinsey, R.N., M.S., C.N.S.N., Department of Nursing

F. Kleinberg, M.D., Department of Pediatrics—Neonatology

B.A. Kottke, M.D., Department of Cardiology

T.E. Kottke, M.D., Department of Cardiology, Department of Health Sciences Research—Clinical Epidemiology

D.E. Larson, M.D., Division of Gastroenterology and Internal Medicine

T.S. Larson, M.D., Division of Nephrology and Internal Medicine

N.F. LaRusso, M.D., Division of Gastroenterology and Internal Medicine

J.T.C. Li, M.D., Division of Allergic Disease and Internal Medicine

K.D. Lindor, M.D., Division of Gastroenterology and Internal Medicine

M.R. Litzow, M.D., Division of Hematology and Internal Medicine

C.L. Loprinzi, M.D., Department of Oncology

E.G. Lufkin, M.D., Division of Endocrinology, Metabolism and Internal Medicine

J.K. Martin, Jr., M.D., Department of Surgery, Mayo Clinic, Jacksonville, Florida

J.T. McCarthy, M.D., Division of Nephrology and Internal Medicine

D.B. McGill, M.D., Division of Gastroenterology and Internal Medicine

D.C. McIlrath, M.D., Department of Surgery—Gastroenterologic and General Surgery

M.M. McMahon, M.D., Division of Endocrinology, Metabolism and Internal Medicine

T.C. Merritt, M.D., Department of Psychiatry and Psychology, Mayo Clinic, Jacksonville, Florida

P.P. Metzger, M.D., Department of Surgery—Colon and Rectal, Mayo Clinic, Jacksonville, Florida

V. Michels, M.D., Department of Medical Genetics

D.E. Midthun, M.D., Division of Thoracic Diseases and Internal Medicine

D.S. Milliner, M.D., Division of Nephrology and Internal Medicine

B.Z. Morgenstern, M.D., Department of Pediatric and Adolescent Medicine—Nephrology

M.J. Murray, M.D., Department of Anesthesiology—Intensive Care and Respiratory Therapy

R.L. Nelson, M.D., Division of Endocrinology, Metabolism and Internal Medicine

Y. Newborn, M.S., R.D., Dietetics, Mayo Clinic, Scottsdale, Arizona

A.D. Newcomer, M.D., Division of Gastroenterology and Internal Medicine

T.T. Nguyen, M.D., Division of Endocrinology and Internal Medicine

M.K. O'Connor, M.D., Department of Psychiatry and Psychology

P.L. Ogburn, M.D., Department of Obstetrics and Gynecology

P.J. Palumbo, M.D., Division of Endocrinology, Metabolism and Internal Medicine

K. Parent, M.D., Division of Gastroenterology and Internal Medicine, Mayo Clinic, Scottsdale, Arizona

J. Perrault, M.D., Division of Gastroenterology and Internal Medicine

S.F. Phillips, M.D., Division of Gastroenterology and Internal Medicine

M.K. Porayko, M.D., Division of Gastroenterology and Internal Medicine

J. Rakela, M.D., Division of Gastroenterology and Internal Medicine

M.E. Rassier, M.D., Division of Nephrology and Internal Medicine

R.A. Rizza, M.D., Division of Endocrinology and Internal Medicine

T.D. Rizzo, Jr., M.D., Department of Physical Medicine and Rehabilitation, Mayo Clinic, Jacksonville, Florida

M.I. Sachs, D.O., Department of Pediatric and Adolescent Medicine—Allergy

M.G. Sarr, M.D., Department of Surgery—Gastroenterology and General Surgery

R.T. Schlinkert, M.D., Department of Surgery, Mayo Clinic, Scottsdale, Arizona

W.F. Schwenk, M.D., Department of Pediatric and Adolescent Medicine—Endocrinology and Metabolism

M.S. Shapiro, M.D., Division of Gastroenterology and Internal Medicine, Mayo Clinic, Scottsdale, Arizona

P.J. Sheridan, D.D.S., Department of Dentistry, Periodontics

M. Sinaki, M.D., Department of Physical Medicine and Rehabilitation

L.H. Smith, M.D., Division of Nephrology and Internal Medicine

W.A. Smithson, M.D., Department of Pediatric and Adolescent Medicine—Hematology and Oncology

L.A. Solberg, Jr., M.D., Division of Hematology, Oncology and Internal Medicine, Mayo Clinic, Jacksonville, Florida

R.J. Spencer, M.D., Department of Surgery, Colon and Rectal Surgery, Mayo Clinic, Scottsdale, Arizona

R.W. Squires, Ph.D., Department of Cardiology

S. Sterioff, M.D., Department of Surgery, Transplantation Surgery

N. Stevens, R.D., Dietetics, Mayo Clinic, Jacksonville, Florida

M.J. Stuart, M.D., Department of Orthopedics

J.A. Swanson, M.D., Department of Pediatric and Adolescent Medicine—Community Pediatric Service

N.J. Talley, M.D., Division of Gastroenterology and Internal Medicine

E.G. Tangalos, M.D., Division of Community Internal Medicine

V. Tarrosa, R.D., Dietetics, Saint Lukes Hospital, Jacksonville, Florida

V.F. Trastek, M.D., Department of Surgery

C. Trcalek, R.D., St Lukes Hospital, Jacksonville, Florida

W.J. Tremaine, M.D., Division of Gastroenterology and Internal Medicine

M. Valentino, M.S., R.D., St Lukes Hospital, Jacksonville, Florida

R.G. VanDellen, M.D., Division of Allergic Disease and Internal Medicine

J.A. Velosa, M.D., Division of Nephrology and Internal Medicine

G. Vockley, M.D., Ph.D., Department of Medical Genetics

W.H. Weidman, M.D., Department of Pediatric and Adolescent Medicine—Cardiology

J.R. Wesley, M.D., Division of Pediatric Surgery

A. Williams, M.D., Division of Nephrology and Internal Medicine

R.L. Wilson, R.N., Department of Nursing

D.N. Wochos, M.D., Division of Nephrology, Hypertension and Internal Medicine, Mayo Clinic, Scottsdale, Arizona

M.W. Yocum, M.D., Division of Allergic Disease and Internal Medicine

B.R. Zimmerman, M.D., Division of Endocrinology, Metabolism and Internal Medicine

Marjorie G. Durhman from Mayo's Visual Information Service designed the cover for this manual reflecting the celebration of 75 years of Dietetics at Mayo Medical Center. Her creative contribution is appreciated.

Patricia J. Erwin, M.A., L.S., from Mayo's Medical Library, provided invaluable assistance in locating countless references. Her contributions are especially noted and have greatly contributed to this manual's completeness.

Jean M. Peterson provided complete manuscript preparation, including typing and proofreading. We are grateful for her dedication to this project.

The publisher is Mosby–Year Book. We appreciate the assistance of Laura DeYoung, Developmental Editor, who guided this project into published form.

Sincere appreciation is given to one and all who have directly and indirectly contributed to this seventh ("75th anniversary") edition of the *Mayo Clinic Diet Manual*.

The Editorial Board

Jennifer K. Nelson
Karen E. Moxness
Michael D. Jensen
Clifford F. Gastineau

Foreword

The Section of Dietetics and Clinical Nutrition of the Mayo Clinic and its integrated hospitals, the Rochester Methodist Hospital and Saint Marys Hospital, continue their commitment to the excellent tradition of providing the *Mayo Clinic Diet Manual* (seventh edition) as a resource for current nutrition practices in preventive and therapeutic medicine and in clinical research. This manual is a comprehensive and expanded resource for healthful nutrition from infancy through adulthood and for the evaluation and management of nutrition problems in clinical practice and in the research setting.

Mayo has had a long-standing tradition in nutrition in clinical practice, in education, and in research, dating back 75 years and has long recognized the important role of the dietitian in the healthcare team. The *Mayo Clinic Diet Manual* has served as a resource for dietitians and for practicing physicians, initially at Mayo, and now throughout many institutions across the United States and even internationally.

This seventh edition of the *Mayo Clinic Diet Manual* coincides with the 75th anniversary of Mayo Dietetics. What a truly remarkable and unique role dietetics and nutrition practice has played at the Mayo Medical Center. Beginning in 1917 with Dr. David Berkman's development of the diabetes service at Saint Marys Hospital, and with Ms. Daisy Ellithorpe as the first hospital dietitian, the formal role of dietetics and clinical nutrition in the management of patients at Mayo began. Since that time the roster of individuals in dietetics and clinical nutrition represents a hall of fame of pioneers in this discipline: Dr. R. M. Wilder (established the nutrition service and brought the first dietitian to Mayo); Dr. W. Boothby (first explored indirect calorimetry and energy expenditure); Dr. J. Berkson (led efforts in treatment of eating disorders); Dr. C. Code (established the Fellowship in Nutrition for advanced degrees in dietetics through a joint Mayo Clinic–University of Minnesota collaboration); Ms. M. Foley (created an ambulatory feeding center for management of patients with diabetes—prior to discovery of insulin); Ms. F. Smith (President of the American Dietetic Association and first editor of the *Journal of the American Dietetic Association*); and Sister M. V. Fromm (established the Saint Marys Hospital Dietetic Internship, author of the first *Mayo Clinic Diet Manual*). The Clinical Research Center was opened at Saint Marys Hospital in 1940 and is currently funded by the National Institutes of Health. The metabolic kitchen in this center provides high quality, precise diets for research subjects. Approximately 6,000 meals per year are provided for research diets. The Rochester Diet Kitchen was established in 1922 for outpatients requiring special nutrition programs, such as patients with diabetes mellitus and gastrointestinal diseases. In 1983 the diet kitchen was renamed the Nutrition Education and Dining Center and subsequently the eponym for it became NEDs Cafeteria. These changes in the diet kitchen reflect the broader scope of providing preventative and therapeutic nutrition for patients and their families other than just for patients needing diet for treatment of diseases. The first edition of the *Mayo Clinic Diet Manual* was published in 1949. Subsequent editions have been translated into Spanish and Italian.

The dietetic staff of the Mayo Clinic has grown from less than five in the 1940s to 12 times that number of registered dietitians in the ambulatory care and inpatient settings including Clinical Dietetics and Food Service. Over 1,000 dietetic interns have graduated from the Saint Marys Hospital dietetics internship program. Sections of Dietetics have been established at the Mayo group practices in Jacksonville, Florida, and Scottsdale, Arizona, and their respective hospitals. Nutrition support teams have been developed at the integrated and affiliated hospitals of the Mayo Clinic with staff physician nutritionists participating along with registered dietitians, pharmacists, and nursing staff. Nutrition programs for executives, sports medicine, and the Cardiovascular Health Center have also been developed in ambulatory care at Mayo Clinic.

This seventh edition of the *Mayo Clinic Diet Manual* includes the following new and expanded sections:
Food Guide Pyramid
National Cholesterol Education Program Guidelines
Food Facts, Fads, and Fallacies
Food Allergy and Intolerance
Diarrhea
Irritable Bowel Syndrome
Sclerotherapy
Parkinson's Disease
Nutrition Management after Transplantation including:
   Nutrition and Transplantation
   Low Bacteria Diets
   Kidney Transplantation
   Pancreas, Pancreas-Kidney Transplantation
   Liver Transplantation
   Thoracic Organ Transplantation
Expanded Appendices including:
   Dietetic Food Labeling
   The Scope of Practice for Diabetes Educators and the
   Standards of Practice for Diabetes Educators

Position Papers of the American Dietetic Association
USDA, USDHHS Suggested Weights for Adults
Multiple Vitamin Preparations
Vitamin Sources, Functions, Deficiency and Toxic Effects

It is clear that the field of Clinical Nutrition and Dietetics continues to expand, and with it, nutrition practices continue to evolve for prevention of disease, for the therapeutic management of illness, and for the search for nutrient modifications in the research setting which may be beneficial to both prevention and treatment of disease. The manual looks at nutrition modulation of well-known metabolic pathways that are disturbed such as phenylketonuria due to an enzyme defect in the metabolism of phenylalanine. But there are other areas for nutrition modification to be explored beyond just providing adequate calories and nutrients in nutrition support for patients whose illness or stress may benefit from nutrient modification of metabolic pathways and immune function. Nutrition modulation through improved substrates, trace minerals, low infusion enteral feedings, and other such interventions may further modify metabolic pathways. Healthful and palatable nutrition combined with fitness offers the best and safest prevention for disease without the adverse side effects associated with pharmacologic treatments. The future holds the promise of better and more healthful foods in abundant supply through proper genetic engineering and cultivation. As I stated in my Foreword to the sixth edition, this manual has something for everyone and it is the hope of the staff of the Section of Dietetics and Clinical Nutrition at the Mayo Clinic, its integrated hospitals and group practices, that those who have this resource will use it well.

P. J. Palumbo, M.D.
Section of Clinical Nutrition
Mayo Clinic

Preface and Acknowledgments

The publication of the seventh edition of the *Mayo Clinic Diet Manual* highlights the 75th anniversary of dietetics at Mayo. Since the beginning, nutrition has been essential to the medical and surgical care of Mayo's patients. Dietetics has also played a vital part in Mayo's integrated group practice. This practice recognizes authorities in their specialty areas and fosters the sharing of knowledge with one another for the benefit of the patient. This is done in a coordinated, noncompetitive atmosphere within all facets of patient care, staff education, and research.

The recognition that optimal nourishment contributes positively to health and to the successful treatment of diseases is not new. Major developments in nutrition science and food technology have found fertile application within all facets of health care. The result is a vibrant and ever changing nutrition practice.

The need for ensuring quality nutrition care within all health care settings is the objective of dietitians within every institution. It has also become an objective for numerous regulatory agencies governing health care at the local, state, and national levels. Diet manuals have historically served to help standardize the planning of meals served to hospitalized patients. Today's diet manuals must serve multiple functions and are intended to guide nutritional assessment and intervention. They are not to be regarded as a collection of diets to be used without further thought or modification.

The goal of the seventh edition of the *Mayo Clinic Diet Manual* is to integrate the major developments in nutrition science and food technology with the application of quality nutrition practices within its health care settings.

The *Mayo Clinic Diet Manual* provides guidelines for nutritional care practices in the Mayo Medical Center. However, it is recognized that other health care organizations may also use this manual. Because of this, the *Mayo Clinic Diet Manual* purposely documents the indications and rationale behind nutrition interventions. This way institutions and their nutritionists can use this background to develop menus, intervention strategies, and nutrition eduction materials that meet the needs of their unique patient population. This approach allows greater latitude for ongoing continuous improvement efforts in all facets of nutrition care. With the manual serving as a foundation, patient care protocols, menus, and nutrition education materials can be continuously updated in an effort to improve health outcome.

The manual is intended as a reference tool for dietitians, and medical and healthcare staff, as well as for students of nutrition and diet therapy. It is to be used in providing nutritional care for both hospitalized and ambulatory patients.

The manual is not intended for use by the lay public or as an educational tool to be used for patient counseling. When nutrition education materials are needed, we recommend the use of those that are designed specifically for that purpose. Mayo has developed a wide array of education materials with varying levels of complexity and scope. These are available for purchase. For further information a card at the end of this manual may be sent to:

> Section of Clinical Dietetics
> Mayo Clinic
> Rochester, MN 55905

As in previous editions, chapters are written based upon the blending of current scientific literature with Mayo's nutrition research and practices. Each chapter has been carefully written by dietitians who practice in each area. It has been reviewed by physicians and others with interests and expertise in the same area. As with other Mayo publications, and in particular, the *Mayo Clinic Diet Manual* is a repository of the collective knowledge Mayo dietitians have gained over the past 75 years. In addition, for the first time this manual reached to and benefitted from the new Mayo practices: Mayo Clinic and Saint Lukes Hospital, Jacksonville, Florida, and Mayo Clinic, Scottsdale, Arizona.

For their collective efforts, sincere appreciation is extended to the dietitians and physicians for the sections they contributed.

The Editorial Board

Jennifer K. Nelson
Karen E. Moxness
Michael D. Jensen
Clifford F. Gastineau

Contents

PART I NORMAL NUTRITION AND THERAPEUTIC DIETS FOR ADULTS

1   **Introduction to Nutritional Care, 3**

2   **Guidelines for Meal Planning and Promotion of Wellness, 5**
Dietary Guidelines for Americans, 5
Food Guide Pyramid, 6
American Heart Association Dietary Guidelines, 9
National Cholesterol Education Program Guidelines for Treatment of
        Hyperlipidemia, 9
Diet and Cancer Risk, 15
Recommended Dietary Allowances, 18
Food Labeling, 21
Food Facts, Fads, and Fallacies, 23

3   **Nutritional Screening and Assessment, 29**

4   **Normal Nutrition, 39**
Pregnancy and Lactation, 39
Nutritional Needs for Physical Performance, 51
Geriatric Nutrition, 58
Vegetarian Diet, 70
Jewish Dietary Practices, 75

5   **Hospital Diet Progressions, 77**
Modifications in Consistency and Texture, 77
    General Hospital Diet, 77
    Clear Liquid Diet, 79
    Full Liquid Diet, 81
    Pureed Diet, 82
    Consistency Modified Diets, 82
    Mechanical Soft Diet, 84
    Soft Diet, 86

xix

Transitional Feeding Progression, 88
   Preoperative, 88
   Postoperative Diet, 88
   Tonsillectomy and Adenoidectomy (T & A) Diet Progression, 89
   Intermaxillary Fixation, 89
   Dysphagia, 91

PART II   NUTRITIONAL MANAGEMENT OF DISEASE AND DISORDERS FOR ADULTS

6   Food Allergy and Intolerance, 97

Introduction, 97
Food Allergies, 100
   Corn allergy, 101
   Egg allergy, 102
   Fish and shellfish allergy, 103
   Milk allergy, 104
   Peanut and soy allergy, 107
   Wheat allergy, 108
Food Intolerance, 110
   Aspartame, 111
   Benzoates and parabens, 112
   Butylated hydroxyanisole (BHA) and butylated hydroxytoluene
     (BHT), 113
   Mold, 114
   Monosodium glutamate, 115
   Nickel restricted diet, 116
   Nitrates and nitrites, 117
   Penicillin, 118
   Sulfites, 119
   Tartrazine and acetylsalicylic acid, 121

7   Cardiovascular Diseases, 123

Hypertension, 123
Hyperlipidemia, 133
Cardiac Surgery, 146
Congestive Heart Failure, 148
Myocardial Infarction, 150

8   Endocrine/Metabolism Diseases and Disorders, 153

Diabetes Mellitus, 153
   Food exchange lists, 169
Hypoglycemia, 183
Obesity, 185
Bariatric Surgery, 195
Osteoporosis, 204

9   Gastrointestinal Diseases and Disorders, 213

Abdominal Gas and Flatulence, 213
Delayed Gastric Emptying, 217
Diarrhea, 222

Esophageal Reflux, 226
Fat Malabsorption, 229
Fiber and Residue Modifications, 233
   High Fiber Diet, 233
   Restricted Fiber Diet, 240
   Low Residue Diet, 242
Gluten Sensitivity: Celiac Sprue and Dermatitis Herpetiformis, 244
Inflammatory Bowel Disease, 250
Irritable Bowel Syndrome, 261
Lactose Intolerance, 264
Peptic Ulcer Disease, 268
Postgastrectomy Dumping Syndrome, 270

10   Hepatobiliary Diseases, 275
Hepatobiliary Diseases, 275
Copper Metabolism, 282
Sclerotherapy, 286

11   Neurologic Diseases, 287
Parkinson's Disease, 287

12   Oncologic Diseases, 293
Cancer, 293

13   Psychological Disorders, 303
Anorexia Nervosa and Bulimia Nervosa, 303
Tyramine Controlled Diet, 311

14   Renal Diseases and Disorders, 315
Acute Renal Failure, 315
Chronic Renal Failure, 317
Hemodialysis, 322
Peritoneal Dialysis, 327
   Continuous ambulatory peritoneal dialysis and
      continuous cyclic peritoneal dialysis, 327
Nephrotic Syndrome, 333
Urolithiasis, 335
   Calcium control, 336
   Oxalate restriction, 339
   Phosphate restriction, 343
   Purine restriction, 344
   Other dietary considerations: acid-ash
      and alkaline-ash diets, 346
Food Exchange Lists for Protein, Sodium, and Potassium Control,
   348
Potassium Control, 356
Food sources of potassium, 357

15   Nutritional Management and Transplantation, 363
Nutrition in Transplantation, 363
Low Bacteria Diets, 367
Kidney Transplantation, 369

Pancreas Transplantation and Pancreas-Kidney Transplantation, 372
Liver Transplantation, 374
Thoracic Organ Transplantation, 377
Bone Marrow Transplantation, 380

16   Nutritional Support of Adults, 385

Enteral Nutritional Support of Adults, 385
Parenteral Nutritional Support of Adults, 399

17   Diets in Preparation for Diagnostic Tests, 411

Breath Hydrogen Concentration, 411
Carbohydrate Metabolism, 412
Fat Absorption, 413
5-HIAA, 415

PART III   NORMAL NUTRITION AND THERAPEUTIC DIETS FOR INFANTS, CHILDREN, AND ADOLESCENTS

18   Pediatric Nutritional Assessment, 419

19   Normal Nutrition, 427

Healthy Infants, Children, and Adolescents, 427
Young Athletes, 442
Vegetarian Diet , 447

20   Other Nutritional Considerations, 453

Developmental Disability, 453
Failure to Thrive, 459
Low Birth Weight Infant, 463
Sick Infants, Children, and Adolescents, 469

PART IV   NUTRITIONAL MANAGEMENT OF DISEASES AND DISORDERS FOR INFANTS, CHILDREN, AND ADOLESCENTS

21   Allergy in Children, 477

22   Cardiovascular Diseases in Childhood, 483

Hypertension, 483
Hyperlipidemia, 487
Pediatric Cardiac Surgery, 491

23   Endocrine Metabolism Diseases and Disorders in Children, 495

Diabetes Mellitus, 495
Inborn Errors of Metabolism, 501
   Glycogen storage diseases, 508
   Maple syrup urine disease, 519
   Nutritional therapy for phenylketonuria (PKU), 524
Weight Control, 539

24 Gastrointestinal Diseases and Disorders in Children, 547
Constipation and Encopresis, 547
Diarrhea, 550
Gluten-Sensitive Enteropathy: Celiac Disease, 555
Inflammatory Bowel Disease, 557
Fat Absorption Test Diet, 559

25 Neurological Disease in Children, 561
Ketogenic Diet, 561

26 Oncologic Disease in Children, 575
Cancer, 575

27 Pulmonary Disease in Children, 579
Cystic Fibrosis, 579

28 Renal Disease and Disorders in Children, 585
Chronic Renal Failure, 585
Hemodialysis and Continuous Ambulatory Peritoneal Dialysis, 589
Nephrotic Syndrome, 595

29 Nutritional Support in Pediatrics, 599
Enteral Nutrition , 599
Parenteral Nutrition, 605

PART V   APPENDICES

A   General Appendices, 617

1   Standards of Practice for Nutrition Support Dietitians, 617
2   Interactions between Drugs, Nutrients, and Nutritional Status, 625
3   Nutritive Values for Alcoholic Beverages and Mixes, 645
4   Adult Weight for Height Tables, 647
         Metropolitan Weight and Height Tables (1983), 648
         USDA and USDHHS Acceptable Weights for Adults (1990), 649
5   Mayo Clinic Normal Physiological Values, 651
6   Nomogram for Estimating Caloric Requirements, 655
7   Nomogram for Body Mass Index, 657
8   Food Labels, 659
9   Characteristics of Nutritive and Nonnutritive Sweeteners, 661
10 Enteral Nutrition Formulas, 665
11 Physician's Adult Enteral Nutrition Order Sheet, 685
         Considerations for ordering adult enteral nutrition formulas, 687

12   Parenteral Nutrition Solutions, 689

13   Parenteral Nutrition Order Form (Adults), 699

      Guidelines for ordering adult parenteral nutrition solutions, 702

14   Conversion of Milligrams to Milliequivalents, 705

15   Approximate Conversions to and from Metric Measures, 707

16   Medical Abbreviations, Prefixes, and Suffixes, 709

17   Cholesterol, Triglyceride, and Lipoprotein Levels in the United Staes, 717

18   The Scope of Practice for Diabetes Educators and the Standards of Practice for Diabetes Educators, 723

19   Position Papers of The American Dietetic Association, 733

20   Multiple Vitamin Preparations, 735

21   Vitamin Sources, Functions, Deficiency, and Toxic Effects, 741

22   Fat Substitutes, 747

23   Caffeine, 757

24   Phosphorus Content of Common Foods, 761

B   Pediatric Appendices, 763

25   Infant Formulas and Feedings , 763

26   Exchange Values for Commercial Baby Foods, 797

27   Common Carbohydrates in Foods (per 100 g Edible Portion), 807

28   National Center for Health Statistics (NCHS) Growth Graphs, 819

29   Baldwin-Wood Tables, 829

30   Growth Charts for Children with Down's Syndrome, 833

31   Growth Chart for Premature Infants, 843

32   Triceps Skinfold Percentiles, 845

33   Nomogram for Anthropometry for Children, 847

34   Arm and Arm Muscle Circumference Percentiles, 849

35   Arm Fat Area and Arm Muscle Area Percentiles, 851

36   Selected References for Pediatric Laboratory Values, 853

37   Tanner Height for Age and Height Velocity Graphs—Girls and Boys, Birth through 19 Years, 855

38   Oral Rehydration Solutions, 861

MAYO · CLINIC
Diet Manual
A Handbook of Nutrition Practices

Normal Nutrition and Therapeutic Diets for Adults

1 / *Introduction to Nutritional Care*

Nutritional care includes (1) assessment of the patient's needs relative to his or her health status; (2) development of a nutritional care plan; (3) implementation of that plan, which includes provision of nutrients via oral, enteral, or parenteral routes; (4) education of the patient; and (5) evaluation of the effectivenesss of the intervention. This manual is designed to assist the healthcare provider in all aspects of nutritional care.

This is a manual of therapeutic nutrition. Nutritional recommendations for a particular disease or disorder are often complex and multifaceted. In order to address the often numerous considerations, many of the chapters in the manual are organized by disease, by disorder, or by health state rather than by dietary constituents. Reference to other sections is made throughout the text because of the overlap of nutritional practices among disorders.

Normal nutrition serves as the foundation for therapeutic diet modifications. Essential references for normal nutrition are included in addition to a more detailed discussion of the needs at life cycle stages within sections on Pregnancy and Lactation; Normal Nutritional Requirements of Infants, Children, and Adolescents; and Geriatrics.

A nutritional assessment is a necessary antecedent to intervention. Therefore, chapters on nutritional assessment precede both the adult and the pediatric sections and are referred to in the subsequent sections.

Many of the chapters are organized under the headings General Description, Nutritional Inadequacy, Indications and Rationale, Goals of Dietary Management, Dietary Recommendations, and Physicians: How to Order Diet.

The General Description section is intended as a brief summary of the key aspects of nutritional intervention or dietary modifications.

The section titled Nutritional Inadequacy identifies those diet plans that have the potential for producing nutrient deficiencies if adhered to for a long period of time. The Recommended Dietary Allowances (RDA) are used as the reference standard. The National Research Council states that the RDA were not intended to fill the needs of those who are ill.[1] However, for lack of more suitable guidelines, the RDA were used in evaluating the therapeutic diets that are presented in this manual.

The Indications and Rationale for dietary modifications section is provided so that nutritional practices can be chosen with the degree of control of dietary components that is appropriate to the individual situation. We have stated when diet regimens are based on traditional practices rather than on documented scientific evidence.

The section Goals of Dietary Management is intended as a brief summary of the key objective or purpose of nutritional intervention.

The Dietary Recommendations section includes a discussion of the aspects of assessment that are unique to a particular disease or disorder and presents specific guidelines for diet modification and for development of a nutritional care plan. This section expands on the practices and philosophy of the Mayo Medical Center. Tables that summarize food composition are included in many sections. As compared to previous editions of the Mayo Clinic Diet Manual, the seventh edition provides fewer standard meal patterns or sample menus. The science of nutrition is rarely so exacting or so accurate that a single ideal plan is advised for all persons.

The section titled Physicians: How to Order Diet gives the preferred terms for requesting a particular nutritional assessment and intervention. The diet order should convey the treatment modality or the goal of dietary treatment and may be general or specific. Altering food habits is often a difficult task. Adequate time for education is essential. Requests for education and counseling should be made as early in the patient's stay as possible.

Note: Various terms are used throughout this text to indicate the degree of restriction or the quantity of a dietary constituent. The term "minimum" indicates that the diet provides as small an amount of the substance as possible without making the diet distinctly inconvenient or unpalatable. "Low," "limited," and "restricted" are used to indicate an intermediate reduction in the amount of the substance in the diet. The term "high" indicates an increase of the substance in the diet that can be achieved with reasonable convenience. When practical, a range for the quantity, which is implied by these general terms, is specified with the diet.

Owing to the nature of some nutritional interventions, brand names of certain products must be stated in the manual. This is not intended as an endorsement of a specific product when an equivalent one exists.

Reference

1. Food and Nutrition Board, Commission on Life Sciences, National Research Council. Recommended Dietary Allowances, 10th ed. Washington, DC: National Academy of Press, 1989.

2 / *Guidelines for Meal Planning and Promotion of Wellness*

DIETARY GUIDELINES FOR AMERICANS

The United States Senate Select Committee on Nutrition and Human Needs issued the Dietary Goals for the United States in 1977 with the intent of encouraging healthy eating habits.[1] In 1980 the United States Department of Agriculture and the United States Department of Health and Human Services issued *Nutrition and Your Health: Dietary Guidelines for Americans*[2] to provide practical dietary advice based on current research. In addition, the United States Senate Appropriations Committee requested that a Dietary Guidelines Advisory Committee be established to periodically review comments that are received and to incorporate new pertinent scientific data, thereby maintaining key references from which to derive the guidelines. The latest revision of the Dietary Guidelines for Americans occurred in 1990.[3] These guidelines along with their indications and rationale appear below. They are for healthy people 2 years of age and over, and are not for people who need special diets because of diseases and conditions that interfere with normal nutrition.

1. **Eat a variety of foods**. The body needs more than 40 nutrients for good health. These nutrients should come from a variety of foods, not from a few highly fortified foods or supplements. A varied diet is defined by a daily food guide with suggested numbers of servings from vegetables, fruits, grain products, dairy products, and meat/meat substitutes.
2. **Maintain healthy weight.** A "healthy" body weight depends on the percentage of body weight as fat, the location of fat deposition, and the existence of any weight-related medical problems. Currently, there are no precise ways to describe healthy weight. However, using tables with suggested weight-for-height-and-age and/or measuring waist-to-hip ratios are popular methods of estimating fat distribution and body weight.
3. **Choose a diet low in fat, saturated fat, and cholesterol.** The numerical goals given for limiting fat and cholesterol are consistent with those of the National Cholesterol Education Program (NCEP). (See Chapter 2—NCEP

5

Guidelines for Treatment of Hypercholesterolemia, p. 9.) These state that fat intake should be limited to 30% of calories, with less than 10% of calories from saturated fat. Most people can keep their blood cholesterol at a desirable level by eating plenty of vegetables, fruits, and grain products; choosing lean meats, fish and poultry without the skin, and low fat dairy products; and using fats and oils sparingly. Individuals interested in assessing their diets for fat content should be encouraged to seek more information from their physicians, registered dietitians, or other healthcare professionals.

4. **Choose a diet with plenty of vegetables, fruits, and grain products.** Consuming more vegetables, fruits, and grain products is emphasized especially for their complex carbohydrates, dietary fiber, and other components linked to good health. It is stressed that some of the benefits from a high fiber diet may be from the food that provides the fiber, not from fiber alone, so fiber from foods is recommended over fiber obtained from supplements.

5. **Use sugars only in moderation.** Sugars should be used in moderate amounts and sparingly if calorie needs are low. Because sugars can contribute to tooth decay, excessive snacking should be avoided and teeth should be brushed and flossed regularly.

6. **Use salt and sodium only in moderation.** Most Americans consume much more salt and sodium than they actually need. A reduction in salt and sodium intake will benefit those people whose blood pressure rises with salt intake.

7. **If you drink alcoholic beverages, do so in moderation.** Drinking alcoholic beverages has no net health benefits and is linked to many health problems and accidents. Therefore, individuals who drink alcoholic beverages are advised to use moderation. Moderate drinking is defined as no more than one drink per day for women and two drinks per day for men. One drink may be 12 oz of beer, 5 oz of wine, or $1^{1}/_{2}$ oz of distilled spirits (80 proof).

For more information on how to put the guidelines into practice, contact the Human Nutrition Information Service, U.S.D.A., Room 325-A, 6505 Belcrest Rd, Hyattsville, MD 20782.

References

1. U.S. Senate Select Committee on Nutrition and Human Needs. 1977a. Dietary goals for the United States. Washington, DC: U.S. Government Printing Office. February 1977.
2. USDA and USDHHS. Nutrition and your health: Dietary guidelines for Americans, 2nd ed., Rev. August 1985. Home and Garden Bulletin No. 232, Washington, DC: USDA/USDHHS. August 1985.
3. USDA and USDHHS. Nutrition and your health: Dietary guidelines for Americans, 3rd ed., Rev. November 1990. Home and Garden Bulletin No. 232, Washington, DC: USDA/ USDHHS. November 1990.

FOOD GUIDE PYRAMID

The Basic Four Food Guide or the Four Food Groups were developed by the United States Department of Agriculture (USDA) in the mid-1950s.[4] These food

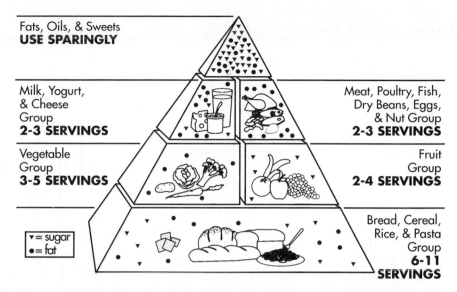

FIGURE 2-1 Food Guide Pyramid. A guide to daily food choices.

TABLE 2-1   How Many Servings Are Needed Each Day?

	Women and Some Older Adults	Children, Teen Girls Active Women, Most Men	Teen Boys and Active Men
CALORIE LEVEL*	**About 1600**	**About 2200**	**About 2800**
Bread group	6	9	11
Vegetable group	3	4	5
Fruit group	2	3	4
Milk group	2–3†	2–3†	2–3†
Meat group	2, for a total of 5 oz	2, for a total of 6 oz	3, for a total of 7 oz

*These are the calorie levels if you choose low fat, lean foods from the 5 major food groups and use foods from the fats, oils, and sweets group sparingly.

†Women who are pregnant or breastfeeding, teenagers, and young adults to age 24 years need 3 servings.

groups were designed to aid individuals in their selection of appropriate types and amounts of foods that would form the foundation of an adequate diet.[4] A subsequent revision took place in 1979 when the USDA added a fifth food group that allowed for increased energy needs that are essential for growth, activity, and for the maintenance of a desirable weight.[5] There has been some debate about whether or not this food guide, if followed, provides the essential amounts of all nutrients, and whether the guide functions as an effective communication tool in nutrition education programs today.

TABLE 2-2   What Counts as a Serving?

FOOD GROUPS

Bread, Cereal, Rice, and Pasta

| 1 slice of bread | 1 oz of ready-to-eat cereal | $^1/_2$ cup of cooked cereal, rice, or pasta |

Vegetable

| 1 cup of raw leafy vegetables | $^1/_2$ cup of other vegetables, cooked or chopped raw | $^3/_4$ cup of vegetable juice |

Fruit

| 1 medium apple, banana, orange | $^1/_2$ cup of chopped, cooked, or canned fruit | $^3/_4$ cup of fruit juice |

Milk, Yogurt, and Cheese

| 1 cup of milk or yogurt | $1^1/_2$ oz of natural cheese | 2 oz of processed cheese |

Meat, Poultry, Fish, Dry Beans, Eggs, and Nuts

| 2–3 oz of cooked lean meat, poultry, or fish | $^1/_2$ cup of cooked dry beans, 1 egg or 2 tbsp of peanut butter count as 1 oz of lean meat |

As a result of that debate, a new educational device, the Food Guide Pyramid, was unveiled in 1991, and in 1992, the pyramid was actually adopted and published by the United States Department of Agriculture.[6]

The Food Guide Pyramid (see Figure 2-1) lists a range for number of servings in each of five food groups based on age, sex, and activity level. Serving sizes are also defined (see Tables 2-1 and 2-2).

One problem with the Food Guide in the past was that it had not focused on the excesses of the American diet—total and saturated fat, cholesterol, sodium, and sugar. However, the Food Guide Pyramid brochure includes a listing of the Dietary Guidelines for Americans and addresses the fat, cholesterol, sodium, and sugar issues. Copies of the Food Guide Pyramid are available from:

The Superintendent of Documents
Consumer Information Center
Department 159-Y
Pueblo, CO 81009

References

4. Agricultural Research Service. Essentials of Adequate Diet, USDA, Home Economics Report No. 3, United States Department of Agriculture, 1957.
5. Science and Education Administration. Food, home and garden bulletin No. 228. United States Department of Agriculture. Superintendent of Documents. U.S. Government Printing Office, Washington, DC, 1980.
6. USDA's Food Guide Pyramid, Stock number 001-000-04587-3. U.S. Government Printing Office, Washington, DC, 20402, 1992.

TABLE 2-3   American Heart Association Dietary Guidelines

1. Total fat intake should be less than 30% of calories.
2. Saturated fat intake should be less than 10% of calories.
3. Polyunsaturated fat intake should not exceed 10% of calories.
4. Cholesterol intake should not exceed 300 mg/day.
5. Carbohydrate intake should constitute 50% or more of calories, with emphasis on complex carbohydrates.
6. Protein intake should provide the remainder of the calories.
7. Sodium intake should not exceed 3 g/day.
8. Alcoholic consumption should not exceed 1–2 fluid oz of ethanol per day. Two oz of 100 proof whisky, 8 oz of wine, or 24 oz of beer each contain 1 oz of ethanol.
9. Total calories should be sufficient to maintain the individual's recommended body weight.*
10. A wide variety of foods should be consumed.

*Metropolitan Tables of Height and Weight, Table of Desirable Weights for Men and Women. Metropolitan Life Insurance Company, New York, 1959.

Reproduced with permission."Dietary guidelines for healthy American adults," 1988, copyright American Heart Association.

AMERICAN HEART ASSOCIATION DIETARY GUIDELINES

Since 1961 the American Heart Association (AHA) has provided dietary guidelines that are intended to prevent or reduce the incidence of coronary heart disease and other atherosclerotic diseases. Periodic literature reviews and subsequent recommendations have been the responsibility of the American Heart Association Nutrition Committee. Statements from the AHA that regard diet and heart disease generally appear every 3 to 5 years. The 1988 AHA Dietary Guidelines for Healthy American Adults appear in Table 2-3.[7,8]

These guidelines are offered to all healthy American adults as safe and prudent. The AHA no longer recommends the three phase approach to diet for treatment of hyperlipidemia. It has adopted the step-one and step-two guidelines endorsed by the National Cholesterol Education Program (NCEP). Refer to Chapter 2—NCEP guidelines.

References

7. American Heart Association. Rationale of the diet-heart statement of the American Heart Association. Report of Nutrition Committee, American Heart Association. Dallas, TX 1982.
8. American Heart Association. Dietary guidelines for healthy American adults. A statement for physicians and health professionals by the Nutrition Committee, American Heart Association, Dallas, TX, 1988.

NATIONAL CHOLESTEROL EDUCATION PROGRAM GUIDELINES FOR TREATMENT OF HYPERLIPIDEMIA

The National Cholesterol Education Program (NCEP) is a treatment and education program of the National Heart, Lung and Blood Institute (NHLBI) of the

National Institutes of Health (NIH). This program, since its inception in the fall of 1985, has sought to develop screening and treatment strategies (as well as educational materials) in order to educate lay individuals and professionals about cholesterol control and risks associated with elevated blood cholesterol levels. This program was put in place as a result of the large body of research that has shown that reducing serum cholesterol level reduces the risk of heart attacks as well as other cardiovascular disease consequences.[9]

The first "Report of the Expert Panel on the Detection, Evaluation and Treatment of High Blood Cholesterol in Adults" provided the structure for the program's goal of decreasing the prevalence of high blood cholesterol in the United States.[9] Initially, only guidelines for adults age 20 years and older were addressed. Subsequent reports and recommendations have been released to address other age and socioeconomic groups as well as the issue of treatment in the face of multiple cardiovascular risk factors.[10-12]

In June 1993, the "Second Report of the National Cholesterol Education Program (NCEP) Expert Panel on Detection, Evaluation and Treatment of High Blood Cholesterol in Adults (Adult Treatment Panel II)" was issued.[13] This second report (referred to as the ATP2 report) provided updated recommendations for the treatment of both individuals and populations. The ATP2 report specifies new cholesterol cutoff points for treatment decisions. It also clarifies and delineates specific major coronary heart disease (CHD) risk factors (RF) and the increased importance of these RF in making treatment decisions about blood cholesterol management.

The NCEP guidelines provide for a two-pronged approach to the task of lowering cholesterol in the United States. The first approach is aimed at identifying and treating hypercholesterolemia in individuals who are at high risk of cardiovascular disease. The second approach of the NCEP is a total population or public health strategy aimed at decreasing the average cholesterol concentration in the entire United States population. It is important to note that the NCEP recommendations are directed at the treatment of high blood cholesterol (specifically total cholesterol and low density lipoprotein [LDL] cholesterol) and not at the treatment of cardiovascular disease per se. However, the ATP2 report does present a more *global* approach to the treatment of elevated cholesterol inasmuch as it now links treatment decisions to a much heavier emphasis on risk factors for CHD than in the previous report. "Dietary therapy remains the first line of treatment of high blood cholesterol . . . and drug therapy is reserved for patients considered to be at high risk for CHD."[14]

The ATP2 report has increased emphasis on and more clearly defines *major* risk factors. In particular, there is a greater emphasis now on the level of high density lipoprotein cholesterol (HDLC) as a CHD risk factor. In fact, due to the effect of a high level of HDLC as being protective *against* CHD, the concept of a high level of HDLC as a *negative risk factor* has been added. For additional information on primary and secondary treatment decisions and risk factor identification, one should consult the full ATP2 report since treatment decisions differ depending on primary versus secondary cardiovascular disease. Finally, the ATP2 report places greater emphasis on weight control and physical activity as major facets of the nonpharmacological treatment of high serum cholesterol.

The guidelines for treatment of high blood cholesterol classify individuals over 20 years old based on an initial screen of *total* serum cholesterol concentration as well as CHD risk factors. Table 2-4 shows the recommended initial classification based on this measurement.[9] Once a decision has been made to treat an individual for high blood cholesterol, Table 2-5 shows the basis for treatment decisions based on subsequent LDL cholesterol determination.

Dietary treatment of elevated cholesterol is the first line of treatment recommended by NCEP-ATP2. Dietary treatment remains as an adjunctive therapy if the individual is progressed to drug therapy for hypercholesterolemia. The NCEP recommendations for dietary modifications are presented in a two-step program. The NCEP two-step dietary program modifications are outlined in Table 2-6. It is recommended that the step-one diet shown should be tried for at least three months before progressing to the more stringent step-two diet.

Once initial dietary therapy with the NCEP step-one diet has been started, serum total cholesterol, LDL and HDL cholesterol (estimated or measured) levels should be checked and further treatment recommendations made. The NCEP-

---

TABLE 2-4   Initial Classification Based on Total Cholesterol and HDL-Cholesterol

TOTAL CHOLESTEROL

< 200 mg/dl	Desirable blood cholesterol
200-239 mg/dl	Borderline high blood cholesterol
≥ 240 mg/dl	High blood cholesterol

HDL-CHOLESTEROL

< 35 mg/dl	Low HDL-cholesterol

From NIH, NHLBI: Second Report of the Expert Panel on Detection, Evaluation, and Treatment of High Blood Cholesterol in Adults (Adult Treatment Panel 2). NIH Publication #933095; June, 1993.

TABLE 2-5   Treatment Decisions Based on LDL-Cholesterol

	Initiation Level	LDL Goal
DIETARY THERAPY		
Without CHD and with fewer than 2 risk factors	≥ 160 mg/dl	< 160 mg/dl
Without CHD and with 2 or more risk factors	≥ 130 mg/dl	< 130 mg/dl
With CHD	> 100 mg/dl	≤ 100 mg/dl
DRUG TREATMENT		
Without CHD and with fewer than 2 risk factors	≥ 190 mg/dl	< 160 mg/dl
Without CHD and with 2 or more risk factors	≥ 160 mg/dl	< 130 mg/dl
With CHD	≥ 130 mg/dl	≤ 100 mg/dl

From NIH, NHLBI: Second Report of the Expert Panel on Detection, Evaluation, and Treatment of High Blood Cholesterol in Adults (Adult Treatment Panel 2). NIH Publication #933095; June, 1993.

TABLE 2-6   Dietary Therapy of High Blood Cholesterol

Nutrient*	Recommended Intake	
	Step-I Diet	**Step-II Diet**
Total fat	30% or less of total calories	
Saturated fatty acids	8–10% of total calories	Less than 7% of total calories
Polyunsaturated fatty acids	Up to 10% of total calories	
Monounsaturated fatty acids	Up to 15% of total calories	
Carbohydrates	55% or more of total calories	
Protein	Approximately 15% of total calories	
Cholesterol	< 300 mg/day	< 200 mg/day
Total calories	To achieve and maintain desirable weight	

*Calories from alcohol not included.

From NIH, NHLBI: Second Report of the Expert Panel on Detection, Evaluation, and Treatment of High Blood Cholesterol in Adults (Adult Treatment Panel 2). NIH Publication #933095; June, 1993.

ATP2 guidelines for these treatment decisions have been divided into two separate categories of decisions. Those categories are "Primary Prevention of CHD" (no prior history of CHD in the individual) and "Secondary Prevention of CHD" (documented past history of CHD in individual or evidence of existence of atherosclerotic occlusion). Figures 2-2 and 2-3 show the flow of treatment decisions in both of these categories. Additional guidance in drug treatment choices is also covered.

If LDL cholesterol is calculated, the Friedewald equation may be used:

$$\text{LDL cholesterol} = \text{total cholesterol} - \left[\frac{\text{triglycerides}^*}{5} + \text{HDL cholesterol} \right]$$

In this equation, dividing the triglyceride level by five estimates the very low density lipoprotein particle's contribution of cholesterol. However, as triglycerides (which are carried primarily by the very low density lipoproteins) approach and exceed 400 mg/dl, the accuracy of this equation declines.[13]

Hypertriglyceridemia

Additionally, the NCEP-ATP2 report discusses those individuals with hypertriglyceridemia (HTG) as a "special group." As the guidelines now stand, the NCEP agrees with the 1992 National Institutes of Health Consensus Development Conference on Triglycerides, HDL and Coronary Heart Disease on the definition of "borderline HTG" as fasting plasma triglycerides of 200 to 400 mg/dl and "high triglycerides" as fasting plasma triglycerides of 400 to 1,000 mg/dl and "very high triglycerides" as greater than 1,000 mg/dl.[14] To treat HTG, NCEP recommends changes in lifestyle that are general rather than specific or quantitative. It is encouraged that treatment focus on weight control, increased exercise, smoking cessation, and limitation of alcohol, in addition to a low saturated fat and choles-

*It is recommended by NCEP-ATP2 that this equation not be used if triglycerides exceed 400 mg/dl.[13]
Mayo Laboratories recommends measuring LDL cholesterol if triglyceride values exceed 200 mg/dl.

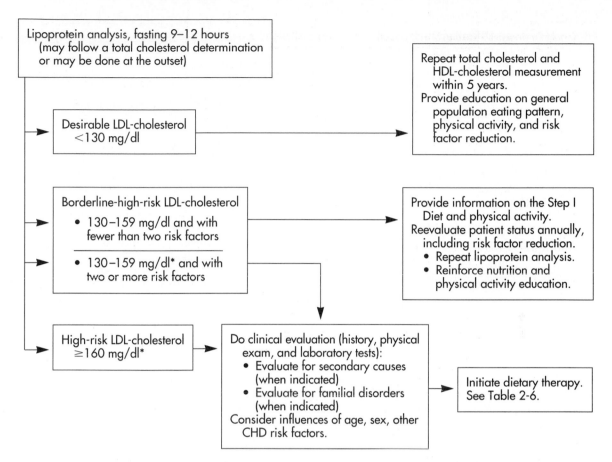

*On the basis of the average of two determinations. If the first two LDL-cholesterol tests differ by more than 30 mg/dl, a third test should be obtained within 1 to 8 weeks and the average value of the three tests used.

FIGURE 2-2 Primary Prevention in Adults without Evidence of CHD: Subsequent Classification Based on LDL-cholesterol. (From NIH, NHLBI: Second Report of the Expert Panel on Detection, Evaluation, and Treatment of High Blood Cholesterol in Adults [Adult Treatment Panel 2]. NIH Publication #933095; June, 1993.)

terol diet.[13] Treatment of any underlying causes of HTG (for example, hypothyroidism, diabetes mellitus) should be the basis of improving secondary HTG. The NCEP-ATP2 acknowledges that drug therapy may also be needed in some cases of HTG—particularly in familial HTG.

HDL Cholesterol

The NCEP's definition of a reduced serum level of HDL cholesterol is a concentration of less than 35 mg/dl. It recognizes a low serum HDL cholesterol as a major risk factor for coronary heart disease (CHD) and recommends that the HDL cholesterol be checked in all patients with high blood cholesterol and in

Please note that in this section the word "blood" is synonymous with "serum."

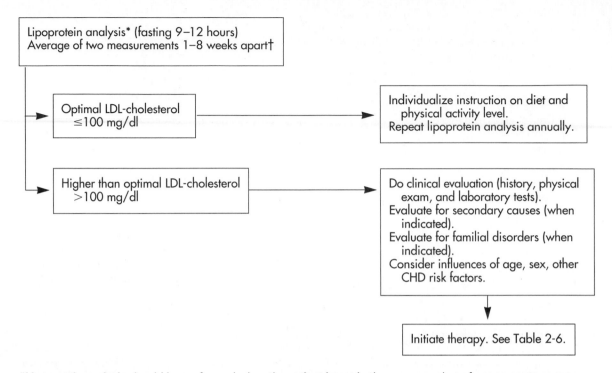

*Lipoprotein analysis should be performed when the patient is not in the recovery phase from an acute coronary or other medical event that would lower their usual LDL-cholesterol level.
†If the first two LDL-cholesterol tests differ by more than 30 mg/dl, a third test should be obtained within 1 to 8 weeks and the average value of the three tests used.

FIGURE 2-3 Secondary Prevention in Adults with Evidence of CHD: Classification Based on LDL-cholesterol. (From NIH, NHLBI: Second Report of the Expert Panel on Detection, Evaluation, and Treatment of High Blood Cholesterol in Adults [Adult Treatment Panel 2]. NIH Publication #933095; June, 1993.)

those patients with borderline high blood cholesterol if two other major risk factors for CHD or if CHD itself is present.[13] Recommended treatment includes cessation of cigarette smoking, weight control, and an increase in physical activity if the individual has a sedentary lifestyle. The concept of a "negative risk factor" of extra protection against CHD in those persons with HDL cholesterol levels greater than or equal to 60 mg/dl is introduced in the NCEP-ATP2 guidelines.[13]

Chapter 7, on Hyperlipidemia for adults, and Chapter 22, on Hyperlipidemia for children provide further guidelines for approaching dietary management of individuals.

References

9. NIH, NHLBI: Report of the Expert Panel on Detection, Evaluation and Treatment of High Blood Cholesterol in Adults. NIH Publication #88-2925; January, 1988.
10. NHBPEP-NCEP. Working group report on management of patients with hypertension and high blood cholesterol. NIH Publication #90-2361; August, 1990.

11. NCEP. Report of the Expert Panel on Blood Cholesterol Levels in Children and Adolescents. NIH Publication #91-2732; 1992.
12. NCEP. Report of the Expert Panel on Population Strategies for Blood Cholesterol Reduction. NIH Publication #90-3046; November, 1990.
13. NCEP, NHLBI: Second Report of the Expert Panel on Detection, Evaluation, and Treatment of High Blood Cholesterol in Adults (Adult Treatment Panel 2). NIH Publication #933095; June, 1993.
14. Consensus Development Conference. Treatment of hypertriglyceridemia. JAMA 1984;251:1196–1200.

DIET AND CANCER RISK

Over the past two decades considerable attention has been given to the potential role of dietary factors in the etiology and prevention of cancer.[15,16] Evidence linking diet and cancer comes from animal and epidemiological studies. It is estimated, from a variety of epidemiological studies, that 35% of cancer deaths may be related to diet.[15,17,18] There is no conclusive evidence that a specific food or nutrient in itself causes or prevents cancer in humans. Rather, scientists believe that an interplay of genetics and a variety of environmental factors, one of which is diet, are responsible.

A variety of mechanisms by which diet might influence cancer are proposed. Despite uncertainties regarding the exact contribution of diet and specific nutrients to cancer risk, there is growing evidence that changes in lifestyle, particularly changes in dietary patterns, may reduce the risk for certain types of cancer. Consistent with this philosophy, the National Cancer Institute (NCI) and the American Cancer Society (ACS) have issued a set of dietary guidelines.[17,18] These guidelines are consistent with the dietary recommendations of other health organizations including the United States Department of Health and Human Services, the Surgeon General's office, the National Academy of Sciences, the American Heart Association, and several others.[17,19] In 1990, the American Cancer Society joined with eight other voluntary and government organizations to issue a report about diet and disease that all the participating agencies could support. It was hoped that these guidelines would be of help in reducing the cancer rate as well as the risks of heart disease, stroke, and diabetes. These are summarized in Table 2-7.

TABLE 2-7 Dietary Guidelines to Reduce Cancer Risk[17,18]

1. Maintain a desirable body weight
2. Eat a varied diet
3. Include a variety of both vegetables and fruits in the daily diet
4. Eat more high fiber foods, such as whole grain cereals, legumes, vegetables, and fruits
5. Cut down on total fat intake (to 30% or less of total calorie intake)
6. Limit consumption of alcoholic beverages if you drink at all
7. Limit consumption of salt-cured and nitrite-preserved foods

These recommendations are designed for adults in good health, and are not meant to be applied indiscriminately to children, pregnant women, convalescents, or the elderly, who may have special nutritional needs or that should be supervised by physicians.

It is important when implementing these guidelines to encourage patients to consider *all* of them for maximum benefit. Emphasis should be placed on variety, moderation, and maintenance of desirable weight. Indiscriminate use of vitamin and/or mineral supplements should be discouraged due to their potential toxicity. Patients who have cancer often request advice on a diet to prevent recurrence or progression of their cancer. In advising cancer patients, consideration should be given to their prognosis, nutritional status, and other medical conditions (see Chapter 12, Cancer). Goals and priorities must be set individually. Educational materials on diet to reduce cancer risk are available from the National Cancer Institute and American Cancer Society.[20,21]

1. **Maintain a desirable body weight.** A number of studies indicate an association between excess body weight and several cancers including breast, uterus, colon, gallbladder, and prostate. Prevalence of these cancers increases with the degree of obesity.[17,18,22]

2. **Eat a varied diet.** Because of the large number of "nutritional" and "non-nutritional" components in foods in the average diet and the complex interplay among them, it is difficult to isolate causative or inhibitory factors for cancer. For example, diets high in fiber contain less fat and fewer calories and usually more vegetables and fruits which contain vitamins and minerals. Thus, it may be difficult to separate the effects of fiber from the confounding effects of fat, calories, vitamins and minerals. An overall change in eating habits to a varied diet, eaten in moderation, offers the best hope for lowering cancer risk.[18,23]

3. **Include a variety of both vegetables and fruits in the daily diet.** Consumption of vegetables and fruits is associated with a decreased risk of lung, prostate, bladder, esophageal, and stomach cancers.[17,18,24] These foods contain vitamins, minerals, fiber, and non-nutritive compounds that, alone or together, may be responsible for reducing cancer risk.[15,16] Clinical trials testing the preventive qualities of carotenoids are under way. It is unknown whether vitamin C per se or other constituents of vitamin C-rich foods have a potentially protective effect against cancers of the stomach and esophagus. More research is needed before the role of vitamin C in human cancer prevention can be assessed. Likewise, the evidence that selenium may be protective is still too limited to justify a recommendation for increasing its consumption, especially with the potential hazard of selenium toxicity.[18,25]

4. **Eat more high fiber foods, such as whole grain cereals, legumes, vegetables, and fruits.** Colon cancer is low in populations who live on a diet high in fiber.[17,18,23] Several mechanisms hypothesizing the preventive role of fiber have been proposed. Fiber may exert its effects by diluting the concentration of carcinogens in the colon, by reducing their contact time through more rapid transit, or by reducing their formation by altering the bacterial flora.[15,16,26] Another theory is that a high fiber diet of grains, fruits, and vegetables may be acting indirectly by replacing high calorie, high fat foods.

5. **Cut down on total fat intake.** Of all the dietary factors thought to affect cancer, fat has been the subject of the most research. Substantial evidence suggests that excessive fat intake increases the risk of developing cancers of the breast, colon, and prostate.[15-18,27,28] The NCI and ACS recommend reducing total fat intake from the current average of about 40% to 30% or less of total calorie intake, which is consistent with advice from the National Cholesterol Education Program.[29] This level of fat intake can be readily achieved by a change in eating habits and is also an effective way to reduce total calories.

6. **Limit consumption of alcoholic beverages if you drink at all.** Heavy drinkers are at increased risk for various cancers such as oral cavity, larynx, and esophagus.[15,17,18,30] These risks are greatly magnified in cigarette smokers. Alcohol has also been implicated in the development of cancers of the liver, pancreas, colon, and, most recently, breast. However, these relationships have not yet been established.[17,30,31]

7. **Limit consumption of salt-cured, smoked, and nitrite-preserved foods.** There is limited inferential evidence that salt-cured, pickled, or nitrite-cured foods may increase the risk of stomach and esophageal cancers in countries where these foods are common in the diet.[15,18] This risk in the U.S. diet appears to be small, and the American meat industry has already substantially reduced the amount of nitrite used in processed meats.

Other Dietary Constituents

The following other dietary constituents have received much attention and are under investigation. However, knowledge about the possible effects on cancer risk is insufficient to warrant any recommendations about their use at this time.

Food Additives.   Food additives would probably make, at most, only a small contribution to cancer risk.[18]

Caffeine.   Evidence on caffeine as a risk factor for cancer is inconclusive. Although some studies implicate caffeine in certain types of cancer, others fail to make such a connection. There is no indication that caffeine is a risk factor in human cancer and, thus, there is no recommendation against its moderate use.[18,30]

Artificial Sweeteners.   There is no evidence for an increase in risk of cancer for moderate users of saccharin. The long-term consequences of its consumption by children and pregnant women cannot be predicted. Aspartame is presumed to be safe but its long-term effects have not been studied.[15,16,18,30]

Methods of Food Preparation.   Broiling and grilling of meat at very high temperatures, such as with charcoal grills, may result in the formation of carcinogens.[15,18] This subject is now under intensive investigation.

References

15. Committee on Diet, Nutrition and Cancer. Diet, nutrition and cancer. Washington, DC: National Academy Press, 1982.
16. U.S. Department of Health and Human Services, Public Health Service, National Institutes of Health. Cancer prevention research summary—nutrition. Bethesda, MD: National Cancer Institute, 1985.

17. Butrum RR, Clifford CK, Lanza E. NCI dietary guidelines: rationale. Am J Clin Nutr 1988; 48:888–895.

18. The Work Study Group on Diet, Nutrition, and Cancer: Weinhouse S, Bal DG, et al. American Cancer Society guidelines on diet, nutrition, and cancer. CA 1991;41:334–338.

19. United States Department of Health and Human Services. Healthy people 2000—national health promotion and disease prevention objectives. Washington, DC: Public Health Service, DHHS Publication No. (PHS) 91-50212. 1990:415–440.

20. American Cancer Society, Inc.; 1599 Clifton Road NE; Atlanta, GA 30329;(800) ACS-2345.

21. The National Cancer Institute; Cancer Information Service (CIS); Bethesda, MD 20892; (800) 4-CANCER.

22. Garfinkel MA. Overweight and mortality. Cancer 1986;58:1826–1829.

23. Kritchevsky D. Diet and cancer. CA 1991;41:328–333.

24. Weisburger JH. Nutritional approach to cancer prevention with emphasis on vitamins, antioxidants, and carotenoids. Am J Clin Nutr 1991;53:226S–237S.

25. Oldfield JE. Some implications of selenium for human health. Nutr Today 1991; 26(4):6–11.

26. Bright-See E. Dietary fiber and cancer. Nutr Today 1988;23(4):4–10.

27. Carroll KK. Dietary fats and cancer. Am J Clin Nutr 1991;53:1064S–1067S.

28. Schatzkin A, Greenwald P, Byar DP, Clifford CK. The dietary fat–breast cancer hypothesis is alive. JAMA 1989;261:3284–3287.

29. National Cholesterol Education Program. Report of the Expert Panel on Detection, Evaluation, and Treatment of High Blood Cholesterol in Adults. Bethesda, MD: U.S. Department of Health and Human Services, Public Health Service, National Institutes of Health, National Heart, Lung and Blood Institute, NIH Pub. No. 88-2925, January 1988.

30. Sherwin R. Beverages and cancer. Clin Nutr 1990;9:56–61.

31. Kelsey JL, Gammon MD. The epidemiology of breast cancer. CA 1991;41:146–165.

RECOMMENDED DIETARY ALLOWANCES

The Recommended Dietary Allowances (RDAs) were first established in 1941 by the National Research Council of the National Academy of Sciences as a "guide for advising on nutrition problems in connection with national defense" and to "provide standards to serve as a goal for good nutrition." The RDAs are defined as "the levels of intake of essential nutrients that on the basis of scientific knowledge, are judged by the Food and Nutrition Board to be adequate to meet the known nutrient needs of practically all healthy persons." There is a safety factor in the RDAs for each nutrient, reflecting the state of knowledge concerning the nutrient, its bioavailability among food sources, and variations in requirements among individuals in the U.S. population. An attempt is made to publish the RDAs every 5 years in order to allow for possible updating as new scientific data become available. The 10th edition of the RDAs, published in 1989 is presented in Table 2-8.[32]

The function of the RDA has evolved with each revision. They are typically used for:

- Planning and procuring food supplies for population subgroups
- Interpreting food consumption records of individuals and populations
- Establishing standards for food assistance programs
- Evaluating the adequacy of food supplies in meeting national nutritional needs
- Designing nutrition education programs

TABLE 2-8 Food and Nutrition Board, National Academy of Sciences—National Research Council Recommended Dietary Allowances,[a] Revised 1989 (Designed for the maintenance of good nutrition of practically all healthy people in the United States)

Category	Age (yr) Condition	Weight[b] (kg)	Weight[b] (lb)	Height[b] (cm)	Height[b] (in)	Protein (g)	Vitamin A (μg RE)[c]	Vitamin D (μg)[d]	Vitamin E (mg α-TE)[e]	Vitamin K (μg)	Vitamin C (mg)	Thiamin (mg)	Riboflavin (mg)	Niacin (mg NE)[f]	Vitamin B6 (mg)	Folate (μg)	Vitamin B12 (μg)	Calcium (mg)	Phosphorus (mg)	Magnesium (mg)	Iron (mg)	Zinc (mg)	Iodine (μg)	Selenium (μg)
Infants	0.0–0.5	6	13	60	24	13	375	7.5	3	5	30	0.3	0.4	5	0.3	25	0.3	400	300	40	6	5	40	10
	0.5–1.0	9	20	71	28	14	375	10	4	10	35	0.4	0.5	6	0.6	35	0.5	600	500	60	10	5	50	15
Children	1–3	13	29	90	35	16	400	10	6	15	40	0.7	0.8	9	1.0	50	0.7	800	800	80	10	10	70	20
	4–6	20	44	112	44	24	500	10	7	20	45	0.9	1.1	12	1.1	75	1.0	800	800	120	10	10	90	20
	7–10	28	62	132	52	28	700	10	7	30	45	1.0	1.2	13	1.4	100	1.4	800	800	170	10	10	120	30
Males	11–14	45	99	157	62	45	1,000	10	10	45	50	1.3	1.5	17	1.7	150	2.0	1,200	1,200	270	12	15	150	40
	15–18	66	145	176	69	59	1,000	10	10	65	60	1.5	1.8	20	2.0	200	2.0	1,200	1,200	400	12	15	150	50
	19–24	72	160	177	70	58	1,000	10	10	70	60	1.5	1.7	19	2.0	200	2.0	1,200	1,200	350	10	15	150	70
	25–50	79	174	176	70	63	1,000	5	10	80	60	1.5	1.7	19	2.0	200	2.0	800	800	350	10	15	150	70
	51+	77	170	173	68	63	1,000	5	10	80	60	1.2	1.4	15	2.0	200	2.0	800	800	350	10	15	150	70
Females	11–14	46	101	157	62	46	800	10	8	45	50	1.1	1.3	15	1.4	150	2.0	1,200	1,200	280	15	12	150	45
	15–18	55	120	163	64	44	800	10	8	55	60	1.1	1.3	15	1.5	180	2.0	1,200	1,200	300	15	12	150	50
	19–24	58	128	164	65	46	800	10	8	60	60	1.1	1.3	15	1.6	180	2.0	1,200	1,200	280	15	12	150	55
	25–50	63	138	163	64	50	800	5	8	65	60	1.1	1.3	15	1.6	180	2.0	800	800	280	15	12	150	55
	51+	65	143	160	63	50	800	5	8	65	60	1.0	1.2	13	1.6	180	2.0	800	800	280	10	12	150	55
Pregnant						60	800	10	10	65	70	1.5	1.6	17	2.2	400	2.2	1,200	1,200	320	30	15	175	65
Lactating	1st 6 mo					65	1,300	10	12	65	95	1.6	1.8	20	2.1	280	2.6	1,200	1,200	355	15	19	200	75
	2nd 6 mo					62	1,200	10	11	65	90	1.6	1.7	20	2.1	260	2.6	1,200	1,200	340	15	16	200	75

[a]The allowances, expressed as average daily intakes over time, are intended to provide for individual variations among most normal persons as they live in the United States under usual environmental stresses. Diets should be based on a variety of common foods in order to provide other nutrients for which human requirements have been less well defined. See text of reference 32 for detailed discussion of allowances and of nutrients not tabulated.

[b]Weights and heights of Reference Adults are actual medians for the U.S. population of the designated age, as reported by NHANES II. The median weights and heights of those under 19 years of age were taken from Hamill et al. (1979) (see pp. 16 and 17 of reference 32). The use of these figures does not imply that the height-to-weight ratios are ideal.

[c]Retinol equivalents. 1 retinol equivalent = 1 μg retinol or 6 μg β-carotene. See text of reference 32 for calculation of vitamin A activity of diets as retinol equivalents.

[d]As cholecalciferol. 10 μg cholecalciferol = 400 IU of vitamin D.

[e]α-Tocopherol equivalents. 1 mg d-α tocopherol = 1 α-TE. See text of reference 32 for variation in allowances and calculation of vitamin E activity of the diet as α-tocopherol equivalents.

[f]1 NE (niacin equivalent) is equal to 1 mg of niacin or 60 mg of dietary tryptophan.

TABLE 2-9   Estimated Safe and Adequate Daily Dietary Intakes of Selected Vitamins and Minerals*

Age (yr)	Vitamins	
	Biotin (µg)	Pantothenic Acid (mg)
INFANTS		
0–0.5	10	2
0.5–1	15	3
CHILDREN AND ADOLESCENTS		
1–3	20	3
4–6	25	3–4
7–10	30	4–5
11+	30–100	4–7
ADULTS		
	30–100	4–7

Age (yr)	Trace Elements†				
	Copper (mg)	Manganese (mg)	Fluoride (mg)	Chromium (µg)	Molybdenum (µg)
INFANTS					
0–0.5	0.4–0.6	0.3–0.6	0.1–0.5	10–40	15–30
0.5–1	0.6–0.7	0.6–1.0	0.2–1.0	20–60	20–40
CHILDREN AND ADOLESCENTS					
1–3	0.7–1.0	1.0–1.5	0.5–1.5	20–80	25–50
4–6	1.0–1.5	1.5–2.0	1.0–2.5	30–120	30–75
7–10	1.0–2.0	2.0–3.0	1.5–2.5	50–200	50–150
11+	1.5–2.5	2.0–5.0	1.5–2.5	50–200	75–250
ADULTS					
	1.5–3.0	2.0–5.0	1.5–4.0	50–200	75–250

*Because there is less information on which to base allowances, these figures are not given in the main table of RDA and are provided here in the form of ranges of recommended intakes.

†Since the toxic levels for many trace elements may be only several times usual intakes, the upper levels for the trace elements given in this table should not be habitually exceeded.

Reprinted with permission from: Recommended Dietary Allowances, 10th ed. Copyright 1989 by the National Academy of Sciences. Courtesy of the National Academy Press, Washington, DC.

- Developing new products in industry
- Establishing guidelines for nutrition labeling of foods—known as the U.S. Recommended Dietary Allowances (U.S. RDAs)

The ninth edition of the RDAs established the category of safe and adequate intakes for selected vitamins (biotin and pantothenic acid) and minerals (copper, manganese, fluoride, chromium, and molybdenum) when data were sufficient for developing standards. This category is maintained in the tenth edition. It is cau-

TABLE 2-10 Estimated Sodium, Chloride, and Potassium Minimum Requirements of Healthy Persons*

Age	Weight (kg)*	Sodium (mg)*†	Chloride (mg)*†	Potassium (mg)‡
0–5 mo	4.5	120	180	500
6–11 mo	8.9	200	300	700
1 yr	11.0	225	350	1,000
2–5 yr	16.0	300	500	1,400
6–9 yr	25.0	400	600	1,600
10–18 yr	50.0	500	750	2,000
>18 yr§	70.0	500	750	2,000

*No allowance has been included for large, prolonged losses from the skin through sweat.

†There is no evidence that higher intakes confer any health benefit.

‡Desirable intakes of potassium may considerably exceed these values (~ 3,500 mg for adults—see reference 32).

§No allowance included for growth. Values for those below 18 years assume a growth rate at the 50th percentile reported by the National Center for Health Statistics (Hamill et al., 1979) and averaged for males and females. See text of reference 32 for information on pregnancy and lactation.

Reprinted with permission from: Recommended Dietary Allowances, 10th ed. Copyright 1989 by the National Academy of Sciences. Courtesy of the National Academy Press, Washington, DC.

tioned that upper levels for these trace elements should not be habitually exceeded because the toxic level may be only a few times usual intakes. The safe and adequate ranges are presented in Table 2-9.[32]

Safe and adequate ranges are no longer provided for sodium, potassium and chloride, since they are difficult to justify. Estimated minimum requirements for these electrolytes are provided for healthy persons at various ages. These are presented in Table 2-10.[32]

Reference

32. Recommended Dietary Allowances, 10th ed. Subcommittee on the Tenth Edition of the RDAs, Food and Nutrition Board Commission on Life Sciences National Research Council, Washington, DC, 1989.

FOOD LABELING

Since 1973 the Food and Drug Administration (FDA) has developed standards to be used in the labeling of foods for which manufacturers make a nutritional claim or for any food to which a nutrient has been added.[33] In the early 1990s the FDA along with the United States Department of Agriculture (USDA) proposed new regulations to improve the format and content of food labels. The goals of these proposed regulations are to provide reliable information and to aid consumers in making healthier food choices. The proposals being considered include: expansion of nutrition labeling to virtually all food products, full ingredient listing, standardized serving sizes, regulation of health claims and descriptors such as "light," "low fat," etc. The proposed standard label format appears in Figure 2-4.

Nutrition Facts

Serving Size 1 cup (228 g)
Servings Per Container 2

Amount Per Serving

Calories 125   Calories from fat 40

	% Daily Value*
Total Fat 4 g	6%
Saturated Fat 2 g	10%
Cholesterol 10 mg	3%
Sodium 850 mg	35%
Total Carbohydrate 16 g	5%
Dietary Fiber 1 g	4%
Sugars 0 g	
Protein 6 g	

Vitamin A 10%	•	Vitamin C 2%
Calcium 0%	•	Iron 2%

*Percent Daily Values are based on a 2,000 calorie diet.
Your daily values may be higher or lower depending on
your calorie needs:

	Calories:	2,000	2,500
Total Fat	Less than	65 g	80 g
Sat Fat	Less Than	20 g	25 g
Cholesterol	Less than	300 mg	300 mg
Sodium	Less than	2,400 mg	2,400 mg
Total Carbohydrate		300 g	375 g
Dietary Fiber		25 g	30 g

Calories per gram:
Fat 9   •   Carbohydrate 4   •   Protein 4

INGREDIENTS: Water, egg noodles (wheat flour, egg yolks,
salt), chicken, salt, food starch-modified, dextrose, vegetable
oil, monosodium glutamate, natural flavoring, garlic powder,
beta carotene added for color, paprika.

FIGURE 2-4   Standard Label Format.

In accord with the Nutrition Labeling and Education Act (NLEA) of 1990, the FDA is expecting all of the proposals to be finalized by November 1992. New labels will be required on all packaged foods beginning in May 1993.[34] However, at the time of this publication the finalized dates are speculative and it is possible that the FDA may receive a one-year extension date.

The new proposals have established two types of reference values: Reference Daily Intakes (RDIs) and Daily Reference Values (DRVs). The RDIs will replace the U.S. Recommended Dietary Allowances (USRDAs) for protein, 26 vitamins and minerals according to gender and five age groups. There are several food components for which USRDA have not been set but that are important in nutrition and health. These include: fiber, fat, saturated fat, unsaturated fat, cholesterol, carbohydrate, sodium, and potassium. DRV will be guidelines for the general population. Together, the RDIs and DRVs will be known as "Daily Values" and will appear on food labels, thereby providing consumers with reliable information for making food choices.[35,36] (See also Appendix 8—Food Labels-Nutrient Content Claims.)

References

33. Anon. Food Labeling. Fed Reg 1973;38:2124–2164.
34. Foulke JE. Wide sweeping FDA proposals to improve food labeling. FDA Consumer 1992; 26(1):9–13.
35. Dictionary of terms. In: Feeney P, ed. What's in a label? A dietitians handbook for helping consumers demystify food labels. Chicago: The American Dietetic Association and ConAgra Inc, 1990:100–101.
36. What's in a label? An interim labeling report for dietitians. Chicago: The American Dietetic Association and ConAgra Inc, 1992:7.

FOOD FACTS, FADS, AND FALLACIES

Food faddism is a multi-billion dollar industry and is the most widespread form of health quackery in the United States.[37] Unfortunately, nutrition misinformation is widespread for many reasons including false claims, lack of provider credentials, and inadequate nutrition education for health professionals. The Association of American Medical Colleges stated that 60% of medical school graduates did not receive adequate nutrition education.[38] Moreover, some politicians have actively pursued legislation supporting nutrition misinformation and seek Food and Drug Administration (FDA) regulatory exemptions on nutrition supplements.[39] In addition, psychological factors may play their part in promoting misinformation. Often, people using a product may improve on their own no matter what type of intervention was used. When this occurs, the type of therapy may get undeserved credit for the relief (placebo effect). The scientific community tries to account for this through controlled studies.

TABLE 2-11 Characteristics of Fraud

- Its rationale or underlying theory is inconsistent with accepted scientific beliefs
- It has not been demonstrated effective by well-designed studies
- Its use involves deception, misinformation, or significant physical danger

Types of fraud are often categorized as procedures or products and have one or more of the following characteristics that appear in Table 2-11.[39]

Target Groups for Fraud

The target groups for false and misleading nutrition promotions are primarily the elderly, athletes, overweight, and those with chronic illnesses.

Elderly.   The elderly are often a target group for nutrition fraud dealing with potions promising youth and freedom from arthritis. Many people search for the maintenance of health and youth in the form of vitamins and minerals. Unfortunately, few people are aware of the potential problems associated with megadoses (refer to Appendix 21 on Vitamins). For example, the use of vitamin E supplements is often promoted to slow aging on the basis that its antioxidant properties prevent cell damage from free radicals. True vitamin E deficiency is rare. It may occur in premature infants who do not receive vitamin E from the mother, some children who have severe protein-calorie malnutrition, or in some people who have had a long-standing inability to absorb fat secondary to an intestinal disease.[40] The Recommended Dietary Allowance for vitamin E is 8 to 10 IU. The average supplement is 400 IU. However, there are many people who take 1000 IU or more. There are potential harmful effects from megadoses of vitamin E.[40] (See Appendix 21 on Vitamins.)

Forty million persons in the United States suffer from many types of arthritis, such as osteoarthritis, rheumatoid arthritis, or gout.[41] When investigators at the University of Toledo conducted a random telephone survey of 300 people, they found that almost half incorrectly believed that arthritis was caused by poor diet, or cold, wet climate.[42] Of those polled, 76% replied vitamins were a good treatment and 57% stated special diets were useful. Unfortunately because there is no specific cure for arthritis, many sufferers in search of a cure turn to unproven diet manipulations and to megadoses of vitamins and minerals.[41] In actuality, factors that may help arthritis include weight loss for the overweight and a well balanced diet.[41] Chapter 4, Geriatric Nutrition, provides an overview of the nutritional needs of the elderly.

Athletes.   Athletes are often told that their bodies need "extra" vitamins, minerals, and muscle building aids so that they can achieve their desired performance and fitness level. However, there is potential harm in these false claims. Products promoted for the purpose of muscle building include glandular products and the use of anabolic steroids. Glandular products are organ tissues (of undefined origin) that have been dehydrated and processed at low temperatures. This process may not prevent bacterial contamination which may result in potential harm. Glandulars contain no hormones, but claim to "support" the corresponding organs within the body. Since they are tissues, they are made of protein and thus digested before the body absorbs them, therefore adding insignificant amounts of amino acids to the body's pool.

The prevalence of use of anabolic steroids for muscle building is difficult to assess, but is believed to be widespread. It is estimated that the use among weight lifters and body builders is as high as 80%, while among all competitors it is approximately 50%.[43] It is estimated that approximately 80% of the steroids are obtained illegally through a black market involving gyms or mail order sources.[43] The use of steroids for this purpose is condemned by many organizations such as the American Medical Association, the American College of Sports Medicine, the National Collegiate Athletic Association, the National Football League, and the International Olympic Committee. Some potential adverse effects (dependent on sex, age, dose, and duration of use) include impaired liver function, increased aggressiveness, stunted growth, testicular atrophy, decreased sperm count, menstrual irregularities, hypertension, elevated low-density lipoprotein cholesterol, and decreased high-density lipoprotein cholesterol.[43] Chapter 4, Nutrition and Physical Performance, presents an overview of the nutritional requirements for athletes.

Overweight persons.   Weight conscious people also are at a high risk for being victims for nutrition fraud. Many people wishing to lose weight want to lose it fast and effortlessly; therefore there is a market for miracle cures for obesity. Weight loss schemes can be categorized into dietary manipulations, mechanical and electrical devices, and pills. Dietary manipulations include fasts, meal replacement drinks, and high protein diets. High protein (ketogenic) diets tend to have increased amounts of fat as well as protein and thus may lead to hyperlipidemia. Unsupervised (or inappropriately supervised) prolonged use of meal replacement drinks (or repeated fasts) lead to extreme calorie reduction and may result in anemia, impairment of liver function, gallbladder and kidney stones, mineral and electrolyte imbalances, and potential decrease in metabolic rate.[44] The risk of health problems imposed by extremely low calorie regimens are highest in those individuals who are mildly obese.[44] These types of dietary manipulations are potentially dangerous and should have medical supervision.

Mechanical and electrical devices encompass vibration and passive exercise. Vibrators are promoted as spot reducing aids. Claims that vibrators may be effective in treating disease or weight loss are misleading. Passive exercise via motor-driven devices that pull the body through the motions of exercise may slightly improve muscle tone, however, does not effectively burn calories for weight loss.[43] Similarly, electrical muscle stimulators (EMS) provide no benefit for weight loss. EMS devices claim to contour the body through low voltage electrical shocks, causing muscles to contract and shrink. However, there is no evidence that EMS can reshape the body and it may even cause burns if used incorrectly.[44] If used correctly, some EMS devices may be useful in physical therapy to help prevent blood clots or retard muscle wasting in paralyzed muscles.

Diet pills are also promoted for weight loss. Diet pills may be categorized as appetite suppressants, absorption blockers, amphetamines, and diuretics. Appetite suppressant agents include amphetamines, phenylpropanolamine (PPA), fiber, and spirulina. However, there is no scientific evidence that any of these have any long term benefit for weight control.[44] Moreover, there is a fine line between appropriate doses and the amounts that may be unsafe, and cause side effects and even addiction (amphetamines). Absorption blockers such as the "starch blocker," "fat magnet," and "Gymnema Sylvestre" claim to alter absorption. These claims are not substantiated. Additionally, the weight loss tends to be only temporary. Chapter 8, Obesity, presents an overview of accepted treatment for weight loss.

Chronic Illness—Cancer and AIDS.   Chronic illnesses are often associated with major morbidity and mortality even with current medical methods. Thus, many people with a chronic illness (such as cancer or acquired immunodeficiency syndrome [AIDS]) may turn to alternative or unconventional treatments for new hope and "magical" cures. Unfortunately, these treatments may postpone traditional medical methods, thus putting the patient at more risk for harm.

Popular unconventional therapies for cancer include the macrobiotic diet, megavitamins, and laetrile. The macrobiotic diet is a strict vegetarian selection of foods consisting of grains, vegetables, dried beans, and seaweeds. Because of its low calorie content (due to the restriction of fat and sugar) and high fiber content, it may not be adequate for cancer patients with anorexia. In addition, the high fiber content may cause problems in those patients with gastrointestinal problems, such as gas, diarrhea, or obstructions.[45] Although this diet is less restrictive than the Zen Macrobiotic Diet, it still is deficient in niacin, riboflavin, vitamin B_{12}, and vitamin D. It may also be low in bioavailable calcium, iron, and zinc as well as protein.[45]

Megavitamin supplementation is based on the belief that the large doses may strengthen the body's capacity to destroy malignant cells or prevent their growth. Supplements may be provided alone or in conjunction with other treatments. However, megavitamin supplementation is of questionable benefit and may be toxic (refer to Appendix 21 on Vitamins).

Advocates of laetrile claim it can kill tumor cells. Laetrile is also called amygdalin, or vitamin B_{17}. However, laetrile is not a vitamin. The postulated mechanism of laetrile was that an enzyme in cancer cells would change amygdalin into cyanide to kill cancer cells. As a result, cyanide poisoning may occur. Presently it is

---

TABLE 2-12   Resources

AIDS Nutrition Network c/o US Department of Health Services 5600 Fishers Ln Rockville, MD 20857 (303) 443-6364	National Council Against Health Fraud PO Box 1276 Loma Linda, CA 92340
Arthritis Foundation PO Box 1900 Atlanta, GA 30326	President's Council on Physical Fitness and Sports 450 5th Street NW Suite 7103 Washington, DC 20001 (202) 272-3421
American Dietetic Association 216 W Jackson Blvd Suite 800 Chicago, IL 60606-6995 (800) 877-1600	FDA—HFY 40 5600 Fishers Lane Rockville, MD 20857 (800) 238-7332
National Cancer Institute Cancer Information Service Building 31 Room 10A18 Bethesda, MD 20892	

illegal to use laetrile in many states. In 1977, the FDA commissioner stated, "laetrile is a major health fraud in the U.S. and that there is no evidence of its safety and effectiveness."[46] Chapter 12, Cancer, presents an overview of accepted nutrition practices for improving nutrition of cancer patients.

AIDS patients have many complications that have an impact on their nutritional status, thus they are prone to nutrition fraud. Often these patients try alternative nutrition therapies out of frustration and lack of promising medical treatments. AIDS patients may adopt a modified macrobiotic diet, lecithin mixtures, glandulars, or megavitamins. These nutritional practices should be evaluated for harm

TABLE 2-13   Where to Report Nutrition and Health Fraud[50]

Problem	Agencies to Contact
False advertising	FTC Bureau of Consumer Protection Regional FTC office National Advertising Division Chief Postal Inspector, U.S. Postal Service Editor or station manager of media outlet where ad appeared
Product marketed with false or misleading claims	Regional FDA office State attorney general State health department Local Better Business Bureau Congressional representatives
Bogus mail-order promotion	Chief Postal Inspector, U.S. Postal Service Editor or station manager of media outlet where ad appeared National Council Against Health Fraud
Improper treatment by licensed practitioner	Local or state professional society (if practitioner is a member) Local hospital (if practitioner is a staff member) State licensing board National Council Against Health Fraud Task Force on Victim Redress
Improper treatment by unlicensed individual	Local district attorney State attorney general National Council Against Health Fraud Task Force on Victim Redress
Advice needed about questionable product or service	National Council Against Health Fraud Consumer Health Information Research Institute Local, state, or national professional or voluntary health groups

and discouraged if potentially dangerous. However, if the practice is not harmful, a placebo effect may improve the patient's mental and physical well-being.[47] Therefore, it is recommended that patients should not be discouraged from following their diet of choice unless it is harmful or not providing their nutritional goals.[48]

Combating Nutrition Fraud

There are ways to combat nutrition misinformation. The National Council Against Health Fraud has published strategies to help patients avoid being victims.[39] The Food and Drug Administration has published guidelines for evaluating potentially fraudulent television advertisements.[49] Table 2-12 presents resources to contact for questions about purported nutrition claims for treatments or cures. Many professional societies also provide information. Table 2-13 presents a listing of agencies that handle reported nutrition and health fraud claims.[50]

References

37. Kuske TT. Fads and quackery in nutrition. J Med Assoc Georgia 1991;80(3):159–162.
38. Emery EM, McDermott RJ, Ritter GP. Toward a policy on regulation of the weight control industry. J Health Educ 1991;22(3):150–153.
39. Barrett S. Health schemes, scams, and frauds. Mount Vernon, NY: Consumer Reports Books, Consumer Union, 1990:221–237.
40. Marshall CW. Vitamins and minerals help or harm? Philadelphia: George F. Stickley Co, 1985:70.
41. Wolman PG. Management of patients using unproven regimens for arthritis. JADA 1987; 87(9):1211–1214.
42. Jarvis WT. Arthritis: folk remedies and quackery. Nutrition Forum 1990;7(1):1–3.
43. Council of Scientific Affairs. Medical and nonmedical uses of anabolic-androgenic steroids. JAMA 1990;264(22):2923–2927.
44. Barrett S. Health schemes, scams, and frauds. Mount Vernon, NY: Consumer Reports Books, Consumer Union, 1990:132–141.
45. Herman-Zaidins M, Mulner I. In: Bloch A, ed. Nutrition management of the cancer patient. Rockville: Aspen Publishers, 1990:362–364.
46. Anon. Unproven methods of cancer management . . . laetrile. CA-A Cancer Journal for Clinicians 1991;41(3):187–192.
47. Anon. Nutrition fraud and AIDS. AJPH 1989;79(3):358–359.
48. Resler SS. Nutrition care of AIDS patients. Journal American Dietetic Association 1988; 88(7):828–832.
49. Department of Health and Human Services. Health fraud kit. Lesson plan: tips for checking proposed broadcast ads. Washington DC: Food and Drug Administration, 1989.
50. Verbal discussion with John H. Renner, MD, President, National Council Against Health Fraud. Consumer Health Information Research Institute, 3521 Broadway, Kansas City, MO 64111; (816) 753–8850.

3 / *Nutritional Screening and Assessment*

The screening and assessment of the patient's nutritional state involves both the initial visit and continued observations during the following days and weeks to determine whether changes in the nutritional status have occurred. Whether this is formalized or less structured, certain elements are involved, such as a review of the medical history, patient interview including a diet history, examination of the patient, anthropometric measurements, review of laboratory data, estimation of nutritional requirements, nutritional intervention, and evaluation of the outcome of the intervention. There is information available on nutritional assessment techniques and on criteria for diagnosing nutritional risks.[1-4] Such methods, however, are open to criticism,[5] and one should understand their limitations when interpreting findings.

In 1990 the American Society for Parenteral and Enteral Nutrition published *Standards of Practice for Nutrition Support Dietitians.*[6] These standards of practice may also be used in conjunction with established protocols for nutritional screening, assessment, and support and appear in Appendix 1.

With these issues in mind, it has been our usual practice to approach nutritional assessment globally rather than by utilizing specific protocols per se.[7] Data that are routinely available are used by the clinician in identifying a nutritional diagnosis rather than utilizing a standard nutritional assessment battery.[8] The following information is a description of this approach to nutritional assessment.

REVIEW OF MEDICAL HISTORY

The initial step in the screening of patients for nutritional problems should be a review of the medical history for high risk conditions that may accompany malnutrition or that may predispose a patient to malnutrition. This permits early intervention in the treatment of established malnutrition and aids in its prevention.

Malnutrition usually results from one or more of the following pathophysiological mechanisms (Table 3-1): alterations in nutrient intake, digestion, absorption,

---

TABLE 3-1   Pathophysiological Mechanisms of Malnutrition

Mechanism	Disorder
Intake	Impairment or inability to regulate ingestion of nutrients. Found in, but not limited to, such diseases or disorders as: Anorexia nervosa — GI motility disorders Bulimia — Hyperemesis Altered level of consciousness — Inability to chew and swallow GI tract obstruction — Iatrogenic and self imposed dietary restrictions
Digestion	Impairment or inability to break down nutrients into absorbable entities. Found in, but not limited to, such diseases or disorders as: Disaccharidase deficiency — Cystic fibrosis Pancreatitis and biliary insufficiency
Absorption	Impairment or inability to assimilate nutrients. Found in, but not limited to, such diseases or disorders as: Inflammatory bowel (Crohn's) disease — Short bowel syndrome Gastrectomy — Radiation enteritis
Excretion or Increased Losses	Impairment or inability to rid the body of waste products of metabolized nutrients or increased losses of nutrients. Found in, but not limited to, such diseases or disorders as: Chronic renal disease — Dialysis Draining abscesses or wounds — Blood loss Fistula
Metabolism	Impairment or inability to utilize assimilated nutrients. Found in, but not limited to, such diseases or disorders as: Inborn errors of metabolism — Chronic obstructive pulmonary disease Liver disease — Chronic renal disease Drug-nutrient interactions
Requirements	Alteration in quantity of nutrients needed to obtain or maintain health that is beyond the ability of the individual to consume. Found in, but not limited to, such conditions as: Trauma — Burns Sepsis — Hypermetabolic states Fever

excretion, metabolism, and/or requirements. Knowledge of medical conditions and of their pathophysiology is helpful in identifying patients who are at risk for malnutrition.

The physical examination of the patient as reported in the medical history may also provide valuable assistance in identifying patients who are malnourished or are at high risk of becoming malnourished. Many of these variable signs can be detected by observation during the interview, such as cachexia, easily plucked hair, poor dentition, depleted fat stores, ascites, skin lesions, glossitis, and skin rashes.[9]

PATIENT INTERVIEW

After reviewing the patient's medical history, the dietitian interviews the patient and, if necessary, the family members.

In general, questions should be directed to (1) the nature and the duration of the illness and their effect on eating patterns; (2) weight loss or gain over the past 3 to 6 months; (3) usual eating habits and food preferences; (4) intake of medications, nutritional supplements, and alcohol.

The method that is selected to obtain the diet history is determined by the time and the personnel available, the setting (e.g., hospital, outpatient clinic), and the degree of accuracy that is needed. After the dietary intake data have been collected and summarized, they may be compared to one of several established nutrient intake guidelines and/or standards to determine nutritional adequacy in meeting the individual's needs.

The dietitian should review medications recently and currently used by the patient, and note those medications that have known drug-nutrient interactions (Appendix 2).[10] The amounts and types of vitamin and/or mineral preparations that are ingested by the patient should be determined and evaluated for potential toxicities (Appendices 20 and 21). If nutritional supplements have been ingested, their nutrient and caloric contribution should be included as a part of the dietary analysis (Appendix 10). Alcohol intake should be noted for its potential effect on nutrient utilization as well as its caloric contribution to the diet. (See Appendix 3.)

ANTHROPOMETRICS

Anthropometrics may be defined as the measurement of size, weight, and proportions of the body. The methods most frequently utilized include height, weight, triceps skinfold thickness, midarm muscle circumference measurements, body mass index, and waist-to-hip ratio. Anthropometric indices may assist in establishing a crude basis for determining body composition and nutritional status. The selection of the most appropriate method depends on whether the intent is for general nutritional screening or for more in-depth nutritional assessment.

Body Height and Weight

An accurate measurement of the patient's height and weight on admission and the weight at regular intervals is important, as these provide crude measures of body fat stores, muscle mass, and, therefore, metabolic fuels as well as changes in hydration status. Such measurements may be utilized in comparison to height and weight norms (Appendix 4). Such norms, however, are often mistakenly considered as an "ideal" weight for height for an individual. These standards do not account for variations in patient age, heredity, degree of athletic training, or possible effect of illness. An individual's preillness weight or usual weight during health can serve as a more realistic norm for determining the effect of illness on body weight.

When there has been a loss of body parts, the estimation of weight loss or gain becomes difficult. Table 3-2 shows the approximate percentage of body weight that is contributed by various body parts. These percentages can be used to adjust body weight norms.[9]

TABLE 3-2   Percentage of Total Body Weight Contributed by Individual Body Parts

Body Part	%
Trunk without limbs	42.7
Hand	0.8
Forearm with hand	3.1
Entire arm with hand	6.5
Foot	1.8
Lower leg with foot	7.1
Entire leg	18.6

With permission and adapted from: Grant A, DeHoog S. Anthropometrics. In: Grant A, DeHoog S, eds. Nutritional assessment and support. 4th ed. Seattle: Grant A, DeHoog S, 1991:19–20.

Weight Change

A history of a very rapid weight loss suggests a catabolic state with a substantial loss of protein tissue, dehydration, or both. Protein tissue with muscle as its prototype represents only about 400 kcal/lb, whereas adipose tissue represents a storage of about 3,500 kcal/lb. Hence, a negative caloric balance from the destruction of protein tissue can be expected to cause a weight loss eight to ten times greater than would be the case if the weight loss from the same negative caloric balance were in the form of only adipose tissue.

The most significant usage of body weight as an index for determining nutritional status is the percent of recent weight change. The following equations are helpful in calculating the degree of weight change:

$$\% \text{ of usual body weight} = \frac{\text{current body weight}}{\text{usual body weight}} \times 100$$

$$\% \text{ of recent weight change} = \frac{\text{usual body weight} - \text{current body weight}}{\text{usual body weight}} \times 100$$

It is difficult to know how much weight loss is significant since one does not know how much of the loss is body tissue rather than fluid loss. Approximately 50 to 60% of a healthy adult is fluid. An unintentional weight loss of 10% in a 6-month period is clinically significant.[11] However, if the patient is or has been edematous, such a weight change may not be of nutritional importance.

BIOCHEMICAL ASSESSMENT

A number of laboratory parameters have been used to assess nutritional status. These are obtained from blood (serum and plasma), urine, feces, or from tissue biopsy (e.g., bone or organ). Although laboratory tests are the most objective measures, their degree of sensitivity and specificity in identifying nutritional status are affected by a number of factors. These include age, gender, physiological state, medications, and nutrient interactions. Hence, there may be questions about the meaning of abnormal values for certain tests. For example, hypoalbuminemia is not an accurate marker of impaired nutritional status per se. Stress and production of cytokines decrease the rate of albumin synthesis. This, coupled with increased catabolism and extravascular extravasation, is the cause of hypoalbuminemia of illness. Therefore, during illness, serum albumin concentration should be viewed as an imperfect measure of nutritional status but as an excellent marker for the injury response.[4] Furthermore, calcium, magnesium, and zinc are bound to albumin, and low levels may be due to reduced serum albumin rather than to malnutrition per se.

Laboratory parameters are more appropriately used to modify the nutritional treatment program. For example, it is essential to assess renal and hepatic function in order to make decisions about provision of protein. In the patient with established diabetes mellitus or stress hyperglycemia, it is important to avoid overfeeding and to limit the dextrose load until glycemic control is achieved. Fluid balance (as determined by fluid intake and output), weight, and serum electrolytes must be monitored closely following the initiation of nutritional support. Refeeding can cause decreased plasma concentrations of potassium, phosphorus, and magnesium unless supplementation is adequate.

In summary, for most clinical purposes, adequate assessment may be achieved by routine blood and urine studies, especially when these studies are combined with a careful nutritional history and physical examination and supported by a systematic analysis of the data so obtained.

ESTIMATION OF NUTRIENT REQUIREMENTS

In arriving at an estimate of nutrient needs, the following must be considered: (1) the requirements for a normal individual; (2) the current nutritional status of the individual; (3) the nature of the disease or injury; (4) the known capacity of the body to store certain nutrients; (5) the known losses through wounds, skin, urine, or intestinal tract; (6) the interactions of drugs and nutrients; and (7) the interre-

TABLE 3-3   Guidelines for Assessing Nutritional Needs

	Intensive Care Unit	Ward	Obese Patient
Kilocalories	Basal Harris Benedict or REE	Basal Harris Benedict to +20% or REE to +20%	Basal Harris Benedict (based on current weight)
Protein	1.5 g of protein per kilogram (intact renal and hepatic function)	1.0–1.5 g of protein per kilogram	1.5 g of protein per kilogram of estimated lean weight
Fat	30% of total calories and infused over a 24-hr period	30% of total calories and infused over a 24-hr period	—

REE = Resting energy expenditure.

lationships of various nutrients. Table 3-3 presents a summary of guidelines for assessing the nutrient needs of individuals in the intensive care unit and in the ward and the adjustments made for obese patients.

Energy Needs

Several methods exist for estimating resting energy requirements. The most widely used formulas are those of Harris and Benedict.[12]

For males:
$$BEE = 66.4 + 13.7(W) + 5(H) - 6.8(A)$$

For females:
$$BEE = 655 + 9.6(W) + 1.8(H) - 4.7(A)$$

BEE is basal energy expenditure, A is age in years, W is actual weight in kilograms, and H is height in centimeters. Various tables, such as the Mayo Clinic Nomogram may also be used (see Appendix 6). Adjustments to the calculated BEE may over- or underestimate the actual resting energy expenditure (REE) when measured by indirect calorimetry.[13] Therefore, for patients who are suspected of having energy requirements that vary greatly from the norm, a measurement of the REE under steady state conditions is recommended.[14-17]

An indirect calorimetric measurement of energy needs may be helpful in the following circumstances: severely stressed (e.g., closed head injury, multiple trauma, sepsis, significant body burn), morbidly obese, severely malnourished, the volume-overloaded patient in whom the "dry weight" estimate is uncertain, the patient receiving nutritional support in whom weaning from mechanical ventilation is difficult, and the elderly.

Energy expenditure is indirectly determined by measuring oxygen consumption and carbon dioxide production, usually at rest. However, REE determinations should not be construed as equivalent to the 24-hour energy requirement. Daily energy fluctuations occur with physical therapy, stress, febrile episodes, and other effectors of metabolic rate. Typically, the intensive care unit patient's energy goal may be calculated at the measured REE provided that steady state conditions have been achieved during the study. It may be appropriate to add 20% for mobile patients in the ward who are not overweight.

One should also consider the respiratory quotient (RQ), which offers information about the degree of over- or underfeeding and the predominant type of fuel

TABLE 3-4   Respiratory Quotient (RQ)

Energy Source	RQ
Fat oxidation (net)	0.7
Protein oxidation (net)	0.80
Mixed substrate oxidation (net)	0.85
Glucose oxidation (net)	1.0
Net fat synthesis (lipogenesis)	> 1.01*

*Ascertain that RQ is not elevated due to hyperventilation.

being used by the body (Table 3-4). An RQ (if not measured during hyperventilation) greater than or equal to 1.0 may reflect net lipogenesis, and the nutrition program must be reviewed to determine if the patient is being overfed.[18]

Energy needs of patients with spinal cord injury are difficult to assess. It has been found that when compared with indirect calorimetry, formulas such as from Harris and Benedict tend to overestimate the energy needs of these patients. It has been found that quadriplegics require approximately 23 kcal/kg of actual body weight per day, and paraplegics require approximately 28 kcal/kg of actual body weight per day.[19] Weekly monitoring of weights of patients with spinal cord injury is helpful. However, one must consider that muscle mass will be depleted in the postinjury course, and weight loss should be expected at this time. For obese patients, basal calories are calculated on the basis of current weight rather than any fraction thereof. Basal calories, as calculated, are provided.

Protein Needs

The recommended dietary allowance (RDA) of protein for normal healthy adults is 0.8 g/kg of body weight. The minimum requirement for the maintenance of nitrogen balance in healthy adults is between 0.4 and 0.5 g/kg. Fever, sepsis, surgery, trauma, and burns increase protein catabolism, and therefore greater amounts of specific amino acids and/or protein may be needed.

Most hospitalized patients can be adequately maintained on protein intakes between 1.0 and 1.5 g/kg of actual body weight per day. For obese patients, protein needs are calculated on the basis of 1.5 times the estimated lean weight (for women, 100 lb for first 5 ft in height and 5 lb for each inch thereafter; for men, 106 lb for first 5 ft in height and 6 lb for each inch thereafter).[20]

Vitamins

Vitamin allowances for healthy persons are well standardized, but the altered needs that are associated with specific disease states remain poorly defined. Supplemental vitamins should be provided to ensure the RDA when the quantity or quality of the intake does not provide adequate vitamins. Appendix 20 presents the composition of various oral multiple vitamin products; multiple vitamin products formulated for intravenous use for adults appear in Appendix 21.

Minerals and Trace Elements

As with vitamins, mineral requirements have been established for healthy adults, but less is known about the need for them during the stress of disease and trauma. An adequate supply of minerals is essential for anabolism. Levels of potassium and phosphorus, the major intracellular ions, fall during nutritional repletion. As nutritional repletion occurs, insulin response shifts these ions intercellularly and into energy pathways. Serum levels may fall if potassium and phosphorus are not supplied in sufficient amounts. Likewise, serum calcium, magnesium, and zinc should be interpreted in light of the albumin concentration. Calcium, magnesium, and zinc are bound to albumin, and low levels may be due to reduced serum albumin. As with vitamins, the mineral intake should assure 100% of the RDA, and supplements should be provided when there are increased requirements, losses, or inadequate intake.

NUTRITIONAL CARE PLAN

After the goals of nutritional therapy are determined, the nutritional care plan can guide the selection of appropriate nutritional support. A nutritional care plan should consist of a completed nutritional assessment, the identification of any nutritional problems, and a statement of realistic and quantifiable nutritional objectives. Therapeutic measures to provide estimated nutrient needs may include oral feeding, enteral tube feeding, and/or parenteral nutrition. Monitoring or reassessment of the nutritional status should be performed at appropriate intervals to evaluate the effectiveness of the nutritional intervention. Documentation in the medical history of the findings from nutritional screening/assessment as well as the plan of intervention and the effectiveness of the intervention should occur according to regulatory and institutional guidelines.

References

1. Bistrian BR, Blackburn GL, Vitale B, Cochran D, Naylor B. Prevalence of malnutrition in general medical patients. JAMA 1976;230:1567–1570.
2. Dreblow DM, Anderson CF, Moxness KE. Nutritional assessment of orthopedic patients. Mayo Clin Proc 1981;56:51–54.
3. Konstantinides FN, Konstantinides NN, Li JC, Myaya ME, Cerra FB. Urinary urea nitrogen: too insensitive for calculating nitrogen balance studies in surgical clinical nutrition. JPEN 1991;15(2):189–193.
4. McMahon MM, Bistrian BR. The physiology of nutritional assessment and therapy in protein-calorie malnutrition. Dis Mon 1990;36(7):373–417.
5. Grant JP. Nutritional assessment in clinical practice. Nutr Clin Pract 1986;1:3–11.
6. Standards Committee. Standards of practice for nutrition support dietitians. Nutr Clin Pract 1990;5(2):74–78.
7. Murray MJ, Marsh M, Wochos DN, Moxness KE, Offord KP, Callaway CW. Nutritional assessment of intensive care unit patients. Mayo Clin Proc 1988;63:1106–1115.
8. Jeejeebhoy KN, Detsky AS, Baker JP. Assessment of nutritional status. JPEN 1990;14(5): 1935–1965.
9. Grant A, DeHoog S. Anthropometrics. In: Grant A, DeHoog S, eds. Nutritional assessment and support. 4th ed. Seattle: Grant A, DeHoog S, 1991:19–20.
10. Smith CH, Bidlade WR. Dietary concerns associated with the use of medications. J Am Diet Assoc 1984;84:901–914.
11. Jeejeebhoy KN. Assessment of nutritional status. In: Rombeau JL, Caldwell MD, eds. Clinical nutrition—enteral and tube feeding. Philadelphia: WB Saunders, 1990:118–126.
12. Harris JA, Benedict FG. A biometric study of basal metabolism in man. Washington, DC: Carnegie Institution, 1919 (Carnegie Institution of Washington, Publication No. 279).
13. Ireton-Jones CS, Turner WW. Actual or ideal body weight: which should be used to predict energy expenditure? J Am Diet Assoc 1991;91(2):193–195.
14. Anderson CF, Loosbrock LM, Moxness KE. Nutrient intake in critically ill patients: too many or too few calories? Mayo Clin Proc 1986;61:853–858.
15. Clark HD, Hoffer LJ. Reappraisal of the resting metabolic rate of normal young men. Am J Clin Nutr 1991;53:21–26.
16. Hunter DC, Jaksic T, Lewis D, Benotti PN, Blackburn GL, Bistrian BR. Resting energy expenditure in the critically ill: estimations versus measurement. Br J Surg 1988;75:875–878.
17. Isbell TR, Klesges RC, Meyers AW, Klesges LM. Measurement reliability and reactivity using repeated measurements of resting energy expenditure with a face mask, mouthpiece and ventilated canopy. JPEN 1991;15:165–168.

18. Ireton-Jones CS. Indirect calorimetry. In: Skipper A, ed. Dietitian's handbook of enteral and parenteral nutrition. Rockville, MD: Aspen Publishers, 1989:205–217.

19. Cox SA, Weiss SM, Posuniek EA, Worthington P, Priolea M, Heffley G. Energy expenditure after spinal cord injury: an evaluation of stable rehabilitating patients. J Trauma 1985;25:419–423.

20. Davidson JK. Symposium: controlling diabetes mellitus with diet therapy. Postgrad Med 1976;59(1):114–122.

4 / *Normal Nutrition*

PREGNANCY AND LACTATION

General Description

The diet for pregnancy and lactation should be well balanced and calorie controlled. Specific attention should also be given to dietary sources of calcium and iron. Also to be considered are the special nutritional needs of pregnant teens, those with diabetes and gestational diabetes, and those who breast-feed.

Nutritional Inadequacy

The diet for pregnancy and lactation is not inherently lacking in nutrients as compared to the recommended dietary allowance (RDA). However, the mother's needs may exceed her ability to consume a quantity of food adequate to meet her established nutrient levels. Research has shown that supplemental vitamins and minerals, especially folic acid, calcium, and iron, may be necessary to provide an adequate intake because these nutrients are often difficult to attain.

PREGNANCY

Indications and Rationale

Many studies have shown that the nutritional quality of the diet affects the course and outcome of pregnancy. Nutritional status before pregnancy is also a major factor that affects the health of a pregnant woman and of her infant.

The characteristics of women considered at nutritional risk during pregnancy are listed in Table 4-1. Pregnant women in these situations should have a more extensive evaluation of their nutritional status and of the adequacy of their dietary intake.

In addition, women who have been taking oral contraceptives, especially long-term users with poor dietary habits, may be at risk for folic acid and vitamin B_6 defi-

39

TABLE 4-1   Women Defined as Nutritionally "At Risk" during Pregnancy

- Do not ordinarily consume an adequate diet
- Carry more than one fetus
- Use cigarettes, alcohol, illicit drugs
- Have lactose intolerance
- Are underweight or overweight at conception or gain inadequate or excessive weight during pregnancy
- Are adolescents
- Have poor knowledge about nutrition or have insufficient financial resources to purchase adequate food

ciency.[1] After terminating use of oral contraceptives, women may be best advised to wait several months and to improve overall diet before attempting pregnancy.

NORMAL PREGNANCY

Weight Gain.   Weight management during pregnancy should promote optimum nutrition for the mother and for the child. An inadequate maternal weight gain may result in low birth weight (less than 2,500 g) of the infant and an increase in perinatal mortality.

Recommendations for optimum weight gain during gestation have been a source of much discussion and controversy since the early 1900s. Prior to the 1960s the recommendation was to restrict total weight gain to less than 15 lb. Since then research has suggested that more liberal weight gains have been associated with improved fetal growth.[2] Recommendations from the American College of Obstetrics and Gynecology have encouraged adult women of normal weight to gain 24 to 27 lb.[3] Most recently the National Academy of Sciences has put forth more specific recommendations for weight gain during gestation, focusing on desirable ranges of weight gain rather than a single target weight to gain. They have also broadened their recommendations by providing ranges of weight gain for five different categories of women, as summarized in Table 4-2.[4]

Although no studies have yet been conducted to determine what rates of weight gain are most conducive to favorable fetal outcomes, it is well established that a healthy pattern of weight gain is one of gradual, steady increments.[4] Short-term fluctuations in weight are more likely to be associated with excessive fluid retention. The recommended rate of weight gain is approximately 2 to 4 lb during the first trimester and 0.8 to 1 lb per week thereafter, for normal weight women.[4]

Energy Intake.   It is well recognized that extra energy is required during pregnancy to meet the demands of both mother and fetus. However, limited data from human studies do not allow a precise definition of reproductive demands. Estimates of the total energy cost of pregnancy, based on dietary intake by pregnant women and resting energy expenditure measurements, have ranged from 45,000 to 80,000 kcal.[5] Recommendations for daily increases in caloric needs have

TABLE 4-2 Recommended Ranges for Weight Gain Based on Prepregnancy Weight

	Weight Gain (lb)
Underweight women (< 90% of desirable*)	28–40
Normal weight women	25–35
Overweight women (> 120% of desirable*)	15–25
(> 135% of desirable*)	15
Women carrying twins (target total weight gain at term)	35–45

Note: Young adolescents and Afro-American women should strive for gains at the upper end of the recommended range. Short women (less than 157 cm or 62 in) should strive for gains at the lower end of the range.

*Desirable weight is based on the 1959 Metropolitan Life Insurance Company weight for height standards.

been estimated by dividing 80,000 kcal by 240 days of gestation, yielding approximately 300 kcal per day above a woman's nonpregnant energy needs.

Studies conducted with women in industrialized nations have concluded that it is possible to gain enough weight to support fetal growth on an energy level only slightly higher than in the nonpregnant state.[5] It is speculated that this is due to a combination of decreased activity during pregnancy and more efficient energy utilization. Energy needs for healthy, well-nourished women may only need to be increased by 200 to 300 kcal/day toward the last half of pregnancy. In order to best determine a woman's energy requirements, nutritional assessment should include analysis of her activity patterns.

Protein. Altogether 925 g of protein are deposited in a normal fetus and maternal accessary tissues. An increase of 10 g of protein per day over the RDA for a nonpregnant woman is adequate to meet these needs.[6]

Calcium. It is recommended that calcium intake be 1,200 mg/day throughout pregnancy and lactation for adult women.[6] There is no clear relation between a mother's bone health and the number of pregnancies or lactation history for those who consume recommended amounts of calcium.[6]

Iron. An increase in the body stores of iron of about 1,200 mg is needed for expansion of the maternal red blood cell volume and for the synthesis of fetal and placental tissues. In order to satisfy the demands of pregnancy the average woman needs to absorb approximately 3 mg/day of iron. To ensure sufficient absorbed iron to satisfy the demands of pregnancy, a total intake of 30 mg/day of iron (an increase of 15 mg/day above what is recommended for nonpregnant women) should be adequate.[4] Since this increase may not regularly be met by the average American diet or by the iron stores of most women, it is recommended that pregnant women receive an oral iron supplement of 30 mg/day of elemental iron during the second and third trimesters, in the form of simple ferrous salts.[4] This amount should maintain hemoglobin levels for most pregnant women. Women who are anemic when they enter the pregnancy need a larger dose.

Folic Acid. The RDA for folic acid during pregnancy is 400 µg.[6] The issue of oral supplementation of folic acid during pregnancy is still controversial.[7]

Folic acid is not stored in the body, but it can be supplied by an appropriate diet that contains fruits, juices, whole-grain or fortified cereals, and green vegetables. The U.S. Public Health Service recently recommended that all women of childbearing age consume 400 µg of folic acid daily to reduce the risk of neural tube defects. Because the effects of high intakes are not well known (but include complicating the diagnosis of vitamin B_{12} deficiency), care should be taken to keep total folate consumption under 1 mg/day except under the supervision of a physician.[8] It has been further recommended that consumption of folic acid at 400 µg/day should be without specification—all dietary, all pill, or part diet and part pill. Also that all potentially pregnant women should have measurements made of serum and red cell folate plus serum homocysteine levels as a marker of folate status. Only if folate is low or homocysteine levels high should a woman increase her folic acid intake.[9] These specific concerns about the risks of taking supplemental folate should not apply to most patients who show no signs of pre-existing anemia and are not at risk for vitamin B_{12} deficiency. For these normal, healthy individuals, the supplementation of folate in a multivitamin form containing vitamin B_{12} should be safe enough not to require the testing suggested above. For folate supplementation to prevent fetal neural tube defects, it may need to be initiated before attempting or achieving pregnancy.

Other Supplemental Vitamins. With the exception of iron and folic acid, routine dietary supplementation with other vitamin and mineral preparations is not necessary. During pregnancy women should be encouraged to disregard vitamin and mineral preparations as corrective measures for inadequate dietary habits and instead consider food as the optimal vehicle for delivery of nutrients.[4] For pregnant women who do not consume an adequate diet and for those in high risk cate-

TABLE 4-3   Daily Vitamin/Mineral Supplementation for Pregnancy

For Those with Inadequate Diets or in High Risk Categories (More Than One Fetus, Heavy Smokers, Alcohol and Drug Abusers)

Vitamin B_6	2 mg	Iron	30 mg
Folate	300 µg	Zinc	15 mg
Vitamin C	50 mg	Copper	2 mg
Vitamin D	5 µg	Calcium	250 mg

In Special Circumstances

Vitamin D	10 µg (400 IU): complete vegetarians, low intake of vitamin D fortified milk, minimal exposure to sunlight
Calcium	600 mg: women under age 25 with daily dietary intake less than 600 mg
Vitamin B_{12}	2 µg: complete vegetarians
Zinc	15 mg: those receiving iron (>30 mg daily) to treat anemia
Copper	2 mg: those receiving iron (>30 mg daily) to treat anemia

gories, the daily vitamins and minerals listed in Table 4-3 are recommended beginning in the second trimester.[10]

Sodium.   During pregnancy, there is a cumulative retention of about 950 mEq of sodium that is distributed between the products of conception—the fetus (290 mEq), the placenta (57 mEq), and the amniotic fluid (100 mEq)—and the maternal extracellular volume, which includes the uterus (80 mEq), the breasts (35 mEq), the plasma (140 mEq), and the edema fluid (240 mEq). The pregnant woman's volume receptors sense these gains as normal.

Since there is no evidence to suggest that increased sodium intake is associated with an increased incidence of toxemia, and since sodium restriction neither helps to prevent or reverse it once it is present, sodium restriction during pregnancy is not recommended. Furthermore, the sodium requirement for pregnancy is usually met by the typical diet.[6]

Alcohol.   Fetal alcohol syndrome, which consists of congenital malformations, growth failure, and central nervous system effects, may result from the excessive consumption of alcohol during pregnancy.[11-14]

The exact mechanism of cause and effect is not yet known. It is uncertain whether the damage is a direct toxic effect from alcohol or from its metabolites. The defects and the growth deficiency may be the result of reduced number of fetal cells (especially brain cells). The effect upon the fetus may be dose related. A high blood alcohol level during a critical time in the fetal development may be as devastating as a continually high intake of alcohol throughout the pregnancy. This presents the possibility that fetal damage may occur shortly after conception before the woman even knows that she is pregnant.

Since no one knows for sure if there is a safe level of alcohol consumption during pregnancy, it is prudent to recommend total abstinence from alcohol for the pregnant woman.[14]

Caffeine.   Caffeine can cross the placenta. It is considered to be a stimulant drug. Few studies have examined the effects of caffeine on reproductive outcomes in humans. In studies where animals were exposed to extremely high doses of caffeine, there were increased incidences of fetal deaths, low birth weights, small litters, delayed bone development, and limb abnormalities.[11] Since caffeine is metabolized differently by humans and animals, data derived from animal studies cannot reliably be extrapolated to humans. In epidemiological studies where women consumed in excess of 8 cups of coffee per day, there was an association with increased frequency of early abortions.[11]

In general it is best to advise pregnant women to avoid or limit their consumption of foods and drugs that contain caffeine. (Sources of caffeine are listed in Appendix 23.) At present it is felt that caffeine consumption equivalent to 2 to 3 cups of regular coffee per day during pregnancy is safe.[11]

Artificial Sweeteners.   Currently the most widely used artificial sweetener is aspartame, more commonly known as Equal™ or Nutrasweet™. Aspartame is used to sweeten a wide variety of foods including chewing gum, diet soda, gelatins, puddings, yogurts, and frozen desserts. Since aspartame's introduction on the market, there have been many controversies regarding its safety, including the potential teratogenic side effects on the growing fetus.

The acceptable daily intake (ADI) for aspartame is 50 mg/kg of body weight. To meet the ADI, a person weighing 50 kg would need to consume an equivalent of 12 cans of diet soda sweetened with 100% aspartame or 71 packets of Equal.[15]

Studies conducted with women and animals, in which they were given significantly more than the ADI for aspartame (200 mg/kg for humans, 100 mg/kg for animals, or the equivalent of 100 to 200 cans of diet soda for a 68 kg person) did not appear to have adverse effects on the growing fetus.[13] Based on research that has been done, it is best to advise pregnant women who regularly consume aspartame sweetened products to ingest no more than 2 to 3 servings of aspartame sweetened products per day.

For women who have phenylketonuria, the use of artificial sweeteners containing aspartame (as well as other sources of phenylalanine) should be avoided in pregnancy to avoid profound mental retardation in the infants born.[16]

ADOLESCENT PREGNANCY

The adolescent age group is beginning to represent a statistically greater percentage of total pregnancies in the United States.[17] The frequency of perinatal problems, such as toxemia, anemia, premature births, infants with low birth weight (less than 2,500 g), and increased maternal and neonatal mortality, has remained significantly higher for teenagers than for adult women. The average birth weight of infants rises as the maternal age increases, and the percentage of infants with low birth weight decreases as the maternal age rises from less than 15 years to 19 years of age.[17,18] Numerous studies that investigate the causes of increased perinatal risks suggest that they are related more to factors such as delayed prenatal care, low socioeconomic status, poor health habits, greater incidence of prematurity, and lower prepregnancy weight than to maternal biological immaturity.[19-22] Thus, factors that are amenable to intervention, such as nutrition, early prenatal care, and improved health habits, gain more importance in assuring a better outcome among pregnant teenagers.[23]

The average age of menarche today is 12 to 13 years. Growth usually continues for 4 years postmenarche although at a much slower rate than during prepuberty. Teenage girls who become pregnant within 4 years of menarche are generally considered biologically immature. Thus, the girls' nutritional needs for pregnancy must be estimated in addition to their needs for growth. After growth is complete (more than 4 years postmenarche or at about 17 years of age), the adolescent's nutritional requirements are similar to the adult pregnant woman's requirements. The dietary intake of nutrients must meet not only the pregnancy requirement, but also the individual needs of the patient at the different stages of growth. Thus, the nutritional requirements for the immature pregnant teenager can be estimated by summing the RDA's for the specific age and the additional recommendations for pregnant adults.[6,24]

The total estimated average energy requirement for an adolescent woman is 2,500 to 2,700 kcal/day.[24] However, since energy expenditure is variable, the best assurance of an adequate intake is a satisfactory weight gain. This should be accomplished by individual counseling on the basis of estimates of body size, growth rate, age, and activity level. Many young girls in today's society limit their food intake severely to be fashionably slim. This presents an additional nutritional risk for pregnant teenagers, both in terms of having a low prepregnancy weight, which is associated with higher perinatal risks, and in terms of their ability to meet their nutritional needs for growth.[25]

Protein. Protein needs in the pregnant teenager are understandably high. Jacobson estimates the protein recommendations for girls 15 to 18 years of age to be 1.5 g of protein per kilogram of pregnant body weight and to be 1.7 g of protein per kilogram of pregnant body weight for girls who are less than 15 years of age.[24] Adequate caloric intake is essential in order for protein to be used for nitrogen retention and for growth.[26,27]

Calcium and Iron. Special attention to the calcium and iron needs of pregnant teenagers is required because the increased needs for these nutrients are not regularly met by the average American teenager's diet. The National Research Council recommends an intake of 1,600 mg/day of calcium for a growing pregnant adolescent.[6] This level is believed necessary to provide sufficient calcium for normal fetal development and maintain stores for maternal bone growth. The iron needs of the growing adolescent are high because of their enlarging muscle mass and blood volume. The National Research Council's recommendation of a daily supplement of 30 mg of elemental iron during pregnancy should be adequate for the pregnant adolescent.[6] Pregnant adolescents who are anemic when they begin the pregnancy may need a larger dose.

Nutritional assessment and education for the pregnant teenager necessitates ongoing individual counseling. Assessment should include the present height and

TABLE 4-4   Suggested Minimum Daily Dietary Intake during Pregnancy and Lactation

Food Group (Servings)	Normal Pregnancy (No. of Servings)	Pregnant Adolescent (No. of Servings)	Lactation (No. of Servings)
DAIRY GROUP (1 cup or calcium equivalent)	4	5	4
MEAT GROUP (2–3 oz or protein equivalent)	3	3	3
FRUIT AND VEGETABLE GROUP (about 1/2 cup edible portion) 1 rich source of vitamin A 2 rich sources of vitamin C	4	≥ 4	5
STARCH GROUP (1 slice bread or 1/2 cup enriched or whole grain)	≥ 4	≥ 5	≥ 4
Other Foods	To meet caloric needs	To meet caloric needs	To meet caloric needs

weight, the gynecological age (the chronological age minus the age at menarche),[21] the dietary intake history, and activity patterns. Attention should be given to the adequacy of dietary intake prior to the pregnancy, to any unusual dietary patterns, to amount of snacking, to meals being skipped, to low intakes of nutrient-dense foods, and to habitual caloric restriction. Vitamin and mineral supplements should be used when the diet is suspected to be inadequate (Table 4-4).[10]

PREGNANCY AND OBESITY

Obesity in pregnancy is associated with an increased risk for gestational diabetes, hypertension, pre-eclampsia, perinatal mortality, and the need for induced labor, or cesarean section.

Lower weight gains are acceptable for overweight women because the fetus can receive part of its needed kilocalories from the maternal energy stores. Studies have shown that obese mothers have the best pregnancy outcomes when they gain approximately 7 kg (15.4 lb) during the pregnancy.[28] Therefore, it is recommended that obese women strive for a weight gain of approximately 15 lb. This allows for the products of conception plus the increase in maternal blood volume and breast size.

Weight management in the overweight pregnant woman should be flexible and personalized. Weight reduction during pregnancy should be avoided, even if the woman is obese. Decreasing one's calorie intake during pregnancy may result in a deficiency in nutrients needed to support the pregnancy, cause protein to be used as an energy source rather than for tissue synthesis, and cause the production of ketones, which can impair fetal neurological development.[29]

PREGNANCY AND DIABETES

Women with previously diagnosed diabetes mellitus account for 0.1 to 0.5% of all pregnancies; an additional 3 to 5% of pregnant women develop gestational diabetes.

Gestational Diabetes.   It has been recommended that all pregnant women be screened between 24 and 28 weeks gestation with a measurement of plasma glucose 1 hour after a 50 g oral glucose challenge. A 3-hour oral glucose tolerance test is indicated if the plasma glucose is greater than 140 mg/dl; however, depending on the institution, other levels for the 1-hour test may be advocated (ranging from 130 to 150 mg/dl).[30] The criteria for the diagnosis of gestational diabetes include two or more of the following plasma glucose concentrations met or exceeded following a 100 g glucose load: (1) fasting plasma glucose of 105 mg/dl; (2) at 1 hour, 190 mg/dl; (3) at 2 hours, 165 mg/dl; and (4) at 3 hours, 145 mg/dl.[31] If the fasting plasma glucose levels of the gestational diabetic cannot be kept below 95 mg/dl and below 120 mg/dl 2 hours after a meal by diet alone, insulin therapy should be started. Sulfonylureas are contraindicated during pregnancy.

Insulin Dependent Diabetes.   Good control of the blood glucose levels during pregnancy for patients with insulin dependent diabetes is critical to the health of both the mother and the fetus. Studies have shown that perinatal mortality rates have dropped to within normal ranges for those patients who demonstrate good glycemic control (i.e., plasma glucose levels between 70 and 100 mg/dl prior to meals and near normal glycosylated hemoglobin levels) during their pregnancy. Increased blood glucose levels during the first 6 to 8 weeks after conception increase the chances of fetal malformations, and increased blood glucose levels later in the pregnancy are associated with macrosomia, fetal hypoglycemia, and respiratory distress syndrome. On the other hand, the fetus does not seem to be adversely affected by transient maternal hypoglycemia.

Dietary recommendations follow the basic principles of the standard diabetic diet (see Chapter 8, Diabetes Mellitus). The caloric level of the diet is based on the number of kilocalories that are required to maintain the woman's prepregnancy weight with an increase of approximately 200 to 300 kcal/day beginning in the second half of pregnancy, or the number of kilocalories that are sufficient to achieve a weight gain, based on the mother's prepregnancy weight. A weight loss during the pregnancy is to be avoided because of the need for adequate fetal nutrition and because maternal ketonuria is associated with very low kilocalorie diets.[31] To minimize fluctuations in the plasma glucose and reduce the risk of ketosis, the calories should be divided into 3 meals and 3 snacks (a midmorning, a midafternoon, and a bedtime snack). Since blood glucose levels tend to be elevated following breakfast, it is recommended that a smaller breakfast be consumed. Breakfast should consist of no more than 1 to 2 starches, and/or 4 oz of milk or 1 meat serving. Fruit and fruit juices should be omitted at breakfast and instead be used for a midmorning snack or at other meals.[32] Artificial sweeteners may be used to add variety to the diet, but women should be advised to use products sweetened with artificial sweeteners in moderation.

The diet should be reviewed frequently and adjusted to reflect maternal weight gain, changes in activity, and food tolerances and preferences. Two important goals are an adequate weight gain and an absence of urinary ketones. Most diabetic women will measure their own blood glucoses 4 to 6 times per day during pregnancy using meters. By keeping a running log of these glucoses, very precise control of glucose levels is made possible as the woman adjusts her insulin (and sometimes her diet and activity).

LACTATION

Maternal nutritional status and the diet can influence the quantity and the quality of human milk. A moderate to severe caloric restriction or actual starvation reduces the milk volume more than the nutrient composition, although the latter is reduced as well.[33] An adequate weight gain during pregnancy and a normal infant birth weight are indirect indicators of good maternal nutritional status and can improve the likelihood of successful lactation.

Kilocalories. It is almost impossible to propose an exact energy level required for milk production for all women since, a woman's energy requirement is highly dependent upon her metabolic and activity needs as well as her tissue reserves. However, it is prudent to encourage an energy intake of at least 1800 kcal/day.[34] Women who have a low pregnancy weight gain, who have decreased weight for height, who nurse longer than 3 months, and who nurse more than one infant most likely need additional kilocalories during lactation. Severe caloric restriction to achieve rapid weight reduction should be discouraged. Intakes below 1,500 kcal/day are not recommended at any time during lactation.[34]

The caloric requirement for a lactating woman is related to the amount of milk that is produced and to the amount of caloric reserve found in the mother's body fat. The National Research Council recommends an extra 500 kcal/day over the prepregnancy needs for the first 3 months and more according to maternal needs after that (see Chapter 2, Recommended Dietary Allowances, Table 2-8). Breast milk has a caloric content of 70 kcal per 100 ml but because of an 80% efficiency in energy conversion, approximately 15 extra kilocalories or 85 total kilocalories are required for the production of 100 ml of milk. The average amount of milk produced per day during the first 6 months of lactation is 750 ml, which necessitates an additional 640 kcal/day. Normally during pregnancy about 3 kg of body fat are stored, which can be mobilized to provide 200 to 300 kcal/day for 3 months. Therefore, the average nonpregnant diet should be increased by 500 kcal/day for the first 3 months, then 800 kcal/day after that. A gradual weight reduction for the mother is compatible with successful lactation. Additional energy recommendations should be adjusted to meet the individual woman's needs. More recently, it has been recommended that energy intakes not fall below 1,500 kcal/day at any time during lactation.[34]

Protein.   Protein requirements are also related to the amount of milk produced. Since the efficiency of the conversion of dietary protein to milk protein is about 70%, and accounting for individual variations, the recommended allowance for lactation is 65 g of protein per day during the first 6 months of lactation and 62 g of protein per day thereafter.[6]

Other Nutrients.   The requirements for other nutrients are all increased and reflect the need for milk production and the need to replenish maternal stores.[33] Human milk levels generally reflect maternal intake and vitamin and fat stores. The mineral content of human milk remains relatively constant with maternal intakes. Deficits in maternal intake are made up for by maternal stores. The RDAs for calcium and for vitamin D involve an additional 400 mg/day and 10 µg/day, respectively, to prevent maternal demineralization.[6]

The lactating woman should be counseled to add 2 cups of milk or the equivalent, an extra serving of vitamin C rich food, and raw fruits and vegetables to her diet to provide adequate folic acid. Vitamin supplementation is not necessary, and lactating women should be encouraged to obtain their nutrients from a well-balanced, varied diet rather than relying on supplements. When the mother's iron status is in question, supplement of 30 mg of elemental iron per day should be taken for the first 2 to 3 months of lactation to replete maternal iron stores. Breast milk concentrations of iron, of fluoride, and of vitamin D can be low and are not affected by dietary supplementation; therefore, supplementation to the infant is advisable.

When assessing the adequacy of the diet of the vegetarian woman who is lactating, special attention should be given, to including adequate kilocalories, iron, protein, calcium, vitamin D and zinc. (Zinc may be poorly absorbed from a vegetarian diet.) A vitamin B_{12} supplement of up to 2.6 µg/day is also recommended.[34]

Fluids. An increase in fluid intake does not increase milk volume; however, additional fluid is needed to maintain a normal maternal fluid balance. Mothers should be encouraged to drink when they are thirsty.

Caffeine, Alcohol, and Drugs. Most chemicals ingested by the lactating woman cross into her milk. Therefore, the mother should seek the advice of her physician before taking any dietary supplement, any medication, or any drug. Caffeine and alcohol also pass into the milk. Although excess caffeine may make the infant irritable and wakeful, research indicates that moderate amounts of caffeine (1 to 2 cups of coffee per day) will not harm or upset the infant.[34] Ethanol appears in human milk in a similar concentration to the maternal blood, although acetaldehyde, which is the major toxic breakdown product of ethanol, does not appear in the milk. Alcohol may impair the milk ejection reflex; therefore it is prudent to limit alcohol intake when lactating. This equates to 0.5 g of alcohol per kilogram of maternal body weight per day. For a 60 kg woman this corresponds to 2.0 to 2.5 oz of liquor, 8 oz of table wine, or 2 cans of beer.[34]

Goals of Dietary Management

The goals of the diet are to support an optimal pregnancy and lactation. This includes energy to support recommended weight gain patterns, adequate protein, vitamins, minerals, and fluids. Whenever feasible food should be the source of nutrients, and self-initiated vitamin and mineral supplements should be avoided. The physician should be made aware of a potential need for supplements and should be the one to recommend the type and quantity. Dietary intake of sodium, caffeine, artificial sweeteners, and alcohol should also be addressed when tailoring the diet for pregnancy and lactation.

Dietary Recommendations

Table 4-4 summarizes the dietary recommendations for pregnancy and lactation.

Physicians—How to Order Diet

The diet order should indicate *diet for pregnancy*. In the case of a gestational diabetic, the diet order should indicate *diet for pregnancy/gestational diabetes*. The dietitian will determine appropriate calorie needs for pregnancy and evaluate the need for vitamin/mineral supplements. The diet order for an individual who is nursing should indicate *diet for lactation*.

References

1. Tyrer LB. Nutrition and the pill. J Reprod Med 1984;29(Suppl 7):547–550.
2. Taffel SM, Keppel KG. Advice about weight gain during pregnancy and actual weight gain. Am J Publ Health 1986;76:1396–1399.
3. American Academy of Pediatrics and American College of Obstetrics and Gynecology. Guidelines for perinatal care. Evanston, IL: AAP, 1983.
4. Subcommittee on Nutritional Status and Weight Gain During Pregnancy. Nutrition during pregnancy. Nutr Today 1990;July/Aug:13–22.
5. Durnin JVGA, Grant S, McKillop FM, Fitzgerald G. Is nutritional status endangered by virtually no extra intake during pregnancy? The Lancet 1985;Oct:823–825.

6. National Research Council, National Academy of Sciences, Committee on Dietary Allowances, Food and Nutrition Board. Recommended dietary allowances. 10th ed. Washington, DC: National Academy Press, 1989:60–62,201.

7. Baily LB. Evaluation of a new recommended dietary allowance for folate. JADA 1992;April: 463–468.

8. Centers for Disease Control. Morbidity and Mortality Weekly Report, vol. 41, no. RR-14.

9. Herbert V. Folate and neural tube defects. Nutr Today 1992;27(6):30–33.

10. Subcommittee on Nutritional Status and Weight Gain During Pregnancy, from the National Academy of Sciences Committee on Nutritional Status During Pregnancy and Lactation. Summary. In: Nutrition during pregnancy. Washington DC: National Academy Press, 1990: 1–23.

11. Subcommittee on Nutritional Status and Weight Gain During Pregnancy from the National Academy of Sciences Committee on Nutritional Status During Pregnancy and Lactation. Substance use and abuse. In: Nutrition during pregnancy. Washington DC: National Academy Press, 1990:390–411.

12. Suter C, Ott D. Maternal and infant nutrition recommendations: a review. J Am Diet Assoc 1984;84:572.

13. Rosett HL, Weiner L. Alcohol and pregnancy. Annu Rev Med 1985;36:73–80.

14. Council on Scientific Affairs, American Medical Association. Fetal effects of maternal alcohol use. JAMA 1983;249:2517–2521.

15. Carroll P. Safe ingestion of aspartame during pregnancy. Top Clin Nutr 1990;5(4):1–5.

16. Lamon JM, Lenke RR, Levy HL, Schulman JD, Shih VE. Selected metabolic diseases— phenylketonuria. In: Schulman JD, Simpson JL, eds. Genetic diseases in pregnancy. New York: Academic Press, 1981:1–47.

17. National Center for Health Statistics. Trends in teenage childbearing, United States 1970–1981. Hyattsville, MD: National Center for Health statistics, Sept 1984. (Vital and health statistics. Series 21, No. 41) (DHHS Pub No. [PHS] 84–1919).

18. Vital statistics of the United States, 1978. Vol 1: Natality. DHHS Pub No. (PHS) 81–1100. Hyattsville, MD: U.S. Department of Health and Human Services, 1982:1–61.

19. Zuckerman B, Alpert JJ, Dooling E, Hingson R, Kayne H, Morelock S, Oppenheimer E. Neonatal outcome: is adolescent pregnancy a risk factor? Pediatrics 1983;71:489–493.

20. Elster AB. The effect of maternal age, parity, and prenatal care on perinatal outcome in adolescent mothers. Am J Obstet Gynecol 1984;149:845–847.

21. Horon IL, Strobino DM, MacDonald HM. Birth weights among infants born to adolescent and young adult women. Am J Obstet Gynecol 1983;146:444–449.

22. Hollingsworth DR, Katchen JM. Gynecologic age and its relation to neonatal outcome. Birth Defects Original Article Series 1981;17:91–105.

23. Committee on Adolescence, American Academy of Pediatrics. Statement on teenage pregnancy. Pediatrics 1979;63:795–797.

24. Worthington-Roberts BS. Nutritional needs of the pregnant adolescent. In: Worthington-Roberts BS, Vermeersch J, Williams SR, eds. Nutrition in pregnancy and lactation. St Louis: Mosby–Year Book, 1981:135–154.

25. Jacobson HN. Nutritional risk of pregnancy during adolescence. Birth Defects Original Article Series 1981;17:69–83.

26. King JC, Calloway DH, Margen S. Nitrogen retention, total body 40K and weight gain in teenage pregnant girls. J Nutr 1973;103:772–785.

27. Calloway DH. Recommended dietary allowances for protein and energy. J Am Diet Assoc 1974;64:157–162.

28. Naeye RL. Weight gain and the outcome of pregnancy. Am J Obstet Gynecol 1979;135:3.

29. Boyne L. Nutrition during pregnancy and lactation. Nutr News 1992;Feb:1–9.

30. Carpenter MW. Testing for gestational diabetes. In: Reece EA, Coustan DR, eds. Diabetes mellitus in pregnancy—principles and practice. New York: Churchill Livingstone, 1988:423–439.

31. Franz M, Cooper N, Mullen L, Birk R. Gestational diabetes guidelines for a safe pregnancy and a healthy baby. Wayzata, MN: International Diabetes Center, 1988:8–13.

32. Fagen C. Nutritional guidelines for management of gestational diabetes. Dietitians in General Clinical Practice Newsletter 1991;9(1):4.

33. Subcommittee on Nutrition During Lactation, from the National Academy of Sciences Committee on Nutritional Status During Pregnancy and Lactation. Nutrition during lactation. Nutr Today 1991;May/June:28–31.

34. Subcommittee on Nutrition During Lactation, from the National Academy of Sciences Committee on Nutritional Status During Pregnancy and Lactation. Summary, conclusions, and recommendations. In: Nutrition during lactation. Washington, DC: National Academy Press, 1991:1–19.

NUTRITIONAL NEEDS FOR PHYSICAL PERFORMANCE

The current dietary recommendations for athletes are similar to recommendations for the general population for protein and fat but are different for fluid, electrolytes, and carbohydrate. Protein should contribute 10 to 20% of calories and fat 30%. There are wide variations in fluid, electrolyte, and carbohydrate requirements. Athletes involved in prolonged, strenuous endurance training require additional fluid and electrolytes and may need up to 70% of calories as carbohydrate, while the "weekend" athlete needs approximately 50 to 60% of calories as carbohydrate. Dietary goals should include not only optimization of athletic performance but also long term health. This implies the need for a dietary plan that will help guard against developing atherosclerosis and hypertension. Hence the characteristics of a desirable diet for the general population should be considered in planning the athlete's diet (see Chapter 2, Guidelines for Meal Planning and Promotion of Wellness).

Fluid and Electrolyte Replacement

The most important nutritional considerations for the athlete are adequate intake of fluid and electrolytes. A very serious consequence of heavy sweating, which may accompany exercise, is the loss of body water. A replacement of fluids during exercise of at least 50% of the predicted weight loss is adequate to prevent heat illnesses.[35] Table 4-5 offers guidelines for fluid replacement to prevent dehydration, before, during, and after exercise.[36-39]

For the athlete, thirst is not considered a reliable indicator of water needs.[38,40] Therefore it is suggested that athletes weigh themselves before and after an event, then drink 1 pint of fluid (16 oz) for every pound lost.[38] After recreational activity, it may be more practical to drink a greater amount of water than might be necessary to satisfy thirst.

Consumption of carbohydrate-containing beverages during prolonged exercise tends to maintain blood glucose levels and spare muscle glycogen, the depletion of which appears to be a limiting factor leading to fatigue during prolonged aero-

TABLE 4-5   Suggested Times and Intervals for Fluid Ingestion before, during, and after Exercise[37-39]

Time or Interval of Ingestion for Competition or Workout	Estimated Amount of Fluid (oz)*
2 hr before competition or workout	16–20
10 to 20 min before competition or workout	16–20
At 10–15 min intervals during competition or workout	4–6
After competition or workout	Replace each pound of weight lost with 16 oz of fluid

*Smaller individuals or cooler environments may lower these estimates.

TABLE 4-6   Composition of Commercial Sport Drinks

Product (8 oz)	% Carbohydrate	Carbohydrate Type*	Kilocalories	Sodium (mg)	Potassium (mg)	Carbohydrate (g)
Bodyfuel 450™	4.5	GP, FR	40	80	20	10
Exceed Fluid Replacement™	7.0	GP, FR	70	50	45	17
Gatorade™	6.0	SU, GL	50	110	25	14
Sqwincher™	6.8	GL, FR	60	55	45	16
Recharge™	7.6	FR, GL	50	15	25	13

*GP = Glucose polymers; FR = fructose; SU = sucrose; GL = glucose.

Bodyfuel 450, Vitex Foods, Los Angeles; Exceed Fluid Replacement, Ross Laboratories, Columbus, Ohio; Gatorade, Quaker Oats Co., Chicago; Sqwincher, Universal Marketing Corp., Columbus, Mo; Recharge, Knudsen & Sons, Chico, California.

From Hoffman CJ, Coleman E. An eating plan and update on recommended dietary practices for the endurance athlete. Copyright the American Dietetic Association. Reprinted by permission from J Am Diet Assoc 1991;91(3):328.

bic exercise. This may be of benefit to the endurance athlete exercising for 60 minutes or longer. Care should be taken, however, not to exceed a 6 to 8% sugar concentration so that gastric emptying and essential fluid replacement are not limited.[39] Improvements in performance have been observed when the rate of carbohydrate consumed averaged about 24 g every 30 minutes. This requires the athlete to drink 8 oz of a 5% carbohydrate solution or 5 oz of an 8% solution every 15 minutes during exercise. (Refer to Table 4-6 for composition of commercial sport drinks.) Drinks should be cool (5° to 10° C or 40° to 50° F) to help promote more rapid gastric emptying.[35]

Sweat is hypotonic and contains sodium at approximately 40 mEq/L (920 mg/L) and potassium at approximately 3 mEq/L (117 mg/L).[41] If a person is exposed to higher environmental temperatures over a period of several weeks to a few months, some tolerance can be achieved. The principal mechanism by which the body achieves this tolerance is to make an even more hypotonic sweat, thus conserving electrolytes. In most situations, both sodium and potassium losses can be easily replaced by eating a variety of foods after competition. Salt tablets are not recommended because they can irritate the gastric mucosa and cause nausea and vomiting. High concentrations of sodium can draw water into the gastrointestinal tract, further exacerbating dehydration.[42] However, in extreme situations where fluid losses exceed 3 L/day, sodium and other electrolytes should be individually assessed and replaced.[35] Ultraendurance athletes who participate in 50-mile runs, 100-mile cycling, or triathalons may benefit from a sport drink that contains electrolytes, which reduces the risk of hyponatremia.[38]

Kilocalories

Specific kilocalorie needs depend on a number of variables, such as body size, age, sex, body composition (determinants of basal metabolic rate), and type, intensity, frequency, and duration of activity. Methods of estimating kilocalories are included in the Nutritional Assessment section of this manual (Chapter 3).

Endurance athletes who are involved in intense activities of more than 3 hour's duration, such as marathons, cross-country skiing, distance swimming, and cycling, have increased energy needs. Three balanced meals and between-meal fluids and snacks are recommended as energy needs dictate. During the training phase, most athletes can best meet their body's demands for energy by following a high carbohydrate diet that provides 65 to 70% of energy from carbohydrate. A threshold of 500 to 800 g (2,000 to 3,200 kilocalories) of carbohydrate per day, regardless of the total daily energy intake, may be necessary to maintain maximal muscle glycogen stores.[39] Because exact kilocalorie recommendations vary with climate and athletic event, the energy needs of each athlete must be considered individually.[38] The endurance athlete requires more kilocalories and a higher percentage of carbohydrate than the athlete who participates in nonaerobic activities.

When an athlete wants to increase muscle strength and embarks on a weight-gaining program, the aim should be to increase the lean body mass at about 0.5 lb/week. The primary stimulus for increasing muscle mass is vigorous resistance type exercise with a gradual increase in food intake.

Athletes who are involved in sports with weight classifications, such as wrestling, should be advised against fasting and very low kilocalorie diets before competition. To reduce the possibility of acute weight loss and dehydration, the American College of Sports Medicine (ACSM) recommends that each wrestler's body composition be assessed several weeks prior to the competitive season to determine an acceptable minimum wrestling weight. If the athlete needs to lose weight, it should be accomplished during the off season. A safe weight loss should not exceed 2 lb/week. A lower limit of 5% body fat is proposed by the ACSM as the lowest acceptable level for safe wrestling competition.[36,43] Because the accuracy of body composition measurements is questionable and dependent on the method and/or equipment used, body fat measurements should not be interpreted as absolute.

Carbohydrate

Carbohydrate is the preferred fuel for working muscles. In general, the diet should obtain 60 to 65% of kilocalories from a variety of carbohydrate sources. Athletes who train exhaustively on successive days or who compete in prolonged endurance events should consume a diet that provides 65 to 70% of energy from carbohydrate.[39] Carbohydrate loading or "glycogen packing" of muscles may be beneficial for endurance athletes who exercise at an intensity between 65 and 85% of VO_2max (maximal aerobic capacity) for longer than 80 minutes.[44] However, the classic two-phase procedure of carbohydrate loading (consisting of glycogen depletion followed by loading) has been abandoned for a modified approach that is safer, yet effective. It is now recommended that athletes follow a high carbohydrate diet throughout the training period. Activity should be tapered about 7 days before an endurance event, with complete rest the day of the event. During the 72 hours preceding competition, athletes should consume 70% of kilocalories as complex carbohydrates or 800 g/day of carbohydrate (6 to 10 g of carbohydrate per kilogram of bodyweight per day), whichever is greater.[39] This procedure will maximize glycogen deposition, and may be followed numerous times throughout the year without health risks.[37,39]

Because many athletes exercise vigorously on the days after an event, the replenishment of muscle glycogen is important. It is recommended that athletes consume at least 1.5 g of carbohydrate per kilogram of body weight immediately after the event and again 60 minutes later.[38] Meals that are rich in carbohydrate can restore muscle glycogen to pre-exercise levels within 24 hours.[44]

Protein

Athletes, like nonathletes, should consume 10 to 20% of their daily kilocalories from protein. The RDA for protein is 0.8 g of protein per kilogram of body weight. Needs might be higher (1 to 1.5 g per kilogram of body weight) for periods of intense training (greater than 70% VO_2max), but there is little evidence that indicates a need for larger increases.[35] Most athletes, assuming they eat a nutritionally balanced diet, have no need for extra protein except perhaps during periods of intense training.[35]

Many athletes are under the impression that consuming a high protein diet will increase muscle mass. However, research suggests that the quantity of dietary protein needed to achieve maximal protein deposition is 1.5 g per kilogram of body weight, and that the limiting factor for muscle protein deposition is energy intake, not protein. Therefore, athletes who wish to increase muscle mass should meet their energy requirements first, through an adequate intake of carbohydrate, and then check that they have met their protein needs.[39] In addition, when protein intake exceeds the amount that is needed for maintenance of body tissue, the protein is used as energy or may be converted to fat and stored as adipose tissue. It should also be noted that high protein diets containing meat and high fat dairy products may deliver an increased percentage of kilocalories from fat.[45] For this reason, athletes should be advised to select sources of high protein foods that contain low amounts of fat, such as skim milk, low fat yogurt, lean meats, fish and poultry, dried beans, legumes, and egg whites.

Fat

Since fatty foods are slow to leave the stomach, they sometimes cause nausea and indigestion if eaten shortly before competition. High fat, low carbohydrate diets can also deplete muscle and liver glycogen stores and compromise endurance and muscle strength. Active persons should be advised on how to identify and how to avoid high carbohydrate foods that contain large amounts of hidden fat.

Kilocalories from fat should not exceed 30% of total energy requirements, especially for elite athletes involved in highly competitive sports.[39,46] For these athletes, it is recommended that 70% of calories come from complex carbohydrate to help provide a winning edge.[46] The exception to the above recommendation of 30% fat is the endurance athlete who does not engage in competitive athletics and may do well on a higher fat intake due to increased calorie needs.

Vitamins and Minerals

There is little evidence to suggest that vitamin-mineral supplementation, in the absence of a specific deficiency, is necessary for active individuals.[47] Therefore, athletes as well as nonathletes should avoid taking large doses of vitamins and minerals and be encouraged to eat nutritionally balanced meals. There are two minerals, however, that warrant further discussion.

Adequate iron status is crucial for optimal exercise performance. An iron deficiency can impair physical performance, and manifests itself most often in distance runners or in endurance athletes.[48] Strenuous physical exercise may create a state of hemodilution and low hemoglobin concentration as a normal physiological response.[48] This low hemoglobin level should be carefully distinguished from a true anemia. Rigorous running regimens may cause small intestinal losses of blood that may, over time, result in iron depletion. Losses of iron through sweat, feces, and urine are also elevated in the endurance athlete. It is important to identify athletes who are at high risk for developing iron deficiency, such as menstruating females, endurance athletes, children, vegetarians, and other individuals who do not meet their iron needs through diet. Treatment includes modification of the usual diet to maximize absorbable iron intake. This will include consumption of foods that are high in iron. The iron in meats (heme iron) is more readily available than iron from plant sources (nonheme iron). Citrus fruit or juice with a meal will facilitate iron absorption from foods through its ascorbic acid content. Iron supplementation as ferrous sulfate may also be advisable. However, the need for iron supplementation should be determined by a physician after an evaluation of the hematology status and diet history.[45]

The calcium needs of the athlete are no greater than the needs of the nonathlete.[49] However, since calcium intake is frequently inadequate for many people, the athlete should also be advised regarding sufficient dietary calcium to promote proper bone growth and to maintain adequate bone density (see Chapter 8, Osteoporosis). Counseling should determine individual calcium requirements after assessing the person's intake and needs.

Drugs and Special Dietary Supplements

During endurance activities, the availability of muscle glycogen is a critical factor. Although certain studies have shown that caffeine may facilitate the use of fats stored in the muscle as an energy source during exercise, its ability to improve performance by sparing muscle glycogen stores is not clearly documented.[50] Most investigators suggest that any seemingly improved endurance may be due to enhanced psychological factors that lead to greater work output or increased tolerance to fatigue. Research has also shown that individuals respond differently to caffeine.[50] Since a high caffeine intake may trigger adverse physiological responses (i.e., fluid loss, polyuria, increased heart rate, and an increased anxiety level), these factors may outweigh any positive effects on fuel utilization.[37]

The ACSM and the American Orthopedic Society for Sports Medicine do not advocate caffeine tablets or caffeine-containing stimulants to enhance performance.[51] Because caffeine is an ingredient in beverages and foods commonly consumed by athletes, its use is permitted by the International Olympic Committee (IOC) but only in limited amounts. The IOC allows an upper limit of 12 µg/ml of urine tested. Over a 2- to 3-hour period, a dose of 100 mg of caffeine will result in a urine concentration of 1.5 µg/ml. Thus, 800 mg of caffeine, which could be obtained from 5 to 6 cups of strong coffee, could exceed the allowable limit.[50]

Depending on the individual, a range of 100 to 300 mg of caffeine is considered a therapeutic dose. Therefore, a dose of 5 mg/kg of body weight would provide a stimulant effect and yet still be allowable according to IOC rules. Thus, for athletes who feel that they may benefit from caffeine, a recommended allowable dose for a 130 lb (59 kg) person would be 295 mg (approximately 2 to 3 cups of coffee).[50]

Although illegal, anabolic steroids are popular among many athletes who desire a large muscle mass. Anabolic steroids do, in fact, enhance anaerobic capacity. There is little scientific evidence, however, that anabolic steroids enhance aerobic work capacity.[52,53] In addition, such steroids may lead to liver damage, liver cancer, cardiovascular disease, mood changes, masculinizing effects in women, and testicular atrophy with temporary sterility in men.[54]

Amino acids are often marketed as legal alternatives to steroids for increasing muscle mass. Athletes should be aware that there are potential risks when taking amino acid supplements. Problems that may occur from excessive protein or amino acid intakes include excessive weight gain, dehydration, gout, and excessive loss of urinary calcium. High protein intakes may impose a heavy burden on the liver and kidneys to secrete excess nitrogen, and may damage those organs.[55]

Some athletes have used amino acid supplements that are touted as growth hormone stimulants. Growth hormone is a powerful anabolic hormone that affects all body systems and influences muscle growth.[55] Growth hormone injection causes muscle hypertrophy in animals but does not increase muscle strength. Excess growth hormone causes acromegaly, in which muscles become larger but functionally weaker.[50] Growth hormone use, like steroid use, is unethical, dangerous, and against the IOC rules.

Athletes should realize that single amino acid supplements in large doses may cause amino acid imbalances and toxicities. There have not been studies conducted on human subjects on large doses of amino acid supplements, and therefore no margin of safety is known. Amino acids taken in large doses are essentially drugs with unknown physiological effects.[50,55]

There is no evidence that "ergogenic" foods such as wheat germ, wheat germ oil, lecithin, bee pollen, gelatin, honey, kelp, brewer's yeast, pangamic acid, ginseng, or sunflower seed improve physical performance.[37] However, when athletes are convinced that certain foods, dietary regimens, or supplements improve performance, those substances or techniques may provide psychological rather than proven physiological benefits. It is when these practices replace a sound nutritional program that health and performance may be compromised, resulting in serious consequences.[37,39]

The Precompetition Meal

Departing from past recommendations, which advised eating 3 to 4 hours before competition,[35,37] the state-of-the-art thinking now is that a carbohydrate meal or beverage can be consumed from 4 hours before exercise up to minutes before the event without any detrimental effect on performance.[38,56] Consuming 1 to 5 g of carbohydrate per kilogram of body weight from 5 minutes to 4 hours before exercise has been found to enhance endurance greatly.[38] To reduce potential gastrointestinal distress, the carbohydrate content of the meal should be reduced as the time remaining before exercise decreases. For example, a carbohydrate feeding of 1 g/kg of body weight is appropriate immediately (within an hour) before exercise, whereas 4 g/kg can be safely consumed 4 hours before exercise.[56]

References

35. Sports and Cardiovascular Nutritionists Dietetic Practice Group. In: Marcus JB, ed. Sports nutrition. Chicago: American Dietetic Association, 1986.
36. McArdle WD, Katch FI, Katch VL. Exercise physiology, energy, nutrition, and human performance, 2nd ed. Philadelphia: Lea & Febiger, 1986:517.
37. Nutrition for physical fitness and athletic performance for adults: technical support paper. J Am Diet Assoc 1987;87:934–939.
38. Hoffman CJ, Coleman E. An eating plan and update on recommended dietary practices for the endurance athlete. J Am Diet Assoc 1991;91:325–330.
39. Smith-Plomden M, Benardot D. Position of the American Dietetic Association and the Canadian Dietetic Association: nutrition for physical fitness and athletic performance for adults. J Am Diet Assoc 1993;93(6):691–696.
40. O'Neil FT, Hynak-Hankinson MT, Gorman J. Research and application of current topics in sports medicine. J Am Diet Assoc 1986;86:1007–1015.
41. Nelson R. Nutrition and physical performance. Presentation for the 22nd AMA National Conference on the medical aspects of sports. Jan 24, 1981.
42. Food power: a coach's guide to improving performance. Rosemont, Ill: Nat Dairy Council, 1984.
43. American College of Sports Medicine: Weight loss in wrestlers. Med Sci Sports 1976;8:xi.
44. Sherman W. Carbohydrate, muscle glycogen, and improved performance. Phys Sports Med 1987;15:157–164.
45. Burke LM, Read RSD. Sports nutrition, approaching the nineties. Sports Med 1989;8(2):80–100.
46. Grandjean AC. Macronutrient intake of U.S. athletes compared with the general population and recommendations made for athletes. Am J Clin Nutr 1989;49:1070–1076.
47. Grandjean AC. Vitamins, diet and the athlete. Clin Sports Med 1983;2:105–115.
48. Selby GB, Eichner ER. Endurances swimming, intravascular hemolysis, anemia, and iron depletion: new perspectives on athlete's anemia. Am J Med 1986;81:791–794.
49. A statement by the American Dietetic Association. Nutrition and physical fitness. J Am Diet Assoc 1980;76:437–483.

50. Benning JR, Steen SN, eds. Sports nutrition for the 90s: the health professional's handbook. Frederick, MD: Aspen Publishers, 1991:11,115–199.
51. Sherman W, Costill DL. The marathon: dietary manipulation to optimize performance. Am J Sports Med 1984;12:44–50.
52. Lamb DR. Anabolic steroids in athletics: how well do they work and how dangerous are they? Am J Sports Med 1984;12:31–36.
53. Haupt HA, Rovere GD. Anabolic steroids: a review of the literature. Am J Sports Med 1984;12:469–483.
54. Martikainen H, Alen M, Rahkila P, Vihko R. Testicular response to human chorionic gonadotrophin during transient hypogonadotrophic hypogonadism induced by androgenic/anabolic steroids in power athletes. J Steroid Biochem 1986;25:109–112.
55. Slavin JL, Lanners BS, Engstrom MA. Amino acid supplements: beneficial or risky? Phys Sports Med 1988;16:221–224.
56. Sherman WM, Wright DA. Pre-event nutrition for prolonged exercise. In: Grandjean AS, Storlie J, eds. The theory and practice of athletic nutrition: bridging the gap. Report of the Ross Symposium. Columbus, OH: Ross Laboratories, 1989:30–46.

GERIATRIC NUTRITION

General Description

The aging process is a continuum throughout adult life marked by a progressive deterioration in bodily functions and by an accumulation of chronic disabilities and diseases. The rate of aging is influenced by genetic and environmental forces and differs among individuals from physiological, chronological, psychological, and social viewpoints. Thus, a single measure of aging is an unreliable index for judging the nutritional needs of an elderly individual.[57]

The elderly should be subdivided into several groups and not considered as a whole. By age 65 people vary greatly in how old their bodies appear and how much they have changed. Some of the subdivisions often used when considering the nutritional status and needs of the elderly are healthy versus frail and institutionalized versus independent-living.

Factors Affecting Nutritional Status of the Elderly

Metabolic, Physiological, and Biochemical Factors.   There is a general agreement that metabolic, physiological, and biochemical processes change with increasing age, and these changes tend to have an adverse effect on the nutritional status of the elderly (Table 4-7). A decrease in the acuity of taste, smell, vision, and hearing may interfere with the act of eating and with the enjoyment of food. Loss of teeth and poorly fitting dentures further interfere with eating. The digestion and absorption of nutrients are affected by a decline in gastrointestinal function. The kidneys' mass and the number of functioning nephrons decrease with age, which in many may cause a diminished capacity to eliminate metabolic waste products. Liver size also decreases with a progressive loss in the liver's functional capacity. Changes in body composition also occur with age. Lean body mass, total body water, and bone mass decrease, while adipose tissue and plasma volume usually

TABLE 4-7   Physiological Changes with Aging

Physiologic Changes	Potential Impact on Nutritional Status
Decreased volume and viscosity of saliva secretion; atrophy of taste buds	Dry mouth, difficulty chewing and initiating swallow, decreased taste sensation, anorexia, pain, and irritation from foodstuffs → avoidance of many food items → decreased food intake
Atrophy of olfactory receptors	Decreased sense of smell and taste sensation, foods lose appeal → decreased food intake
Missing teeth, periodontitis	Poorly fitting dentures cause difficulty chewing → restricted variety of food or decreased food intake. Dentures interfere with sense of taste → food loses appeal → decreased food intake
Impaired vision and hearing	Interferes with socialization at mealtimes, difficulty in food preparation → diminished enjoyment of food → decreased intake
Decreased secretion of acid in stomach, enzymes in small intestine, and decreased peristalsis	Diminished digestion and absorption of some nutrients
Decreased capacity of kidney to concentrate urine	Dehydration and need for increased water to prevent azotemia
Decreased intestinal motility, weakened abdominal and pelvic muscles, and decreased sensory perception	Chronic constipation → decreased or altered food intake
Decreased lean body mass, increased adipose tissue, lower metabolic rate	Vulnerable to obesity
Decreased breathing capacity	Limited activity → decreased caloric expenditure → obesity or decreased food intake → wasting
Decline in glucose tolerance	Vulnerable to development of diabetes → restricted dietary selections → decreased food intake

increase. A lower metabolic rate and a decline in tolerance of carbohydrate render the older person more vulnerable to obesity and diabetes.[58,59]

Socioeconomic and Psychological Factors.   Social isolation, limited financial resources, lack of education regarding nutrition, lack of family support, loss of significant other(s) or care giver(s), and the decreased mobility that results from physical disabilities or from social isolation can lessen the availability of a selection of foods.[60,61] The elderly at highest risk are most often dependent on others for care, and this dependency may result in the potential for abuse, such as the withholding of food or the providing of inadequate or unacceptable food. Food items in large packages and information labels that are difficult to read and to interpret can contribute to inappropriate food purchasing. The elderly are also susceptible to the misleading claims of advertisers and may unnecessarily use nutritional supplements and over-the-counter therapies, which can be costly and may lead to adverse effects.[62]

Psychological factors that can affect nutritional status include depression, grief, and dementia. Decreased appetite is one of the most reported symptoms of depres-

TABLE 4-8	Prescription and Over-the-Counter Drugs Frequently Consumed by Older Americans with Potential to Negatively Impact Nutritional Status

Alcohol	***Central Nervous System Agents***
	Antidepressants
Analgesics	Antipsychotics
Aspirin	Antiseizure medications
Antibiotics	***Endocrine and Metabolic Agents***
	Oral hypoglycemics
Anti-inflammatory Agents	
Corticosteroids	***Gastrointestinal Agents***
Nonsteroidal anti-inflammatory drugs (NSAIDS)	Antacids
	Laxatives
Cardiovascular Agents	H-2 receptor antagonists
Antiarrhythmics	
Antihypertensives	
Cardiac glycosides	
Potassium supplements	

See Appendix 2 for effect the drug may have on nutritional status.

Reprinted with permission: Prescription and over-the-counter drugs frequently consumed by older persons with potential to negatively impact nutritional status. Reprinted with permission: Nutrition Screening Initiative, a project of the American Academy of Family Physicians, the American Dietetic Association, and the National Council on Aging, Inc., and funded in part by a grant from Ross Laboratories, a division of Abbott Laboratories. Washington, DC; 1991.

sion. The decrease in appetite can result from decreased activity, increased isolation, the loss of food's symbolism of warmth and sharing, and the use of food as a weapon (refusing to eat as a subconscious death wish). Altered levels of neurotransmitters such as norepinephrine have been documented in depression and can affect appetite. Persons with dementia may not be interested in eating, often do not remember if they have eaten, and may not recognize the need to eat. For those in institutions, time provided by staff for assistance with feeding is generally less than that provided by family members for similar individuals living at home.[60,63]

Chronic Disease.   The presence of chronic diseases, such as diabetes, hypertension, chronic obstructive pulmonary disease, heart disease, or arthritis, and associated diet or drug therapy further contribute to the potential for inadequate nutrition in the elderly. Alcohol abuse may be another contributor to malnutrition in the elderly, affecting nutrient absorption and displacing nutrient-dense foods in the diet. The elderly are particularly susceptible to the effects of alcohol abuse. The risk of developing a poor nutritional state is greater in the elderly since they tend to have reduced caloric requirements. The adverse consequences of moderate alcohol consumption are still being debated.[58,64,65]

Many commonly used drugs may interfere with the digestion, absorption, utilization, or excretion of essential nutrients. Drugs may also have an effect on appetite, taste, and smell (see Appendix 2).

Older Americans make up approximately 12% of the population, but they use approximately 25% of the prescription drugs dispensed each year. It has also been found that 40% of persons over age 60 years use over-the-counter preparations every day.[66] This practice of "polypharmacy" can lead to adverse effects of the prescribed drugs. Furthermore, changes in the metabolism of drugs in the elderly have been well documented. See Table 4-8 for drugs frequently taken by the elderly with potential for a negative impact on nutritional status.[67]

The appropriate choice of drugs, proper dose adjustment, and thorough education of the patient and family (or caregivers) can often improve the medical status of the patient. One should obtain an accurate drug history in assessing nutritional status, since vitamin, mineral, and other dietary supplements are widely used by the geriatric population as a form of "nutritional insurance," and generally considered safe by them. However, little consideration may have been given to potential adverse interactions between these supplements and prescribed drugs.

Special Dietary Considerations

Physician-prescribed and self-imposed diets are common in the elderly population because of the frequency of chronic diseases. However, each therapeutic dietary modification limits the selection of foods available to the individual. The psychological effects of having favorite foods restricted, the loss of flavor caused by the elimination of customary seasonings, and required alterations in meal preparation methods may have an adverse effect on the desire to eat. Dietary modifications should be imposed only when such an intervention can be expected to result in a significant health improvement.

Poor dentition and dysphagia often lead to the use of texture-modified diets. Individuals with dysphagia secondary to neurological impairments may have difficulty with pureed foods since these foods lack sufficient taste, texture, temperature, and pressure requirements to elicit an adequate swallow.[60] (See Chapter 5, Dysphagia.)

Coronary heart disease (CHD) is the number one cause of death in the United States for both men and women.[68] It accounts for nearly half of the total mortality in those age 65 or greater.[69] Prevention, delay in onset, or reversal of CHD, therefore, can potentially benefit a large segment of the elderly population.

Hypercholesterolemia has been regarded as one of the three major risk factors for CHD for many years. Previous studies, including Framingham and the Multiple Risk Factor Intervention Trial (MRFIT) found that the relative risk for the disease due to elevated blood cholesterol levels is much lower in those greater than 60 years of age.[70] However, more recent studies, including an updated version of the Framingham results, show that although the relative risk of CHD due to elevated serum cholesterol levels declines with increased age, the attributable risk resulting from rises in cholesterol levels increases with age.[71] Simply put, an elevated serum cholesterol level contributes to more cases of CHD in older individuals than in younger ones. Based on National Cholesterol Education Program (NCEP) guidelines, 36% of all adults in the United States are considered candidates for medical advice and intervention.[72] That level jumps to 60% of individuals age 60 and older. Since total blood cholesterol determination is still one of the most common screening methods with lipids, it may be appropriate to treat an elevated total serum cholesterol in the elderly the same way as in the middle-aged. The individual's willingness and ability to comply with dietary and other treatment methods must be considered. (For additional information, refer to Chapter 7, Hyperlipidemia.)

Anemia is the most common hematological disorder in elderly patients. There is controversy about whether or not an age-related decline in hematological parameters occurs. Proponents believe that normal blood values should be lowered for elderly patients. Opponents contend that while anemia is prevalent in the elderly, it should not be regarded as a normal result of the aging process, and other causes should be excluded.[73,74]

Anemia in the elderly population may be classified into three types: disorders associated with decreased red cell production (hypoproliferative anemias); disorders associated with ineffective hematopoiesis (megaloblastic and sideroblastic anemias); and disorders associated with decreased red cell survival time (hemolytic anemias).[73]

An inadequate iron supply for hemoglobin synthesis is the most common cause of the first type of anemia. This usually occurs secondary to blood loss, but may also occur as a result of chronic inflammation or malnutrition. There is no evidence to suggest that iron intake is deficient or that iron absorption is impaired in elderly people. In addition, after the menstrual years, the daily iron needs of women decrease to those of men. The RDA for iron is thus the same for elderly women and men—10 mg/day.[73,75]

The megaloblastic anemias are almost exclusively due to vitamin B_{12} or folate deficiency. Vitamin B_{12} deficiency may be dietary in origin or the result of bacterial overgrowth. However, more often it is a result of pernicious anemia. In this disorder, vitamin B_{12} must be administered parenterally on a monthly basis for the rest of a person's life. Folate deficiency anemia is rare in the elderly but is most likely to occur in conjunction with alcohol abuse, celiac disease, nontropical sprue, and the use of certain medications. The cause of sideroblastic anemias usually remains unknown, but these may occur secondary to alcohol or drug use or a number of diseases, including infections, neoplasms, and inflammatory disorders.[73]

The third major group of anemias in elderly patients, the hemolytic anemias, are the least common and not related to nutrient deficiencies. The cause is usually idiopathic.

A very common disease seen in the elderly is osteoporosis. This form of osteopenia, characterized by reduced bone mass and impaired skeletal function, affects 15 to 20 million people in the United States and is most commonly seen in women. Adequate intake of calcium along with a balanced diet throughout the life cycle may protect against the development of osteoporosis. Supplements may also be used to assure an adequate intake of calcium.[76,77] For additional information, refer to Chapter 8, Osteoporosis.

Aging, even without the presence of disease, causes physiological changes, which can alter some laboratory test results. Interpreting laboratory values in the elderly can be difficult. It is vital to understand the changes in physiology with aging and the effect they may have on laboratory results when assessing this population.[78] See Table 4-9 for the effects of aging on various laboratory values.[79]

TABLE 4-9   Effects of Aging on Various Laboratory Values[79]

Values That Do Not Change with Age	*Values That Change and Have Clinical Significance*
Hemoglobin/hematocrit/RBC indices	Erythrocyte sedimentation rate
Platelet count	Arterial oxygen pressure
WBC count and differential	Postprandial blood glucose
Serum electrolytes (sodium, potassium, chloride, bicarbonate, and magnesium)	Serum lipid profile
Coagulation profile	*Value That Does Not Change but Has Clinical Significance*
Liver function tests	Serum creatinine
Thyroid function tests	
Values That Change Statistically but Have No or Minimal Clinical Significance	
Serum albumin	
Serum calcium	
Serum uric acid	

RBC = Red blood cell; WBC = white blood cell.

With permission from Duthie EH, Abbasi AA. Laboratory testing: current recommendations for older adults. Geriatrics 1991; 46:41–50.

Nutritional Needs of the Elderly

As the American population ages, there is much concern over the nutritional needs of the elderly. However, the information available to determine the specific requirements for essential nutrients is inconclusive.[59,80-83] More research is needed in this area, especially in regard to adults over the age of 70. Based on the data available, the elderly have altered requirements for some nutrients when compared to younger adults. Whether all current RDAs, based on adults 51 years of age and older, are adequate to meet the needs of all elderly continues to be studied.[80-82,84,85] See Chapter 2, Recommended Dietary Allowances.

There are diminished energy needs with aging because of decreases in lean body mass, metabolic rate, and physical activity. However, a concern for the very old is that the amounts of food consumed are not enough to meet even these decreased energy requirements. The lower energy requirement, coupled with the same RDAs as for younger adults, has been used as an argument for a more nutrient dense diet, but if the convention were to express RDA per 1,000 kcal expended by the individual, the apparent need for a greater nutrient density would disappear.

As the body ages, daily albumin synthesis and serum albumin levels decrease along with lean body mass, while an increase in total body fat is seen. Although there is controversy as to how this may affect the protein needs of the elderly, there is some evidence that an increased need for protein exists above the current RDA level of 0.8 g/kg of body weight. This level may also need to be adjusted for those individuals with suboptimal dietary intake or chronic disease.[82,85,86]

National surveys report that elderly individuals often have decreased intakes of vitamins A, B_2, B_6, and C. Other studies have reported low intakes of vitamins B_1, B_{12}, D, folate, niacin, zinc, and calcium.[57,59,87,88] Although vitamin and mineral deficiencies are seen, there is little experimental data on which to estimate the exact dietary requirements for the micronutrients. With age, an increased need for vitamins and minerals may result from less efficient intestinal absorption, more frequent illness, use of certain medications, poor dentition, poor dietary intake, living alone, and the housebound state.

Current research indicates that vitamin needs may also change with advancing age. While specific levels of change have not been identified, it has been suggested that the RDAs for vitamins B_6, B_{12}, D and calcium may need to be increased, while vitamin A is decreased.[59,82-88] There are few data available to indicate that trace element and macronutrient requirements are different for the elderly than for younger adults.[82,89,90] The administration of specific vitamin or mineral supplements should be based on need and defined by clinical and biochemical assessment of the nutritional status.

Adequate intake of dietary fiber is helpful in alleviating constipation, one of the most frequent gastrointestinal complaints of the elderly. Fiber helps offset the effects of diminished muscle tone and peristalsis. In order to avoid abdominal discomfort, dietary fiber should be increased gradually while adequate amounts of liquid are consumed. Refer to Chapter 9, Fiber and Residue Modifications. Mineral oil should be avoided since it may contribute to decreased absorption of vitamins A and D.

Adequate fluid intake can help prevent dehydration. Dehydration may be due in part to a decreased thirst response and decreased concentrating capacity of the kidney. Alcohol and some medications (i.e., diuretics) can increase fluid excretion. Basic free water needs can be estimated for healthy elderly adults at 1 ml per kilocalorie ingested or 30 ml per kilogram of body weight per day.[59,82,86]

Conclusion

The heterogeneity of the older population must not be overlooked. Nutritional assessment of the elderly and recommendations for nutritional care should consider individual abilities, capabilities, and levels of function. The presence or absence of chronic diseases, the general health, and the amount of physical activity may also affect dietary requirements of the older person. Additional consideration must be given to the individual's level of independence, functional status, and place of residence. The American Dietetic Association has proposed a continuum of nutritional care for older adults based on their level of independence (Table 4-10).

The 1991 Consensus Conference of the Nutrition Screening Initiative (NSI) has led to increased professional awareness of poor nutritional status and better definitions and indicators of poor nutritional status in the elderly population. (See Table 4-11.)[67] A public awareness checklist and two screening levels have been developed to allow one to recognize these risks and indicators.

The checklist, Determine Your Nutritional Health (Fig. 4-1), is designed to help the elderly or those who interact with them to recognize food and lifestyle habits, diseases, and conditions that may adversely affect nutritional health. The checklist

TABLE 4-10   Continuum of Nutrition Care for Older Americans

Community-Based Long-Term Care	
Obstacle to Adequate Intake	**Nutrition Service**
Lack of socialization, motivation, income, or physical strength to prepare meals	—Congregate nutrition program (1 hot lunch 5–7 days) —Nutrition education: importance of nutrition; motivational activities; easy, inexpensive, and nutritious meals; special requirements (e.g., low sodium, ethnic)
Limited income	—Congregate meals + Food Stamps or other income supplement —Congregate meals + nutrition education: increasing food purchasing power, low-cost and nutritious meals
Limited access to food stores, inability to carry groceries	—Congregate meals + transportation (with assistance) to food stores
Physical inability to food shop	—Congregate meals + food shopping services —Congregate meals + delivery of basic food supplies every 2 weeks
Inability to participate in congregate nutrition program, limited ability to prepare foods; can reheat foods	—Home delivery of prepared frozen or shelf-stable foods every two weeks or once a month —Nutrition education: maintaining intake at home —Home health aide for meal preparation —Home delivery of chilled prepared foods every 2–3 days
Limited socialization	—Telephone assurance, friendly visitors, or equivalent program
Inability to safely prepare foods	—Home-delivered nutrition services: hot, daily delivery of 1 meal; provision of ready-to-eat food for remainder of meals or home health aide/neighbor/family assistance —Nutrition education for family/caregivers —Adult day care programs with nutrition services
Severe physical or mental debilitation	—Home health aide assistance with feeding —Nutrition education for family/caregivers —Hospice care including dietary counseling
Institutionalization	

With permission: Anon. ADA takes proactive stance, testifies on Older Americans Act Reauthorization. Copyright The American Dietetic Association. Reprinted with permission from J Am Diet Assoc 1984;84:822–835.

refers those with scores that indicate nutritional risk to organizations or individuals that provide services that can help improve their nutritional health.

The screening levels are designed to help formalize and systematize an approach to nutritional screening and assessment for trained persons in various disciplines of healthcare. The Level 1 Screen includes height, weight, Body Mass

---

TABLE 4-11   Major Indicators of Poor Nutritional Status in Older Americans

---

*Significant Weight Loss over Time**

- 5.0% or more of prior body weight in 1 month
- 7.5% or more of body weight in 3 months
- 10.0% or more of body weight in 6 months or involuntary weight loss of 10 lb in 6 months

Significantly Low or High Weight for Height

- 20% below or above desirable weight for that individual (considering loss of height due to vertebral collapse, kyphosis, and deformity)

Significant Reduction in Serum Albumin

- Serum albumin of less than 3.5 g/dl

Significant Change in Functional Status

- Change from "independent" to "dependent" in two of the ADLs or one of the nutrition-related IADLs†

Significant and Sustained Inappropriate Food Intake

- Failure to consume the recommended minimum from one or more of the food groups suggested in the Dietary Guidelines for Americans (e.g., groups such as milk and milk products, cereals and grains, fruits, vegetables, meat/poultry/fish/eggs/legumes) or sufficient variety of foods for a period of 3 months or more
- Excessive consumption of fat, saturated fat, and/or alcohol (alcohol: >1 oz/day, women; 2 oz/day, men)

Significant Reduction in Mid-Arm Circumference

- To less than 10th percentile (NHANES standards)‡

Significant Increase or Decrease in Triceps Skinfolds

- To less than 10th percentile or more than 95th percentile (NHANES standards)

Significant Obesity

- More than 120% of desirable weight or Body Mass Index (BMI) over 27 or triceps skinfolds above 95th percentile (NHANES standards)

Other Nutrition-related Disorders

- Presence of osteoporosis, osteomalacia, folate deficiency, or vitamin B_{12} deficiency

---

*Significant increase in weight requires similar documentation examination and interpretation.

†ADL = Activities of Daily Living; IADL = Instrumental Activities of Daily Living.

‡NHANES = National Health and Nutrition Evaluation Survey.

Reprinted with permission from Nutrition Screening Initiative, a project of the American Academy of Family Physicians, The American Dietetic Association, and the National Council on Aging, Inc., and funded in part by a grant from Ross Laboratories, a division of Abbott Laboratories. Washington, DC; 1991.

Index, and checklists for use in evaluation of eating habits and socioeconomic and functional status. The Level 2 Screen includes the components of Level 1 as well as anthropometric measurements, laboratory tests, cognitive assessment, emotional status assessment, functional status assessment, chronic medication use, living environment, and clinical signs of nutrient deficiency.[91-93]

The warning signs of poor nutritional health are often overlooked. Use this checklist to find out if you or someone you know is at nutritional risk.

Read the statements below. Circle the number in the yes column for those that apply to you or someone you know. For each yes answer, score the number in the box. Total your nutritional score.

DETERMINE YOUR NUTRITIONAL HEALTH

	YES
I have an illness or condition that made me change the kind and/or amount of food I eat.	2
I eat fewer than 2 meals per day.	3
I eat few fruits or vegetables, or milk products.	2
I have 3 or more drinks of beer, liquor or wine almost every day.	2
I have tooth or mouth problems that make it hard for me to eat.	2
I don't always have enough money to buy the food I need.	4
I eat alone most of the time.	1
I take 3 or more different prescribed or over-the-counter drugs a day.	1
Without wanting to, I have lost or gained 10 pounds in the last 6 months.	2
I am not always physically able to shop, cook, and/or feed myself.	2
TOTAL	

Total Your Nutrition Score. If it's —

0–2   **Good!** Recheck your nutritional score in 6 months.

3–5   **You are at moderate nutritional risk.** See what can be done to improve your eating habits and lifestyle. Your office on aging, senior nutrition program, senior citizens center or health department can help. Recheck your nutritional score in 3 months.

6 or more   **You are at high nutritional risk.** Bring this checklist the next time you see your doctor, dietician or other qualified health or social service professional. Talk with them about any problems you may have. Ask for help to improve your nutritional health.

These materials developed and distributed by the Nutrition Screening Initiative, a project of:

AMERICAN ACADEMY OF FAMILY PHYSICIANS

THE AMERICAN DIETETIC ASSOCIATION

NATIONAL COUNCIL ON THE AGING, INC.

Remember that warning signs suggest risk, but do not represent diagnosis of any condition. Turn the page to learn more about the Warning Signs of poor nutritional health.

FIGURE 4-1 Checklist for Identifying Elderly Individuals at Nutritional Risk. (Reprinted with permission: Nutrition Screening Initiative, a project of the American Academy of Family Physicians, The American Dietetic Association, and the National Council on Aging, Inc., and funded in part by a grant from Ross Laboratories, a division of Abbott Laboratories. Washington, DC; 1991.)

Continued.

**The Nutrition Checklist is based on the Warning Signs described below.
Use the word _DETERMINE_ to remind you of the Warning Signs.**

DISEASE

Any disease, illness or chronic condition which causes you to change the way you eat, or makes it hard for you to eat, puts your nutritional health at risk. Four out of five adults have chronic diseases that are affected by diet. Confusion or memory loss that keeps getting worse is estimated to affect one out of five or more older adults. This can make it hard to remember what, when or if you've eaten. Feeling sad or depressed, which happens to about one in eight older adults, can cause big changes in appetite, digestion, energy level, weight and well-being.

EATING POORLY

Eating too little and eating too much both lead to poor health. Eating the same foods day after day or not eating fruit, vegetables, and milk products daily will also cause poor nutritional health. One in five adults skip meals daily. Only 13% of adults eat the minimum amount of fruit and vegetables needed. One in four older adults drink too much alcohol. Many health problems become worse if you drink more than one or two alcoholic beverages per day.

TOOTH LOSS/MOUTH PAIN

A healthy mouth, teeth and gums are needed to eat. Missing, loose, or rotten teeth or dentures which don't fit well or cause mouth sores make it hard to eat.

ECONOMIC HARDSHIP

As many as 40% of older Americans have incomes of less than $6,000 per year. Having less — or choosing to spend less — than $25–30 per week for food makes it very hard to get the foods you need to stay healthy.

REDUCED SOCIAL CONTACT

One third of all older people live alone. Being with people daily has a positive effect on morale, well-being and eating.

MULTIPLE MEDICINES

Many older Americans must take medicines for health problems. Almost half of older Americans take multiple medicines daily. Growing old may change the way we respond to drugs. The more medicines you take, the greater the chance for side effects such as increased or decreased appetite, change in taste, constipation, weakness, drowsiness, diarrhea, nausea, and others. Vitamins or minerals when taken in large doses act like drugs and can cause harm. Alert your doctor to everything you take.

INVOLUNTARY WEIGHT LOSS/GAIN

Losing or gaining a lot of weight when you are not trying to do so is an important warning sign that must not be ignored. Being overweight or underweight also increases your chance of poor health.

NEEDS ASSISTANCE IN SELF CARE

Although most older people are able to eat, one of every five have trouble walking, shopping, buying and cooking food, especially as they get older.

ELDER YEARS ABOVE AGE 80

Most older people lead full and productive lives. But as age increases, risk of frailty and health problems increase. Checking your nutritional health regularly makes good sense.

Reprinted with permission: Nutrition Screening Initiative, a project of the American Academy of Family Physicians, the American Dietetic Association, and the National Council on Aging, Inc., and funded in part by a grant from Ross Laboratories, a division of Abbott Laboratories. Washington, DC; 1991.

FIGURE 4-1—cont'd Checklist for Identifying Elderly Individuals at Nutritional Risk.

References

57. Morley JE. Nutritional status of the elderly. Am J Med 1986;81:679–695.
58. Granieri E. Nutrition and the older adult. Dysphagia 1990;4:196–201.
59. Mobarhan S, Trumbore LS. Nutritional problems of the elderly. Clin Geriatr Med 1991;7:191–214.
60. Curran J. Overview of geriatric nutrition. Dysphagia 1990;5:72–76.
61. Henderson CT. Approaches to nutritional care in the elderly. Compr Ther 1989;15(6):25–30.
62. Bidlack WR. Nutrition misinformation: health fraud in the elderly population—creation of food fads for profit. In: Morley JE, Glick Z, Rubenstein LZ, eds. Geriatric nutrition: a comprehensive review. New York: Raven Press, 1990:397–417.
63. Silver AJ. Anorexia of aging and protein-energy malnutrition. In: Morley JE, Glick Z, Rubenstein LZ, eds. Geriatric nutrition: a comprehensive review. New York: Raven Press, 1990:105–115.
64. Jacques PF, Sulsky S, Hartz SC, Russell RM. Moderate alcohol intake and nutritional status in nonalcoholic elderly subjects. Am J Clin Nutr 1989;50:875–883.
65. Goodwin JS. Social, psychological and physical factors affecting the nutritional status of elderly subjects: separating cause and effect. Am J Clin Nutr 1989;50:1201–1209.
66. Council on Scientific Affairs, American Medical Association white paper on elderly health. Arch Intern Med 1990;150:2459–2472.
67. White JV, Ham RJ, Lipschitz DA, Dwyer JT, Wellman NS. Consensus of the Nutrition Screening Initiative: risk factors and indicators of poor nutritional status in older Americans. J Am Diet Assoc 1991;91:783–787.
68. American Heart Association and National Heart, Lung, and Blood Institute. The cholesterol facts: a summary of the evidence relating dietary fats, serum cholesterol, and coronary heart disease. Circulation 1990;81:1721–1733.
69. Benfante R, Reed D. Is elevated serum cholesterol level a risk factor for heart disease in the elderly? JAMA 1990;263(3):393–396.
70. Allred JB, Gallagher-Allred CR, Bowers DF. Elevated blood cholesterol: a risk factor for heart disease that decreases with advanced age. J Am Diet Assoc 1990;90:574–576.
71. Castelli WP, Wilson PWF, Levy D, Anderson K. Cardiovascular risk factors in the elderly. Am J Cardiol 1989;63:12H–19H.
72. Sempos C, Fulwood R, Haines C, Carroll M, Anda R, Williamson DR, Remington P, Cleeman J. The prevalence of high blood cholesterol levels among adults in the United States. JAMA 1989;262:45–52.
73. Daly MP. Anemia in the elderly. Am Fam Physician 1989;39:129–136.
74. Garry PJ, Goodwin JS, Hunt WC. Iron status and anemia in the elderly: new findings and a review of previous studies. J Am Geriatr Soc 1983;31:389–399.
75. Subcommittee on the Tenth Edition of the RDAs. Recommended dietary allowances, 10th ed. Washington, DC: National Academy Press, 1989:201.
76. Public Health Service, National Institutes of Health, and National Institute of Arthritis and Musculoskeletal and Skin Diseases. Osteoporosis: cause, treatment, prevention. NIH publication no. 86-2226. Washington, DC: US DHHS, May 1986.
77. Barth RW, Lane JM. Osteoporosis. Orthop Clin North Am 1988;19(4):845–858.
78. Garner BC. Guide to changing lab values in elders. Geriatr Nurs 1989;May/June:144–145.
79. Duthie EH, Abbasi AA. Laboratory testing: current recommendations for older adults. Geriatrics 1991;46:41–50.
80. Subcommittee on the Tenth Edition of the RDAs. Recommended dietary allowances, 10th ed. Washington, DC: National Academy Press, 1989:1–9,19,30,57–60.
81. Roe DA. Geriatric nutrition, 2nd ed. Englewood Cliffs: Prentice Hall,, 1987:64–86.
82. Bidlack WR. Nutritional requirements of the elderly. In: Morley J, Glick Z, Rubenstein L, eds. Geriatric nutrition: a comprehensive review. New York: Raven Press, 1990:41–72.

83. Suter PM, Russell RM. Vitamin requirements of the elderly. Am J Clin Nutr 1987;45:501–512.

84. Lehr D, Roe DA, Rosenberg IH, Geronymo K, Butler RN. Practical nutritional advice for the elderly. Part I: evaluation, supplements, RDAs. Geriatrics 1990;45:26–34.

85. Klein S, Rogers R. Nutritional requirements in the elderly. Gastroenterol Clin North Am 1990;19:473–491.

86. Schneider EL, Vining EM, Hadley EC, Farnham SA. Recommended dietary allowances and the health of the elderly. N Engl J Med 1986;314:157–160.

87. Johnson LE. Vitamin disorders in the elderly. In: Morley J, Glick Z, Rubenstein L, eds. Geriatric nutrition: a comprehensive review. New York: Raven Press, 1990:117–147.

88. Andres R, Hallfrisch J. Nutrient intake recommendations needed for the older American. J Am Diet Assoc 1989;89:1739–1741.

89. Bunker VW, Clayton BE. Research review: studies in the nutrition of elderly people with particular reference to essential trace elements. Age and Ageing 1989;18:422–429.

90. ADA takes proactive stance, testifies on Older Americans Act Reauthorization. J Am Diet Assoc 1984;84:822–835.

91. White JV, Dwyer JT, Posner BM, Ham RJ, Lipschitz DA, Wellman NS. Nutrition Screening Initiative: development and implementation of the public awareness checklist and screening tools. J Am Diet Assoc 1992;92:163–167.

92. Greer, Margolis, Mitchell, Grunwald, and associates. Nutrition screening manual for professionals caring for older Americans. Washington, DC: Nutrition Screening Initiative, 1991.

93. White JV, Ham RJ, Lipschitz DA. Report of nutrition screening I: toward a common view. Washington, DC: Nutrition Screening Initiative, 1991.

VEGETARIAN DIET

General Description

Vegetarianism is practiced by an increasing number of people for reasons of health, of economy, of religion, of ecology, or of philosophy. This term embraces a variety of dietary practices. Vegetarian diets are most frequently classified (Table 4-12) according to the extent by which animal foods are excluded. It has become increasingly apparent that individuals consuming certain vegetarian diets come closer than their omnivore counterparts to achieving the recommended dietary goals of reduced fat intake and increased fiber consumption.[94]

TABLE 4-12   Classification of Vegetarian Diets

- Total vegetarians or "vegans" eat only foods of plant origin.
- Fruitarians consume only fresh or dried fruits and nuts, honey, and olive oil.
- Lactovegetarians eat plant foods plus milk and dairy products.
- Lacto-ovovegetarians consume plant foods, milk and dairy products, and eggs.
- Semivegetarians or partial vegetarians consume some groups of animal foods but not all. Meat is usually excluded; poultry or fish and seafood may also be excluded. These individuals are non-red meat-eaters and/or may exclude some animal food groups completely; because of this, semivegetarians often consider themselves vegetarians.

The reader is referred to Chapter 19, Vegetarian Diet, for a discussion on vegetarian diets for infants, for children, and for adolescents.

Nutritional Inadequacy

The American Dietetic Association recognizes that well-planned vegetarian diets can be consistent with a good nutritional intake.[94] The extent to which food selection and feeding patterns meet the dietary recommendations for an individual is dependent upon the type of vegetarian diet chosen and upon the degree of food selection and meal planning. Nutrients that may be limited or lacking in vegetarian diets are high quality protein, vitamin B_{12}, vitamin D, riboflavin, calcium, zinc, and iron. An individual's intake should be assessed for nutritional adequacy and supplemented accordingly.

In addition, there are times when individuals may be at nutritional risk if vegetarian diets are not carefully planned. Such periods include pregnancy and lactation, growth, and when health problems or disease limit the intake or increase the nutrient requirements beyond normal.

Goals of Dietary Management

The nutritional goal in vegetarianism is to achieve an intake that meets all known nutrient needs. A well-planned diet that consists of a variety of largely unrefined plant foods supplemented with some milk and eggs (lacto-ovovegetarian diet) meets all known nutrient needs. A total dietary intake of plant foods can be made adequate by careful planning. Attention should be given to sources of specific nutrients that may be in a less available form or in a lower concentration or absent in plant foods. Caloric intake should also be sufficient to meet energy needs.[94]

Dietary Recommendations

Lacto-ovovegetarian and lactovegetarian diets are nutritionally sound, but a conscious effort must be made to select the proper foods in sufficient amounts to maintain optimal weight and health. If selected appropriately, these diets are also adequate in meeting the needs induced by the stress of growth, pregnancy, and lactation.

Care must be taken in planning "pure" vegetarian diets since these diets lack concentrated sources of proteins with desirable proportions of essential amino acids. They are also limited in calcium, iron, zinc, riboflavin, vitamin B_{12}, and vitamin D.

Protein.   Plant proteins have a lower biological value than do proteins of animal origin. The biological value of a protein is defined as its ability to support growth and to maintain body structure, and this ability depends on the number, the proportion, and the type of amino acids the protein contains. The proteins of legumes, whole grains, nuts, and vegetables contain all the essential amino acids but yield certain ones at lower levels than do proteins of animal origin. The lower biological value of plant proteins is the result of low levels of one or more of the essential amino acids. However, when plant proteins from a variety of sources are consumed, there is a higher likelihood that a mixture of all essential amino acids in proportions similar to those found in proteins of animal origin occurs. Food combinations that supply the essential amino acids in appropriate proportions are as efficient as proteins of animal origin in meeting the protein needs at minimal levels of intake.[94] In fact when different proteins are combined in appropriate ways, plant proteins cannot be distinguished nutritionally from those of animal origin. Therefore, the amino acid profile that is derived from the mixture of proteins, and not the origin or "value" of a single protein, should be the criterion in deciding whether protein needs are being met in vegetarian diets.

The sources of protein must be combined in such a way that the amount and the proportion of amino acids that result support normal growth and maintenance. To supply enough derived protein to contain all the essential amino acids in desirable proportions, meals should consist of a combination of grains and legumes, of grains and nuts or seeds, or of grains and vegetables.

In 1991 E.C. Henley proposed a Protein Digestibility Corrected Amino Acid Score as a method for measuring protein quality in diets for humans above the age of 1 year.[95] On the basis of this formula, properly processed soy products can be considered as equivalent to protein of animal origin.

Vitamin B$_{12}$.   The lacto-ovovegetarian and lactovegetarian categories, in general, have an adequate intake of vitamin B$_{12}$. Vitamin B$_{12}$ is not present in plant foods in large enough amounts for them to be considered a significant dietary source, however. Some persons eating pure vegetarian or vegan diets appear to remain in good health for many years, or nearly a lifetime, without developing symptoms of deficiency. Others are forced to use supplementary vitamin B$_{12}$ or to adopt a lactovegetarian or lacto-ovovegetarian diet after a few months or a few years. The reason for this variation is not clear, and the results of nutritional studies are not uniform. Supplementary vitamin B$_{12}$ for the pure vegetarian can be obtained from fortified breakfast cereals, soybean milk (fortified with vitamin B$_{12}$) or commercial meat analogs (fortified with vitamin B$_{12}$). Vitamin B$_{12}$ is also available as cyanocobalamin (the physiologically active form for humans) in vitamin supplements.[94]

Riboflavin, Calcium, Vitamin D, Iron, and Zinc.   The lacto-ovovegetarians are able to meet their needs for calcium and riboflavin from dairy products, while the pure vegetarian's intake of these nutrients may only be marginal. Sources of calcium for the vegetarian include dark green leafy vegetables (foods high in oxalic acid, such as spinach, chard, and beet greens may lessen calcium availability), some nuts and seeds, and fortified soybean milk. Those individuals who do not consume milk or soybean milk in adequate quantities may need supplemental calcium (see Chapter 8, Osteoporosis). Vitamin D may be obtained by the exposure of the skin to sunlight or by supplementation.

The absorptional availability of iron and of zinc can be influenced by a number of dietary maneuvers. One can increase the use of fortified grains and cereals, but one must also limit those high in bran and in phytates since phytic acid tends to reduce iron and zinc absorption. The proportion of iron that is available for absorption can be increased by including a source of ascorbic acid at the same meal. It is important to recommend good food sources of iron (enriched cereals and grains, legumes, dates, prunes and raisins, greens) and of zinc (leavened breads, legumes and nuts, spinach) and to emphasize their inclusion in each meal.

Planning and Evaluating Vegetarian Diets

Table 4-13 presents a scheme for planning a nutritionally adequate vegetarian diet. It can also be utilized to evaluate the adequacy of vegetarian dietary practices.[96]

TABLE 4-13   AD-BAC Protein Complement Guide

	D Vegetable	
B Legumes	A Whole Grains and Cereals	C Nuts and Seeds

Four Groups	Limiting Amino Acids*
"A"—Whole Grains and Cereals	Lysine, threonine
Wheat	(sometimes tryptophan)
Rye	
Barley	
Corn	
Millet	
Oats	
Rice	
Buckwheat	
Triticale	
Bulgur	
"B"—Legumes	Methionine, tryptophan
Peanuts	
Peas	
Mung beans	
Broad beans	
Black-eyed peas	
Lentils	
Lima beans	
Soybeans	
Black beans	
Kidney beans	
Garbanzos (chick peas)	
Navy beans	
"C"—Nuts and Seeds	Lysine
Cashews	
Pistachios	
Walnuts	
Brazil nuts	
Almonds	
Pecans	
Pumpkin seeds	
Squash seeds	
Sunflower seeds	
Sesame seeds	
Filberts	
Pine nuts	
"D"—Vegetables	Methionin
Potato	
Dark green vegetables	
Other vegetables	

*Essential amino acid present in disproportionately small amounts.

TABLE 4-14   Modified Food Guide for Vegetarian Diets[98,99]

Food Group	Serving Size	Number of Servings Adult*	Number of Servings Pregnancy or Lactation
Legumes, nuts, and seeds (including nut butters)	2 tbsp or $\frac{1}{2}$ cup cooked	1	4
Milk, milk products fortified soybean milk, or meat analogs	1 cup or 1 item	2+	4
Vegetables (emphasis on dark green)	1 cup raw or $\frac{1}{2}$ cup cooked	3	8
Fruit (rich in Vitamin C)	1 item or $\frac{1}{2}$ cup canned	4	
Whole-grain products and enriched cereals		5	6

*The adult meal plan falls short in calcium and energy requirements for women and in calcium, protein, and energy requirements for men. The use of larger serving sizes helps to bridge this gap.

Whole grains and their products (category "A") should be used in generous amounts in any vegetarian diet. They are sources of protein, iron, and riboflavin in addition to being the complementary protein to legumes (category "B"), nuts and seeds (category "C"), and vegetables (category "D"). In order to yield a balance of amino acids, a meal pattern should include food from the "A" category and a supplementing protein from the "B," "C," or "D" category. Different types of foods whose proteins complement one another should be eaten over the course of the day. Amino acids from exogenous and endogenous sources combine in the body's protein pool; therefore, it is not necessary to have precise complemention at each meal.[94,97]

Table 4-14 is a modification to the basic four food guide that may be useful in planning vegetarian diets, including a diet for pregnancy and for lactation.[98,99]

Physicians: How to Order Diet

The diet order should indicate *vegetarian diet*. The dietitian determines food preferences and establishes a nutritionally adequate diet.

References

94. ADA Reports. Position of the American Dietetic Association: vegetarian diets. J Am Diet Assoc 1993;93(11):1317–1349.
95. Henley EC. FDA proposed labeling rules for protein. J Am Diet Assoc 1992;92(3):293–296.
96. Pemberton CM, Moxness KE, German MJ, Nelson JK, Gastineau CF. Vegetarian diet. In: Pemberton CM, Moxness KE, German MJ, Nelson JK, Gastineau CF, eds. Mayo Clinic diet manual, 6th ed. Toronto: BC Decker, 1988:29–33.
97. Dwyer J. Nutritional consequences of vegetarianism. Annu Rev Nutr 1991;11:61–91.
98. King JC, Cohenour SH, Corruccini CG, Scheneeman P. Evaluation and modification of the basic four food guide. J Nutr Ed 1978;10:27–29.
99. Mutch PB. Food guides for the vegetarian. Am J Clin Nutr 1988;48:913–919.

JEWISH DIETARY PRACTICES

The following discussion of Jewish dietary habits is presented to promote better understanding and to facilitate service to the patient who follows kosher practices. The Mayo Clinic and its associated hospitals do not have a kosher food service. However, commercially prepared frozen kosher dinners (regular and salt-free) are available.

"Kosher" means "fit." The term refers to foods that can be eaten in accordance with Jewish dietary laws, which include specific foods and food combinations that are allowed or prohibited. These laws assign all foods to one of three general categories:

1. Inherently kosher food such as grains, fresh fruits and vegetables
2. Foods that can be processed to be kosher
3. Foods inherently not kosher such as pork, shellfish, and fish without scales and fins

The following are guidelines for a kosher diet:

1. Beef and poultry must be slaughtered by a licensed Jewish slaughterer and processed in a specified manner to be kosher. Proper kosher procedure involves soaking the meat or poultry in water for at least 30 minutes and then salting with kosher salt; an alternative method is to broil the meat until it is well done. Kosher meat may come only from cloven-hoofed animals (such as cows and sheep) that graze and chew their cud. Pork is not allowed. Kosher poultry includes properly slaughtered and prepared chicken, turkey, duck, goose, and Cornish game hen.
2. Only fish with fins and true scales are permitted; shellfish and eels are not allowed.
3. Dairy and meat products may not be eaten at the same meal. After eating meat, there should be an interval of up to 6 hours before dairy products may be consumed again. Dairy foods may be eaten immediately up to a meal that contains meat.
4. In a kosher food service, separate facilities for food preparation and separate serving dishes and utensils are used for meat and for dairy foods. In a nonkosher food service, previously unused disposable dishes and utensils may be used for serving the food; previously unused disposable foil containers may be used for heating foods.
5. Products leavened with yeast are not allowed for 8 days during Passover. During Passover, bread products are unleavened or are leavened with eggs or with steam and are made from specially approved flour.
6. Foods that are "pareve" (neither meat nor dairy) may be eaten in any combination with other foods and in their usual form. Therefore, grains, fresh fruits and vegetables, and soy products may be included in meals that contain either meat or milk products. (Grape juice and any jams or jellies that contain grapes are kosher only if the product has kosher certification.) Nondairy creamers and margarines that are truly milk-free are considered pareve only if the label has kosher certification.
7. Symbols are used on processed foods to certify that the food is kosher. These include the emblem Ⓤ, copyrighted by the Union of Orthodox

Jewish Congregations; the emblem Ⓚ, copyrighted by the Organized Kasrus (O.K.) Laboratories; Ⓥ️Ⓗ, the emblem used by Vaad-Harobonim of Massachusetts; Ⓜ️Ⓚ, the emblem used by Montreal Vaad-Hair; Ⓒ.Ⓞ.Ⓡ, copyrighted emblem of the Council of Orthodox Rabbis of Toronto; and △C.R.C., emblem of the Chicago Rabbinical Council.

8. Some therapeutic food products and some dietary supplements are permissible for those who follow kosher practices. For information on the acceptability of a particular product, ask a rabbi or the Union of Orthodox Jewish Congregations of America, 84 Fifth Avenue, New York, NY.

9. There is a toll-free information line for questions on Jewish dietary practices:
   1 (800) 843-8825 (outside New York)
   1 (914) 667-1007 (inside New York)
           through
   Union for Traditional Judaism
   261 East Lincoln Avenue
   Mount Vernon, NY 10552

10. Nonkosher food products may be used if they are considered to be essential to the treatment of an extremely ill person. A rabbi should be consulted on this or on any similar matter.

5 / *Hospital Diet Progressions*

MODIFICATIONS IN CONSISTENCY AND TEXTURE

GENERAL HOSPITAL DIET

General Description

The general diet utilizes the Food Guide Pyramid,[1] Dietary Guidelines for Americans,[2] the American Diabetes Association and American Dietetic Association Exchange Lists,[3] or other guides for meal planning (Chapter 2) to provide a nutritionally adequate diet. Menus are either selected by or planned for the patient according to food preferences.

Nutritional Inadequacy

The general diet is planned to be consistent with the Recommended Dietary Allowances (RDAs).[4] Nutritional adequacy depends on the patient's selection of food as well as the patient's intake of food. In the hospital setting, the dietitian may evaluate the selection of foods to ensure adequate nutritional intake. The dietitian monitors food selections and nutrient intakes and modifies the diet if the patient is malnourished or at risk for developing malnutrition (see Chapter 3, Nutritional Screening and Assessment).

Indications and Rationale

The general diet is intended for the hospitalized patient whose medical condition does not warrant a therapeutic modification.

There are two general philosophies guiding the composition of a general hospital diet. One focuses on educating the patient in the principles of good nutrition by example, and the other focuses on providing food the patient is willing and is able to eat. Usually, a compromise is reached between these philosophies, with the emphasis adjusted to meet the needs of a particular patient.

The general diet is designed to provide for the control of sodium, cholesterol, and fat intake and to increase fiber and complex carbohydrate in order to foster advantageous health practices. If the patient is able to eat adequately, hospitalization may provide an opportune time to teach these principles to the patient. Either the Dietary Guidelines for Americans[3] or the American Heart Association Dietary Guidelines[5] (Chapter 2) may be used as a guide.

In many instances, hospitalization is not an appropriate time to impose undue dietary restrictions, especially if the modifications keep the patient from consuming enough protein and calories to meet the nutritional needs of convalescence from illness, injury, or surgery. The importance of an adequate and appropriate food intake at these times may warrant compromise in traditional meal planning practices.

Meal Plan

The meal plan in Table 5-1 uses portion sizes that are approximately equal to those of the American Diabetes Association and American Dietetic Association Exchange Lists with additional groupings for desserts and for sweets. It represents the typical or usual content of the general hospital diet on a daily basis.

Approximate Composition

The approximate composition of the general diet will vary depending on specific food choices. The approximate composition appears in Table 5-2.

Physicians: How to Order Diet

The diet order should indicate *general diet.*

TABLE 5-1   General Hospital Meal Plan

Food Category	Quantity
Meat or meat substitute	5–7 oz
Milk or dairy products	2–4 servings
Cereals or starches	6–11 servings
Vegetables	3–5 servings
Fruits	2–4 servings
Fats	4–6 servings
Sweets	0–2 servings
Desserts	0–2 servings

TABLE 5-2   Composition of the General Hospital Diet

Kilocalories (kcal)	Protein (g)	Fat (g)	Carbohydrate (g)
1,600–2,200	60–80	60–80	200–300

References

1. U.S. Department of Agriculture. Food guide pyramid. Stock No. 001-000-04587-3. Washington, DC: U.S. Government Printing Office, 1992.
2. U.S. Department of Agriculture and U.S. Department of Health and Human Services. Nutrition and your health: dietary guidelines for Americans, 3rd ed. Home and Garden Bulletin No. 232. Washington, DC: USDA/USDHHS, Nov 1990.
3. American Diabetes Association and American Dietetic Association. Exchange lists for meal planning. Alexandria, VA/Chicago, IL: ADA/ADA, 1986.
4. Subcommittee on the Tenth Edition of the RDAs. Recommended dietary allowances, 10th ed., Washington, DC, National Academy Press, 1989.
5. American Heart Association. Dietary guidelines for healthy American adults: statement for physicians and health professionals by the Nutrition Committee. Dallas, TX: AHA, 1988.

CLEAR LIQUID DIET

General Description

The clear liquid diet provides foods and fluids that are clear and liquid at room temperature. The type of liquid provided may vary depending upon the clinical condition of the patient, the diagnostic test or procedure, or specific surgery a patient is undergoing.

Nutritional Inadequacy

The diet is inadequate in calories and in essential nutrients. It should seldom be used for more than 1 to 3 days as the sole source of nourishment. If a residue-free liquid diet is required for longer periods of time, a commercially prepared nutritional supplement is advised (see Chapter 16, Enteral Nutritional Support), or intravenous nutritional support may be considered (see Chapter 16, Parenteral Nutritional Support).

Indications and Rationale

The purpose of the diet is to provide an oral source of fluids that are easily absorbed and leave minimal residue in the gastrointestinal tract. The clear liquid diet also minimizes stimulation of the gastrointestinal tract. Certain liquids, particularly carbonated beverages and specific juices, are not tolerated by some surgical patients.

The diet is used as an initial feeding progression between intravenous feeding and a full liquid diet or a solid diet that follows surgery, as a dietary preparation for bowel examination or for surgery, for an acute disturbance of gastrointestinal function, and for a severely debilitated patient as a first step in oral feeding.

Meal Plan

The meal plan in Table 5-3 is used for the clear liquid diet. Types of foods recommended for the clear liquid diet appear in Table 5-4.

Approximate Composition

The approximate composition of the clear liquid diet will vary depending upon the types and amounts of liquids provided and consumed by the patient. The approximate composition appears in Table 5-5.

Physicians: How to Order Diet

The diet order should indicate *clear liquid diet*. The diet order should also indicate if modifications are desired following a particular surgical procedure or if additional supplements are desired. If it is anticipated that the patient will require therapeutic diet modifications, such as diabetic or sodium restrictions, these modifications should be indicated on the diet order.

TABLE 5-3   Clear Liquid Meal Plan

Breakfast	Noon	Evening
Juice	Broth	Broth
Gelatin	Juice	Juice
Coffee or tea	Fruit ice	Gelatin
	Coffee or tea	Coffee or tea

Between-meal feedings: available if desired

TABLE 5-4   Clear Liquid Diet—Recommended Foods

Food Group	Items
Soup	Clear fat-free broth, bouillon
Beverages	Coffee, tea, decaffeinated coffee and tea, cereal beverages, carbonated beverages,* artificially flavored fruit drinks
Fruit	Fruit juice* (except juice with pulp, nectars, tomato, and prune juice)
Dessert	Gelatin, fruit ice, Popsicle™
Sweets	Sugar, hard candy, honey, Polycose™
Miscellaneous	Salt
Supplements	Residue-free, high calorie oral supplements (see Chapter 16, Enteral Nutritional Support)

*Carbonated beverages and certain fruit juices may not be tolerated by some surgical patients.

TABLE 5-5   Composition of the Clear Liquid Diet

Kilocalories (kcal)	Protein (g)	Fat (g)	Carbohydrate (g)	Sodium (mEq)	Potassium (mEq)
600	8	3	130	38	16

FULL LIQUID DIET

General Description

The full liquid diet provides foods and fluids that are liquid or semiliquid at room temperature. The type of food provided may vary depending upon the clinical condition of the patient.

Nutritional Inadequacy

The diet is inadequate in all nutrients except protein, calcium, and ascorbic acid. If the full liquid diet is used for more than 2 to 3 days, liquid nutritional supplements (see Chapter 16, Enteral Nutritional Support) or blenderized foods should be used to improve nutritional adequacy.

Indications and Rationale

The purpose of the diet is to provide an oral source of fluids for individuals who are incapable of chewing, swallowing, or digesting solid food.

The full liquid diet is also used as an intermediate progression to solid foods following surgery, in conjunction with parenteral nutrition, in the presence of chewing or swallowing disorders, in the presence of esophageal or gastrointestinal strictures, during moderate gastrointestinal inflammations, and for acutely ill patients.

Meal Plan

The meal plan in Table 5-6 is used for the full liquid diet. Types of foods recommended for the full liquid diet appear in Table 5-7.

Approximate Composition

The approximate composition of the full liquid diet will vary depending upon the types and amounts of liquids provided and consumed by the patient. The approximate composition appears in Table 5-8.

Physicians: How to Order Diet

The diet order should indicate *full liquid diet*. If it is anticipated that the patient will require therapeutic diet modifications, such as a diabetic or a sodium restriction, these modifications should be indicated on the diet order.

TABLE 5-6   Full Liquid Meal Plan

Breakfast	Noon	Evening
Juice	Juice	Juice
Refined Cooked Cereal	Strained cream soup	Strained cream soup
Milk or Cream	Pudding	Ice cream
Coffee or Tea	Milk	Milk
Sugar or Honey	Coffee or tea	Coffee or tea
	Sugar or honey	Sugar or honey
	Salt, pepper	Salt, pepper

TABLE 5-7   Full Liquid Diet—Recommended Foods

Food Group	Items
Soup	Broth, bouillon, strained or blenderized cream soup‡
Beverages	Coffee, tea, decaffeinated coffee and tea, cereal beverages, carbonated beverages,* artificially flavored fruit drinks
Meat	None
Fat	Butter, margarine, cream
Milk	Milk and milk beverages,‡ yogurt without seeds, nuts, or fruit pieces, cocoa
Starch	Refined cooked cereal
Vegetables	Vegetable juice, vegetable puree in soups
Fruit	Fruit juices*
Dessert†	Gelatin, sherbet, ice cream, custard‡, pudding‡, Popsicle™, fruit ice
Sweets	Sugar, honey, hard candy, Polycose™, flavorings
Miscellaneous	Salt, pepper, mild seasonings as tolerated
Supplements	All liquid meal replacement enteral formulas; see Chapter 16, Enteral Nutritional Support

*Carbonated beverages and juices may not be tolerated by some surgical patients.

†Without seeds, nuts, or fruit pieces.

‡Some patients exhibit a temporary lactose intolerance postoperatively. The diet may be modified by substituting lactose-hydrolyzed milk or lactose-free products.

TABLE 5-8   Composition of the Full Liquid Diet

Kilocalories (kcal)	Protein (g)	Fat (g)	Carbohydrate (g)	Sodium (mEq)	Potassium (mEq)
1,100	40	30	170	66	57

CONSISTENCY MODIFIED DIETS

PUREED DIET

General Description

The pureed diet includes strained, pureed, and liquid foods.

Nutritional Inadequacy

The diet is not inherently lacking in nutrients in comparison with the RDA providing that the patient is able to consume adequate amounts of food. The dietitian monitors the nutrient intake and modifies the diet with supplements or between meal feedings if the intake is insufficient.

TABLE 5-9   Pureed Diet Meal Plan

Breakfast	Noon and Evening
Juice	Cream soup
Refined cooked cereal	Strained meat or poultry
Milk	Mashed potato with gravy
Coffee or tea	Pureed vegetable
Sugar	Pureed fruit
	Dessert
	Milk
	Juice
	Coffee or tea
	Sugar, salt, pepper

TABLE 5-10   Pureed Diet—Recommended Foods

Food Group	Items
Soups	Broth, bouillon, strained or blenderized cream soup
Beverages	All
Meat	Strained or pureed meat or poultry
Cheese	Used in a sauce, soup or blended casserole; blended cottage cheese
Fat	Butter, margarine, cream substitute, cream, oil, gravy, white sauce, whipped topping
Milk	Milk; milk beverages; yogurt without seeds, nuts, or fruit pieces; cocoa
Starch	Refined cooked cereal; mashed potatoes
Vegetables	Strained or pureed; vegetable juice
Fruit	Strained or pureed; fruit juice
Desserts	Gelatin; sherbet; ice cream without seeds, nuts, or fruit pieces; custard; pudding; fruit ice; Popsicle™
Sweets	Sugar, honey, jelly, candy, flavorings
Miscellaneous	Seasonings, condiments

Indications and Rationale

The purpose of the diet is to provide foods that do not require mastication and that are easily swallowed.

The diet is used for patients with inflammation, ulceration, or structural or motor deficits of the oral cavity and the esophagus, or for patients without teeth. The diet may also be used following esophageal or oral surgery or after radiation of the oral or pharyngeal region.

Extreme temperatures are generally not well tolerated. The dietitian evaluates the individual's acceptance and tolerance of the diet and adjusts the consistency of the foods as necessary. If a syringe or straw is required to feed the patient, additional liquid may be needed to thin the foods.

TABLE 5-11 Composition of the Pureed Diet

Kilocalories (kcal)	Protein (g)	Fat (g)	Carbohydrate (g)	Sodium (mEq)	Potassium (mEq)
1,700	60	55	250	100	95

Meal Plan

The meal plan in Table 5-9 is used for the pureed diet. Types of foods recommended for the pureed diet appear in Table 5-10.

Approximate Composition

The approximate composition of the pureed diet will vary depending upon the types and amounts of foods provided and consumed by the patient. The approximate composition appears in Table 5-11.

Physicians: How to Order Diet

The diet order should indicate *pureed diet*. The diet order should also indicate if the patient requires other therapeutic diet modifications such as diabetic or sodium restrictions.

MECHANICAL SOFT DIET

General Description

The mechanical soft diet is a general diet that is modified only in texture for ease of mastication. Initially, it includes ground meat and canned fruits and soft-cooked vegetables. The dietitian modifies the texture to include soft, easy to chew foods in accordance to the patient's tolerance and acceptance.

Nutritional Inadequacy

The diet is not inherently lacking in nutrients in comparison with the RDA providing the patient is able to consume adequate amounts of food. The dietitian monitors the nutrient intake and modifies the diet with nutritional supplements or between meal feedings if the nutrient intake is insufficient.

Indications and Rationale

The purpose of the diet is to provide moist foods that are easy to chew and to swallow.

The mechanical soft diet may be appropriate for: patients with poorly fitting dentures or with no teeth; severely debilitated patients who are unable to chew; patients with dysphagia that is secondary to neurologic, esophageal, oral, or laryngeal disorders or surgeries; patients with strictures of the intestinal tract; patients after laser or radiation treatment to the oral cavity; and patients who are progressing from enteral or parenteral nutrition to solid food.

TABLE 5-12 Mechanical Soft Diet Meal Plan

Breakfast	Noon	Evening
Juice	Soup	Soup
Cooked cereal	Ground meat, poultry, fish	Casserole
Milk	Mashed potato with gravy	Cooked vegetables
Canned fruit	Cooked vegetable	Canned fruit or juice
Coffee or tea	Dessert	Dessert
Sugar	Butter or margarine	Butter or margarine
	Milk	Milk
	Coffee or tea	Coffee or tea
	Sugar, salt, pepper	Sugar, salt, pepper

TABLE 5-13 Mechanical Soft Diet—Recommended Foods

Food Group	Items
Soups	Broth, bouillon, cream or broth-based soup
Beverages	All
Meat	Ground or finely diced, moist meats or poultry; flaked fish; eggs; cottage cheese; cheese; creamy peanut butter; soft casseroles
Fat	Butter, margarine, cream substitute, cream, oil, gravy, salad dressing
Milk	Milk, milk beverages, yogurt without seeds or nuts, cocoa
Starch	Cooked or refined ready-to-eat cereal; potatoes; rice; pasta; white, refined wheat, or light rye bread or rolls; graham crackers as tolerated
Vegetables	Soft, cooked, without hulls or tough skin (e.g., peas and corn); juice
Fruit	Cooked or canned fruit without seeds or skins, banana, fruit juice, citrus fruit without membrane
Desserts	Gelatin, sherbet, ice cream without nuts or fruit, custard, pudding, fruit ice, Popsicle™
Sweets	Sugar, honey, jelly, candy, flavorings
Miscellaneous	Seasonings, condiments

Bread and bread products may not be well tolerated and therefore are not routinely served to patients who have difficulty swallowing until the dietitian evaluates the patient's tolerance.

Meal Plan

The meal plan in Table 5-12 is used for the mechanical soft diet. Types of foods recommended for the mechanical soft diet appear in Table 5-13.

Approximate Composition

The approximate composition of the mechanical soft diet will vary depending upon the types and amounts of foods provided and consumed by the patient. The approximate composition appears in Table 5-14.

TABLE 5-14   Composition of the Mechanical Soft Diet

Kilocalories (kcal)	Protein (g)	Fat (g)	Carbohydrate (g)	Sodium* (mEq)	Potassium (mEq)
1,700	70	60	220	130	90

*Value is for the amount of sodium in usual foods and does not include salt added in preparation.

Physicians: How to Order Diet

The diet order should indicate *mechanical soft diet*. The diet order should also indicate if the patient requires other therapeutic diet modifications such as diabetic or sodium restrictions.

SOFT DIET

General Description

The soft diet provides soft whole food that is lightly seasoned and moderately low in fiber. Small volume meals are offered until the patient's tolerance to solid food is established.

Nutritional Inadequacy

The diet is not inherently lacking in nutrients in comparison with the RDA providing the patient is able to consume adequate amounts of food. Supplements or between meal feedings may be used, if needed, to increase intake. The dietitian monitors food selections and nutrient intakes and modifies the diet if the patient is malnourished or at risk for developing malnutrition (see Chapter 3, Nutritional Screening and Assessment).

Indications and Rationale

The soft diet provides a transition between a liquid and a general diet. The soft diet may be used for debilitated patients who are unable to consume a general diet or for patients with mild gastrointestinal problems.

The soft diet should be individualized according to the clinical diagnosis, surgery, the patient's appetite, food tolerances, previous nutritional status, and chewing and swallowing ability.

Meal Plan

The meal plan in Table 5-15 is used for the soft diet. Types of foods recommended for the soft diet appear in Table 5-16.

Approximate Composition

The approximate composition of the soft diet will vary depending upon the types and amounts of foods provided and consumed by the patient. The approximate composition appears in Table 5-17.

TABLE 5-15   Soft Diet Meal Plan

Breakfast	Noon	Evening
Juice or fruit	Soup	Soup
Cereal	Meat	Casserole
Egg	Mashed potatoes	Cooked vegetable
Toast	Cooked vegetable	Canned fruit
Butter or margarine	Canned fruit or juice	Bread
Milk	Bread	Butter or margarine
Beverage	Butter or margarine	Dessert
Cream and sugar	Dessert	Milk (optional)
Jelly or honey	Milk (optional)	Coffee or tea
	Beverage	Cream and sugar
	Cream and sugar	

TABLE 5-16   Soft Diet—Recommended Foods

Food Group	Items
Soups	Broth, bouillon, cream soup, mildly seasoned soup
Beverages	All
Meat	Moist, tender meat, fish, or poultry; eggs; cottage cheese; mild flavored cheese; creamy peanut butter; soft casseroles
Fat	Butter, margarine, cream substitutes, cream, oil, gravy, crisp bacon, salad dressing
Milk	Milk, milk beverages, yogurt without seeds or nuts, cocoa
Starch	Cooked or ready-to-eat cereal; potatoes; rice; pasta; white, refined wheat, light rye, or graham bread, rolls, or crackers
Vegetables	Soft, cooked, vegetables; lettuce and tomatoes; limit gas-forming vegetables and whole kernel corn
Fruit	Cooked or canned fruit, soft fresh fruit, fruit juice
Desserts	Gelatin, sherbet, ice cream without nuts, custard, pudding, cake, cookies without nuts or coconut, fruit ice, Popsicle™
Sweets	Sugar, honey, jelly, candy without nuts or coconut, flavorings
Miscellaneous	Seasonings, mildly seasoned condiments

TABLE 5-17   Composition of the Soft Diet

Kilocalories (kcal)	Protein (g)	Fat (g)	Carbohydrate (g)	Sodium* (mEq)	Potassium (mEq)
1,800	65	75	225	150	90

*Value is for the amount of sodium in usual foods and does not include salt added in preparation.

Physicians: How to Order Diet

The diet order should indicate *soft diet*. The diet order should also indicate if the patient requires other therapeutic diet modifications such as diabetic or sodium restrictions.

TRANSITIONAL FEEDING PROGRESSION

PREOPERATIVE DIET

A general diet may be ordered the night before surgery. Usually nothing is permitted by mouth after this evening meal.

If it is necessary to limit foods that produce residue in the gastrointestinal tract, a diet that is controlled in residue (see Chapter 9, Fiber and Residue Modification) may be used before the surgery. A clear liquid diet may also be preferred for patients having colon surgery.

POSTOPERATIVE DIET

General Description

Diets that are included in the standard postoperative regimens are clear liquid, full liquid, soft and general diets. The rate of progression depends on the type of surgery and the response of the patient.

Indications and Rationale

Oral intake of food should be resumed as soon as possible, although intravenous glucose and electrolyte solutions may be sufficient to sustain most patients for short periods of time postsurgically without serious depletion of body protein or other stored nutrients. Oral intake of a liquid diet can begin when the gastrointestinal tract is functioning. Commonly, feedings are not begun until peristaltic sounds are heard and there is passage of flatus. In all instances, one should be ready to discontinue feeding or to revert to an earlier stage in the dietary progression if there is abdominal distention, cramping, or other evidence of intolerance.

Alternative methods of feeding, such as peripheral or central parenteral nutrition or enteral nutrition, should be considered for patients who are severely debilitated, malnourished, or for prolonged periods are unwilling or unable to eat adequately. See Chapter 16, Nutritional Support of Adults, and Chapter 29, Nutritional Support in Pediatrics, for a discussion of supplements, enteral feedings, and parenteral nutritional support.

General Postoperative Dietary Progressions

The diet progressions listed in Table 5-18 permit the surgeon to designate how rapidly the feeding is to be resumed after surgery. The dietitian evaluates each patient's acceptance and tolerance of the diet and may adjust the rate of progression.

TABLE 5-18 Diet Progression

Start with a clear liquid diet (first meal) and advance to a general diet by the meal indicated for the rate of progression desired.

Example of rapid progression: Breakfast—clear liquids; Noon meal—full liquid or soft; Evening meal—general diet.

Progression	Meal
Rapid	Third
Regular	Sixth
Slow	Ninth

TONSILLECTOMY AND ADENOIDECTOMY (T & A) DIET PROGRESSION

The diet progression following a tonsillectomy or adenoidectomy is a modification of the full liquid and the mechanical soft diets. Foods that are considered nonirritating following throat surgery are provided. The dietitian will meet with the patient to determine individual tolerances and preferences. In general, citrus fruits and juices, dry items (such as toast), and very hot liquids may not be tolerated. The use of straws is usually prohibited because suction may provoke bleeding.

Standard Progression

The first meal is a T & A full liquid diet. The second and third meals are a mechanical soft diet, and subsequent meals are a general diet as tolerated.

Physicians: How to Order Diet

The diet order may indicate either the rate of progression (rapid, regular, or slow progression) or the specific diet (clear liquid, full liquid, or soft diet) at each stage in the patient's convalescence. Following tonsillectomy or adenoidectomy, the diet order should indicate *T & A diet.*

INTERMAXILLARY FIXATION

General Description

The diet consists of liquids and other foods that are blenderized to a smooth liquid consistency. Generally, 6 to 8 small meals per day are recommended.

Nutritional Inadequacy

The diet is not inherently lacking in nutrients in comparison with the RDA providing the patient is able to consume adequate types and amounts of food. Special consideration may be needed for patients who are not able to consume adequate food to maintain their weight, for patients whose nutritional requirements are increased because of a traumatic accident, or for patients who are in a compromised nutritional state prior to surgery.

Indications or Rationale

Intermaxillary fixation is a surgical procedure used for craniofacial reconstruction. This includes fixation of fractures of the mandible or the maxilla secondary to trauma or to repair of developmental malocclusions. The jaws are wired together with the aid of arch bars or with braces attached to the teeth. The amount of space between the upper and the lower teeth is minimal unless teeth have been removed to correct the malocclusion of the teeth or unless teeth are missing secondary to facial fractures. Fixation of the jaws is variable in duration and may last 4 to 8 weeks.

Dietary Recommendations

To achieve an adequate caloric intake, 6 to 8 small meals are usually recommended. There is a tendency for a person with a wired jaw to decrease food intake dramatically over the duration of jaw wiring because eating causes fatigue, the taste of liquid meals can become boring, and the increased liquid intake causes a "full feeling." Patients should be encouraged to consume an adequate caloric intake to maintain their weight. Weekly weighing is recommended to evaluate the adequacy of the caloric intake.

A food processor or a blender is required to blenderize foods to a completely smooth mixture. The blenderized liquid should be strained with a wire mesh strainer if particles remain after processing. When consumed, the blenderized liquids pass through the space between the teeth. The consistency that is needed is determined by the individual patient's ability to consume liquids.

Suggestions for Blenderizing Foods

1. Meats need to be well cooked and cubed or ground prior to blenderizing. Generally, straining is required to remove chunks.
2. Liquefying foods with sour cream, milk, half and half, cream, juice, broth, cheese sauce, or tomato sauce instead of water is recommended to enhance the flavor and nutritional value of foods. The liquid should be added gradually because too much liquid may change or dilute the flavor of foods.
3. Whole milk should be used rather than a lower fat milk to improve the texture of the liquid and to increase kilocalories when there are no other therapeutic modifications.
4. The salty or sweet flavor in foods is magnified when foods are blended. Other strong seasonings may also be enhanced when foods are blended. Extremely sweet foods may not be tolerated for an extended time period.
5. The temperature of liquid foods should be lukewarm to prevent burning the mouth. Extremely cold foods are often not tolerated.
6. To increase kilocalories and protein, the following techniques may be used: grate cheese into soups, potatoes, casseroles, and vegetables (processed cheese and cheese spread melt more thoroughly); add powdered milk to casseroles, mashed potatoes, soups, cooked cereals, puddings, or milk drinks at a ratio of 2 Tbsp/C; add creamy peanut butter to puddings or milkshakes; add pasteurized eggs to milk drinks, casseroles, and puddings; add extra butter or margarine to foods.

7. Frozen or pasteurized eggs, such as egg substitutes, are recommended to minimize the risk of salmonella poisoning.

8. For ease and quickness in meal preparation, commercial products and supplements may be used. These include canned casseroles, soups, puddings, instant mashed potatoes or cereals, commercial strained baby foods, and meal replacement liquid supplements (see Chapter 16, Enteral Nutritional Support).

9. *Foods should be refrigerated or frozen within the hour after preparation since blenderized foods are an excellent culture medium for the growth of bacteria.* Extra portions can be frozen in meal size amounts or in covered ice cube trays.

10. If a straw is allowed, plastic straws that have a flexible top are easier to use and are wider in diameter. It may be helpful to cut 1 or 2 inches off the base of the straw because shorter straws require less suction.

Dietary Progression

Once the wires have been removed, a soft textured diet is usually required for a limited time until the jaw muscles regain strength. The progression to regular food varies with the individual.

Physicians: How to Order Diet

The diet order should indicate *diet for wired jaw or intermaxillary fixation.*

DYSPHAGIA

General Description

Dietary adjustments are an important part of therapy for dysphagia. Once dysphagia is diagnosed, the patient must be nourished safely while being taught therapeutic and compensatory strategies for dealing with the swallowing disorder. The patient's nutritional status must be maintained despite any limitations on oral intake. Dietary adjustments such as thickened liquids and changes in food consistency may be needed to ensure an adequate diet that is safe for the patient.[6]

Nutritional Inadequacy

The dietary recommendations for dysphagia are not inherently lacking in nutrients in comparison with the RDA. However, many patients may not be able to consume an adequate intake orally. Supplemental enteral nutritional support may be necessary (see Chapter 16, Enteral Nutritional Support).

Indications and Rationale

Dysphagia, a difficulty in swallowing, can occur in any of the three phases of swallowing: oral, pharyngeal, and esophageal.[7] Its cause may be mechanical or paralytic. The mechanical cause is primarily due to surgical resection or to alteration of one or more of the organs of swallowing owing to trauma, obstruction, cancer, or other disease. The paralytic type results from a lesion in the cerebral cortex or from a lesion of the cranial nerves of the brain stem, in particular the medulla

TABLE 5-19   Nerves That Control Swallowing

Cranial Nerve	Name	Function	Outcome Loss
5th	Trigeminal	Controls muscles of mastication; provides sensation to face, teeth, gums, and tongue	Loss of sensation; inability to move mandible
7th	Facial	Provides the sense of taste; controls the muscles of the face	Increased salivation; pouching of food in cheeks
9th	Glossopharyngeal	Transmits sensation to the tongue, pharynx, and soft palate; influences sense of taste, production of saliva, and swallowing	Decreases sensation of taste and salivation; diminishes or inhibits gag reflex
10th	Vagus	Controls sensation in larynx, base of tongue, pharynx, palate, and their muscles	Increased difficulty in swallowing; nasal regurgitation; reduced or lost gag reflex
12th	Hypoglossal	Controls the extrinsic and intrinsic muscles of the tongue	Inability to position food for chewing, resulting in pouching

With permission from: Donahue P. When it's hard to swallow: feeding techniques for dysphagia management. J Gerontol Nurs 1990;16(4)6–9.

oblongata. The most common cause of dysphagia paralytica is a cerebral vascular accident. Head injury, brain tumors, and diseases such as amyotrophic lateral sclerosis that involve the neurological system may also cause dysphagia.[8]

Five cranial nerves function to control swallowing. Dysphagia may be the result of damage to one or more of these nerves. Since each of these nerves has a different role in controlling swallowing, the nature and the severity of dysphagia depend on which nerve or nerves are damaged (Table 5-19).[7]

Swallowing disorders may also be characterized by weak or uncoordinated muscles of the mouth and of the throat, by reduced sensation of the mouth and of the throat, or by deficits of the motor and the sensory nerves that impede chewing and/or swallowing after neurological damage. Symptoms of dysphagia include facial droop, drooling, oral retention, coughing after swallowing, gurgling voice quality, and a feeling of a "lump in the throat."[9] There is also an increased risk of aspiration and of pneumonia.

Goals of Dietary Management

The goals of dysphagia therapy are to maintain safe feeding, maintain or improve nutritional status, and facilitate independence in meeting nutritional needs.

Dietary Recommendations

A multidisciplinary team approach is essential to the successful management of dysphagia. The patient's physician, nurse, dietitian, and swallowing therapist need to coordinate their efforts to provide the most effective care for the patient with dysphagia.[10]

All patients with swallowing disturbances should undergo a nutritional assessment including nutrition history and review of the medical record.[11]

The effects of dysphagia on nutritional status include inadequate dietary intake, weight loss, vitamin and mineral deficiencies, and consequently, protein-calorie malnutrition. Factors that contribute to an inadequate dietary intake include swallowing difficulties, a decrease in the olfactory and the gustatory senses, a decrease in the appetite and saliva production, psychological factors such as the fear of choking, and the effects of therapy, such as surgery and medication.

If the patient is to be fed orally, the dietitian coordinates efforts with the speech pathologist or the occupational therapist to evaluate the swallowing deficits and to provide the appropriate food consistency.

Feeding Guidelines

Only those foods that can be chewed and swallowed safely should be provided. One must avoid overwhelming the patient with too many food items. Foods at room temperature are usually best tolerated as well as those which are mildly spiced or moderately sweet. Sticky foods that adhere to the roof of the mouth should be avoided because they cause fatigue. Small pieces of food should also be avoided because they can become lost in the mouth and can increase the chance of choking.[11]

Liquid consistencies often cause the greatest problem. Thin liquids can flow into the pharyngeal area without a swallow being triggered and fall into an open airway. To avoid this problem, liquids can be thickened with various thickening agents (Table 5-20). Dual textures may be contraindicated such as broth soup with noodles or chunks, jello with fruit, ground meat with broth or juice, canned fruit with juice, and dry cereal with milk. Foods that form a cohesive bolus within the mouth are the best selections. Those that break apart, such as dry chopped meat or plain rice, are not recommended. Moisten foods by adding gravies to facilitate formation of a bolus.

A variety of food items should be served in an appetizing manner with as many characteristics of a normal diet as possible. Typically, patients progress from pureed to ground to soft textured foods and eventually to all textures of foods.

TABLE 5-20 Instant Food Thickeners*

Product	Composition	Kcal/tbsp	Suggested Uses
Thick-It™ (Milani Food, Inc.)	Modified corn starch, maltodextrin	18	Products such as these aid in thickening liquids (hot or cold) and making pureed foods more cohesive for easier swallowing, thereby decreasing risk of aspiration.
Nutra-Thik™ (Menu Magic Foods)	Modified food starch	18	
Thick 'N Easy™ (American Institutional Products, Inc.)	Modified corn starch, maltodextrin	18	

*This list is not all inclusive.

The transition time from one texture to another will vary depending on the patient's oral motor involvement and cognitive ability. Each patient should be evaluated and managed individually.

To reduce the risk of choking and the use of abnormal reflexes, appropriate positioning is imperative. The patient should be upright at a 90 degree angle with hips flexed, feet flat on the floor, and the head slightly forward. The environment should be pleasant and free from distractions.[7]

Physicians: How to Order Diet

The diet order should indicate *diet as tolerated for dysphagia.*

References

6. Donahue P. When it's hard to swallow: feeding techniques for dysphagia management. J Gerontol Nurs 1990;16(4):6–9.
7. Loustau A, Lee KA. Dealing with the dangers of dysphagia. Nursing 1985;15:47–50.
8. Bruckstein AH. Dysphagia. Am Fam Physician 1989;39(1):147–156.
9. O'Gara J. Dietary adjustments and nutritional therapy during treatment for oral-pharyngeal dysphagia. Dysphagia 1990;4:209–212.
10. Mello L, Schindler, C. Diet and dysphagia. Dietitians in Nutrition Support 1988; X(5):8–11.
11. Martens L, Cameron T, Simonsen M. Effects of a multidisciplinary management program on neurologically impaired patients with dysphagia. Dysphagia 1990;5:147–151.

Nutritional Management of Disease and Disorders for Adults

6 / *Food Allergy and Intolerance*

INTRODUCTION

Food allergy, hypersensitivity, and sensitivity to a food is an abnormal immunological reaction in which the body's immune system overreacts to foods that are ordinarily harmless.[1] The part of a food to which a person reacts is usually a protein and is called an allergen. Reaction may occur a few minutes or several hours after the food is eaten. One or several organ systems may be affected: skin (itchy rash or hives, swelling, or eczema), gastrointestinal tract (itching or swelling of lips and tongue, nausea, cramps, abdominal pain, vomiting, or diarrhea), respiratory tract (runny or stuffy nose, sneezing, coughing, tightness in chest, or shortness of breath and wheezing). The most dangerous allergic reaction is systemic anaphylaxis, which may affect any body system and includes abdominal pain, cyanosis, hypotension, chest pain, urticaria, shock, and/or death. Fortunately, severe anaphylaxis to food is infrequent. Other complaints sometimes attributed to food allergy have included migraine headache, tension-fatigue syndrome, muscle aches and pains, and short attention span. However, little evidence exists to link these problems conclusively with food allergy. The number of people who have a true food allergy is unknown. Many adverse reactions to foods prove not to be true allergic or immunological reactions.

On the other hand, a food intolerance is a nonimmune reaction to food or food additives.[1] For many of these reactions, the exact mechanisms are unknown. Examples of food intolerances include milk intolerance caused by lactase deficiency, intolerance to vasoactive amines (e.g., tyramine in cheese, phenylethylamine in chocolate, caffeine in coffee) causing pharmacological reactions, and intolerance to food additives (e.g., tartrazine, monosodium glutamate, and sulfites). The signs and symptoms of proven food intolerance vary and can be mistaken for those of food allergy.

Diagnosis of a food allergy requires identification of the offending food, proof that it causes the adverse response, and verification of immunological involvement

TABLE 6-1   Food Allergy Assessment[2]

Examination	Findings
History	Provides detailed description of symptoms, time from ingestion of food to onset of symptoms, most recent reaction, quantity of food necessary to produce a reaction, and suspected foods.* Includes family history of allergic disease, enzyme deficiencies, and so forth.*
Physical examination	Includes anthropometric evaluation, assessment of growth and development, and nutritional status.* Assesses other chronic disease. Evaluates allergic conditions like allergic rhinitis, eczema, and asthma.
Food and symptom diary for 2 wk	Provides actual record of food, amount and time when eaten, time of appearance of symptoms, and any medication taken.* Allows assessment of dietary adequacy.*
Immunological testing (skin tests, specific antibody assays)	Yields list of suspect foods. Requires confirmation of positive results by trial elimination diet and food challenge to show clinical sensitivity to food.
Trial elimination diet for 2 to 4 wk or until symptoms clear	Needs to be nutritionally sound.* Requires that patient record all ingested food as the suspect food may be ingested in an alternative form.* Begins with a simple elimination diet. Only foods suspected by history, food diary, and/or immunological testing are eliminated.* Progresses to more extensive elimination diet if symptoms do not clear on simple diet. Only one food in each of four food groups or exotic foods never before eaten are allowed.* May require use of hypoallergenic diet (i.e., Vivonex,† Pregestimil,‡ Nutramigen‡) if symptoms do not clear on an extensive elimination diet.*
Food challenge — use will be determined by severity of response to food	Excludes foods known to cause severe reactions such as wheezing, asthma, or anaphylaxis.* Returns suspect foods to diet one at a time after symptoms have cleared for 2 to 4 wk.* 8 to 10 mg ($^{1}/_{2}$ to 1 tsp) is given for the first dose. The amount is increased until it approximates usual intake. Is repeated following positive reactions as coincident reactions are common.* Is performed as double-blind challenge when uncertainty about reaction persists.*

*Points in the diagnostic process where the dietitian's expertise may be particularly valuable.

†Sandoz Nutrition, Minneapolis, MN.

‡Mead Johnson Nutritional Division, Evansville, IN.

Butkus SN, Mahan LK. Food allergies: immunological reactions to food. Copyright The American Dietetic Association. Reprinted by permission from Journal of The American Dietetic Association 1986;86:601–608.

(Table 6-1).[2] Once the allergy is diagnosed and the offending allergen identified, the treatment is to remove this food from the diet. Each individual's sensitivity will determine the degree to which foods must be eliminated.

Diagnosis of a food intolerance is less straightforward. A trial elimination of a suspected food should occur. Once symptoms are resolved, the food may be reintroduced. If the same symptoms reoccur, then an intolerance has been established.

The dietitian should be prepared to suggest which foods to avoid, how to substitute for restricted foods when planning meals, and how to ensure nutritional adequacy. Vitamin and mineral supplementation may be needed, especially when multiple foods are omitted. The organizations and cookbooks appearing at the end of this section may be helpful resources for both the patient and dietitian.

Food allergies are more common in infants and children than in adults. Children with food allergies should be periodically re-evaluated by a physician since they may "outgrow" allergies and no longer need restricted diets (see Chapter 21, Pediatric Allergy). There is also evidence that adults who eliminate an allergen may on occasion have developed a tolerance to it when it is reintroduced at a later time.

The following sections describe various dietary interventions to food allergy and intolerance.

References

1. Anderson JA. The establishment of common language concerning adverse reactions to food and food additives. J Allergy Clin Immunol 1986;78(1):140–144.
2. Butkus SN, Mahan LK. Food allergies: immunologic reactions to food. JADA 1986;86:601–608.

Suggested Further Reading

• American Academy of Allergy and Immunology. Adverse reactions to foods: a parents' guide to problem foods, food additives, diagnosis and treatment. Milwaukee, WI: AAAI, 1988.
• Metcalfe DD, Sampson HA, Simon RA, eds. Food allergy: adverse reaction to foods and food additives. Boston: Blackwell Scientific Publications, 1991.
• Perkin JE. Food allergies and adverse reactions. Gaithersburg, MD: Aspen Publishers, 1990.
• Sampson HA, Metcalfe DD. Food allergies. JAMA 1992;268(20):2840–2844.
• Sampson HA, Koerner CB. Nutrition guide to food allergies. In: Muñoz-Furlong A, ed. Fairfax, VA: The Food Allergy Network, 1992.

Other Resources

Associations and Organizations

American Academy of Allergy and Immunology
611 East Wells Street
Milwaukee, WI 53202
(414) 272-6071

American Dietetic Association
216 West Jackson Blvd.
Suite 800
Chicago, IL 60606-6995
(312) 899-0040

Asthma and Allergy Foundation of America
1717 Massachusetts Avenue
Suite 305
Washington, DC 20036
(202) 265-0265

The Food Allergy Network
4744 Holly Avenue
Fairfax, VA 22030
(703) 691-3179

National Institute of Allergy and Infectious Diseases
Office of Research Reporting and Public Response
9000 Rockville Pike
Bethesda, MD 20205
(301) 496-5714

Books and Cookbooks

- Frasier C. Coping with food allergy. New York: Random House/Time Books, 1985.
- Meisel J. Your food-allergic child: a parents' guide. Lexington, MA: Mills & Sanderson, 1988.
- Beaudette T. Food sensitivity — a resource including recipes. Chicago: American Dietetic Association, 1985.
- Dobler M. Food allergies. Chicago : American Dietetic Association, 1991.

FOOD ALLERGIES

A true food allergy is an abnormal immunological reaction in which the body's immune system overreacts to food that is otherwise harmless. Foods most frequently reported to cause allergic reactions are cows' milk, eggs, peanuts, soybeans, wheat, corn, fish, and shellfish.[3] The predominate allergies in infancy and early childhood are to milk, eggs, peanuts, and soybeans. Milk and egg allergies generally disappear, while peanut and soybean allergies may remain throughout adulthood.[3] Fish allergies are more prevalent in adults because children are not as likely to eat the more allergenic types (crustacea and mollusks).[3]

Allergen cross-reactivity occurs when a person is allergic to two foods of the same biological family, such as peanuts and soybeans (see Chapter 21, Allergy in Children, Table 21-1, Classification of Foods from Food Families, p. 478). Although its existence is debatable among researchers, significant cross-reactivity has been demonstrated for crawfish, lobster, and shrimp.[4] Another factor under study is the effect of heat and processing on food allergens. Although some allergens, such as that in apple, are destroyed by cooking, the most common allergens appear to be unaffected by denaturation caused by heat and acid; therefore these processes do not affect the allergenicity of most foods.[3] However, many patients report allergy symptoms from a food when raw but not when cooked, or vice versa.

There are two key factors to bear in mind when modifying the diet for someone with an allergy. First is that the food allergen may be "hidden" as an ingredient in other foods. This is especially true for packaged or processed foods with multiple ingredients. Secondly, when food is eliminated from the diet, important nutrients may also be eliminated. Tables in the following sections list key words found on ingredient labels that may indicate the presence of an allergen. The sections also indicate the lost nutrients for the eliminated food.[5]

When educating patients and their families, it is important to help them learn to interpret food labels correctly. It is also important to periodically assess the patient's nutrient intake for adequacy. The following sections give suggestions for managing various types of food allergies.

References

3. Taylor SL. Food allergies and related adverse reactions to foods: a food science perspective. In: Perkin JE, ed. Food allergies and adverse reactions. Gaithersburg, MD: Aspen Publishers, 1990:189–206.
4. Perkin JE. Major food allergens and principles of dietary management. In: Perkin JE, ed. Food allergies and adverse reactions. Gaithersburg, MD: Aspen Publishers, 1990:51–68.
5. Sampson HA, Koerner CB. In: Muñoz-Fulong A, ed. Nutrition guide to food allergies. Fairfax, VA: The Food Allergy Network, 1992:20–21.

CORN ALLERGY

A true corn allergy is extremely rare. A corn elimination diet may be very difficult to follow, especially if the patient has sensitivity to corn sugar and corn syrup. These products as well as cornstarch, are used widely in processed foods.[6]

Nutritional Inadequacy

Corn provides a source of chromium, iron, niacin, riboflavin, and thiamin. These nutrients are also available from other grain products. The effect of corn restriction on nutrient intake is primarily due to the restriction of the many foods that contain corn or corn derivatives. An individual following a corn elimination diet should be periodically assessed for nutritional deficiencies.

Goals of Dietary Management

The goal in the dietary management of corn allergy is to restrict corn and corn-containing products (totally or to a level the patient can tolerate) while providing for nutritional adequacy.

Dietary Recommendations

Corn is used as a major ingredient in baked goods, beverages, candy, canned fruits, cereals, cookies, jams, jellies, lunchmeats, snack foods, and syrups. Alternative sweeteners, thickeners, and leavening agents include fruit juice, beet or cane sugar, maple syrup, honey, aspartame, wheat starch, potato starch, rice

---

TABLE 6-2 Terms Indicating the Presence of Corn

Baking powder (contains cornstarch)
Corn (corn flour, corn alcohol, cornstarch, cornmeal)
Corn sweetener or corn syrup solids
Grits
Hominy
Maize

Corn may be present in the following (check with the manufacturer):
    Starch— including food starch, modified food starch, or vegetable starch
    Vegetable gum

starch, tapioca, baking soda, and cream of tartar. Although many convenience foods are eliminated, there may be some that have no corn sweetener or use the other allowed sweeteners. Health food stores typically carry a variety of baked goods and candies that may be acceptable.[7] Other grain products, such as wheat, barley, oats, rye, and rice can be substituted for corn. Like other grain oils, corn oil is not restricted, because the protein is removed in processing. Labels should be checked closely (Table 6-2).

Physicians: How to Order Diet

The diet order should read: *corn allergy.*

References

6. Perkin JE. Major food allergens and dietary management. In: Perkin JE, ed. Food allergies and adverse reactions. Gaithersburg, MD: Aspen Publishers, 1990:51–68, 259–260.
7. Greenberg LE, Moses NS. Egg-free and corn-free diets. In: Chiaramonte LT, Schneider AT, Lifshitz F, eds. Food allergy: a practical approach to diagnosis and management. New York: Marcel Dekker, 1988:441–452.

EGG ALLERGY

Eggs are a commonly used food as well as an ingredient in many prepared foods. Egg white contains the allergens that may cause food sensitivity: ovalbumin, ovotransferrin (conalbumin), and ovomucoid.[8] However, IgE antibodies can also be directed to egg yolk proteins, and cross-reactivity may exist between egg yolk and egg albumin proteins. It is recommended therefore that both yolk and white be avoided by those with egg allergy.[9]

The administration of vaccines cultured in egg to egg-allergic individuals remains in question. The American Academy of Pediatrics and other medical and public health groups should be consulted when dealing with this issue.

Nutritional Inadequacy

Eggs contain the following nutrients: vitamin B_{12}, folate, biotin, pantothenic acid, riboflavin, and the mineral selenium. Elimination of eggs from the diet does not result in a diet inherently lacking in these vitamins, since eggs do not comprise a major part of ones' intake. However, a wide variety of prepared foods do contain egg. An individual's dietary intake should be periodically assessed, and if found deficient, supplementation may be indicated.

Goals of Dietary Management

The goal in the dietary management of egg allergy is to restrict egg (totally or to the level the patient can tolerate) while providing for nutritional adequacy.

Dietary Recommendations

Egg, by itself, is relatively easy to avoid. It should be noted that although common egg substitutes do contain egg (minus the cholesterol), there are "egg-free" egg substitutes available.

TABLE 6-3 Terms Indicating the Presence of Egg

Albumin
Egg–including egg white and egg yolk
Globulin
Livetin
Ovalbumin
Ovoglobulin
Ovomucin
Ovomucoid
Ovovitellin
Simplesse
Vitellin

Egg may be more difficult to avoid when buying prepared foods. Table 6-3 lists terms that when found on labels, indicate the presence of egg.

The following substitutes may be used in recipes calling for one or two eggs:

- Egg-free egg substitute (check label for quantity)
- 1 tsp baking powder + 1 Tbsp water + 1 Tbsp vinegar
- 1 tsp baking soda + 1 Tbsp oil + 1 Tbsp vinegar + 2 Tbsp baking powder
- ½ tsp cream of tartar + ¼ tsp baking soda + 1 Tbsp oil + 1 Tbsp vinegar

Egg may be present in beverages such as root beer (foaming agent), wine, and coffee (as a clarifier). Baked goods may not only contain egg but also be glazed with egg whites. Any processed food should be checked to verify the presence or absence of egg. Simplesse™, a fat substitute (see Appendix 22), contains egg.

Physicians: How to Order Diet

The diet order should indicate: *egg allergy*.

References

8. Chiarmonte LT, Rao YAK. Common food allergens. In: Chiaramonte LT, Schneider AT, Lifshitz F, eds. Food allergy, a practical approach to diagnosis and management. New York: Marcel Dekker, 1988:89–106.

9. Perkin JE. Major food allergens and dietary management. In: Perkin JE, ed. Food allergies and adverse reactions. Gaithersburg, MD: Aspen Publishers, 1990:51–68, 253–256.

FISH OR SHELLFISH ALLERGY

Fish is the most common food that produces allergic reactions among adults.[10] In Scandinavian countries, fish allergy is common in all age groups. Research continues to study the cross-reactivity among various species of bony fish. It is currently recommended that fish-allergic individuals avoid all species of bony fish.

Allergy to various shellfish, crustacea (shrimp, crab, lobster, crawfish), and mollusks (clams, oyster, scallops) are also common in adults.[11] In practice, individuals allergic to one crustacean should avoid other crustaceans because cross-reactivity is commonly demonstrated by skin testing or radioallergosorbent tests (RASTs). No data are available to support or refute this practice.

Nutritional Inadequacy

Fish provides a source of high biological value protein as well as other key nutrients, including niacin, phosphorus, selenium, vitamin B_6, vitamin B_{12}, iron, magnesium, and potassium. These nutrients are also available in a variety of other foods, so elimination of fish generally does not affect the nutritional quality of the diet.

Goals of Dietary Management

The goal in the dietary management of fish allergy is to restrict fish (all or those that cause reactions) while providing for nutritional adequacy.

Dietary Recommendations

Fish is typically not a hidden ingredient in foods and so is relatively easy to avoid. However, fish may be found in Worcestershire sauce (if it contains anchovies), Caesar salad, caviar, and roe. Be cautious in restaurants because shellfish may be present in Asian foods, and French fries or fried foods may be cooked in the same oil used to fry fish. (See also Table 21-1, Pediatric Allergy for a listing of fish, crustaceans and mollusks.)

Physicians: How to Order Diet

The diet order should read: *fish or shellfish allergy.*

References

10. Yunginger JW. Food antigens. In: Metcalfe DD, Sampson HA, Simon RA, eds. Food allergy: adverse reactions to foods and food additives. Boston: Blackwell Scientific Publications, 1991:36–51.
11. Koerner CB, Sampson HA. Diets and nutrition. In: Metcalfe DD, Sampson HA, Simon RA, eds. Food allergy: adverse reactions to foods and food additives. Boston: Blackwell Scientific Publications, 1991:332–354.

MILK ALLERGY

Allergy to milk may be caused by one of the many proteins found in milk. Whey proteins (β-lactoglobulin and β-lactalbumin) and casein are the proteins that play primary roles in allergic reactions.

It is commonly thought that heat treatment of milk reduces its allergenicity, but the allergens in cows' milk are known to be heat stable. The allergenicity of whey can be reduced with high heat (100° to 115°C for at least 30 minutes); however, the nutritional quality is significantly affected. Condensation, evaporation, drying, and pasteurization have no effect on the allergenicity of cows' milk.[12]

The proteins in goats' milk are closely related to cows' milk proteins. Therefore goats' milk may not be tolerated by individuals with a cows' milk allergy.[13]

Completely hydrolyzed casein and elemental diets have negligible antigenicity and allergenicity.[14] These products include Nutramigen™ (Mead-Johnson

Nutritionals), Alimentum™ (Ross Laboratories), Neocate™—an infant elemental diet (Scientific Hospital Supplies), Criticare HN™ (Mead Johnson Nutritionals), and Tolerex™ (Sandoz Nutrition). See Appendix 10 and Appendix 25 for compositions. Infants with milk allergy may also be sensitive to soy; for this reason many high risk or seriously ill infants may progress directly from a milk-based formula to one containing casein hydrolysates. Whey protein hydrolysates, however, have evoked allergic responses, and products containing these proteins should not be consumed by individuals with milk allergies.[15]

Allergic reactions to milk may occur at any age. The reactions are varied and include gastrointestinal problems (diarrhea, vomiting, abdominal pain, bleeding, and malabsorption), respiratory problems (wheezing, coughing, nasal congestion), and skin problems (urticaria, eczema).[16]

Treatment for milk allergy is to restrict this food and products made with it from the diet.

Nutritional Inadequacy

Cows' milk is a major source of Vitamins B_{12}, D, riboflavin, and pantothenic acid, and the minerals calcium and phosphorus. Individuals who must eliminate milk should be encouraged to consume alternative sources of these nutrients (Table 6-4). If dietary intake of these nutrients is routinely deficient, supplementation may be necessary. A calcium supplement is frequently necessary because it is difficult to achieve an adequate calcium intake when milk and milk products are eliminated (see Chapter 8, Osteoporosis).

Goals of Dietary Management

The goal in the dietary management of milk allergy is to restrict milk (totally or to the level the patient can tolerate) while providing for nutritional adequacy.

Dietary Recommendations

Milk itself may be relatively easy to avoid. Substitutes for milk include soy milk and liquid casein-free cream substitutes. Products labeled "non-dairy" frequent-

TABLE 6-4   Nutrients Found in Milk— Alternative Food Sources

Nutrients	Alternative Sources
VITAMINS	
B_{12}	Eggs, fish, meat, poultry
D	Eggs, fish, liver
Pantothenic acid	Cereals (whole-grain), fish, legumes, meat, poultry
Riboflavin	Leafy green vegetables, poultry, meat, fish
MINERALS	
Calcium	Leafy green vegetables, salmon, sardines
Phosphorus	Eggs, fish, poultry, meat, whole grain products

TABLE 6-5   Terms Indicating the Presence of Milk

Butter—including artificial butter flavor
Buttermilk
Casein or caseinate—including calcium caseinate, magnesium caseinate, potassium
                caseinate, rennet casein, sodium caseinate
Cheese
    Cream—including sour cream, sour cream solids, creamer (casein containing)
    Curd
Dry milk solids
Half and half
Lactalbumin
Lactose
Milk—including milk derivative, milk protein, milk solids
Simplesse™
Whey—including delactosed whey, demineralized whey, whey concentrate
Yogurt

Milk may be present in the following ingredients (check with the manufacturer):
    Caramel color
    Caramel flavor
    Natural flavoring

ly contain sodium caseinate, which may cause a reaction in milk-sensitive persons.[17] Milk may be more difficult to avoid when buying prepared foods. Table 6-5 lists terms that if found on food labels indicate the presence of milk or milk protein.

The designation "pareve" refers to kosher foods, which should contain either no meat or no milk or their derivatives. There have been instances, however, of milk contamination of these products with subsequent allergic reactions.[17] Simplesse™, a fat substitute (see Appendix 22), contains milk protein, and milk-sensitive individuals should be cautioned against its use. Many milk-free tofu-based products exist, which may be used in place of milk-containing items.

Physicians: How to Order Diet

The diet order should read: *milk allergy*. The dietitian will plan the diet within the preceding guidelines.

References

12. Anon. Heat treated cows' milk remains allergenic. Nutr Rev 1983;41:96–97.
13. Bahna SL. Milk allergy. In: Chiaramonte LT, Schneider AT, Lifshitz F, eds. Food allergy, a practical approach to diagnosis and management. New York: Marcel Dekker, 1988: 107–116.
14. Gjesing B, Osterballe O, Schwartz B, Wahn U, Lowenstein H. Allergen-specific IgE antibodies against antigenic components in cow milk and milk substitutes. Allergy 1986; 41:51–56.

15. Businco L, Cantani A, Longhi A, Giampeitro PG. Anaphylactic reactions to a cows' milk whey protein hydrolysate (Alpha-Ré, Nestlé) in infants with cows' milk allergy. Ann Allergy 1989;62:333–335.

16. Perkin JE. Major food allergens and principles of dietary management. In: Perkin JE, ed. Food allergies and adverse reactions. Gaithersburg, MD: Aspen Publishers, 1990:51–68.

17. Jones RT, Squillae DL, Yunginger JW. Anaphylaxis in a milk-allergic child after ingestion of milk-contaminated kosher-pareve-labeled "dairy-free" dessert. Ann Allergy 1992; 68:223–227.

PEANUT AND SOY ALLERGY

Peanuts and soybeans are classified as legumes. Other legumes include dried beans (black, kidney, navy, pinto, soy, and string), carob, chickpeas (garbanzo beans), lentils, peas (dried, green, and black-eyed), and licorice. Peanuts and soybeans, the two most common legumes, are also the most allergenic of the legumes. A reaction to one legume does not mean that the entire legume family must be eliminated unless a reaction to other members has occurred. Reactions include urticaria, asthma, anaphylaxis, and gastrointestinal symptoms.[18,19]

Nutritional Inadequacy

Peanuts are a source of chromium, magnesium, manganese, niacin, and vitamin E. They also provide some biotin, copper, folate, phosphorus, potassium, and vitamin B_6. Since many foods also provide these vitamins, it is not likely that elimination of peanut and peanut products will result in a diet that is nutrient deficient.

Soybeans provide calcium, folate, iron, magnesium, phosphorus, riboflavin, thiamin, vitamin B_6, and zinc. Because of the increased use of soy in so many products, elimination of these foods may result in a nutritionally inadequate diet. An individual's intake should be periodically assessed, and if found deficient, supplementation may be indicated.

Goals of Dietary Management

The goal in the dietary management of peanut-soy allergy is to restrict peanut-soy (totally or to the level the patient can tolerate) while providing for nutritional adequacy.

Dietary Recommendations

Peanuts themselves are relatively easy to avoid. People with a peanut allergy may be able to tolerate nuts grown on trees. These are not legumes and include pecans, walnuts, and almonds. Tree nuts may be substituted in baked goods or as nut-butter spreads. (Note: Although a person who is allergic to legumes may tolerate tree nuts, other individuals may have allergic reactions to these foods.) Most refined peanut oil is not allergenic, because the protein is removed during processing. However, cold-pressed peanut oil may contain peanut protein and cause a reaction. Peanuts or peanut oil may be used as flavor enhancers in Asian foods. Table 6-6 lists terms that when found on labels indicate the presence of peanuts.

Soybeans and other soy products are more readily used in processed foods, and thus their avoidance is more difficult. Eating out will be a problem for individuals

TABLE 6-6 Terms Indicating the Presence of Peanut and Soy

PEANUT

Peanut—including peanut butter, peanut flour, mixed nuts (check label)
Peanut oil—cold-pressed

SOY

Bean curd
Lecithin
Miso
Soy—including soy albumin, soy flour, soy milk, soy nuts, soy oil (cold-pressed), soy
    protein, soy protein isolate, soy sauce
Tempeh
Textured vegetable protein
Tofu

Soy may be present in the following (check with the manufacturer):
    Vegetable broth
    Vegetable gum
    Vegetable starch

with soy allergy. Fast foods may contain soy extenders or soy expanders. Asian food may contain soy sauce or tofu (soybean curd). Individuals will need to check labels of prepared foods carefully for ingredients containing soy (Table 6-6). The ingredient "hydrolyzed vegetable protein" in processed foods usually indicates the presence of soy. The Nutrition and Labeling Education Act of 1993 requires that the source of hydrolyzed protein (e.g., hydrolyzed soy protein) be specified in the ingredient listing of processed foods.[20]

Physicians: How to Order Diet

The diet order should read: *peanut and/or soy allergy.*

References

18. Perkin JE. Major food allergens and dietary management. In: Perkin JE, ed. Food allergies and adverse reactions. Gaithersburg, MD: Aspen Publishers, 1990:51–68.
19. Yunginger JW. Food antigens. In: Metcalfe DD, Sampson HA, Simon RA, eds. Food allergy: adverse reactions to foods and food additives. Boston: Blackwell Scientific Publications, 1991:36–51.
20. Food and Drug Administration. Food labeling: declaration of ingredients. Federal Register, U.S. Government Printing Office, Washington DC 1993;58(3):2850–2887.

WHEAT ALLERGY

The four main fractions of wheat—gliadin, globulin, glutenin, and albumin—are considered to be allergenic.[21] Gliadin, the alcohol-soluble component of gluten, is also responsible for celiac sprue or gluten-sensitive enteropathy (see Chapter 9,

---

TABLE 6-7   Terms Indicating the Presence of Wheat

Farina
Gluten—including high gluten flour, vital gluten, wheat gluten
Graham flour
High protein flour
Wheat—including wheat bran, wheat germ, wheat gluten, wheat starch, whole wheat
        flour
Malt
Cereal extracts

Wheat may be present in the following (check with the manufacturer):
    Starch—including gelatinized starch, modified food starch, modified starch, veg-
            etable starch
    Vegetable gum

Gluten Sensitivity, and Chapter 24, Pediatric Gluten Sensitivity). However, in the case of wheat allergy, the proteins found in wheat are stimulating an allergic response from the immune system. In the case of wheat allergy, wheat in all forms should be avoided. In sprue and celiac disease, gluten from wheat, rye, barley, and oats must be avoided.

Nutritional Inadequacy

Wheat is a source of the vitamins thiamin, niacin, riboflavin, and folate and the minerals magnesium, molybdenum, potassium, iron, and selenium. Wheat is a common food in the Western diet. Therefore a wheat-free diet may severely limit the variety of foods available for consumption. An individual's dietary intake should be periodically assessed, and if found deficient, supplementation may be indicated.

Goals of Dietary Management

The goal in the dietary management of wheat allergy is to restrict wheat and wheat-containing products (totally or to a level the patient can tolerate) while providing for nutritional adequacy.

Dietary Recommendations

Wheat is a major ingredient in most baked products, crackers, cereals, and pastas. Because many of these foods are included at every meal, every day, a wheat-free diet is difficult to maintain. The substitution of other grains, such as barley, corn, oats, rye, and rice, should be encouraged in order to add variety and to provide a similar source of nutrients.[22] The patient should be warned, however, that foods made from these grains may have had wheat or wheat gluten added to them in order to provide structure. Labels should be closely checked (Table 6-7). Other nongrain flour alternatives include buckwheat (a member of the rhubarb family), nut, seed or bean flours, potato flour, soy flour, and amaranth flour. Quinoa is similar to rice and makes an acceptable substitute for wheat noodles in casseroles

TABLE 6-8   Substitutes for Wheat Flour

Substitute	Amount in Place of 1 Cup Wheat Flour	Characteristics
Oat flour	1⅛ cup	Sticky
Rice flour	⅞ cup	Grain
Rye	⅓ cup	Dark color, distinctive flavor
Corn flour (cornmeal	1 cup (¾ cup)	Heavy, crumbly
Barley	½ cup	Mild flavor
Buckwheat	⅞ cup	Mild, mellow flavor, does not thicken well
Potato flour	⅝ cup	Heavy, dense

The following can be used as thickeners in place of wheat flours: cornstarch, potato starch, arrowroot, tapioca (quick cooking), rice flour, and gelatin. (Approximately half the amount, in comparison to wheat flour, is needed.)

and cold salads. Table 6-8 presents a description of these flour substitutes as well as equivalents for 1 cup of wheat flour.

Another source of wheat-free food is special gluten-free products (wheat-, oat-, rye-, and barley-free foods). See Chapter 9, Gluten Sensitivity, for further information on these products.

Foods containing malt and certain alcoholic beverages contain wheat and should be avoided.[22] These include beer, gin, and selected whiskeys.

Physicians: How to Order Diet

The diet order should indicate: *wheat allergy*.

References

21. Yunginger JW. Food antigens. In: Metcalfe DD, Sampson HA, Simon RA, eds. Food allergy: adverse reactions to foods and food additives. Boston: Blackwell Scientific Publications, 1991:36–51.
22. Perkin JE. Major food allergens and dietary management. In: Perkin JE, ed. Food allergies and adverse reactions. Gaithersburg, MD: Aspen Publishers, 1990:51–68, 257–258.

FOOD INTOLERANCE

Food intolerances are symptoms that result from the ingestion of specific foods but do not involve immunological mechanisms. An example would be a milk (lactose) intolerance caused by lactase deficiency (see Chapter 9, Lactose Intolerance). Less common food intolerances may be caused by various additives, which include sulfites, tartrazine, butylated hydroxyanisole (BHA), butylated hydroxytoluene (BHT), and monosodium glutamate (MSG). Other substances in food, such as nickel, aspartame, penicillin, or mold, may also elicit nonimmunological reactions.

In 1938, the Food, Drug and Cosmetic Act (FD&C) gave the Food and Drug Administration (FDA) authority over food and food ingredients. The Food Additive Amendment of 1958 requires FDA approval before an additive can be included in any food.[23] Today thousands of agents are added to the foods we consume. These include preservatives, stabilizers, conditioners, thickeners, colorings, flavorings, sweeteners, and antioxidants. Only a small number have been associated with hypersensitivity reactions.[24] Of these, dyes and preservatives have been found to cause urticaria (hives) or other reactions in people who are sensitive to them. Reactions to some additives have been proven, while others have not. A trial of a diet free of dyes and preservatives is sometimes worthwhile for people with chronic urticaria. The following guidelines may be helpful in selecting foods that do not contain dyes, preservatives, or other additives:

- *Purchase fresh, unprocessed foods.* Many foods that have been canned, frozen, mixed, boxed, and are ready-to-serve may have dyes and preservatives added. Whenever possible, buy fresh, unprocessed foods.
- *Check labels.* Labels may list the presence of additives by name. Patients should be taught to read labels and to identify the presence of the specific additive to which they are intolerant. Only those found to produce reactions should be avoided.

As with a food allergy, if a diet becomes too restricted because of many suspected food intolerances, that diet may become unbalanced and unhealthy. Tolerance to these foods will be unique to each individual and should be checked one food at a time.

The following sections describe various dietary interventions for food intolerances.

References

23. Simon RA. A timely update on adverse reactions to food additives. Advance Plus. Members Bulletin of the Asthma and Allergy Foundation of America, 1717 Massachusetts Ave NW, Suite 305, Washington, DC 20036, Mar/Apr 1991.
24. Adams EJ. Nutritional care in food allergy and food intolerance. In: Mahan LK, Arlin M, eds. Krause's food nutrition and diet therapy. Philadelphia: WB Saunders, 1992:653–670.

Other Readings

•. Metcalfe DD, Sampson HA, Simon RA, eds. Food allergy: adverse reactions to foods and food additives. Oxford: Blackwell Scientific Publications, 1991.
•. Perkin JE, ed. Food allergies and adverse reactions. Gaithersburg, MD: Aspen Publishers, 1990.

ASPARTAME

Aspartame is a nutritive artificial sweetener. It contains about 4 cal/g and is 180 to 200 times sweeter than sucrose.[25] Since the beginning of its use, the safety of aspartame has been controversial. The most commonly reported adverse reaction is headache.[26] Aspartame has also been reported to increase susceptibility to seizures[27] and to increase appetite.[28] Reported allergylike symptoms following the ingestion of aspartame include rash[25] and leg nodules.[29] Individuals with phenylketonuria should avoid aspartame because it is a significant source of phenylalanine (see Chapter 23, Phenylketonuria).

The World Health Organization (WHO) and the FDA have set a maximum level of acceptable intake at 40 to 50 mg/kg of body weight.[27,30] One can of soft drink contains approximately 200 mg of aspartame. Using the guidelines and assuming no other aspartame source is consumed, a 50 kg (110 lb) adult could drink 12.5 cans before reaching the maximum level. In a position paper on sweeteners, the American Diabetes Association cites statistics that indicate most adults consume less than 3.5 mg of aspartame per kilogram of body weight.[31] According to the American Dietetic Association, if aspartame replaced dietary sucrose, aspartame intake would range from 3 to 11 mg/kg/day.[32] There is little solid evidence that aspartame poses a significant health problem. However, it may be advisable for an aspartame-sensitive person to restrict or completely avoid aspartame, depending on the level of sensitivity. Patients should be advised to read labels in order to identify foods containing aspartame. The terms Nutrasweet™ and Equal™ indicate that aspartame is present.

Physicians: How to Order Diet

Diet order should read: *aspartame restricted diet.*

References

25. American Medical Association Council on Scientific Affairs. Aspartame—review of safety issue. JAMA 1985;254(3):400–402.
26. Bradstock MK, Serdula MK, Marks JS. Evaluation of reactions to food additives: the aspartame experience. Am J Clin Nutr 1986;43:464–469.
27. Maher TJ. Natural food constituents and food additives: the pharmacologic connection. J Allergy Clin Immunol 1987;79(3):413–422.
28. Blundell JE, Hill AJ. Paradoxical effects of an intense sweetener (aspartame) on appetite (letter). Lancet 1986;1:1092–1093.
29. Novick NL. Aspartame-induced granulomatous panniculitis. Ann Intern Med 1985;102(2):206–207.
30. Alfin-Slater RB, Xavier Pi-Sunyer F. Sugar and sugar substitutes—comparisons and indications. Postgrad Med 1987;82(2):45–56.
31. American Diabetes Association. Position statement: use of noncaloric sweeteners. Diabetes Care 1987;10(4):526.
32. American Dietetic Association. Appropriate use of nutritive and non-nutritive sweeteners. JADA 1987;87(12):1689–1690.

BENZOATES AND PARABENS

Benzoic acid and sodium benzoate are used as preservatives and antimicrobial agents in foods and pharmaceuticals. Sodium benzoate is also currently used to treat infants with inborn errors of the urea cycle (reduces hyperammonemia) and manage seizures in infants with nonketotic hyperglycinemia. Benzoates have been approved by the FDA, appearing on the "generally recognized as safe" (GRAS) list. With this status, it has become a very common additive to a wide variety of foods and beverages. Current data indicate that adverse reactions to benzoates are extremely rare.[33]

The sodium salt of benzoic acid, sodium benzoate, is the most common antimicrobial additive to foods. Either name may appear on the ingredient label.

Benzoic acid is naturally present in cranberries, prunes, plums, cinnamon, anise, and tea. As a preservative, it may be found in a variety of prepared foods and beverages, including carbonated and noncarbonated beverages, syrups, fruit salads, icings, jams, jellies, preserves, salted margarines, mincemeat, pickles and relishes, sauerkraut, pie and pastry fillings, and cider.[34]

Parabens are also used as preservatives and antimicrobial agents in foods. The later stages of paraben metabolism mimic the metabolism of benzoates. Therefore patients who react to benzoates may also be sensitive to parabens.[33] Parabens do not occur naturally in foods. Terms on food labels indicating the presence of parabens include methyl p-hydroxybenzoate or propyl p-hydroxybenzoate.

Parabens are found in foods such as processed vegetables, baked goods, fats and oils, and seasonings.[34] Parabens may be used to improve the keeping quality of cakes, pie crusts, pastries, icings, toppings, and fillings (fruit jellies and creams). They are used in ciders, carbonated beverages, and beer. Other foods that may contain parabens include fruit products (sauces, juices, salads, syrups, fillings, preserves, and jellies), sucrose syrup, olives, and pickles.[34]

Physicians: How to Order Diet

The diet order should indicate: *benzoate and paraben restricted diet.*

References

33. Jacobsen DW. Adverse reactions to benzoates and parabens. In: Metcalfe DD, Sampson HA, Simon RA, eds. Food allergy: adverse reactions to foods and food additives. Oxford: Blackwell Scientific Publications, 1991:276–287.
34. Chichester DF, Tanner FW. Antimicrobial food additives. In: Furia TE, ed. Handbook of food additives. Cleveland, OH: CRC Press, 1972:115–184.

BUTYLATED HYDROXYANISOLE (BHA) AND BUTYLATED HYDROXYTOLUENE (BHT)

BHA and BHT are antioxidants used to inhibit fat oxidation. They are usually used in combination with other antioxidants. Double-blind, placebo-controlled studies have linked these additives in small quantities with chronic urticaria.[35] The occasional patient who is sensitive to these additives should be advised to read labels and look for these ingredients.

BHA and BHT are the most effective antioxidants used in vegetable oils and shortenings for deep-fat frying. Therefore they may also be present in high fat foods such as potato chips, nutmeats, doughnuts, pastries, and pie crusts. Smaller quantities of BHA and BHT are used for their stabilizing effects in foods containing only 1 to 2% fat, such as dehydrated potatoes, dried fruits, breakfast cereals, and cake mixes. Other products that may contain BHA or BHT include terpene-like flavoring oils (orange, lemon), chewing gum, candy, and yeast.[36]

Physicians: How to Order Diet

The diet order should indicate: *BHA and BHT restricted diet.*

References

35. Bosso JV, Simon RA. Urticaria, angioedema, and anaphylaxis provoked by food additives. In: Metcalfe DD, Sampson HA, Simon RA, eds. Food allergy: adverse reactions to foods and food additives. Oxford: Blackwell Scientific Publications, 1991:288–300.

36. Stuckey BN. Antioxidants as food stabilizers. In: Furia TE, ed. Handbook of food additives. Cleveland, OH: CRC Press, 1972:185–224.

MOLD

General Description

The diet is intended to eliminate molds (Table 6-9). Food sources of molds may be categorized as (1) mold foods (such as mushrooms) and (2) mold-containing foods, which include foods to which molds are added to develop a particular flavor (such as cheese, sour cream, buttermilk, bacon, sausage, and ham). Mold may grow on any food. Therefore, foods should not be stored for extended periods of time.[37,38]

Nutritional Inadequacy

Since food sources of mold are limited, a mold-free diet is not inherently lacking in nutrients when compared to the recommended dietary allowances (RDA). Vitamin or mineral supplementation may be indicated for patients with significant food restrictions due to intolerance.

TABLE 6-9   Guidelines for Avoiding Dietary Mold[37]

1. Eat canned foods immediately.
2. Eat fresh fruits soon after preparation.
3. Do not eat leftover foods.
4. Do not consume meats or fish that have been stored for over 24 hours.
5. Exclude the following foods:
   - Beer
   - Breads, soured or made with large quantities of yeast
   - Buttermilk
   - Cider
   - Cheeses (all types)
   - Dried fruit
   - Mushrooms
   - Sauerkraut
   - Sour cream
   - Soured milk
   - Vinegar and foods that contain vinegar
   - Wine and other alcoholic beverages

With permission from: Perkin JE. Adverse reactions to food additives and other food constituents. In: Perkin JE (ed). Food allergies and adverse reactions. Gaithersberg, MD: Aspen Publishers, Inc., 1990:146.

Indications and Rationale

Although sensitivity to molds in the air and the environment has been recognized, some believe that adverse reaction to ingested molds can also occur.[39] Because this is controversial, dietary mold avoidance is not consistently included in the treatment for adverse reactions to mold.

When inhaled, molds may cause allergic rhinitis (sneezing, runny nose, congestion, and itchy eyes and nose). This can result in increased secretions and may lead to wheezing and difficulty breathing.

Dietary Recommendations

Table 6-9 lists dietary sources of mold, which should be avoided by mold-sensitive individuals.[37]

References

37. Perkin JE. Adverse reactions to food additives and other food constituents. In: Perkin JE, ed. Food allergies and adverse reactions. Gaithersburg, MD: Aspen Publishers, 1990: 145–146.
38. Solomon WR. Common pollen and fungus allergens. In: Bierman CW, Pearlman DS, eds. Allergic diseases from infancy to adulthood. Philadelphia: WB Saunders, 1988:146.
39. Rockwell WJ. Reactions to molds in foods. In: Chiaramonte LT, Schneider AT, Lifshitz F, eds. Food allergy, a practical approach to diagnosis and management. New York: Marcel Decker, 1988:153–168.

MONOSODIUM GLUTAMATE

MSG is a widely used food additive that is valued for its flavor-enhancing properties. Symptoms reported with MSG ingestion include headache, tightness in the chest, stiffness and/or generalized weakness of the limbs, light-headedness, facial flushing, profuse sweating, heartburn, gastric discomfort, and a burning sensation at the back of the neck. These symptoms have been reported after eating Chinese food and have been called the "Chinese restaurant syndrome."[40] In addition, severe exacerbation of asthma following the ingestion of MSG-containing food has been reported.[41,42]

MSG is a sodium salt of glutamic acid, one of the most abundant amino acids found in protein. Glutamic acid (glutamate) is the alleged harmful component of MSG. Besides MSG, glutamic acid can be present in other salts such as calcium glutamate or potassium glutamate. Glutamate is also present naturally in foods such as meat, cheese, peas, mushrooms, and milk. However, the amount of naturally occurring glutamate is unlikely to provoke asthma.[42]

MSG is used as a flavor enhancer in Chinese, Japanese, and other Asian foods. It is also added to many canned, packaged, and prepared foods and is often an ingredient in commercial spice mixtures and bouillon cubes. It is the widespread use of MSG that is of concern when addressing MSG sensitivity.

Research has shown, however, that this intolerance may not be as common as previously thought. Surveys have estimated that 1 to 2% of Americans are at risk for MSG intolerance, and that estimate may be high.[42] In addition, symptoms are usually subjective and transitory, with no documented long-term effects. As a precautionary measure, those who have questionable MSG intolerance or sensitivity should be advised to read the ingredient labels of processed foods to determine the presence of glutamate.

MSG is on the GRAS list of food additives approved by the FDA. Therefore, the FDA places no regulatory restrictions on the use of MSG. In 1994, food labels will be required to indicate the presence of MSG. The phrase "contains glutamate" will appear on labels of foods containing MSG or hydrolyzed protein, which also contains glutamate.[43]

Physicians: How to Order Diet

Diet should read: *MSG restricted diet.*

References

40. Dulce C, Vial T, Verdier F, Testud F, Nicolas B, Descotes J. The Chinese restaurant syndrome: a reappraisal of monosodium glutamates causative role. Adverse Drug React Toxicol Rev 1992;11(1):19–39.
41. Perkin JE. Adverse reactions to food additives and other food constituents. In: Perkin JE, ed. Food allergies and adverse reactions. Gaithersburg, MD: Aspen Publishers, 1990:129–170.
42 Allen DH. Monosodium glutamate. In: Metcalfe DD, Sampson HA, Simon RA, eds. Food allergy: adverse reactions to foods and food additives. Oxford: Blackwell Scientific Publications, 1991:261–266.
43. Food and Drug Administration. Food labeling: declaration of ingredients. Federal Register, U.S. Government Printing Office, Washington, DC; 1993;58(3):2850–2887.

NICKEL RESTRICTED DIET

General Description

Contact with nickel or nickel salts may cause dermatitis in sensitive individuals. This has been observed in miners exposed to nickel-containing ore and persons working in nickel refineries.[44] However, even contact with common objects like coins, clothing fasteners, or stainless steel cookware can induce dermatitis. It has been suggested that limiting the amount of ingested nickel may also help reduce the frequency and duration of eczema as well as gradually diminish its intensity.[45]

A low nickel diet is usually prescribed for patients who experience a flare-up of their dermatitis following the ingestion of a 2.5 mg nickel challenge and are without symptoms following ingestion of a placebo.[45]

Although the nickel content of beer and wine is low, they contain vasoactive substances. Therefore, these substances should also be avoided. Other vasoactive foods include mackerel, herring, tuna, citrus fruits and juices, raw tomatoes, onions, and carrots.[45]

The first quart of water taken from the tap should not be consumed or used in food preparation. Avoid using nickel-plated or stainless steel utensils.[45] Acidic foods should not be cooked in stainless steel.

It is generally recommended that a nickel restricted diet be followed for 1 to 2 months. If good results occur, the patient may begin to try small amounts of foods containing nickel to see if tolerance may be reestablished.

Table 6-10 presents dietary guidelines for restricting nickel.

TABLE 6-10 Nickel Restricted Diet

	Avoid	Allowed
Meat	Shellfish (shrimp and mussels)	All other fish, meat, poultry, eggs
Dairy products	None	Butter, cheese, milk, yogurt, margarine
Vegetables	Beans (green, brown, white), sprouts, kale, leeks, lettuce, peas, spinach	Asparagus, beets, broccoli, brussels sprouts, cabbage, cauliflower, corn, cucumber, dill, eggplant, mushrooms, parsley, peppers, potatoes
Fruit	Figs, pineapple, prunes, raspberries	Peaches, pears, raisins, rhubarb, all other berries
Grains	Buckwheat, millet, oatmeal, wheat bran products, multigrain bread	Rice cereals, cornflakes, macaroni, popcorn, white rice, spaghetti, wheat flour, whole-grain rye and wheat bread in moderation
Drinks	Chocolate and cocoa drinks, tea from dispensers	Coffee and tea (in moderation), soft drinks, alcoholic beverages
Miscellaneous	Almonds, hazel nuts, peanuts, baking powder, lentils, linseed, sunflower seeds, soy powder, sweets containing chocolate, marzipan, nuts, licorice, vitamin/mineral supplements containing nickel	Yeast

Physicians: How to Order Diet

Diet order should read: *nickel restricted diet.*

References

44. Root EJ. Current perspectives on nickel. Nutr Today 1990;May/June:12–15.
45. Vein NK, Menné T. Nickel contact allergy and a nickel restricted diet. Semin Dermatol 1990;9(3):197–200.

Other Reading

Pennington JA, Jones JW. Molybdenum, nickel, cobalt, vanadium, and strontium in total diet. JADA 1987;87(12):1644–1650.

NITRATES AND NITRITES

Nitrates and nitrites are commonly used as preservatives and are known for their flavoring and coloring attributes. They have been shown to provoke vascular headaches in some people. Their consumption has also been associated with increased incidence of certain cancers (see Chapter 2, Diet and Cancer Risk).

Nitrates and nitrites are found in cured or processed meats such as frankfurters and salami.[46] Nitrates or nitrites will be listed on the ingredient label as sodium nitrate, potassium nitrate, sodium nitrite, or potassium nitrite.[47]

Physicians: How to Order Diet

The diet order should indicate: *nitrate and nitrite restricted diet.*

References

46. Bosso JV, Simon RA. Urticaria, angioedema, and anaphylaxis provoked by food additives. In: Metcalfe DD, Sampson HA, Simon RA, eds. Food allergy: adverse reactions to foods and food additives. Oxford: Blackwell Scientific Publications, 1991:288–300.
47. Chichester DF, Tanner FW. Antimicrobial food additives. In: Furia TE, ed. Handbook of food additives. Cleveland, OH: CRC Press, 1972:115–184.

PENICILLIN

General Description

The diet is intended to eliminate penicillin. Milk and all dairy products are to be avoided since they may contain penicillin as a contaminant.[48]

Nutritional Inadequacy

The diet is low in calcium as compared to the RDA. If the diet is to be followed for an extended period, a calcium supplement should be prescribed.

Indications and Rationale

The diet may be useful in the treatment of some types of chronic urticaria or other forms of allergic response attributable to penicillin hypersensitivity. Other than anecdotal case reports, there is little evidence that major dietary manipulations have specific benefit for patients who are allergic to penicillin and have other disorders such as urticaria or asthma.

The contamination of milk occurs when animals with bovine mastitis are treated with penicillin. Although the sale of milk from these animals is legally prohibited for a certain period, due to poor screening tools and regulations small amounts of penicillin may nevertheless be present in milk. Milk processing is not likely to destroy all the penicillin, and it is possible that the degradation products are as sensitizing as penicillin itself, if not more so. Therefore, no dairy products may be used in any form.

There have been instances in which people have had reactions to penicillin found in red meat, poultry, offal (organ meats), and soft drinks.[48-50] Good quality-assurance programs and the fact that beef, pork, and poultry are one-time point-of-sale products reduce the potential for penicillin and other drug residues.[51,52] There is also evidence that penicillin contaminated meat is less likely to provoke an allergic reaction.[53]

An acceptable level of penicillin in the diet has not been determined. The diet is intended to be as free of penicillin and molds as possible.

Food Labeling

The patient should be advised to read product labels carefully and to avoid dairy products (i.e., milk and milk products, cheese and cheese products, cream and cream products, milk solids, casein, lactalbumin, curds, and whey).

Medications

Antibiotics that are related to penicillin may have the same effect as penicillin itself. Caution should be exercised in the prescription and administration of medications.

The diet should not be followed for a prolonged period without adequate medical supervision and evaluation of symptomatic response.

Physicians: How to Order Diet

The diet order should indicate: *penicillin restricted diet.*

References

48. Ormerod AD, Reid MS, Main RA. Penicillin in milk—its importance in urticaria. Clin Allergy 1987;17:229–234.
49. Schwartz HJ, Sher TH. Anaphylaxis to penicillin in a frozen dinner. Ann Allergy 1984; 52:342–343.
50. Teh WL, Rigg AS. Possible penicillin allergy after eating chicken. Lancet 1992;339:620.
51. Gloyd JS. Residue screening tests: a solution in search of a need? J Am Vet Med Assoc 1989;195:1686.
52. Fuhrmann T. Overview of residue concerns of the dairy industry. J Am Vet Med Assoc 1991;198:836–838.
53. Lindemayr H, Knobler R, Kraft D, Baumgartner W. Challenge of penicillin-allergic volunteers with penicillin-contaminated meat. Allergy 1981;36:471–478.

SULFITES

Sulfites and sulfiting agents are additives used to prevent browning, modify dough texture, control microbial growth, and bleach certain foods.[54] In 1986 the FDA banned the use of sulfites from sources of fresh fruits and vegetables (other than potatoes). The FDA has also attempted to ban sulfite use on potato products served or sold unpackaged or unlabeled. However, this has not yet gone into effect. If food or alcoholic beverages contain sulfites in greater than 10 parts per million, it must be listed on the label according to rulings by the FDA and the Bureau of Alcohol, Tobacco and Firearms.[55,56]

Table 6-11 lists foods that contain sulfites.

According to some studies, asthmatics who require steroid-type medications may experience a reaction after ingesting sulfites.[54] The most common reaction is bronchospasm. Other reported symptoms (not proven) include flushing, hives, gastrointestinal disturbance and possibly anaphylactic shock.

Individuals with sulfite sensitivity should read labels carefully to avoid sulfite containing foods. Names for sulfite containing additives appear in Table 6-12.

TABLE 6-11   Foods Commonly Containing Sulfites*

Bakery products	Cookies, crackers, pie crusts, pizza crusts, quiche crusts, flour tortillas. All bakery products containing dried fruits or vegetables
Beverage	Beer, cocktail mixes, dried citrus fruit, beverage mixes, wine, wine coolers
Dairy products	Filled milk (skim milk enriched in fat content with vegetable oil)
Fish and shellfish	Canned clams; dried cod; fresh, frozen, canned, and dried shrimp; frozen lobster; scallops
Fruit	Processed fruit including canned, bottled, or frozen fruit juices, dried fruit, canned, bottled, or frozen "dietetic" fruit or fruit juices, maraschino cherries, glazed fruit
Vegetables	Fresh, precut potatoes
Other	Condiments and relishes (horseradish, onion and pickle relish, pickles, olives, salad dressing mixes, wine vinegar)
Sweets	Confections and frostings containing brown, raw, powdered, or white sugar derived from sugar beets

*This list is not inclusive. Check labels of all foods for the presence of sulfite-containing ingredients.

TABLE 6-12   Sulfite-Containing Additives

Sulfur dioxide
Sodium sulfite
Sodium or potassium bisulfite
Sodium or potassium metabisulfite

Physicians: How to Order Diet

The diet order should read: *sulfite restricted diet.*

References

54. Taylor SL, Bush RK, Nordlee JA. Sulfites. In: Metcalfe DD, Sampson HA, Simon RA, eds. Food allergy: adverse reactions to foods and food additives. Oxford: Blackwell Scientific Publications, 1991:239–260.
55. Perkin JE. Adverse reactions to food additives and other food constituents. In: Perkin JE, ed. Food allergies and adverse reactions. Gaithersburg, MD: Aspen Publishers, 1990:129–170.
56. Food and Drug Administration. Food labeling: declaration of ingredients. Federal Register 1993;58(3):2850–2887.

TARTRAZINE AND ACETYLSALICYLIC ACID

General Description

Tartrazine (FD & C Yellow No. 5) is a certified coloring dye used in foods, drugs, and cosmetics.[57] Manufacturers are required to identify tartrazine on food product labels if it is used in the product.[58] Patients should check product ingredient labels for the words "FD & C Yellow No. 5" or "Yellow No. 5."

Tartrazine has been associated with intolerance. Instances of cross-sensitivity between tartrazine and salicylate in the form of acetylsalicylic acid (as aspirin) have also been reported. The incidence of aspirin-sensitive patients reacting to tartrazine has been shown to be from 0 to 25%.[59] Salicylate (not acetylsalicylic acid) does occur naturally in food but has not been found to be a cause of reactions. Daily consumption of dietary salicylate is estimated to be 10 to 200 mg/day. Aspirin provides 600 to 625 mg of acetylsalicylic acid depending upon the dose, with potential for more taken during the day. This, in addition to the different forms of salicylate in aspirin and food, leaves it unclear whether dietary salicylates are involved in this adverse cross-reaction. Acetylsalicylic acid (aspirin) is the only proven allergenic salicylate.

Nutritional Inadequacy

The tartrazine free diet can be planned to meet nutritional needs.

Indications and Rationale

Chronic Urticaria. The fraction of patients with chronic urticaria actually sensitive to tartrazine and acetylsalicylic acid is uncertain, and many physicians do not use a restricting diet as a form of treatment.[57] The mechanisms by which these compounds induce or aggravate urticaria have not been established.

Asthma. In some patients with asthma, particularly those with nasal polyps, the ingestion of aspirin may cause severe asthmatic reactions. In a very small percentage of these patients, asthmatic attacks may also follow the ingestion of tartrazine.[57] Asthmatic patients who are sensitive to aspirin or tartrazine, however, can often ingest the salicylate naturally present in food without difficulty. There are no well-controlled studies that show that dietary manipulation of dietary salicylate (other than avoidance of the drug aspirin) has important effects on the course of the asthma. In the tartrazine-reactive patient, however, it does seem reasonable to exclude tartrazine from the diet.

A food is acceptable only if it has been established that it does not contain tartrazine. By law, product ingredient labels must list the words "FD & C Yellow No. 5" or "Yellow No. 5."[58] Patients should be advised to check labels of foods and to avoid those products containing tartrazine.

Physicians: How to Order Diet

The diet order should read: *tartrazine-free diet.*

References

57. Stevenson DD. Tartrazine, azo and nonazo dyes. In: Metcalfe DD, Sampson HA, Simon RA, eds. Food allergy: adverse reactions to foods and food additives. Oxford: Blackwell Scientific Publications, 1991:267–275.

58. Food and Drug Adminstration. Food labeling: declaration of ingredients. Federal Register 1993;58(3):2850–2887.

59. Virchow C, Szczeklik A, Bianco S. Intolerance to tartrazine in aspirin-induced asthma: results of a multicenter study. Respiration 1988;53:20–23.

7 / *Cardiovascular Diseases*

HYPERTENSION

General Description

The dietary management of hypertension focuses on weight reduction and on restriction of sodium and alcohol intake. Other dietary factors that have been implicated in hypertension may be considered as well: potassium, calcium, magnesium, fat, and fatty acids.

Nutritional Inadequacy

The diet for hypertension is not inherently lacking in nutrients when compared to the Recommended Dietary Allowances (RDA). However, for those diets restricted to 1,200 kcal or less, it is difficult to meet the RDA consistently. A daily multiple vitamin that provides nutrients at a level equivalent to the RDA is recommended for persons who consume 1,200 kcal or less.

Indication and Rationale

Hypertension is defined as a sustained elevation of systemic blood pressure. "Primary" or "essential" hypertension is elevation of blood pressure that is unrelated to any identifiable cause. The term "secondary" hypertension is used when a cause can be identified. It is much less common. Possible causes of secondary hypertension include renal insufficiency, renovascular diseases, coarctation of the aorta, Cushing's syndrome, primary aldosteronism, and pheochromocytoma.[1] According to the Joint National Committee on Detection, Evaluation, and Treatment of High Blood Pressure, hypertension should not be diagnosed on the basis of a single blood pressure measurement. Initial elevated readings should be confirmed by at least two subsequent blood pressure determinations. An average level of diastolic pressure of 90 mm Hg or greater or an average systolic pressure of 140 mm Hg or greater is required for diagnosis.[1] (Table 7-1 presents the classifications of

TABLE 7-1   Classification of Blood Pressure for Adults Age 18 Years or Older*

Category	Systolic (mm Hg)	Diastolic (mm Hg)
Normal†	< 130	< 85
High normal	130–139	85–89
Hypertension‡		
Stage 1 (Mild)	140–159	90–99
Stage 2 (Moderate)	160–179	100–109
Stage 3 (Severe)	180–209	110–119
Stage 4 (Very severe)	≥ 210	≥ 120

*Not taking antihypertensive drugs and not acutely ill. When systolic and diastolic pressure fall into different categories, the higher category should be selected to classify the individual's blood pressure status. For instance, 160/92 should be classified as Stage 2, and 180/120 should be classified as Stage 4. Isolated systolic hypertension (ISH) is defined as SBP ≥140 mm Hg and DBP <90 mm HG and staged appropriately (e.g., 170/85 mm Hg is defined as Stage 2 ISH).

†Optimal blood pressure with respect to cardiovascular risk is SBP <120 mm Hg and DPB <80 mm Hg. However, unusually low readings should be evaluated for clinical significance.

‡Based on the average of two or more readings taken at each of two or more visits following an initial screening.

Note: In addition to classifying stages of hypertension based on average blood pressure levels, the clinician should specify presence or absence of target-organ disease and additional risk factors. For example, a patient with diabetes and a blood pressure of 142/94 mm Hg plus left ventricular hypertrophy should be classified as "Stage 1 hypertension with target-organ disease (left ventricular hypertrophy) and with another major risk factor (diabetes)." This specificity is important for risk classification and management.

From National Institutes of Health. The fifth report of the Joint National Committee on Detection, Evaluation, and Treatment of High Blood Pressure. NIH Publication No. 93-1088. Washington, DC, October, 1992.

TABLE 7-2   Lifestyle Modifications for Hypertension Control and/or Overall Cardiovascular Risk

Lose weight if overweight.
Limit alcohol intake to no more than 1 oz of ethanol per day (24 oz of beer, 8 oz of wine, or 2 oz of 100 proof whiskey).
Exercise (aerobic) regularly.
Reduce sodium intake to less than 100 mEq per day (<2.3 g of sodium or <6 g of sodium chloride).
Maintain adequate dietary potassium, calcium, and magnesium intake.
Stop smoking and reduce dietary saturated fat and cholesterol intake for overall cardiovascular health. Reducing fat intake also helps reduce caloric intake— important for control of weight and Type II diabetes.

From National Institutes of Health. The fifth report of the Joint National Committee on Detection, Evaluation, and Treatment of High Blood Pressure. NIH Publication No. 93-1088. Washington, DC, October, 1992.

blood pressure in adults.) According to these definitions, as many as 50 million people in the United States have elevated blood pressure or are taking antihypertensive medication. The prevalence of hypertension increases with age and is higher for black Americans than for white Americans.[1,2] Differences in blood pressure among other ethnic groups have also been reported, but data are insufficient to

TABLE 7-3   Other Dietary Factors Not Yet Conclusive for Treatment of Hypertension

Dietary Factor	Selected References
• Adequate potassium	1,2,6,11,13,14
• Increase in total potassium to sodium ratio	2,20
• Adequate calcium	1,2,4–7,11,13,21
• Adequate magnesium	1,2,6,11,13
• Variation in total fat and proportions of fatty acids	1,2,11,22-26

Note: Caffeine may temporarily increase blood pressure, but tolerance usually develops quickly. Therefore, unless cardiac or other forms of excessive sensitivity to caffeine are present, no limitation of consumption of caffeine-containing beverages is needed for control of hypertension.[1]

permit firm conclusions to be drawn.[3] Hypertension is a major risk factor for development of atherosclerotic cardiovascular diseases (i.e., myocardial infarction, coronary heart disease, congestive heart failure, stroke, and peripheral arterial diseases) as well as kidney disease.[1-3]

Prescribed treatment regimens vary because hypertension varies in its degree of severity. Because of the attendant risks and costs of pharmacological therapy, one should initially look to the use of nonpharmacological means of treatment.[1-13] Table 7-2 presents lifestyle modifications found to be supportive to reduction in blood pressure and/or overall cardiovascular risk. Three diet-related therapies recommended for hypertension that are well supported by scientific evidence are weight reduction, sodium restriction, and alcohol restriction.[1,2] In Stage 1 (mild) hypertension, diet and exercise may serve as the primary approaches to treatment.[1,4-6,9,13,14] Additionally, the use of diet therapy as an adjunct to the pharmacological treatment of Stage 2 (moderate) to Stage 3 (severe) hypertension has been shown to enhance the effectiveness of the drug treatment and, in some cases, eliminate the need for or reduce the quantity of the medications needed for blood pressure control.[6,8,9,10,12]

Dietary modifications are a major part of the nonpharmacological treatment of existing hypertension and have also gained support as having a role in the prevention of high blood pressure—particularly for those individuals at high risk.[1,2,9] At present, research on the effect of other dietary factors on the control of hypertension, in addition to weight control and restriction of sodium and alcohol, is suggestive but not conclusive. See Table 7-3.

Weight Reduction.   While not all obese individuals become hypertensive, obesity and blood pressure are closely associated. A strong correlation exists between increases in body weight and subsequent development of hypertension.[1,2,3,15] Independent of other variables (e.g., sodium restriction), weight loss in hypertensives has been shown to decrease blood pressure and aid in its control.[1-4,12,15] Blood pressure tends to rise in a stepwise fashion according to the degree of obesity or magnitude of weight gain. Associations between body weight and blood pressure demonstrate a striking correlation, as do associations between body build and blood pressure. Studies suggest that fat deposits in the abdominal region may also pose a higher risk of hypertension.[1,3]

Weight reduction reduces blood pressure in a large proportion of hypertensive individuals who are more than 10% above ideal weight.[1] It has been shown that an average weight loss of approximately 10 to 15 lb can decrease blood pressure.[4,5,11] The effects of sustained weight loss on blood pressure have not yet been determined. If using weight reduction as a sole therapy for hypertensives, blood pressures should be followed closely since not all patients will respond to weight loss.[4]

The specific mechanisms and factors by which obesity might be involved in the development of hypertension are being studied. Specific characteristics of obesity (e.g., the distribution of body fat and the adipose cell morphology) as well as hemodynamic and hormonal-based theories (e.g., increased secretion of catecholamines due to a hyperactive sympathetic nervous system) have been proposed as possible explanations for the hypertensive effects of obesity.[3,6,11,15]

Sodium.   Blood pressure response to sodium restriction varies in degree from patient to patient.[1,2,9,10,11] Numerous clinical studies have concluded that moderate sodium restriction does reduce blood pressure for sodium-sensitive individuals. On the other hand, moderate sodium restriction does not reduce blood pressure for sodium-resistant individuals. It is estimated that approximately 50 to 60% of hypertensives are sodium-sensitive.[16] However, a means of prospectively identifying sodium-sensitive individuals is unavailable at the present time.

Factors associated with a blood pressure fall in response to sodium restriction have been identified and include a low plasma renin activity, age, race, initial blood pressure level, and degree of sodium restriction.[2,4,9,11,13] A moderate sodium restriction, to approximately 70 to 100 mEq/day, can be of therapeutic value for hypertensive patients whether medications are used or not.[1,2,7,9,11,14]

For those patients on diuretic therapy, dietary sodium restriction lessens the risk of hypokalemia by preventing excessive urinary losses of potassium and may reduce the dosage needed for blood pressure control. The antihypertensive effect of sodium restriction is particularly additive to vasodilators, to converting enzyme inhibitors, and to adrenergic inhibitors.[17] See Appendix 2 for drug-nutrient interactions.

Alcohol.   There is a positive association between amounts of alcohol consumed and blood pressure levels.[2,13] This effect appears to be independent of age, obesity, exercise, smoking status, and sex. It also seems unrelated to the type of alcoholic beverage drunk but is presumed to be due to the ethanol per se.[2,13] The effect of alcohol is more marked for those averaging more than 30 g/day of ethanol (e.g., 2 oz of 100-proof whiskey, 8 oz of wine, or 24 oz of beer).[1] The effect on blood pressure of less than 30 g/day of ethanol is not clear.[5]

Goals of Dietary Management

The goal of treating hypertension is to prevent the morbidity and mortality associated with high blood pressure by sufficiently lowering and maintaining the blood pressure level in accordance with standards set by the Joint National Committee on Detection, Evaluation, and Treatment of High Blood Pressure.[1] Dietary management alone may be effective in accomplishing this goal in some individuals. In addition, dietary modifications are valuable as an adjunct to pharmacological therapy. The risk of cardiovascular disease is also lessened by controlling the blood pressure with dietary and/or drug treatment.[2,3]

Dietary Recommendations

Table 7-2 presents a summary of dietary and other lifestyle modifications for control of hypertension from the Joint National Committee on Detection, Evaluation, and Treatment of High Blood Pressure.[1] This table includes those dietary features that are possible to quantify and that are viewed as the primary considerations of dietary management. The concomitant use of a low total fat, low saturated fat, and low cholesterol diet may be necessary if hypertensive patients are hyperlipidemic as well. (See Chapter 7, Hyperlipidemia, for dietary recommendations.)

Weight Reduction.   It is advisable for hypertensive patients who are more than 110% of ideal body weight to reduce weight.[1] It may not be possible or advisable to reduce to the level indicated in common height-weight tables (Appendix 4). However, it has been shown that weight reduction results in a lowered blood pressure in the overweight hypertensive patient even when the ideal body weight is not achieved.[1] Weight loss to a level that results in a lowering of blood pressure should be the goal in management of hypertension. Weight reduction in the obese patient should be pursued even if blood pressure is not lowered. (See Chapter 8, Obesity, for further discussion of the risks associated with obesity and for determination of goal weights.)

The diet for weight control should provide a specific kilocalorie restriction in order to achieve goal weight. Patient food preferences and guidelines for portion sizes of foods will not only accomplish kilocalorie control but also control sodium intake. Aerobic exercise should also be encouraged. A regular exercise program facilitates weight reduction and may be beneficial for treatment of hypertension. Health practitioners should advise hypertensive patients who are initiating an exercise program to do so gradually and after appropriate clinical evaluation.[1,5]

Sodium.   Estimates of the average sodium content of the daily American diet range from 4 to 6 g (175 to 265 mEq).[2] The estimated minimum requirement for sodium is 0.5 g/day.[18] A moderate dietary sodium reduction to a level of less than 2.3 g/day (100 mEq) is recommended for hypertension control.[1]

Sources of dietary sodium are table salt; foods to which salt or sodium compounds have been added; foods that inherently contain sodium; bottled, tap, or chemically softened waters that contain sodium salts; and some medications. In the United States, sodium added during processing and manufacturing of foods provides approximately 75% of the sodium intake. An additional 15% is added by the individual during cooking and at the table in the form of sodium chloride (table salt). The remaining 10% is from the natural sodium content of foods.[19] Table salt is 40% sodium by weight; 1 tsp of table salt contains approximately 2,000 mg of sodium (87 mEq).

Sodium Calculations.   The amount of sodium calculated by the dietitian when formulating the diet plan for control of hypertension should be no more than 10% above the level of sodium that is prescribed by the physician. However, it is acceptable for the calculated level of sodium to be more than 10% below the prescribed level. In most situations, one should not add extra table salt to bring the sodium intake up to the prescribed level.

For those patients with high normal or borderline high blood pressure, a no extra salt (NES) or no added salt diet is recommended. This diet is a noncalculated

TABLE 7-4   Approximate Sodium Content of Selected Foods

Foods by Group	Approx. Portion	Approx. Sodium (mEq)	(mg)
MEAT AND MEAT SUBSTITUTES			
Unsalted	1 oz	1	20
Salted	1 oz	3†	70
Cottage cheese (dry curd)	1/4 cup	1	20
Egg	1 med	3	70
Peanut butter, salted	2 Tbsp	6	130
Mild aged cheddar cheese	1 oz	8	180
Cottage cheese, creamed	1/4 cup	10	230
Ham	1 oz	12–18	270–410
Processed American cheese food	1 oz	12–15	270–350
Cold cuts or deli meats	1 oz	14–18	320–410
Smoked link sausage	1 oz	18	410
Frankfurter, small	1 1/2 oz	20	460
Tuna, canned, water-packed	1/4 cup	14	130
MILK			
Whole	8 oz	5	120
Skim, nonfat or 1%	8 oz	6	140
Yogurt	8 oz	5-8	120–180
Buttermilk (from skim milk)	8 oz	14	320
STARCH			
Puffed ready-to-eat cereal	1 1/2 cups	0–1.5	0–30
Low sodium bread	1 slice	0.5	10
Cooked potatoes, cereals, pasta, rice (unsalted)	1/2 cup	0.5	10
Regular bread	1 slice	5	120
Unsalted top saltine crackers	six 2" sq	6	140
Graham crackers	three 2 1/2" sq	6	140
Chips, corn, potato, or tortilla	1 oz	5–10	120–240
Regular saltine crackers	six 2" sq	11	250
Cooked potatoes, cereals, and other starches (salted)	1/2 cup	10†	230
Corn or wheat flake cold cereal	3/4 cup	10*	230
Pancake, biscuit, waffle (from mix)	1 med	10–15*	230–350
Pretzels	25 small	13	300
Commercial soup	1 cup	20–50*	500–1200
VEGETABLES			
Unsalted (most kinds)	1/2 cup	Trace–1	0–20
Raw celery	3 stalks	3	70
Reg. canned tomato paste (unsalted)	1/2 cup	4	90
Reg. canned (except tomatoes)	1/2 cup	10†	230
Reg. canned tomatoes, sauce or puree	1/2 cup	7–12	160–270
Reg. canned tomato juice	1/2 cup	19	440
Reg. vegetable juice cocktail	1/2 cup	19	440
Sauerkraut	1/2 cup	34	780
Dill pickle	1 medium	40	930
FRUIT			
Most kinds, fruit or juice	1/2 cup	Trace#	0–10

TABLE 7-4 Approximate Sodium Content of Selected Foods—cont'd

Foods by Group	Approx. Portion	Approx. Sodium (mEq)	Approx. Sodium (mg)
FAT			
Cream (any weight)	1 Tbsp	Trace#	0–10
Vegetable oil	1 tsp	Trace#	0–10
Unsalted butter, margarine	1 tsp	Trace#	0–10
Peanuts, unsalted	10 large	<1	0–20
Regular mayonnaise	1 tsp	1	20
Regular butter, margarine	1 tsp	2	50
Mayonnaise type salad dressing	2 tsp	3	70
Tartar sauce, commercial	1½ tsp	4	80–90
Peanuts, salted	10 large	3	70
Regular pourable salad dressing (average)	1 Tbsp	7	160
Bacon	1 medium strip	7	160
Commercial gravy or gravy mix	2 Tbsp	7	160
Green olives	9–10 small	40	930
BEVERAGES			
Beer, liquor, or wine	12 oz, 1½ oz, or 4 oz	0–0.5	0–10
Coffee (reg. or decaf)	8 oz	Trace	0–10
Carbonated drinks	12 oz	Trace–3	0–70
Tea, instant	8 oz	Trace	0–10
Tea, brewed	8 oz	1	20
Tang, orange	12 oz	1	20
Hawaiian punch	12 oz	1–2	20–40
Tonic water	8 oz	1	20
Club soda	12 oz	3	70
Instant cocoa	1 pkt	7	160
Tang, grape	12 oz	10	230
Bouillon	1 cube	40–65	900–1500
DESSERTS			
Fruit ice	⅓ cup	1	20
Cooked pudding (mix, but not instant)	¼ cup	1–2	20–40
Ice cream, sherbet, frozen yogurt	½ cup	2–4	40–90
Flavored gelatin (average)	½ cup	2–4	40–90
Angel food cake (homemade, no ring)	1/16	3‡	70
Cookies, assorted plain	two 2" diam.	1–10	20–230
Instant pudding from mix	¼ cup	5–10	120–240
Pie, fruit or cream (homemade)	⅛ of 9" pie	8–15	180–350
SEASONINGS AND CONDIMENTS			
Prepared mustard	1 tsp	3	70
Regular catsup	1 Tbsp	7	160
"Light" salt	¼ tsp	12	280
Regular meat tenderizer	¼ tsp	19	440
Garlic or onion salt	¼ tsp	17–20*	390–460
Salt	¼ tsp	25	580
Regular soy sauce	1 Tbsp	37–45*	850–1040

*Actual sodium content of commercially prepared items varies with manufacturer.

†"Salted" = ¼ tsp salt per pound of meat; or ⅛ tsp salt per ½ cup serving potato or substitute, cooked vegetable, and cooked cereal.

‡Wide variations depending on recipe.

#Trace is <0.5 mEq (12 mg) sodium.

diet in which the primary objective is to limit highly concentrated sources of sodium and to avoid added salt. The actual sodium content of a NES diet is variable and usually ranges from 90 to 150 mEq depending on the caloric level of the diet and the sodium content of the foods consumed. Guidelines for a NES diet are as follows:
1. Limit the amount of salt added to food in cooking or at the table to a total of no more than ½ tsp/day.
2. Avoid or limit high sodium foods. See Tables 7-4 and 7-5.

The sodium that is inherent in some foods must be calculated as part of the sodium allowance. Animal foods, such as meats, eggs, and dairy products, and some vegetables contain natural sodium and should be used in controlled amounts. Sodium compounds are also used in food processing for various reasons. For example, sodium benzoate is a preservative used in relishes, sauces, and margarine. Another additive, sodium citrate, enhances the flavor of gelatin desserts and some beverages. Although there are many low sodium products on the market, such items should be used in controlled amounts. If such a product contains no more than 10 mg (0.4 mEq) of sodium per serving, it is considered to contribute negligible amounts of sodium to the diet.

Table 7-5 presents guidelines for categorizing foods based on sodium content. This table can serve as a guide in determining the use of various foods for different levels of sodium-restricted diets. The food groups and portions sizes are based on the Exchange Lists for Meal Planning developed by the American Diabetes Association and the American Dietetic Association (see Chapter 8, Diabetes Mellitus). The approximate sodium content, especially of processed or convenience foods, varies. The values given in Table 7-5 represent averages. When tailor-

---

TABLE 7-5   Guidelines for Categorizing Foods Based on Sodium Content

MEAT AND MEAT SUBSTITUTES
Low: 0–2 mEq (0–46 mg)
Moderate: 2–10 mEq (46–230 mg)
High: 10 mEq (>230 mg)

FATS
Low: 0–2 mEq (0–46 mg)
Moderate: 2–8 mEq (46–184 mg)
High: >8 mEq (>184 mg)

MILK
Low: 0–7 mEq (0–161 mg)
Moderate: 7–12 mEq (161–276 mg)
High: >12 mEq (>276 mg)

BEVERAGES
Low: 0–3 mEq (0–69 mg)
High: >3 mEq (>69+ mg)

STARCHES
Low: 0–9 mEq (0–207 mg)
High: >9 mEq (>207 mg)

FRUITS AND VEGETABLES
Low: 0–3 mEq (0–69 mg)
Moderate: 3–10 mEq (69–230 mg)
High: >10 mEq (>230 mg)

DESSERTS
Low: 0–10 mEq (0–230 mg)
High: >10 mEq (>230 mg)

SEASONINGS AND CONDIMENTS
Low: 0–3 mEq (0–69 mg)
Moderate: 3–9 mEq (69–207 mg)
High: >9 mEq (>207 mg)

Refer to Appendix 12 for conversion of milligrams to milliequivalents.

ing a diet to an individual's needs, it may be necessary to consult food composition tables, the manufacturers' analyses, or product labels for more specific information on the sodium content. Some foods noted in the table may be difficult or impossible to include in sodium-restricted diets.

Food Labeling. It is important to read labels on packaged foods when modifying sodium in the diet. Federal regulations have been formulated by the Food and Drug Administration to control the terms used in sodium labeling. These terms can be helpful in determining the sodium content of specific foods and their use in a sodium-controlled diet. The terms used on labels that refer to the sodium content are as follows:[19]

1. "Sodium-free" means less than 5 mg (0.2 mEq) of sodium per serving.
2. "Very low sodium" means 35 mg (1.5 mEq) or less of sodium per serving.
3. "Low sodium" means 140 mg (6 mEq) or less of sodium per serving.
4. "Reduced sodium" means that foods are altered to reduce the usual level of sodium by at least 25%.
5. "Without added salt,""Unsalted," and "No salt added" are terms used for foods once processed with salt but now processed without it. Products labeled with these terms must list the amount of sodium in milligrams per serving.
6. "Lite" and "Light" are terms for products that may be reduced in calories, fat, or sodium. Check the label. "Light in sodium" terminology indicates that the sodium content has been reduced by at least 50%.

Medications. Antacids, laxatives, cough medicines, and other medications may contain significant amounts of sodium. One should check the label or ask a local pharmacist or manufacturer for the sodium content.

Water. Drinking water, either natural, bottled, or softened, may be a significant source of sodium. Those interested in knowing the sodium content of the local water supply are advised to ask the public health department. The public health department may report sodium content in terms of parts per million. One part per million is equivalent to 1 mg of sodium/L of water. Depending on the sodium content and quantity of water used, it may be necessary for the patient to use distilled water for drinking and for cooking.

Alcohol. It is difficult to quantify an acceptable level of alcohol use for all persons with hypertension. It has been suggested that during the initial treatment of hypertension, the patient abstain from alcohol in order to determine its effect on blood pressure levels.[6] The Joint National Committee on Detection, Evaluation, and Treatment of High Blood Pressure recommends that those who drink should do so in moderation (i.e., no more than 1 fl oz [30 g] of ethanol daily, which is contained in approximately 2 oz of 100-proof whiskey, 8 oz of wine, or 24 oz of beer).[1] The caloric content of alcohol should also be considered, especially for overweight hypertensives needing to lose weight (Appendix 3).

Physicians: How to Order Diet

The diet order should indicate *diet for hypertension*. It may include those parameters that the physician wishes to be addressed (weight reduction, restriction of sodium and alcohol intake). If a specific amount of sodium or other dietary component is ordered, the dietitian plans a diet that does not exceed that amount by more than

10%. The physician should also specify any additional factors needing to be modified (e.g., fat and cholesterol control for hyperlipidemia).

Supplementary Information

Additional information (both patient and professional) is available upon request from the sources listed below.

National Heart, Lung, and Blood Institute
National Institutes of Health Information Center
PO Box 30105
Bethesda, MD 20824-0105

American Heart Association—consult your local affiliate or
7320 Greenville Avenue
Dallas, TX 75231

American Dietetic Association
216 West Jackson Blvd.
Suite 800
Chicago, IL 60606-6995

References

1. National Institutes of Health. Fifth report of the Joint National Committee on Detection, Evaluation, and Treatment of High Blood Pressure. NIH Publication No. 93-1088. Washington, DC, NIH, Oct 1992.
2. U.S. Dept. of Health & Human Services. Surgeon General's report on nutrition and health. DHHSA (PHS) Publication No. 88-50210. Washington, DC: USDHHS 1988; Chapter 3:139–175.
3. Committee on Diet and Health, Food and Nutrition Board, Commission on Life Sciences, National Research Council. Diet and health: implications for reducing chronic disease risk. Washington DC: National Academy Press, 1988:107,112,113,549–561,572,659.
4. Langford HG. Nonpharmacological therapy of hypertension: commentary on diet and blood pressure. Hypertension 1989;13(Suppl I):I-98–I-102.
5. Kaplan NM. Nonpharmacological control of high blood pressure. Am J Hypertens 1989;2(2):55S–59S.
6. Haynie R. Nonpharmacological therapy for hypertension. Compr Ther 1989;15(11):33–37.
7. Chapman KM, Nelson, RA. The case for dietary management of the older hypertensive. Geriatrics 1990;45(Apr):69–76.
8. Aberg H, Tibblin G. Addition of non-pharmacological methods of treatment in patients on antihypertensive drugs: results of previous medications, laboratory tests and life quality. J Intern Med 1989;226:39–46.
9. Elliott P. The INTERSALT study: an addition to the evidence on salt and blood pressure, and some implications. J Hum Hypertens 1989;3:289–298.
10. Weinberger MH, Cohen SJ, Miller JZ, Luft FC, Grim CE, Fineberg NS. Dietary sodium restriction as adjunctive treatment of hypertension. JAMA 1988;259(17):2561–2565.
11. Beilin L. Diet and hypertension: critical concepts and controversies. State of the art lecture. J Hypertens 1987;5(Suppl 5):S447–S457.
12. Kumanyika SK. Weight reduction and sodium restriction in the management of hypertension. Clin Geriatr Med 1989;5(4):769–789.
13. Beilin LJ. Diet, alcohol and hypertension. Clin Exper Hypertens Theory Pract 1989; A-11(5 and 6):991–1010.

14. Stamler J, Prineas RJ, Neaton JD, Grimm RH, McDonald RH, Schnaper HW, Schoenberger JA, Elmer PJ, Cutler JA. Background and design of the new U.S. trial on diet and drug treatment of "mild" hypertension (TOMHS). Am J Cardiol 1987;59:51G–60G.

15. Singh RB, Rastogi SS, Singh DS, Mehta PJ. Effect of obesity and weight reduction in hypertension. Acta Cardiologica 1990;XLV(1):45–56.

16. Williams GH, Hollenberg NK. Sodium-sensitive essential hypertension: emerging insights into an old entity. J Am Coll Nutr 1989;8(6):490–494.

17. MacGregor GA. Sodium is more important than calcium in essential hypertension. Hypertension 1985;7:628-637.

18. Subcommittee on the Tenth Edition of the RDAs, Food and Nutrition Board, Commission on Life Sciences, National Research Council. Recommended dietary allowances, 10th ed. Washington, DC: National Academy Press, 1989:253.

19. Anon. The new food label. FDA backgrounder. 1992;Dec 10:1–10.

20. Tobian L. Potassium and sodium in hypertension. J Hypertens 1988;6(Suppl 4):S12–S24.

21. Grobbee DE, Wall-Manning HJ. The role of calcium supplementation in the treatment of hypertension: current evidence. Drugs 1990;39(1):7–18.

22. Sacks FM. Dietary fats and blood pressure: a critical review of the evidence. Nutr Rev 1989;47(10):291–300.

23. Knapp HR, FitzGerald GA. The antihypertensive effects of fish oil: a controlled study of polyunsaturated fatty acid supplements in essential hypertension. N Engl J Med 1989; 320:1037–1043.

24. Wing LMH, Nestel PJ, Chalmers JP, Rouse I, West MJ, Bune AJ, Tonkin AL, Russell AE. Lack of effect of fish oil supplementation on blood pressure in treated hypertensives. J Hypertens 1990;8:339–343.

25. Bonaa KH, Bjerve KS, Straume B, Gram IT, Thelle D. Effect of eicosapentaenoic and docosahexaenoic acids on blood pressure in hypertension: a population-based intervention trial from the Tromso Study. N Eng J Med 1990;322:795–801.

26. Knapp HR. Omega-3 fatty acids, endogenous prostaglandins, and blood pressure regulation in humans. Nutr Rev 1989;47(10):301–313.

HYPERLIPIDEMIA

General Description

Dietary management is the primary treatment for most types of hyperlipidemia. Recommendations for the levels of intake of fat, cholesterol, carbohydrate, and alcohol are determined by which lipids are elevated in the bloodstream. For persons above desirable body weight, caloric restriction and exercise are emphasized.

Nutritional Inadequacy

Diets for the management of hyperlipidemia are generally adequate in nutrients when compared to the RDA. However, for diets that emphasize caloric restriction to 1,200 kcal or less, it is difficult to meet the RDA consistently. A daily multiple vitamin supplement that provides nutrients at a level equivalent to the RDA is recommended for persons who consume 1,200 kcal or less. A multiple vitamin supplement may also be warranted for persons who have food aversions or intolerances that greatly limit the variety of food choices.

Indications and Rationale

Hyperlipidemia or dyslipidemia are general terms that refer to abnormal levels of lipids (cholesterol and/or triglycerides). Hyperlipoproteinemia is an abnormal elevation of one or more lipoproteins in the blood. Lipoproteins transport cholesterol, triglycerides, and phospholipids in the blood. Some lipoproteins may be regulators of cholesterol accumulation in the arterial wall as well.

The elevation of serum cholesterol, particularly low density lipoprotein cholesterol (LDLC), is of concern because of its association with the predisposition to atherosclerosis. Treatment is based on the assumption that normalization of the serum lipid values will reduce the risk of atherogenesis and cardiovascular events.

Diagnosis.   The diagnosis of hyperlipidemia is based on laboratory determination of the total cholesterol and total triglyceride concentration in the plasma. Measurement of lipoproteins should be done to determine the type of abnormal lipoproteins present.

Lipoproteins are classified by their density, their composition, and their electrophoretic mobility into classes as shown in Table 7-6.[27] Lipoprotein fractions are evaluated and used as screening tools for atherosclerosis.

Cholesterol.   Cholesterol is synthesized primarily in the liver from the intermediary metabolism of carbohydrates, fats, and proteins. Primary hypercholesterolemia is a result of genetic abnormalities, a high fat diet, or a combination of both. Elevated serum cholesterol levels that are above 200 mg/dl are associated with an increased risk of developing coronary heart disease (CHD). The risk increases when cholesterol levels are significantly above 240 mg/dl. For each 1% increase in blood cholesterol, there is a 2% increase in incidence of CHD in populations.[28-30]

Low Density Lipoprotein Cholesterol (LDLC).   Increased serum levels of LDLC have been shown to be associated with increased atherosclerosis.[30-33] Genetic predisposition may play a major role in the elevation of LDLC, but dietary fat and cholesterol may also increase LDLC.

LDLC is better than total cholesterol for assessing the risk of cardiovascular disease and is therefore preferred for clinical decisions about intervention. It may be measured in the laboratory or calculated. If the values for total cholesterol, high density lipoprotein cholesterol (HDLC), and triglycerides are available, the LDLC can be calculated using the Friedewald Formula (see top of next page):[31,34]

TABLE 7-6   Classification of Lipoproteins

Classification	Major Lipid Components
Chylomicrons	Triglycerides
Chylomicron remnants	Triglycerides
Very low density lipoprotein (VLDL)	Triglycerides
Intermediate density lipoprotein (IDL)	Triglycerides and cholesterol
Low density lipoprotein (LDL)	Cholesterol
High density lipoprotein (HDL)	Phospholipids

$$LDLC = \text{total cholesterol} - \left(\frac{\text{triglycerides}}{5} + HDLC \right)$$

According to the National Cholesterol Education Program, Adult Treatment Panel guidelines, LDLC estimation by the above formula cannot accurately predict LDLC if the triglyceride value is above 400 mg/dl.[35] Mayo Laboratories recommends measuring LDLC if triglyceride value exceeds 200 mg/dl, as the accuracy of the calculation is variable. Therefore, in making treatment decisions, if triglycerides are greatly elevated, in addition to total cholesterol, LDLC blood levels should be measured directly. A general optimal goal for LDLC level is 130 mg/dl or less. (Appendix 17 provides percentile rankings for serum LDLC values according to age and sex.)

High Density Lipoprotein Cholesterol (HDLC). HDLC levels have been shown to have an inverse relationship with CHD.[29,31] A reduced serum level of HDLC is defined as a concentration below 35 mg/dl for males and 45 mg/dl for females. (See Appendix 17 for percentile rankings for serum HDLC values according to age and sex.) A reduced HDLC increases the risk for CHD and hence is classified as a major risk factor.[29,31] The common causes of a reduced serum HDLC are listed in Table 7-7.[31,36] Low levels of HDLC are often associated with hypertriglyceridemia, and normalization of triglycerides usually results in a rise in HDLC levels. To simplify understanding of which patients are at risk, the total cholesterol to HDLC ratio or the LDLC to HDLC ratio may be used (Tables 7-8 and 7-9).[37]

Triglycerides. Triglycerides are lipid molecules (triacylglycerol) derived primarily from endogenous or dietary fat or conversion from any form of excess calories. They are transported on very low density lipoproteins (VLDL) (endogenous) or chylomicrons (dietary) to tissues for use as fuel or to adipose tissue for stor-

TABLE 7-7 Common Causes of Reduced Serum HDLC Levels

Cigarette smoking	Starvation
Obesity	Hypertriglyceridemia
Lack of exercise	Genetic factors
Poorly controlled diabetes mellitus	Drugs
Chronic renal failure	Progestational agents
Hypothyroidism	Androgenic and related steroids
Liver disease	Anabolic steroids
	Beta-adrenergic blocking agents

TABLE 7-8 Ratio of Total Cholesterol to HDLC

	Average	Optimal
Males	≤ 5.0	≤ 3.5
Females	≤ 4.5	≤ 3.5

TABLE 7-9   Ratio of LDLC to HDLC

	Average	Optimal
Males and females	≤ 3.0	≤ 2.5

TABLE 7-10   Possible Causes of Elevated Triglycerides[31,35,40-43]

Obesity	Simple sugars in sensitive individuals
Alcohol	Drugs
Uncontrolled diabetes mellitus	Thiazide diuretics
Hypothyroidism	Beta-adrenergic blocking agents
Chronic renal disease	Corticosteroids
Genetic factors	Estrogenic hormones (including oral
Liver disease	contraceptives)
Dysproteinemia	Retinoids (e.g., cis-retinoic acid or
	accutane)

age.[38,39] A major cause of elevated triglycerides is obesity. Dietary fat may increase triglyceride levels, and there are some individuals in whom simple sugars and/or excessive alcohol may increase triglycerides.[38] Other causes of elevated triglycerides are listed in Table 7-10.[31,35,40-43]

Triglycerides are measured after a 12 hour fast and a 48 hour abstinence from alcohol.

The relationship between elevated serum triglycerides and coronary artery disease is controversial.[31,38,39] Hypertriglyceridemia does not appear to be an independent risk factor for men but has been shown to be an independent risk factor for women and for patients with diabetes.[39,40] In addition, elevated triglyceride levels equal to 250 mg/dl or more appear to be a risk factor for peripheral vascular disease if other risk factors are present.[40,44] Hypertriglyceridemia is generally associated with low levels of HDLC, which is an independent risk factor for CHD.[31,39,40,44] For patients who do not respond adequately to diet and/or other lifestyle modifications, pharmacological intervention may be necessary.

Classification and Typing. The National Cholesterol Education Program (NCEP) Guidelines (Chapter 2)[44] and Tables 7-11 and 7-12 are often used for classification of hypercholesterolemia in adults over age 20. Although these guidelines were not correlated to age or sex, they are most appropriate for middle-aged men 30 to 60 years of age. The algorithm may not work as well for women or for men and women over 60 years of age. The plasma cholesterol values by percentiles (Table 7-11) may be more helpful in classifying and treating women and nonmiddle aged men. The 75th percentile for serum cholesterol values is used as the upper limit of normal.[45] An abnormal level of triglycerides is considered to be above the 95th percentile.[43] (Note: Appendix 17 provides Lipid Research Clinics [LRC]

TABLE 7-11   Upper Limits of Normal Cholesterol and Triglycerides[45]

The following set of values by percentiles has been determined at the Mayo Clinic for a defined population of healthy persons and with analytic systems that have been standardized for accuracy with the Lipid Standardization Laboratory of the Centers for Disease Control, Atlanta, GA. We recommend use of the 75th percentile values as upper limits for serum cholesterol and the 95th percentile values for serum triglycerides.

Values are in milligrams per deciliter.*

Serum cholesterol and triglycerides are dependent on age and sex. The 75th percentile values are proposed as guidelines for significant hypercholesterolemia and the 95th percentile for significant triglyceridemia. This should not be construed to imply that values below these percentiles are without risk in the development of atherosclerosis, particularly coronary artery disease. The risk of coronary artery disease apparently is present at lower lipid levels and increases stepwise with increments in serum lipid values.

The predictive value of blood lipid concentrations diminishes with increasing age. Hypertension and cigarette smoking augment the cardiac risk attendant on hyperlipidemia.

	Female (mg/dl)			Male (mg/dl)	
Age (yr)	Cholesterol (upper 75th percentile)	Triglyceride (upper 95th percentile)	Age (yr)	Cholesterol (upper 75th percentile)	Triglyceride (upper 95th percentile)
0–5	not established	not established	0–5	not established	not established
6–9	173	76	6–9	172	102
10–14	174	121	10–14	179	103
15–19	175	122	15–19	167	124
20–24	181	97	20–24	185	137
25–29	190	100	25–29	202	157
30–34	199	106	30–34	216	171
35–39	209	110	35–39	226	182
40–44	219	117	40–44	235	189
45–49	229	122	45–49	242	193
50–54	241	128	50–54	246	195
55–59	253	134	55–59	250	197
60–64	265	140	60–64	253	198
65–69	278	147	65–69	255	199
70–74	291	154	70–74	256	199
75+	306	162	75+	257	199

*CONVERSIONS:

To convert total cholesterol, HDLC or LDLC:

$$mg/dl \text{ to } mM/L = mg/dl \times 0.02586 = mM/L$$
$$mM/L \text{ to } mg/dl = mM/L \times 38.68 = mg/dl$$

To convert triglycerides:

$$mg/dl \text{ to } mM/L = mg/dl \times 0.01129 = mM/L$$
$$mM/L \text{ to } mg/dl = mM/L \times 88.57 = mg/dl$$

TABLE 7-12 Typing of Hyperlipoproteinemias

Fredrickson Type	Lipid Abnormality	Elevated Lipoproteins
I	Hyperchylomicronemia	Chylomicrons
IIa	Hypercholesterolemia	LDL
IIb	Combined hypercholesterolemia and endogenous hypertriglyceridemia	LDL, VLDL
III	Dysbetalipoproteinemia (broad beta pattern)	IDL
IV	Hypertriglyceridemia	VLDL
V	Hypertriglyceridemia	VLDL, chylomicrons

LDL = Low density lipoproteins; VLDL = very low density lipoproteins; IDL = intermediate density lipoproteins.

Prevalence Study Values, which are cited by NCEP and may be used by many institutions. Table 7-11 provides Mayo Clinic Laboratory values, which vary slightly from LRC Prevalence Study values.) These levels are proposed as guidelines for significant hypercholesterolemia and hypertriglyceridemia. This does not imply that values below these levels are without risk of atherosclerosis. The risk of coronary artery disease still exists at lower lipid levels especially if other risk factors are present.

Fredrickson's classification (Table 7-12) is another classification scheme.[46] However, this type of classification is not uniformly employed.

A third classification scheme is often referred to as the European guidelines. These guidelines use a combination of total cholesterol, triglyceride, and other risk factors and the presence or absence of coronary disease in their algorithm.[47]

Cardiovascular Risk Factors. Risk factors are conditions and habits that have been demonstrated to be associated with an increased probability of cardiovascular disease.[37,48] Genetic factors greatly influence the risk of developing premature CHD. If one or more close relative suffered a heart attack before the age of 55 years or has a primary form of hyperlipidemia, the likelihood of other family members having hyperlipidemia is greater. The patient's family should be screened for hyperlipidemia if a primary lipid abnormality is identified in a patient.

The four most important modifiable risk factors are elevated serum lipids, elevated blood pressure, abuse of tobacco products, and a sedentary lifestyle. The significance of the risk factors varies with individuals, and the presence of more than one risk factor tends to greatly increase the risk. (See Chapter 2, National Cholesterol Education Program Guidelines for Treatment of Hypercholesterolemia.) Elevated blood pressure is a risk factor that frequently accompanies hyperlipidemia. Medical management includes sodium (salt) restriction, weight reduction if obesity exists, regular exercise, and reduction of excessive alcohol intake (see Chapter 7, Hypertension).

Cigarette smoking is a major independent risk factor for a heart attack, manifested as both fatal and nonfatal myocardial infarction and sudden cardiac death. Smoking also increases the risk of heart attack recurrence among survivors of a myocardial infarction.[49] It deserves special attention in the prevention of cardiovascular disease and should be given a high priority in risk factor reduction and the treatment of cardiovascular disease.

Obesity is also an independent risk factor for CHD and may be associated with an elevated LDLC, elevated triglycerides, reduced HDLC, increased arterial blood pressure, and impaired glucose tolerance. Weight reduction frequently results in improvement in all these abnormalities.

An objective of weight reduction in the person who is obese and has hyperlipidemia is the normalization of the lipid profile, glucose, and blood pressure. For some individuals, this may occur with a modest reduction in weight; but for other persons, the achievement of a distinctly lean weight may be necessary. Various indices of obesity can be used. Body Mass Index is easily calculated (see Appendix 7). The percent of body weight as fat is perhaps the best, but the measurement requires rather complex procedures such as underwater weighing. Percent body fat can be approximated by skinfold measurements and has been helpful in the serial follow-up of patients. The sum of axilla, triceps, and suprailium skinfolds for men and women can be used for predicting body fat levels. Desirable values are 16 to 19% of body weight as fat for men and 23 to 26% of body weight as fat for women.[50,51]

Regular aerobic physical activity (for a minimum of 20 to 30 minutes 3 times per week) offers some protection from the complications of cardiovascular disease by raising the HDLC. Regular aerobic activity may also have a lowering effect on the total serum cholesterol, LDLC levels, and triglycerides, when coupled with a weight reduction program.[52] Exercise also reduces blood pressure, decreases blood platelet activity, and reduces the sympathetic nervous system's response to mental stress.

Psychological, social, cultural, and religious factors indirectly influence the risk of CHD by their effects on the kinds and amounts of foods eaten, on cigarette and alcohol use, and on exercise. Persons who are impatient, highly competitive, and live with a sense of time urgency are greater candidates for cardiovascular disease than persons who live in a more relaxed fashion. Stress management, relaxation skills, and biofeedback may aid in the reduction of overall risk factors.[53]

Other Dietary Factors Associated with Heart Disease.   There are a variety of interactions between fiber and cholesterol, from altering gastric emptying to interfering with cholesterol bile acid and triglyceride absorption. The insoluble fibers seem to have less benefit than the soluble fibers (see Chapter 9, Fiber and Residue Modifications). Although the benefit of increasing dietary fiber intake has not been proven, an increase in the total fiber (soluble and insoluble) intake is recommended. Along with the increased consumption of high fiber plant foods, a proportionately greater consumption of complex carbohydrates and thus a proportionately lower consumption of fat and cholesterol is recommended.[54]

Several studies support the theory that certain polyunsaturated fish oils can reduce the incidence of CHD.[55,56] Particular attention has been given to the omega-3 essential fatty acids, especially eicosapentaenoic acid (EPA) and docosahexaenoic acid (DHA). Ocean fish and shellfish, which contain high concentrations of omega-3 fatty acids, are known to suppress the synthesis of triglycerides when given in large quantities to humans and animals, but they do not lower LDLC or specifically raise HDLC.[57] Based on these findings, along with the potential for undesirable side effects associated with supplementation of the diet, fish oil capsules are not recommended. Rather, the recommendation is for consumption of fish 2 or 3 times per week.

A moderate intake of alcohol (1 to 2 alcoholic beverages per day) may not be harmful, but a high consumption of alcohol is known to affect lipoprotein metabolism in several ways. The effect on LDLC is negligible, but alcohol can elevate triglycerides and HDLC. It is unclear if the rise in HDLC induced by alcohol is of benefit. Because of these uncertainties and because of the potential for other deleterious effects from chronic daily use, the use of alcohol is not advocated as a means of improving blood lipid levels.[31]

Coffee has been linked with heart disease, but studies have reported conflicting results. At the time of this publication, no specific recommendations regarding coffee consumption for the management of hyperlipidemia have been made.[33] Although it is thought that caffeine does not play a causal role in the development of atherosclerosis, caffeine can cause tachycardia, arrhythmias, and palpitations in some people. For these persons, it is wise to limit use of caffeine.

Recent studies suggest that regular consumption of garlic may aid in lowering LDLC and prevent blood from clotting. However, more convincing evidence is necessary before specific recommendations can be made.[58]

Treatment.   Lipid disorders are treated first by modification of the diet and instituting a repetitive aerobic exercise program. After an average time span of 3 to 6 months, drugs may be prescribed in addition to diet and exercise if the hyperlipidemia persists. The effects of diet and of drugs are additive; thus the dietary modification should be continued during the drug therapy. Continuation of the diet is advised even with the normalization of the blood lipids and the lipoprotein pattern.

Goals of Dietary Management

The goals of dietary management (alone or in conjunction with exercise or with lipid lowering medications) are to reduce total fat, saturated fat, and cholesterol intake. This is in an attempt to reduce total cholesterol, LDLC and triglyceride levels, thus also reducing the risk of atherosclerosis or modifying its progression in patients with the disease.

Dietary Recommendations

Various approaches to dietary management have been proposed. Current practice is to tailor the recommendations to the abnormalities of the specific lipid components.

The NCEP and the American Heart Association (AHA) provide a two-step approach that addresses elevated total cholesterol levels.[35,44] (See Chapter 2, American Heart Association Dietary Guidelines, and National Cholesterol Education Program Guidelines for Treatment of Hypercholesterolemia, Table 2-6.) This two-step approach may be justified in some situations but may impose unnecessary restrictions for some patients or fail to address other concerns, such as hypertriglyceridemia and low HDLC. A reasonable approach is to use the AHA and NCEP guidelines with additional considerations to modify recommendations for areas not covered, such as elevated triglycerides. (See Tables 7-13 and 7-14 for general dietary guidelines. An individualized meal plan with specific recommendations for portion sizes will be necessary for dietary intervention for those with hyperlipidemia.)

TABLE 7-13 Dietary Guidelines for Patients with High Cholesterol

Cholesterol can usually be decreased by:
- Decreasing total fat intake
- Decreasing saturated fat intake
- Using unsaturated fats in recommended amounts
- Decreasing high cholesterol food intake
- Reducing weight or maintaining a desirable body weight

| | **How to Decrease Your Cholesterol and Fat Intake** | | |
	Avoid	**Decrease**	**Use Instead**
Milk	Whole milk, cheese, or yogurt made from whole milk. Ice cream, nondairy substitutes	2% milk, ice milk, creamed cottage cheese (4%), part skim milk cheeses, low fat yogurt (1–2%)	Skim or 1% milk, nonfat yogurt, no-fat or fat-free cheese,* low fat cottage cheese (1–2%),* pot cheese
Meat Limit to no more than 6 oz (cooked) per day.	Organ meats, fatty and heavily marbled meats, regular cold cuts, frankfurters, sausage, bacon, friedmeats, canned meats or meat mixtures	Egg yolks, peanut butter, nuts, fish canned in oil, oysters, shrimp	Lean meats, fish, poultry without the skin, egg whites or egg substitutes, water-packed tuna or salmon, low fat cold cuts* and low fat frankfurters,* dried beans
Grain	Rich baked goods—pies, cakes, cookies, donuts, commercial sweet rolls, pastries, and muffins; egg noodles; high fat snack crackers and chips	Crackers, cakes, cookies, muffins, and other bakery products made with unsaturated fat and less than 3 g of fat per serving; check the label	Whole-grain breads and cereals, English muffins, bagels, and bread sticks, rice, pasta, macaroni, potatoes, low fat crackers (such as soda, graham, rye, plain),* angel food cake, plain popcorn, pretzels, vanilla wafers, fig bar cookies
Fat Use fats and oils sparingly.	All fat—especially saturated fats—butter, lard, bacon, fat, gravy and cream sauces, cream, half-and-half, sour cream, cream cheese, hydrogenated margarine and shortening, cocoa butter (found in chocolate), coconut oil, palm oil, palm kernel oil, most nondairy creamers	Mayonnaise, creamy salad dressings, reduced calorie sour cream or cream cheese (not fat-free)	Polyunsaturated oils—safflower, corn, sunflower, soybean, sesame, or cotton-seed; monounsaturated oils—olive, canola or peanut oil; salad dressings made with unsaturated oils listed above; margarine from polyunsaturated oil or margarine where the first ingredient listed is "liquid" oil; no-fat or fat-free spreads, dressings, cream cheeses and sour creams*
Fruit and vegetables	Coconut, fruits and vegetables in cream or creamy sauces, butter, and dips	Avocado, olives	Fresh, frozen, canned, or dried fruits and vegetables

*Low-fat is defined as less than or equal to 3 g of fat per serving. No-fat or fat-free products are defined as 0 to 0.5 g of fat per serving. Check the label.

TABLE 7-14   Dietary Guidelines for Patients with High Triglycerides

Triglycerides can usually be decreased by:
- Reducing weight or maintaining a desirable body weight
- Getting regular physical activity
- Decreasing or avoiding alcohol
- Decreasing sugar and sugar-containing foods

FACTORS HELPFUL IN REDUCING TRIGLYCERIDES
Lose Weight or Maintain a Desirable Weight

- Limit foods high in fat.
- Reduce portion sizes.
- Strive for long-term diet and weight changes.
- Exercise regularly.

Get Regular Physical Activity

- Check with your physician before starting an exercise program.
- Choose an exercise or activity that you enjoy.
- Plan to make exercise a part of your daily routine.

Decrease Your Alcohol Intake

Avoid	Decrease	Use Instead
• Beer, including light beer • Wine • Liquor (i.e., vodka, gin, rum, whiskey) • Liqueurs and cordials	• Low alcohol beer • Wine spritzer (wine and club soda) • Mixed drinks with ½ jigger of liquor	• Club soda and mineral water • Nonalcoholic sparkling fruit juice • Tomato or vegetable juice • Fruit juice (unsweetened) • Fruit juice spritzers (juice and club soda) • Sugar-free carbonated beverages

Decrease Your Sugar Intake

Avoid	Decrease	Use Instead
• Regular sweetened carbonated beverages, lemonade and fruit drinks • Beverages containing sugar or corn sweeteners • Cake, pie, donuts, pastries, ice cream, sherbet, sweetened gelatin • Sugar frosted or highly sweetened cereals • Candy, chocolates, sugar, honey, jam, jelly	• Plain donuts, plain cookies (such as vanilla wafers), plain cakes (such as angel food cake)	• Fruit juices (unsweetened) and spritzers • Sugar free carbonated beverages • Fresh or unsweetened fruit for dessert • Sugar-free hot chocolate • Sugar-free gelatin • Sugar-free pudding • Fruit or foods from the grain group, such as crackers, muffins, bread sticks, or pretzels for snacks

Dietary programs for each of the Fredrickson types of hyperlipidemia have been developed. Difficulties exist in the use of this approach because typing is not universally done and because the lipid profile, and therefore typing category, of an individual may change over time.

Assessment.   A diet history should be taken prior to the formulation of a diet plan. The approximate intake of cholesterol, total fat, saturated fat, unsaturated fat, alcohol, and simple and complex carbohydrate should be determined. In the clinical setting, it is generally sufficient to make an approximation of the intake. For individuals who are overweight, assessment should include a review of the weight history, any previous weight reduction efforts, eating-related behaviors, exercise history, and current medications.

Hypercholesterolemia.   Serum cholesterol abnormalities include (1) an elevation of total cholesterol, (2) an elevated LDLC, (3) low HDLC, and (4) a high ratio of total cholesterol to HDLC and of LDLC to HDLC. When these abnormalities exist, the dietary intake of total fat should be restricted to 30% of total calories (less than 10% saturated, no more than 10% polyunsaturated, and the remainder monounsaturated fat) and less than 300 mg/day of cholesterol. Desirable body weight is encouraged. The dietary guidelines are based on those of the NCEP and the AHA.

The reduction in total fat intake to 30% of total calories necessitates a corresponding increase in complex carbohydrates to meet caloric needs. The carbohydrate fraction then usually contributes 50 to 60% of the kilocalories. Whole-grain bread and cereal products, fruits, and vegetables are encouraged to increase the fiber intake.[41] Protein intake is usually 12 to 15% of the caloric intake. In those patients who remain hyperlipidemic after a 3 month trial, a Step Two diet should be followed: 30% of total calories from fat, with less than 7% saturated fat, and cholesterol less than 200 mg/day.

For individuals who are overweight, weight reduction is advised (see Chapter 8, Obesity, for additional information).[33]

Hypertriglyceridemia.   When the predominant lipid abnormality is the elevation of triglycerides, VLDL is found to be elevated and total cholesterol and LDLC only slightly or moderately increased. Hypertriglyceridemia is often found associated with obesity and marginally or distinctly elevated levels of serum glucose. Dietary measures should emphasize the reduction of weight, avoidance of excess calories, and the restriction of fat and cholesterol in the diet.[38] A program of regular physical activity should also be encouraged. In some patients it is necessary to restrict simple carbohydrates and alcohol.[38] Table 7-14 presents dietary guidelines for patients with high triglyceride levels.

For persons with serum triglycerides that are greater than 250 mg/dl, alcohol intake should be substantially reduced or eliminated. For those with elevations in serum triglycerides greater than 500 mg/dl, abstinence from alcohol is advised.[41]

Weight loss is recommended. For some persons, this may necessitate the achievement of a distinctly lean weight.[38,41] (See Chapter 8, Obesity, for additional information on weight reduction.)

A moderate restriction of total fat to 30% of kilocalories, saturated fat to 10% of kilocalories, and cholesterol to less than 300 mg/day may be helpful in lowering triglyceride levels in many patients. This results in a kilocalorie distribution of approximately 12 to 15% from protein, approximately 30% from fat, and 50 to 60% from carbohydrates. The diet should provide complex carbohydrates, which contain more fiber and fewer calories.[38]

Dietary carbohydrates in large amounts stimulate the synthesis of triglycerides in the liver and promote the secretion of triglyceride-rich VLDL. It appears that this may be exaggerated in patients with hypertriglyceridemia. Some patients may initially experience an increase in triglycerides on Step One and Step Two diets; however, these patients should have more favorable lipoprotein profiles and therefore a lower risk of CHD. Therefore, the diet recommendations regarding limitation of carbohydrates are debatable.[59] The diet should emphasize complex carbohydrates and fiber (inherent in the Step One and Step Two regimens) for the treatment of elevated triglyceride levels.[38]

Some individuals with hypertriglyceridemia are sensitive to simple sugars. This is believed to be due to an exaggerated insulin response to a sucrose load. These individuals can reduce triglyceride levels when they lower their sucrose intake to less than 5% of total calories. The beneficial effects appear to be greater for men than women.[41]

Hypercholesterolemia and Hypertriglyceridemia.   Individuals with both hypercholesterolemia and hypertriglyceridemia should be counseled about measures to reduce both lipid fractions. Modification in intake of fat and cholesterol should be used with additional restrictions of alcohol and possibly reduction of simple carbohydrate levels.

Hypertriglyceridemia (Chylomicrons).   Increased levels of chylomicrons is a rare syndrome in children and adults. The total fat intake should be restricted to very low levels (30 g or less); medium chain triglycerides may be used as a kilocalorie source. (See Chapter 9, Fat Malabsorption, for information on medium chain triglycerides.)

Physicians: How to Order Diet

The diet order should specify *low fat, low cholesterol, and no alcohol or low simple sugar,* if appropriate. The dietitian determines the caloric level and whether or not further modifications (e.g., sodium) are necessary.

References

27. Mahley RW. Atherogenic hyperlipoproteinemia. Med Clin North Am 1982;66:375–402.
28. Davis CE, Rifkind BM, Brenner H, Gordon DJ. A single cholesterol measurement underestimates the risk of coronary heart disease: an empirical example from the Lipid Research Clinic's mortality follow-up study. JAMA 1990;264:3044–3046.
29. Gordon DJ, Rifkind BM. High density lipoprotein: the clinical implications of recent studies. N Engl J Med 1989;321:1311–1316.
30. Lipid Research Clinic. The Lipid Research Clinic's coronary primary prevention trial results: I. Reduction in incidence of coronary heart disease. JAMA 1984;251:351–364.
31. Report of the Expert Panel of Detection, Evaluation, and Treatment of High Blood Cholesterol in Adults. U.S. Department of Health and Human Services, National Institutes of Health; Washington, D.C. NIH Publication No. 89-2925. 1989.
32. Lipid Research Clinic. The Lipid Research Clinic's coronary primary prevention trial results: II. The relationship of reduction in incidence of coronary heart disease to cholesterol lowering. JAMA 1984;251:365–374.

33. Segal DL. The rationale for controlling dietary lipids in the prevention of coronary heart disease. Bull Pan Am Health Organ 1990;24(2):197–209.

34. Friedwald WT, Levy RI, Fredrickson DS. Estimation of the concentration of low density lipoprotein cholesterol in plasma without use of the preparation ultracentrifuge. Clin Chem 1972;18(6):499–502.

35. National Cholesterol Education Program. Second Report of the Expert Panel on Detection, Evaluation, and Treatment of High Blood Cholesterol in Adults (Adult Treatment Panel II). U.S. Department of Health and Human Services, National Institutes of Health, Washington, D.C. NIH Publication No. 93-3093. June 13, 1993.

36. Grundy SM, Goodman DS, Rifkind BM, Cleeman JI. The place of HDL in cholesterol management: a perspective from the National Cholesterol Education Program. Arch Intern Med 1989;149:505–510.

37. Kannel WB. High density lipoproteins: epidemiologic profile and risks of coronary artery disease. Am J Cardiol 1983;52:9B–12B.

38. National Institutes of Health Consensus Development Panel. Triglyceride, high-density lipoprotein, and coronary heart disease. JAMA 1993;269(4):505–510.

39. Austin MA. Plasma triglyceride as a risk factor for coronary heart disease: the epidemiological evidence and beyond. Am J Epidemiol 1989;129(2):249–259.

40. Castelli WP. The triglyceride issue: a view from Framingham. Am Heart J 1986;112(2): 432–437.

41. Reiser S. Metabolic risk factors associated with heart disease and diabetes in carbohydrate-sensitive humans when consuming sucrose as compared to starch. In: Reiser S, ed. Metabolic effects of utilizable dietary carbohydrates. New York: Marcel Dekker, 1982: 239–259.

42. Grundy SM. Management of hyperlipidemia of kidney disease. Kidney Intern 1990;37: 847–853.

43. Hagan J, Wylie-Rosett J. Lipids: impact on dietary prescription in diabetes. J Am Diet Assoc 1989;89(8):1104–1111.

44. Margolis S, Dobs AS. Nutritional management of plasma lipid disorders. J Am Coll Nutr 1989;8(Suppl):33s–45s.

45. Laevelle DE, ed. 1991 Mayo Medical Laboratories test catalog. Rochester, MN: Mayo Medical Laboratories, 1990:279–287.

46. The dietary management of hyperlipoproteinemia: a handbook for physicians and dietitians. DHEW Publication No. (NIH) 80–110. Bethesda, MD: US Department of HEW, 1980.

47. Assmann G, Betteridge DJ, Gotto AM Jr, Steiner G. Management of hypertriglyceridemic patients, treatment classifications and goals. Am J Cardiol 1991;68(3):30A–34A.

48. Grundy SM, Bilheimer D, Blackburn H. Rationale of the diet-heart statement of American Heart Association. Circulation 1982;65:839A–854A.

49. Surgeon General. Reducing the health consequences of smoking: 25 years of progress. U.S. Department of Health and Human Services, National Institutes of Health, Washington, DC, USHH, 1989.

50. Jackson AS, Pollock ML. Generalized equations for predicting body density of men. Br J Nutr 1978;40:497-504.

51. Jackson AS, Pollock ML, Ward A. Generalized equations for predicting body density of women. Med Sci Sports Exerc 1980;12:175–182.

52. Tran ZV, Weltman A. Differential effects of exercise on serum lipid and lipoprotein levels seen with changes in weight. JAMA 1985;254:919–924.

53. Williams JK, Vita JA, Manuck SB, Selwyn AP, Kaplan JR. Psychosocial factors impair vascular response of coronary arteries. Circulation 1991;84(5):2146–2153.

54. Kris-Etherton PM, Krummel D, Dreon D, Mickey S, Wood PD. The effect of diet on plasma lipids, lipoproteins and coronary heart disease. J Am Diet Assoc 1988;88(11): 1373–1400.

55. Nestel PJ. Fish oil attenuates the cholesterol induced rise in lipoprotein cholesterol. Am J Clin Nutr 1986;43:752–757.

56. Dyerberg J. Linolenate-derived polyunsaturated fatty acids and prevention of athero-sclerosis. Nutr Rev 1986;44:125–133.

57. Herold PM, Kinsella JE. Fish oil consumption and decreased risk of cardiovascular disease: a comparison of findings from animal and human feeding trials. Am J Clin Nutr 1986;43:566–598.

58. Mansel P, Reckless JP. Garlic effects of serum lipids, blood pressure, coagulation, platelet aggregation and vasodilation. BMJ 1991;303:379–380.

59. Carmena R, Grundy SM. Management of hypertriglyceridemic patients, dietary management of hypertriglyceridemic patients. Am J Cardiol 1991;68(3):35A–37A.

CARDIAC SURGERY

General Description

The dietary progression for routine and elective postoperative cardiac surgery patients is more rapid than the progression for abdominal surgery. In addition, the diet is controlled in sodium and, when indicated, fat and cholesterol.

Nutritional Inadequacy

The diet for cardiac surgery patients is not inherently lacking in nutrients as compared to the RDA. However, with an actual intake or with weight reduction diets of 1,200 kcal or less, it is difficult to meet the RDA consistently. A daily multiple vitamin supplement that provides nutrients at a level equivalent to the RDA is recommended for persons who consume 1,200 kcal or less or for those who have food aversions or intolerances that greatly limit the variety of their food choices.

Indications and Rationale

Sodium is controlled as a precaution against congestive heart failure. The degree and the duration of the sodium restriction varies with the individual diagnosis and with the response of the patient. The patient follows the sodium restricted diet postoperatively until his or her dismissal from the hospital or for several weeks after dismissal. (See Chapter 7, Hypertension, and Tables 7-4 and 7-5 for the approximate sodium content of foods.) The diet is then advanced to a lesser degree of sodium restriction and followed for several weeks or longer. After this time, many patients resume their usual dietary practices.

The control of cholesterol and total fat intake post surgery serves as an educational tool for those individuals who have a history of hyperlipidemia. It encourages diet modification for reduction of risk factors for CHD. (See Chapter 7, Hyperlipidemia.) Blood cholesterol and triglyceride levels may be altered after cardiac surgery. Therefore, levels of plasma lipids should be rechecked 3 months after surgery for a better measure of long-term trends.

Goals of Dietary Management

The dietary management of individuals who have had cardiac surgery is aimed at providing a diet that will optimize nutritional intake and support the healing process while restricting sodium to help prevent congestive failure. Modification of the diet to reduce hyperlipidemia is prescribed for individuals who have or are at risk for CHD.

Dietary Recommendations

Table 7-15 summarizes the general types of heart surgery and the dietary recommendations that are usually prescribed.[60-64]

Postsurgical cardiac patients may experience complications of gastrointestinal distress and of decreased appetite. Medications such as Persantine™, Digoxin™, and Procainamide™, as well as the cardiotonic, diuretic, and antibiotic drug groups, may have a tendency to result in nausea and intolerance to many foods. This may make it difficult to achieve recommended kilocalorie and protein intake.[65]

Monitoring of dietary intake and the nutritional plan of care needs close attention during hospitalization in order to assist patients in choosing a varied and an adequate intake within the limits of the prescribed dietary modifications.

While it is unlikely that the patient will eat more than the planned amounts, it should be remembered that eating a large meal may have an adverse effect on the heart that has only marginal functional capacity. Larger meals can interfere with breathing by impairing diaphragmatic motion through abdominal distention and by increasing the demand for cardiac output through increasing the metabolic rate. Therefore, some patients may benefit from adjustments in their meals, such as small, frequent feedings. Cool items are

TABLE 7-15   Cardiac Surgery and Dietary Recommendations[60-64]

Surgical Procedure	Diet and Progression
Repair of complex forms of congenital heart defects	Begin with 20 mEq of sodium; advance to 90 mEq of sodium or a No Extra Salt diet (usually 90 to 120 mEq of sodium daily)
Prosthetic valve replacement	Begin with sodium restriction (levels range from 20 to 90 mEq at discretion of physician); advance to 90 mEq of sodium or a No Extra Salt diet (usually 90 to 120 mEq of sodium daily)
Repair of simpler forms of congenital heart defects (e.g., atrial septal defect, isolated pulmonary stenosis)	Begin with sodium restriction (levels range from 20 to 90 mEq at discretion of physician); advance to usual diet
Coronary artery bypass grafting	Begin with sodium restriction (levels range from 90 to 120 mEq at discretion of physician); low fat, low cholesterol

often more acceptable (e.g., cottage cheese and fruit plates, milk drinks, fruits and juices, sherbet or pudding). Meat, potatoes, and vegetables are added gradually as tolerated.

Physicians: How to Order Diet

The diet order should specify *initial level of sodium*. This is automatically continued throughout each stage of the postoperative series (clear liquid, full liquid, and soft diets). The physician should also indicate if the diet should be modified to help prevent hyperlipidemia.

Requests for instruction in the home diet should also indicate the level of sodium restriction and the estimated time duration that sodium restriction will be necessary.

References

60. Kris-Etherton PM, ed. Cardiovascular disease: nutrition for prevention and treatment. Chicago: American Dietetic Association, 1990:155–157.
61. Blankenhorn DM, Johnson RL, Mack WJ, Elzein HA, Vailas LI. The influence of diet on the appearance of new lesions in human coronary arteries. JAMA 1991;263:1646–1652.
62. Driscoll DJ. Evaluation of the cyanotic newborn. In: Gillette PC, ed. The pediatric clinics of North America. Philadelphia: WB Saunders, 1990:1–23.
63. Kern LS, O'Brien P. The Fontan Procedure. Heart Lung 1985;14:457–467.
64. O'Brien P, Elizson M. The child following the Fontan Procedure: nursing strategies. AACN Clin Iss Crit Care Nurs 1990;14:457–467.
65. U.S. Pharmacopeial Convention. Drug information for the health care professional, Rockville MD, U.S. Pharmacopeial Convention, 1991.

CONGESTIVE HEART FAILURE

General Description

The diet for congestive heart failure is restricted in sodium. The diet is restricted more stringently for more severe degrees of failure. Occasionally, fluids are restricted as well. Smaller, more frequent meals are provided in order to minimize abdominal distention and lessen the demand for cardiac output through control of the thermic effect of food. For the obese patient, weight reduction is also necessary to aid in reduction of cardiac workload. In some cases, however, the patient is underweight with poor nutritional status. The severe form of this condition is called cardiac cachexia, and the development of cardiac cachexia is multifactorial. Contributing factors may include reduced food intake secondary to anorexia, increased circulating levels of tumor necrosis factor, possible hypermetabolism, and drug-nutrient interactions.[66,67] Special consideration and nutritional intervention are important for those patients who are at nutritional risk.

Nutritional Inadequacy

The dietary management of congestive heart failure is not inherently lacking in nutrients. Nutritional assessment of each patient and appropriate supplementation is recommended. Individuals with intakes of 1,200 kcal or less would benefit from a multiple vitamin supplement.

Indications and Rationale

Congestive heart failure stems from a mechanical inadequacy of the heart to maintain the circulation of blood to the tissues. Congestion and edema develop in the tissues, particularly in the lungs, liver, bowel, and legs. The condition is characterized by decreased blood flow to the kidneys and by retention of both sodium and water. Edema of the lower legs and shortness of breath are both common manifestations of congestive failure.[68]

To minimize the sodium and fluid retention, the hospitalized patient in severe cardiac failure may be given a diet that contains 45 mEq or less of sodium per day. For the patient who is in moderate failure, a 90 mEq or less sodium-restricted diet may be specified. Upon dismissal from the hospital, usually 90 to 150 mEq of sodium in the diet each day is recommended, and close compliance is encouraged. Potassium supplementation may be prescribed for patients treated with diuretics, which induce potassium depletion. However, for patients treated with potassium-sparing diuretics and angiotensin-converting enzyme inhibitors, which tend to elevate serum potassium levels, there should be caution against the use of potassium-containing salt substitutes.[69] Fluids may be restricted if hyponatremia occurs. A fluid restriction of 1.5 to 2.0 L/day is common; however, for the patient in acute or severe failure, a fluid restriction of less than 1.0 L/day may be required. Smaller, frequent feedings are usually better tolerated and help to decrease cardiac workload.[70] Limiting caffeine-containing beverages lowers the risk of increased heart rate or dysrhythmia.[70]

Energy requirements for the patient with congestive heart failure may be 30 to 50% above basal needs because of increased cardiac and pulmonary expenditure.[66] The cachectic patient needs additional calories in order to prevent further catabolism. Because of the difficulties that may occur with overfeeding, it is important to proceed with caution when attempting to increase calories in order to replete patients' stores. Food preferences of the patient should be accommodated and oral intake encouraged. Liquid nutritional supplements of high nutrient density may be provided to increase the calorie and protein content of the diet. For the patient who cannot meet nutritional needs through oral intake, enteral or parenteral nutrition may be necessary.

Physicians: How to Order Diet

The diet order should indicate a *specific level of sodium* (45 or 90 mEq of sodium) or a NES diet (90 to 150 mEq of sodium). The physician should specify the *level of fluid restriction,* if necessary, and additional dietary modifications that may be required.

References

66. Poindexter SM, Dear WE, Dudrick SJ. Nutrition in congestive heart failure. Nutr Clin Pract 1986;1:83–88.
67. Levine B, Kalman J, Mayer L, Fillet HM, Packer M. Elevated circulating levels of tumor necrosis factor in severe chronic heart failure. N Engl J Med 1990;323:236–241.

68. Wright SM. Pathophysiology of congestive heart failure. J Cardiovasc Nurs 1990;4(3):1–16.

69. Arai AE, Greenberg BH. Medical management of congestive heart failure. Western J Med 1990;Oct:406–414.

70. Klatsky AL. Coffee use prior to myocardial infarction: heavier intake may increase the risk. Am J Epidemiol 1990;132(3):479–488.

MYOCARDIAL INFARCTION

General Description

The dietary program for patients in the coronary care unit routinely consists of the control of sodium, cholesterol, fat, kilocalories, and the restriction of caffeine-containing beverages.

Nutritional Inadequacy

The dietary recommendations for patients in the coronary care unit are not inherently lacking in nutrients when compared to the RDA. A daily multiple vitamin that provides nutrients at a level equivalent to the RDA is recommended for persons requiring a long-term diet of 1,200 kcal/day or less.

Indications and Rationale

The diet is intended to reduce cardiac workload and initiate modification of diet-related cardiac risk factors.

During the first several days or weeks after a myocardial infarction, the patient may experience congestive heart failure. The control of sodium in the diet lessens the cardiac workload, a precaution against congestive failure, and favors the control of hypertension if that is a factor.[71] (See Chapter 7, the sections on Hypertension and Congestive Heart Failure.) For patients with normal cardiac function after a myocardial infarction and no hypertension, sodium restriction is less of a concern.

In the intensive care unit or post myocardial infarction, caffeine is totally restricted in order to avoid myocardial stimulation.[72] However, for the long-term dietary care of patients who have had myocardial infarction and hence are vulnerable to second attacks, it is prudent to recommend that caffeine-containing beverages be limited to no more than 3 c/day.[73,74]

Ingestion of food significantly increases heart rate, blood pressure, and cardiac output. Large feedings may increase myocardial oxygen demand by increasing splanchnic blood flow. Smaller, frequent feedings are usually better tolerated[75] and are therefore recommended during the acute postinfarction period.

The control of cholesterol and total fat intake postinfarction serves to prepare the patient for lifelong adherence to a low cholesterol, low fat diet and encourages diet modification for reduction of cardiac risk factors (see Chapter 7, the section on Hyperlipidemia).

General Dietary Recommendations

Mayo patients with myocardial infarction are often placed in a three-phase Cardiac Rehabilitation Program.

Phase I (Inpatient). The diet is low in sodium (less than or equal to 90 mEq each day), cholesterol, and fat. It begins with liquids during the first 24 hours and progresses as tolerated to a normal consistency diet. The meals are small. Caffeine-containing beverages are restricted. If weight reduction is indicated, kilocalorie needs are assessed with a view toward the dismissal diet. Prior to dismissal, the patient is educated in an appropriate individualized diet.

Phase II (Outpatient—Monitored). Phase II is approximately 8 weeks in duration. The diet information provided during Phase I is reviewed, reinforced, and modified as necessary. The patient returns at 3, 6, and 9 month intervals for the evaluation of serum lipids and for reinforcement of diet and exercise compliance. (See Chapter 7, the sections on Hyperlipidemia and Hypertension.)

Phase III (Outpatient—Lifelong, Nonmonitored). Phase III is a minimum of 6 months beyond Phase II. It is community based and provides education, prevention, support, and rehabilitation.

Physicians: How to Order Diet

The diet order should indicate *postmyocardial infarction diet.* The standard diet order is usually 90 mEq of sodium, low cholesterol. Alternatively, the individual dietary components may be specified: level of sodium, cholesterol, fat, and caffeine restriction. Any additional dietary or nutritional modifications (e.g., diabetes, fluid restriction) should also be indicated.

References

71. Kaplan NM. Nonpharmacological control of high blood pressure. Am J Hypertension 1989;2:555–595.
72. Meyers MG, Harris L. High dose caffeine and ventricular arrhythmias. Can J Cardiol 1990;6:95–98.
73. Klatsky AL, Friedman GD, Armstrong MA. Coffee use prior to myocardial infarction restudied: heavier intake may increase the risk. Am J Epidemiol 1990;132:479–488.
74. Grobbee DE, Rimm EB, Giovannucci E, Colditz G, Stampfer M, Willett W. Coffee, caffeine and cardiovascular disease in men. N Engl J Med 1990;323:1026–1032.
75. Bagatell CJ, Heymsfield SB. Effect of meal size on myocardial oxygen requirements: implications for postmyocardial infarction diet. Am J Clin Nutr 1984;39:421–426.

8 / *Endocrine/Metabolism Diseases and Disorders*

DIABETES MELLITUS

General Description

The diets that are used as part of the management of diabetes mellitus are controlled in kilocalories, protein, fat, and carbohydrate. Additional dietary considerations include consistency in the timing of meals, in the distribution of kilocalories and/or carbohydrate among the meals, and in control of the intake of kilocalories, saturated fat, and cholesterol. The nature of the specific dietary recommendations and the importance of additional considerations vary with the type of diabetes mellitus and with the total medical management program.

Nutritional Inadequacy

The diet recommended for diabetes mellitus is adequate in nutrients when compared to the Recommended Dietary Allowance (RDA). However, for diets of 1,200 kcal or less, it is difficult to meet the RDA consistently. A daily multiple vitamin supplement is recommended for persons who consume diets of 1,200 kcal or less.

Indications and Rationale

Diabetes is a heterogeneous disease with no single cause and no standard treatment. It is necessary to individualize the care of each person according to the nature and severity of the disease.

The following is a summary of the classification of diabetes and other categories of glucose intolerance. All categories are associated with hyperglycemia, but the cause, severity, and other clinical characteristics vary. Almost all persons with diabetes can be considered to have either noninsulin-dependent diabetes (NIDDM) or insulin-dependent diabetes (IDDM), although many distinct diabetic states exist that do not strictly fit in either classification.[1,2]

Insulin-Dependent Diabetes Mellitus.   IDDM accounts for 10 to 15% of persons with diabetes and usually appears before the age of 40 but may develop at any age. Classic symptoms include polydipsia, polyphagia, and polyuria. Sudden onset of these symptoms is common, with a progression to ketoacidosis and coma in a short period of time if untreated. IDDM is associated with a total or near total loss of the capacity of beta cells to secrete insulin. Insulin therapy, rather than the use of oral hypoglycemic agents, is required to prevent ketosis. Conventional insulin therapy usually consists of one or two injections daily of an intermediate, or a mixture of intermediate and regular insulin. The diet therapy emphasizes good nutrition with modifications of the diet to reduce wide glucose swings and hopefully to reduce the risk of atherosclerotic and microvascular complications. Special modifications are tailored to the specific insulin program.

An intensive insulin therapy program for IDDM is a program of treatment intended for individuals with unstable patterns of glycemia who are ready to comply with a relatively elaborate mode of treatment. The plasma glucose level in the nondiabetic is maintained within relatively narrow limits. The pancreas secretes a larger amount of insulin during and immediately after meals and supplies a lower level of insulin between meals and at night. The intensive insulin therapy program seeks to imitate this pattern of delivery of insulin by an injection of rapidly acting (regular) insulin before meals and an injection of longer acting (ultralente or NPH) once or twice daily. The premeal injections of regular insulin are adjusted according to the capillary blood glucose level, which is determined prior to the injection. Insulin pumps may be used as an alternative to the manual injection of insulin. They are worn externally, with a needle placed subcutaneously, and are programmed to deliver a bolus of regular insulin before each meal and a continuous basal infusion of regular insulin.

A weight gain follows the initiation of intensive insulin therapy for IDDM because of the diminished glycosuria and its associated caloric wastage. Therefore, the caloric allowance may require an adjustment downward. If changes in meal size or composition are made, the program of intensive insulin therapy provides instructions for adjusting the premeal dose of regular insulin. With intensive insulin therapy, usually only 15 g of carbohydrate (or 1 starch exchange) is needed for a bedtime snack; midmorning and midafternoon snacks are usually not necessary.

Non–Insulin-Dependent Diabetes Mellitus.   NIDDM accounts for 85 to 90% of persons with diabetes. Although it usually develops in the middle-aged, overweight individual, it occasionally occurs in persons who are under age 40 and who are not overweight. The onset is usually gradual, characterized by subtle or no symptoms, and is often detected by screening blood tests. Since polyuria, polydipsia, and weight loss or polyphagia are a consequence of the large amounts of glucose in the urine, these symptoms may be absent in NIDDM. Persons having NIDDM have some pancreatic insulin production and do not require injected insulin to prevent ketosis. However, the person with NIDDM may need to use oral hypoglycemic agents or insulin for the correction of symptomatic or persistent hyperglycemia. A common diagnostic mistake is to assume that all patients receiving insulin have IDDM. Mild ketosis may develop under special circumstances, such as in episodes of infection or stress. Individuals who have NIDDM, particularly those who are obese, may have resistance to both endogenous and injected insulin.

In the obese individual with NIDDM, glucose tolerance may improve with weight loss. Control of the total kilocalorie intake is the most important dietary measure in NIDDM. Often, glucose values improve remarkably within days after a kilocalorie restriction has begun, and further improvement results with weight loss in some individuals. Further modification of the diet may be recommended in an attempt to reduce the risk of atherosclerotic and microvascular complications.

Secondary Diabetes Mellitus. Diabetes may occur as the result of pancreatitis, surgical removal of the pancreas, Cushing's disease, pheochromocytoma, and pharmacological doses of glucocorticoids (e.g., Prednisone) or other diabetogenic hormones or drugs. Diabetes may resolve if the primary disorder or the cause is corrected. Dietary recommendations are dependent on the treatment modality, whether the diabetes is controlled by diet alone or by diet in conjunction with diabetes medication.

Impaired Glucose Tolerance (IGT). Persons diagnosed with IGT are generally asymptomatic. Subtypes of IGT include nonobese, obese, and those associated with pancreatic disease, diabetogenic hormones or drugs, and insulin receptor abnormalities. Insulin resistance has been implicated as one of the underlying abnormalities causing IGT.[3] IGT may represent a risk factor in the development of NIDDM leading to neuropathy, coronary heart disease, and macrovascular disease. Screening for IGT alone is not justified, but, a fasting plasma glucose level greater than 115 mg/dl is an indication for diagnostic testing for diabetes.[4] Further measurements of fasting and postprandial plasma glucose should resolve the question of whether the person with marginal values and findings, such as neuropathy that might suggest the presence of diabetes, does indeed have diabetes.[5] Glucose tolerance tests are less used for this purpose than in previous years. Diet therapy and a regular exercise program should be initiated with emphasis on the correction of obesity.

Gestational Diabetes Mellitus (GDM). Gestational diabetes is defined as glucose intolerance that begins or is recognized during pregnancy. Persons with diabetes who become pregnant are not included in this category. GDM is associated with increased perinatal complications and with an increased risk for the progression to diabetes within 5 to 10 years after parturition. The causes of GDM are not completely understood but may be due in part to insulin resistance. Insulin resistance may be related to two factors: (1) increased levels of various hormones, including estrogen, progesterone, and human placental lactogen, and (2) increased weight. Both of these factors increase the requirement for insulin.[6] Good glycemic control is required during pregnancy to prevent fetal complications.[7] Diet therapy emphasizes good nutrition with a controlled intake of kilocalories throughout the day (3 meals and 3 snacks) and an appropriate weight gain. Specific recommendations for a diet during pregnancy are discussed on pp. 167 and 168.

Goals of Dietary Management

The goals of dietary management for diabetes mellitus are: (1) a nutritionally adequate intake with a caloric level that is appropriate for the achievement and/or the maintenance of a desirable weight, (2) the prevention of hyperglycemia and

TABLE 8-1   Priorities for Dietary Management of Insulin-Dependent Diabetes Mellitus (IDDM)

High Priority	Lower Priority
• Consume adequate kilocalories to maintain desirable weight. • Keep the timing of meals and the composition of the diet consistent from day to day, with the carbohydrate content fairly evenly divided from meal to meal. • Limit simple carbohydrate to 10–15% of total kilocalories. • Depending upon the insulin regimen, plan for a bedtime snack to prevent nocturnal hypoglycemia; take midmorning and midafternoon snacks, if needed, to match the food intake to the peak insulin action. • Plan for food to be taken to correct hypoglycemic episodes. • Plan for food and fluids to be taken for periods of increased physical activity and during illness. • Make modifications in the diet for hypertension, hyperlipidemia, and/or renal insufficiency, if present.	• If obese, follow a low kilocalorie diet to reduce weight, then a kilocalorie-controlled diet to maintain a desirable weight (persons with IDDM are usually not obese).

hypoglycemia, and (3) the reduction of the risk of atherosclerosis and microvascular complications. The recently released findings of the Diabetes Control and Complications Trial have shown that intensive insulin therapy along with dietary measures can help contribute to normalization of blood glucose levels. Euglycemia can significantly delay or prevent long-term complications of diabetes.[8] Tables 8-1 and 8-2 list priorities for meal planning. The priorities listed are of equal importance within each group.

Dietary Recommendations

Weight Reduction and/or Maintenance of Desirable Weight.   The adult with IDDM is usually lean and should receive sufficient kilocalories to maintain a desirable body weight. Additional kilocalories and nutrients are warranted for periods of increased requirements (e.g., pregnancy and lactation), as in the nondiabetic individual. Those who are overweight may benefit from weight reduction.

The majority of individuals with NIDDM are overweight. Weight reduction helps to correct cellular resistance to insulin action and may even result in a return of the plasma glucose levels to the normal range. A kilocalorie-restricted diet and regular exercise are of primary importance in achieving desirable weight. Weight control may also reduce the individual's risk for cardiovascular disease through the reduction of blood lipids and blood pressure.

TABLE 8-2 Priorities for Dietary Management for Non–Insulin-Dependent Diabetes Mellitus (NIDDM)

NIDDM Managed by Diet	NIDDM Managed by Diet and Oral Hypoglycemic Agents	NIDDM Managed by Diet and Insulin
HIGH PRIORITY		
• If obese, follow a low kilocalorie diet to reduce weight, then a kilocalorie-controlled diet to maintain a desirable weight.	• If obese, follow a low kilocalorie diet to reduce weight, then a kilocalorie-controlled diet to maintain desirable weight.	• If obese, follow a low kilocalorie diet to reduce weight, then a kilocalorie-controlled diet to maintain a desirable weight.
• Limit simple carbohydrate to 10–15% of total kilocalories.	• Limit simple carbohydrate to 10–15% of total kilocalories.	• Limit simple carbohydrate to 10–15% of total kilocalories.
• Make modifications in the diet for hypertension, hyperlipidemia and/or renal insufficiency, if present.·	• Make modifications in the diet for hypertension, hyperlipidemia, and/or renal insufficiency, if present.	• Keep the timing of the meals and the composition of the diet consistent from day to day, with the carbohydrate content of the diet fairly evenly divided from meal to meal.
	• Keep the timing of the meals and the composition of the diet consistent from day to day with the carbohydrate content evenly divided from meal to meal.	• Plan a bedtime snack to prevent nocturnal hypoglycemia; mid-morning and midafternoon snacks, if needed, to match the food intake to the peak insulin action.
	• Plan a bedtime snack to prevent nocturnal hypoglycemia when a long acting oral hypoglycemic agent (e.g., chlorpropamide, glyburide) is used.	• Depending upon the insulin regimen, plan for food to be taken to correct hypoglycemic episodes.
		• Plan for food and fluids to be taken for periods of increased physical activity or during illness.
		• Make modifications in the diet for hypertension, hyperlipidemia, and/or renal insufficiency, if present.
LOWER PRIORITY		
• Keep the timing of the meals and the composition of the diet consistent from day to day with the carbohydrate content evenly divided from meal to meal.	• Take midmorning or midafternoon snacks if between meal intervals are extended or if there is a history of hypoglycemia.	
	• Plan for food and fluids to be taken for periods of increased physical activity or during illness.	
	• Plan a bedtime snack to prevent nocturnal hypoglycemia when a short acting oral hypoglycemic agent (e.g., acetohexamide, tolbutamide, tolazamide, glipizide) is used.	

The desirable or the goal weight for the person with NIDDM is the same as for other obese persons. (See Chapter 8, Obesity.) Standard height-weight tables can be used as an initial guide. However, other factors, such as the individual's weight history and medical history, should be considered. There is evidence that insulin resistance is related to fat cell morphology and the pattern of body fat distribution.[9] Therefore, some individuals whose weight is within the standards of the height-weight tables may achieve improved plasma glucose control through weight reduction. Individuals who are morbidly obese may normalize their plasma glucose levels at weights that are substantially greater than the statistical norms.

Very Low Calorie Diets (VLCDs).   Recent studies have suggested that VLCDs, which provide only 500 to 800 kcal/day, can be useful in treating selected individuals who are severely obese and have NIDDM. These people continue to secrete some insulin, but have failed to respond to treatment with oral hypoglycemic agents.[10-12] Under professional medical supervision, short-term VLCDs have been found to be safe for rapid weight loss and for improving plasma glucose control. Decreases in blood pressure and plasma lipids have also been seen.[13,14] VLCDs should contain adequate protein of high biological quality and be given in conjunction with multivitamin, mineral, and potassium supplements to meet the RDA. Concern remains over the safety and effectiveness of the long-term use of VLCDs. Sustained weight loss is best achieved through a long-term weight management program with behavior modification. (See Chapter 8, Obesity.)

Meal Timing and Consistency in Composition of Meals.   For persons taking diabetes medication, keeping the number of meals, the scheduled times for eating, and the composition of meals relatively consistent from day to day is important. Food intake should be synchronized with the prescribed insulin program. It is recommended that individuals who receive conventional insulin therapy consume 3 meals per day spaced 4 to 5 hours apart, and a bedtime snack. A consistent distribution of kilocalories, protein, and carbohydrate among the main meals helps to prevent large glucose excursions and curtail hypoglycemia. If there is a consistent tendency toward hyperglycemia or hypoglycemia at a given time of day, adjustments in the timing, size, and number of meals and snacks may improve glycemic control. These adjustments may alleviate the need for changing from a simple to a more complex insulin regimen. Somewhat more flexibility in timing and meal size is possible with intensive insulin therapy. If insulin or hypoglycemic agents are not used, the timing and composition of the meals are less crucial.

Kilocalories.   See Chapter 3, Nutritional and Screening Assessment, for the methods used for estimation of caloric needs. For persons who require weight reduction, see Chapter 8, Obesity, for the determination of caloric level and the recommended rate of weight loss.

Distribution of Kilocalories.   Following the American Diabetes Association guidelines, the recommended distribution of kilocalories is 12 to 20% of kilocalories as protein, 20 to 30% of kilocalories as fat, and 55 to 60% of kilocalories as carbohydrate.[9]

The protein requirements for individuals with diabetes are the same as for other individuals. The amount of protein in the diet meets and may exceed the RDA of 0.8 g/kg of body weight. The percentage of kilocalories from protein may be as much as 20% in diets of 1,200 kcal or less and may decrease to 12% at higher caloric levels.

There is no known advantage associated with a protein intake that is in excess of the RDA. In fact, high levels of protein intake may be disadvantageous.[15] The person with diabetes (both IDDM and NIDDM) is vulnerable to renal complications (diabetic nephropathy) that may progress to chronic renal failure. This process may possibly accelerate with a high protein diet.[16] For the person who has only a slight elevation of creatinine levels (perhaps 1.5 to 2 mg/dl, it is prudent to keep the protein level at approximately the RDA (0.8 g/kg of body weight). Further reductions in protein intake may be necessary with the progression of renal disease (see Chapter 14, Renal Diseases and Disorders).

The person with diabetes is at an increased risk of premature atherosclerosis.[17] Recommendations for fat intake are consistent with the guidelines of the American Heart Association (see Chapter 2). Generally, it is recommended that total daily fat intake be limited to 30% or less of total kilocalories, that polyunsaturated fats be used in preference to saturated fats, and that cholesterol be limited to 300 mg or less. For persons with hypercholesterolemia, further reductions in total fat and cholesterol are warranted (see Chapter 7, Hyperlipidemia). For those who otherwise have a low risk of cardiovascular disease and have blood cholesterol levels less than the 75th percentile, the usual admonitions regarding cholesterol and saturated fat restriction may be liberalized. A less restrictive fat allowance may also be warranted for some individuals in order to obtain compliance with the total management plan. Generally, there is less emphasis on cholesterol and fat restrictions for the very elderly person with diabetes.

Carbohydrates ideally constitute 55 to 60% of total kilocalories. These higher levels of carbohydrate do not impede good glycemic control and generally allow a corresponding decrease in the fat intake, which may be advantageous in reducing blood lipids and the risk of atherosclerosis.[18] An increased use of plant fibers from whole-grain bread and cereal products, legumes, fruits, and vegetables is encouraged because of its beneficial effect on blood glucose and overall health.

Restriction of Simple Carbohydrates. Simple carbohydrates are defined as monosaccharides and disaccharides. Lactose, sucrose, and fructose are those most prevalent as an inherent constituent of usual foods. The most widely used sweeteners (table sugar, corn syrup, and honey) are composed almost exclusively of sucrose and fructose.

It has been common practice to limit the intake of simple carbohydrate, particularly from sweeteners, in the diet of persons with diabetes on the premise that simple carbohydrates are quickly absorbed and cause a rapid postprandial rise in the plasma glucose concentrations. Research, which suggests that some complex carbohydrates produce greater plasma glucose excursions than foods predominantly composed of simple carbohydrates, has prompted reevaluation of long-standing assumptions.[19] Simple carbohydrates have less effect on the blood glucose when ingested as part of a mixed meal. However, more evidence is necessary before radical changes in amounts of sugar allowed can be recommended.

At present, the recommendation remains that simple carbohydrates be limited to 10 to 15% of total kilocalories because they provide suboptimal nutritional value and an excess consumption may impede weight control efforts. The excessive use of simple carbohydrates also has the potential to elevate the blood triglyceride levels.

Glycemic Effects of Carbohydrates. The effects of carbohydrates on plasma glucose levels are not as clear-cut as once believed. Reports have focused attention on the differences in plasma glucose response to simple sugars (mono- and disaccharides) and to complex carbohydrates (polysaccharides).[19-21] While the studies have challenged current concepts and practices, they have not provided final answers.[22,23]

Factors that have been said to lower the glycemic response by delaying the digestion and/or the absorption of food include: (1) fibrous coatings on food such as legumes, (2) raw foods, (3) substances such as pectins, phytates, tannins, and (4) fiber content, particularly of guar and pectin. Carbohydrate eaten over several hours as compared to carbohydrate eaten over a short period of time tends to reduce the glycemic response. Carbohydrates eaten separately or as part of a meal may produce different plasma glucose responses. Each individual may respond differently to various carbohydrates.

At this time there is insufficient information to make a precise appraisal of the glycemic response to foods, especially when they are eaten as part of a mixed meal. Some studies[24,25] indicate that people with NIDDM show little positive response to a mixed meal of low glycemic foods, while other studies[25,26] indicate that there may be some benefit to people with both NIDDM and IDDM. Current recommendations, based on those of the American Diabetes Association,[26] are to place more emphasis, when possible, on the use of carbohydrate-containing foods that produce the smallest rise in the plasma glucose level and less emphasis on those associated with higher glycemic responses. The consumption of a modest amount of sucrose is acceptable, contingent on the maintenance of metabolic control. In addition, regular monitoring of blood glucose level can be an effective tool for assessing individual responses to foods. Further research is necessary before major changes can be made in the Food Exchange Lists.

Fiber. High fiber intake appears to be beneficial for individuals with diabetes.[10,27-30] Studies have suggested that an increase in the intake of soluble dietary fiber can lead to decreases in plasma glucose and glycosuria and a reduction in insulin requirements.[10,27,28,30] Soluble fiber sources include oat products and legumes, dried beans, peas, lentils, fruits, and vegetables. These are thought to delay gastric emptying and prolong intestinal transit time. They appear to have greater effect in lowering plasma glucose[10,27,28,30] and serum cholesterol and triglyceride levels[10,27,28] than insoluble fiber. Soluble fiber supplements (guar gum and pectin) also effectively improve glucose and insulin response.[30] It has been estimated that one needs to consume at least 35 to 40 g of primarily soluble dietary fiber (an amount that may not be tolerated by everyone) to improve glycemic control.[10,27,28] Some studies suggest that diets that include up to 50 g (25 g per 1,000 kcal) of fiber may also be beneficial.[10,27,28] There are conflicting reports regarding the practicality of long-term adherence to such high fiber diets.[28,29]

It is prudent to encourage a reasonable increase in dietary fiber intake through emphasis on the use of whole grains, legumes, and fresh or lightly cooked vegetables and fruits. This is most effectively accomplished if planned as part of a high complex carbohydrate diet (55 to 60% of total kilocalories as carbohydrate).[10,27]

It is important to note that high fiber diets are contraindicated for persons with gastroparesis because of the risk of inducing a gastric bezoar and obstruction.[31]

Further information about the high fiber diet appears in Chapter 9, Fiber and Residue Modifications.

Sweeteners

There is widespread use of sweeteners in the Western diet, and therefore there is a demand by individuals with diabetes for acceptable substitute sweeteners. Although the use of these substitutes is not advocated, a dietitian can advise persons on the appropriateness of their use. Considerations include the characteristics of the desired sweetener, the caloric contribution, the safety of the desired amount, and the individual's glycemic control and lipid status. Alternative sweeteners can be classified as nutritive or non-nutritive.[32]

Nutritive Sweeteners. Nutritive sweeteners are identical in caloric value by weight to sucrose (table sugar).[33] They include sorbitol, fructose, corn syrups, dextrose, mannitol, and xylitol (see Appendix 9).[32]

Persons with diabetes should restrict their intake of nutritive sweeteners because of their caloric content and the resultant elevation of lipids and plasma glucose levels. If they are used in substantial amounts, as in a candy bar or dessert, these sweeteners should be included as part of a meal, with their caloric contribution included in the day's total calories.

Non-nutritive Sweeteners. Non-nutritive sweeteners are characterized by an intensely sweet taste. While some contain calories, non-nutritive sweeteners are generally used in such small quantities that they do not make a significant contribution to caloric intake.[33] The three non-nutritive sweeteners that are currently available in the United States are saccharin, aspartame, and acesulfame K. Cyclamate and stevioside are available in other countries. Other non-nutritive sweeteners awaiting FDA approval are aspartame encapsulate, alitame, and sucralose (see Appendix 9, Nutritive and Non-nutritive Sweeteners).

The American Diabetes Association finds the use of saccharin acceptable for people with diabetes when used within the FDA's established safety levels (500 mg/day for children or 1,000 mg/day for adults).[32,34] However, there is some question about the safety of saccharin, and continued research is needed.[32]

From clinical studies, aspartame demonstrates no adverse effect on diabetes control. The American Diabetes Association has approved the use of foods that contain aspartame for persons with diabetes.[34] The recommended safe limit for aspartame is 50 mg/kg of body weight per day.[32-36] Aspartame is known commercially as Nutrasweet™ or Equal™. There has been concern about the effect of aspartame on people with phenylketonuria due to the phenylalanine content. Therefore products containing aspartame should be avoided by these individuals. It should be noted that there is little information about the effects of non-nutritive sweeteners during pregnancy.[32] Further studies have been recommended to address the safety of aspartame (and other sweeteners) use in children and in pregnant or lactating women.[36,37] At this time the use of any artificial sweetener during pregnancy is not routinely recommended. However, some physicians allow a limit of 2 to 3 artificially sweetened products per day.

Acesulfame K is the newest non-nutritive sweetener available for use in the United States. It is available commercially as Sunette™ or Sweet One™. The safety level established by the World Health Organization is 0 to 9 mg/kg of body weight; by the FDA, 0 to 15 mg/kg.[32]

Dietetic Foods.   Foods for special dietary use are widely available and are of interest to persons with diabetes because of the reduced caloric and/or sugar content. Individuals should be taught to read the nutrition labels in order to recognize the energy and nutritional value of such dietetic products.

A dietetic product that contains less than 20 kcal per serving may be used as a "free food" at meals or as snacks. "Free foods" should be limited to a total of 20 kcal per meal or to a total of 60 kcal maximum distributed throughout the day.

Foods that are represented as useful in the diet of a diabetic must be accompanied by a nutrition label and by the statement "Diabetics: This product may be useful in your diet on the advice of a physician." The use of dietetic products, such as dietetic candy, cookies, chocolate, and ice cream, that are of high caloric density and contain sorbitol or mannitol is generally discouraged. Appendix 8 discusses food labeling. Appendix 9 presents information on nutritive and non-nutritive sweeteners.

Alcohol.   Intake of alcohol should be limited. It is high in kilocalories, lacks essential nutrients, and may promote ketoacidosis, hypertriglyceridemia, and alcohol-induced hypoglycemia.[39,40]

For individuals who consume lower calorie diets to promote weight reduction, alcohol should be used infrequently, if at all, because of its high caloric content. On the other hand, for individuals taking insulin who are at desirable weight and in good glycemic control, alcohol may be consumed occasionally (no more than 2 drinks per week) without altering the meal plan. It is important that no food be omitted, because alcohol may cause hypoglycemia. It is recommended that alcoholic beverages be consumed immediately before, during, or directly following a meal.

If an individual consumes more than 2 drinks per week, alcohol calories should be included as part of the daily intake. This is achieved by exchanging alcohol calories for fat calories. It is important to emphasize that the nutrient content and metabolic characteristics of fat and alcohol differ, but for the purposes of meal planning, they may be used interchangeably. Since diets are generally planned with a modest number of fat exchanges to achieve a total of 30% or less of total calories, limited use of alcohol should be stressed. Appendix 3 presents standard portion sizes for a variety of alcoholic beverages, their nutrient content, and their exchange value for calorie control.[40]

When determining total caloric intake from alcoholic beverages, the carbohydrate composition of the mix should also be considered. Preferred mixes to be used with distilled spirits should be either calorie-free (water, diet soda, or diet tonic) or counted within the meal plan. For example, a cocktail made with 4 oz of unsweetened fruit juice will have 1 fruit exchange in addition to the calories from the alcohol. Sweetened mixes as well as wine coolers, liqueurs, and cordials should be discouraged since they are sources of simple carbohydrates.

Individuals who take the sulfonylurea oral agent chlorpropamide (Diabinese) should be cautioned that this medication may have a disulfiram (Antabuse) effect.

Persons taking chlorpropamide may experience flushing, nausea, tachycardia, and abdominal discomfort after drinking alcohol.[41]

Recommendations for the use of alcohol are left to the judgment of the patient's physician.

Modifications of the Standard Diet for Diabetes

Dietary Recommendations during Illness. The stress of illness, injury, or surgery can raise plasma glucose levels and increase insulin requirements. In IDDM, ketosis may occur if the insulin dose is not appropriately adjusted and if an adequate amount of carbohydrate is not given. Persons who do not require insulin are less likely to develop ketoacidosis, but may develop hyperosmolar nonketotic coma if excessive glycosuria occurs and if an adequate amount of water is not consumed.

If the person is too ill to consume regular foods, a combination of soft and easily digested foods or liquids that gives approximately the same amount of carbohydrate as the regular meal plan should be consumed.

TABLE 8-3 Available Carbohydrate*

Food Groups	Available Carbohydrate from 1 exchange (g)
Meat	5.0
Fat	0.5
Skim milk	17.0
Starch	17.0
Vegetables	6.0
Fruits	15.0

*Available carbohydrate is the proportion of macronutrients that can be converted into glucose by the body (100% of carbohydrate, 60% of protein, 10% of fat).

TABLE 8-4 Carbohydrate Content of Sugar-Containing Foods and Beverages

	Amount	Carbohydrate* (g)
Carbonated beverage, sugar-sweetened (such as 7-Up)	1/2 cup (4 fl oz)	15
Fruit juices		
Apple, orange	1/2 cup (4 fl oz)	15
Grape, cranberry	1/3 cup (3 fl oz)	15
Gelatin, sugar-sweetened	1/2 cup	20
Granulated sugar, corn syrup, or honey	1 Tbsp	15
Hard sugar candy	1/2 oz (3 pieces)	15
Kool-aid, sugar-sweetened	1/2 cup (4 fl oz)	10
Lifesavers	5 pieces	15
Popsicle, double stick	1/2 popsicle	10

*Rounded to the nearest 5 g. Carbohydrate content may vary among brands. Adapted from: Pennington J. Food values of portions commonly used, 15th ed. New York: Harper & Row, 1989.

If nausea or vomiting are present or the person is not able to consume usual foods, the carbohydrate content of the meal plan can be replaced by using sugar-containing liquids. Table 8-3 indicates the amount of available carbohydrate from one exchange from each food group. Table 8-4 indicates the carbohydrate content of some sugar-containing foods and beverages.

For patients who need to consume a clear liquid diet for a clinical procedure or test, the above guidelines may be used in the conversion of the patient's usual dietary intake to clear liquids. A diet history is taken in order to estimate available carbohydrate for each meal and snack, after which clear liquid substitutions are made that approximate the calculated carbohydrate content.

For hospitalized patients who receive clear liquid diets, a precise calculation of the available carbohydrate is not necessary since stress, trauma, and intravenous glucose are likely to alter the insulin requirement. Postoperatively, the diabetic liquid diet is similar to the regular clear and full liquid diets. As the patient's appetite improves, the composition and caloric level of the diet more closely resemble those of a diabetic diet.

Hypoglycemia.   Hypoglycemia in diabetes may occur as a consequence of the action of insulin or of oral hypoglycemic agents. Symptoms tend to occur when the plasma glucose level falls below 60 mg/dl, although the exact level may vary. Hypoglycemic episodes are usually termed "insulin reactions," although these episodes may also occur with the oral agents. A hypoglycemic episode is more likely to occur with a delayed or incompletely consumed meal or an increase in exercise. Hypoglycemia may occur more frequently in persons on intensive insulin treatment programs such as insulin pumps or multiple daily injections.[8,42] To prevent nocturnal hypoglycemia, a bedtime snack is recommended for all persons who take insulin or an oral hypoglycemic agent. Between meal snacks should be included if the span between meals is more than 5 hours. There is no risk of hypoglycemia in the diabetic person who does not receive insulin or oral hypoglycemic agents.

The initial symptoms of a hypoglycemic episode are mainly the results of epinephrine or catecholamine release. These symptoms include feelings of apprehension and anxiety, rapid heartbeat, and cold perspiration.[43] Fortunately, these symptoms ordinarily awaken the person if they occur during sleep. If the person's cardiac status is such that a dysrhythmia may be provoked by a catecholamine excess, such as during the period that follows a myocardial infarction, a hypoglycemic episode could have serious or even fatal consequences. In a long-term diabetic, there may be a deterioration of the function of the autonomic nervous system so that epinephrine-related symptoms are blunted or absent. Symptoms that result from impaired brain function may be the first clue that hypoglycemia is occurring. The brain and the other parts of the nervous system use only glucose for fuel. With prolonged or severe hypoglycemia, cerebral function is disturbed, which results in confusion, a change in personality, and finally coma or seizures.[43] Hypoglycemic episodes pose a particular threat of stroke for those with limited cerebral circulation.

Although plasma glucose levels may rise well above hypoglycemic levels within 5 to 15 minutes after the ingestion of food, symptoms of hypoglycemia may persist for longer periods, particularly the cerebral symptoms. It is important to give enough food to correct the hypoglycemia, but resist giving excessive amounts of food when the symptoms do not resolve promptly. During the next several hours there may be an appearance of excessive lability if the patient takes larger-than-needed amounts of food and has resultant hyperglycemia. In general, the administration of 15 g of a simple carbohydrate is sufficient, but may need to be repeated if the symptoms do not abate within about 15 minutes. At night larger amounts, such as 22.5 g, may be necessary because of the time delay until the next meal. It is particularly important that the person who is vulnerable to insulin reactions take precautions to avoid such episodes while driving a car. A particularly hazardous time is the hour before the evening meal when the person may be driving home from work. If the person has not eaten in the previous 2 hours, the consumption of a fruit, starch, or milk exchange before getting behind the wheel of a car is often a reasonable precaution.

Exercise.   A regular exercise program along with diet and/or medication can aid in the management of diabetes. It may improve glucose homeostasis in the person with NIDDM and may lower insulin requirements in the individual with IDDM. Frequent monitoring of blood glucose levels is helpful in predicting plasma glucose levels before, during, and after exercise.

The plasma glucose response to exercise in the person taking insulin is variable. It depends upon the level of metabolic control before exercise and the level of insulin at the time of exercise. Exercise usually decreases plasma glucose levels when the diabetes is well controlled. In the poorly controlled diabetic with plasma glucose greater than 300 mg/dl, exercise may actually increase glucose levels.[44] The presence of urinary ketones would suggest that current insulin levels are inadequate for glucose transport, forcing energy demands to be met by lipolysis and resulting in ketogenesis. Exercising in this condition would further elevate blood glucose levels and produce high levels of ketones, so exercise is contraindicated.[45]

For individuals with NIDDM, plasma glucose levels usually decrease following exercise. Since many individuals with NIDDM are overweight, regular exercise may be a useful adjunct to diet. Both exercise and weight reduction independently enhance insulin sensitivity and decrease very low-density lipoproteins and low-density lipoprotein cholesterol levels.

For individuals taking insulin, hypoglycemia may occur during or following exercise and may require adjustments in insulin and diet.

Overeating prior to exercise with the intent of preventing hypoglycemia is common and can be avoided. Individuals need to monitor their blood glucose levels and adapt these guidelines to their personal needs. Suggested guidelines for diet and exercise appear in Table 8-5.

Liberalized Diabetic Diet.   A liberalized diet (termed at the Mayo Clinic the Diabetic Diet—No Kilocalorie Restriction) is used for persons with a mildly impaired glucose tolerance. These individuals can often be at an appropriate weight and may benefit from moderate restriction of simple carbohydrate and an improvement in eating habits. This liberalized diet may also be used for the person with diabetes who has a poor food intake or for those persons who cannot or

TABLE 8-5   Diet and Exercise

Types of Exercise and Examples	If Blood Sugar Is:	Increase Food Intake by:	Suggested Foods to Use
Exercise of Short Duration or of Moderate Intensity			
Examples: walking $^1/_2$ mile or leisurely biking for $^1/_2$ hr or less	≥ 80 mg < 80 mg*	• May not be necessary • 15 g of carbohydrate per $^1/_2$ hr	• 1 fruit or 1 starch exchange
Exercise of Moderate Intensity			
Examples: tennis, swimming, jogging, leisure cycling, gardening, golfing, vacuuming for $^1/_2$ hr	80–180 mg < 80 mg*	• 15 g of carbohydrate per hour of exercise • 36–50 g of carbohydrate prior to exercise, then 15 g per hour of exercise	• 1 fruit or 1 starch exchange • $^1/_2$ meat sandwich with $^1/_2$ milk and 1 fruit exchange
	180–300 mg	• Not necessary to increase food	
	≥ 300 mg†	• Exercise is not recommended	
Strenuous Activity or Exercise			
Examples: football, hockey, racquetball, basketball games, tennis (singles), strenuous cycling or swimming, shoveling heavy snow for 1 hr	80–180 mg < 80 mg 180–300 mg ≥ 300 mg†	• 36–50 mg of carbohydrate, depending on intensity and duration • 50 g of carbohydrate, monitor blood sugar levels carefully • 15 g of carbohydrate per hour of exercise • Exercise is not recommended	• $^1/_2$ meat sandwich with $^1/_2$ milk and 1 fruit exchange • 1 meat sandwich (2 slices of bread) with $^1/_2$ milk and 1 fruit exchange • 1 fruit or 1 starch exchange

*When blood sugar is < 80 mg before exercise, a carbohydrate supplement may be needed in addition to the extra food suggested.

†High blood sugar may reflect inadequate insulin therapy, and exercise may cause the blood sugar to increase further.

With permission and adapted from Jensen MD, Miles JM. The roles of diet and exercise in the management of patients with insulin-dependent diabetes mellitus. Mayo Clin Proc 1986;61:813–819.

will not follow the exchange system. (Such individuals may include cancer patients who have significant eating problems, the elderly, and those who have impaired sight or a learning disability.) The principles of the Diabetic Diet—No Kilocalorie Restriction appear in Table 8-6.

Diabetes and Chronic Renal Failure.   In the presence of impaired renal function secondary to diabetic nephropathy, modifications in the dietary protein, sodium, potassium, and/or fluid allowances are often necessary.

As renal failure progresses, the principles of the diabetic diet may need to be modified. The features of the renal diet take priority, especially when very low protein levels are necessary.

TABLE 8-6 Diabetic Diet—No Kilocalorie Restriction

1. This diet does not use food exchanges or measurements.
2. The diet should be varied and nutritionally balanced. It should meet the normal nutritional needs of the person.
3. Sugar and foods high in sugar should be limited. (See Foods to Avoid, p. 170.)
4. Dietetic foods with a significant caloric content should be avoided.
5. Meals and snacks should be eaten at regular intervals, with each meal consistent in quantity.

The decrease in protein requires a corresponding increase in fat and carbohydrate. Low-protein products can be used as a source of kilocalories. To assure adequate kilocalories, simple carbohydrates such as sugar, jellies, and sweetened fruit may also have to be included. If simple carbohydrates are consumed, they should be measured carefully and distributed evenly throughout the day to minimize the fluctuation in plasma glucose levels.[47] The rationale for incorporating simple sugars into the diet must be clearly explained to the patient to ensure compliance. Consistency in the timing and the composition of meals and the use of additional food for increased exercise to prevent hypoglycemic reactions remain necessary.

The renal exchange list should be used in planning the diet for individuals with diabetes and renal failure. (See Chapter 14, Renal Diseases and Disorders.)

Diabetes and Pregnancy. The diet for pregnancy follows the same basic principles as the standard diabetic diet and also includes the necessary requirements for pregnancy.

Of all pregnancies, 0.1 to 0.5% are in women who have been previously diagnosed as having diabetes, an additional 2.5% of pregnant women develop gestational diabetes.[48] Gestational diabetes is defined as an abnormal glucose tolerance that is noted during the course of the pregnancy. All women should be screened at 24 to 28 weeks of gestation. If the fasting plasma glucose levels of the gestational diabetic cannot be kept under 95 mg/dl and a 2-hour postprandial plasma glucose below 120 mg/dl by the diet alone, insulin therapy may be started. Sulfonylureas are contraindicated during pregnancy.[49]

Good control of the plasma glucose levels during pregnancy is critical to the health of both mother and fetus. Studies have shown that perinatal infant mortality rates drop to near normal ranges for those patients who demonstrate good glycemic control (i.e., 80 to 100 mg/dl fasting and before meals) during their pregnancy.[48] An increase in the plasma glucose levels during the first 6 to 8 weeks after conception increases the chances of fetal malformations. An increase in the plasma glucose levels later in the pregnancy is associated with macrosomia, fetal hypoglycemia, and respiratory distress syndrome.

The caloric level of the diet is based on the number of kilocalories that are required to maintain the woman's prepregnancy weight with an increase of approximately 300 kcal/day during the second and third trimesters to achieve a total weight gain of 7 to 13.6 kg (15 to 30 lb).[50] The rate of weight gain during pregnancy should be carefully monitored and similar to that desired for nondiabetic pregnant women. A weight loss during the pregnancy is contraindicated because of the need for adequate fetal nutrition and also because of the increased incidence of maternal ketonuria with very low kilocalorie diets.[51] The fetus acts as a "glucose sink" by constantly removing glucose from the maternal circulation. This renders the woman vulnerable to hypoglycemia before meals and to ketosis. Between meal feedings minimize the fluctuations in plasma glucose levels and help prevent ketosis. The caloric allotment is divided into 3 meals and 3 snacks—a midmorning, a midafternoon, and a bedtime snack. Regularity of meals, exercise, and glucose monitoring are advised to prevent wide fluctuations in the blood glucose levels. Alcohol, artificial sweeteners, and caffeine are not recommended. For further information regarding the diet in pregnancy, see Chapter 4, Pregnancy and Lactation.

   Diet Following Gastroplasty for Weight Reduction.   For persons with diabetes who have undergone gastroplasty for weight reduction, the dietary plan for gastroplasty is ordinarily satisfactory during the first few months. The person is restricted to a very small volume of food at each meal because of the limited gastric capacity. Between meal snacks may be necessary. The diet can be gradually modified toward the standard diabetic diet recommendations. See Chapter 8, Bariatric Surgery, for further information.

   Tube Feeding.   Persons with diabetes who receive tube feeding should be provided with adequate kilocalories and protein to meet their nutritional requirements. Kilocalories should not be spared in order to achieve optimal plasma glucose levels. Rather, insulin regulation and glucose monitoring should be used to achieve glycemic control. In the hospital, continuous feedings are suggested for optimal glycemic control. These continuous feedings help slow gastric emptying and also delay and perhaps reduce the peak glucose response.[52] If continuous feedings are not possible, an intermittent feeding schedule with a small volume at a slow rate is recommended. See Chapter 16, Enteral Nutritional Support, for further information.

Physicians: How to Order Diet

The diet order should indicate *diabetic diet*. If weight reduction is desired, the diet order should indicate *diabetic, weight reduction diet*. The dietitian determines the appropriate caloric level and the other characteristics of the diet based on the previous discussion. If additional therapeutic modifications, such as full liquid or sodium restriction, are desired, they should be indicated in the diet order.

Community Support Programs

   The dietitian should be aware that there are many community support programs and associations available to the person with diabetes. These support systems can provide up-to-date information as well as peer support.

American Diabetes Association
National Service Center
1660 Duke St.
Alexandria, VA 22314

American Dietetic Association
216 West Jackson Blvd., Suite 800
Chicago, IL 60606-6995

National Diabetes Information Clearinghouse
Box NDIC
Bethesda, MD 20892

Juvenile Diabetes Foundation
423 Park Ave. South
New York, NY 10016-8013

Canadian Diabetes Association
78 Bond St.
Toronto, Ontario
Canada M5B 2J8

FOOD EXCHANGE LISTS

The following list is adapted from the 1986 American Diabetes Association and American Dietetic Association (ADA) Exchange Lists for Meal Planning.[53] Modifications to the ADA exchange lists were made in order to include a more comprehensive listing of foods as well as their gram weights. This detailed information is intended as a reference for the dietitian and not necessarily for patient instruction. For patient education, the following exchange lists may be simplified, condensed, or modified depending on the goals of dietary management, the need for other dietary restrictions, and the abilities of the patient. Table 8-7 summarizes the amount of carbohydrate, protein, and fat in one serving from each exchange list.

TABLE 8-7 Summary of Nutrients in One Serving from Each Exchange List

Exchange List	Carbohydrate (g)	Protein (g)	Fat (g)	Kilocalories (kcal)
Meat	–			
Lean	–	7	3	55
Medium fat	–	7	5	75
High fat	–	7	8	100
Milk				
Skim	12	8	Trace	80
Low fat (2%)	12	8	5	125
Whole	12	8	10	170
Starch or bread	15	3	Trace	80
Vegetable	5	2	–	25
Fruit	15	–	–	60
Fat	–	–	5	45

Foods to Avoid

Foods that contain large amounts of sugar generally should be avoided or used in limited amounts.*

Candy	Jam	Sugar coated cereals
Candy bars	Jelly	Sweet rolls
Chewing gum	Marmalade	Sweetened condensed milk
Cookies†	Molasses	Sweetened fruit
Custard	Pastries	Sweetened soft drinks
Granola	Pies	Sweetened yogurt
Granola type bars	Sugar	Syrup
Honey		

*Sugar-containing foods may be recommended for some circumstances, particularly as a caloric source for persons with chronic renal failure or a severely restricted intake because of illness and for treatment of hypoglycemia.

†Exceptions are listed under Special Occasion Foods, see p. 177.

"Free" Foods

The foods listed under "Use as Desired" are relatively free of kilocalories and do not need to be calculated in the meal plan.

The foods listed under "Use in Limited Amounts" contain less than 20 kcal per serving. They do not need to be calculated in the meal plan unless the total sum of their use exceeds 20 kcal per meal or a total of 60 kcal maximum distributed throughout the day. Artificially sweetened foods and beverages are limited because of a general restriction on the quantity of artificial sweeteners used rather than their caloric contribution.

Use as Desired	Use in Limited Amounts
BEVERAGES	
Coffee	Artificially sweetened beverages
Decaffeinated coffee	
Tea	
Water	
Carbonated water	
Club soda	
Mineral water	
Tonic water, sugar-free	
Seltzers, sugar-free	
CONDIMENTS AND SEASONINGS	
Salt, seasoning salts	Ketchup (1 Tbsp)
Pepper	Barbecue sauce (1 Tbsp)
Herbs	Cocktail sauce (1 Tbsp)
Spices	Meat sauces (1 Tbsp)
Flavoring extracts	Taco sauce (1 Tbsp)
Mustard	Dietetic jam or jelly (2 tsp)
Horseradish	Low calorie salad dressing (2 Tbsp)
Lemon juice	Pancake syrup, sugar-free (2 Tbsp)
Lime juice	

Use as Desired	Use in Limited Amounts
CONDIMENTS AND SEASONINGS—cont'd	
Vinegar	
Fat-free butter flavoring	
Worcestershire or soy sauce	
Nonstick pan spray	
OTHER FOODS	
Plain, unflavored gelatin	Artificial sweetener
Fat-free bouillon or broth	Artificially sweetened, flavored gelatin
Dill pickles	Gum, sugar-free (2–3 sticks)
	Hard candy, sugar-free (2–3 pieces)
	Unsweetened cocoa powder (1 Tbsp)
	Unsweetened cranberries (½ cup)
	Whipped topping, low calorie (1 Tbsp)

Group 1—Meat Exchanges

Meat should be weighed after cooking and after the bone, skin, and excess fat have been removed. The use of meats from the lean and medium fat categories is encouraged.

Measure or Weight	Gram Weight	Lean Meat: 7 g Protein, 3 g Fat, 55 kcal
1 oz	30	Beef: baby beef, chipped beef, chuck, flank steak, tenderloin, plate ribs, plate skirt steak, round (bottom, top), all rump cuts, lean spareribs, ground beef (more than 90% lean), USDA good or choice cuts
1 oz	30	Pork: leg (whole rump, center shank), tenderloin, ham (canned, cured, boiled), Canadian bacon
1 oz	30	Veal: leg, loin, rib, shank, shoulder
1 oz	30	Poultry (meat without skin): chicken, turkey, Cornish hen
1 oz	30	Wild game: venison, rabbit, squirrel, pheasant, goose (without skin)
1 oz	30	Fish: any fresh or frozen
1 oz	30	Herring (plain or smoked)
¼ cup	30	Tuna, mackerel (canned in water, drained)
1 oz (2 medium)	30	Sardines, drained
2 oz (½ cup)	60	Clams, crab, lobster (fresh or canned in water)
3 oz (6 medium)	90	Oysters
2 oz (8)	50	Scallops (bay)
2 oz (5–6 medium)	60	Shrimp
¼ cup	60	Egg substitutes, low cholesterol
3 whites	90	Egg whites
1 oz (¼ cup)	30	Cheeses (low fat that contain ≤ 3 g fat per oz)
¼ cup	45	Cottage cheese: any
2 Tbsp	10	Parmesan cheese (grated)
1 oz	30	Luncheon meats, low fat (containing ≤ 3 g fat per oz or > 90% lean)

Measure or Weight	Gram Weight	Medium Fat Meat: 7 g Protein, 5 g Fat, 73 kcal
1 oz	30	Beef: roasts and steaks, ground, round or beef (>80% lean) corned beef (canned), rib eye steak
1 oz	30	Lamb: leg, rib, sirloin, loin (roast and chops), shank, shoulder
1 oz	30	Pork: loin (all tenderloin cuts), shoulder arm (picnic), shoulder blade, Boston butt
1 oz	30	Poultry: chicken and turkey (with skin), ground turkey, capon, domestic duck or goose (well drained of fat)
1 oz	30	Veal: cutlet (ground or cubed, unbreaded)
1 oz	30	Liver, heart, kidney, sweetbreads
1 oz	30	Cheese: mozzarella, ricotta, Neufchatel, farmer cheese
1 oz	30	Luncheon meats, low fat (containing 3–5 g fat per oz or 85–90% lean)
¹/₄ cup	30	Tuna (canned in oil, drained), salmon (canned, drained), mackerel
1	50	Egg (limit 3–4/wk)
4 oz	120	Tofu

Measure or Weight	Gram Weight	High Fat Meat*: 7 g Protein, 8 g Fat, 100 kcal
1 oz	30	Beef: brisket, corned beef (brisket), ground (< 80% lean), ground chuck, rib roasts, club and rib steaks, USDA Prime cuts
1 oz	30	Pork: spareribs, loin (back ribs), ground, country style ham, deviled ham, sausage
1 oz	30	Lamb: breast, ground
1 oz	30	Veal: breast
1 oz	30	Cheese: all regular, including American, blue, cheddar, Monterey, muenster, Swiss
2 Tbsp	30	Cheese spreads
1 slice 4¹/₂ in by ¹/₈ in (1 oz)	45	Cold cuts
1 oz	30	Sausage: Polish, Italian, bratwurst, knockwurst (omit 1 fat)
1 small (1¹/₂ oz)	45	Frankfurter, turkey or chicken (beef, pork, or combination—omit 1 fat)
2 Tbsp	30	Peanut butter (omit 2 fats)

*These meats are high in fat and kilocalories and therefore should be used only occasionally.

Meat Alternatives

If these foods are used as a substitute for meat (as in a vegetarian diet), the carbohydrate content should be accounted for as indicated below.

Measure or Weight	Gram Weight	Meat Alternative	Exchange Value
1 cup	200*	Beans (cooked):	
		Butter	1 meat + 2 starch
		Lima	1 meat + 2 starch
		Pinto	1 meat + 2 starch
		Red	1 meat + 2 starch
		Soy	3 meat + 1 starch
		White	1 meat + 3 starch
1 cup	170	Garbanzo beans, canned (chick peas)	1 meat + 3 starch
1 cup	100	Lentils (cooked)	2 meat + 2 starch
		Peas (cooked):	
1 cup	100	Black-eyed	1 meat + 2 starch
1 cup	200	Split	1 meat + 3 starch
		Nuts and seeds:	
$^{1}/_{4}$ cup (25 nuts)	30	Peanuts	1 meat + 2 fat + 1 vegetable
1 oz (3 Tbsp)	30	Pumpkin seeds	1 meat + 2 fat + 1 vegetable
1 oz (3 Tbsp)	30	Sesame seeds	1 meat + 2 fat
1 oz (4 Tbsp)	30	Soybean nuts, roasted	2 meat + 1 starch
1 oz (3 Tbsp)	30	Squash seeds	1 meat + 2 fat + 1 vegetable
1 oz (3 Tbsp)	30	Sunflower or safflower seeds	1 meat + 2 fat + 1 vegetable
$^{1}/_{4}$ cup	30	Wheat germ (toasted)	1 meat + 1 starch

*Average weight is 200 g.

Group 2—Milk Exchanges

Measure	Gram Weight	Nonfat Fortified Milk: 8 g Protein, 12 g Carbohydrate, Trace Fat, 80 kcal
1 cup	240	Skim or nonfat milk
1/3 cup	25	Powdered milk (nonfat dry, before adding liquid)
1/2 cup	120	Canned, evaporated skim milk
1/4 cup	20	Buttermilk, dry
1 cup	240	Buttermilk made from skim milk
1 cup	240	Yogurt made from skim milk (plain, unflavored)
		1% Fat Fortified Milk: (1 Nonfat Milk + 1/2 Fat Exchange), 8 g Protein, 12 g Carbohydrate, 2.5 g Fat, 102 kcal
1 cup	240	1% milk
1 cup	240	Low fat buttermilk
		2% Fat Fortified Milk: (1 Nonfat Milk + 1 Fat Exchange), 8 g Protein, 12 g Carbohydrate, 5 g Fat, 125 kcal
1 cup	240	2% milk
1 cup	240	Yogurt made from 2% milk (plain, unflavored)
1/2 cup	120	Canned evaporated 2% milk
		Whole Milk: (1 Nonfat Milk + 2 Fat Exchange), 8 g Protein, 12 g Carbohydrate, 10 g Fat, 170 kcal
1 cup	240	Whole milk
1/2 cup	120	Canned, evaporated whole milk
1 cup	240	Buttermilk made from whole milk
1 cup	240	Yogurt made from whole milk (plain, unflavored)

Group 3—Starch Exchanges

Each serving from the starch group contains 3 g protein, 15 g carbohydrate, trace fat, 80 kilocalories.

Measure	Gram Weight	Cereal
$^1/_2$ cup	30	Bran flakes or Chex™
$^1/_3$ cup	25	Other bran cereals
$^1/_2$ cup	100	Cooked cereal
$^1/_2$ cup	100	Grits, cooked
3 Tbsp	20	Grape-Nuts™
$1^1/_2$ cups	20	Puffed cereal, unfrosted
$^1/_2$ cup	110	Oat bran, cooked
$^3/_4$ cup	20	Other ready-to-eat, unsweetened cereal
1 biscuit or $1^1/_2$ cup	25	Shredded Wheat™

Measure	Gram Weight	Bread
$^1/_2$ small	30	Bagel
2	25	Breadsticks, crisp, 4" long by $^1/_2$" diameter
$^1/_2$ cup	20	Croutons (plain or herb seasoned), no fat added
$^1/_2$ small	30	English muffin
$^1/_2$	35	Frankfurter bun
$^1/_2$	35	Hamburger bun
$^1/_2$	30	Pita bread, thin, 6" diameter
1 small	30	Plain dinner roll
1 slice	25	Raisin bread (unfrosted)
1 slice	25	Rye or pumpernickel bread
1	30	Tortilla, 6" diameter
1 slice	25	White, including French and Italian
1 slice	25	Whole wheat
4 Tbsp	20	Dried bread crumbs

Measure	Gram Weight	Other Starches
1/2 cup	100	Barley or bulgur, cooked
2 1/2 Tbsp	20	Cornmeal, dry
2 1/2 Tbsp	25	Cornstarch, dry
3 Tbsp	20	Flour
1/2 cup	100	Pasta: spaghetti, noodles, macaroni (cooked)
3 cups	20	Popcorn (popped, without oil)
1 1/2 cups	20	Popcorn (popped in oil)
1/3 cup	75	Rice, brown or white (cooked)
2 1/2 Tbsp	20	Tapioca, dry
3 Tbsp	20	Wheat germ
1 cup	240	Vegetable or broth based soup

Measure	Gram Weight	Crackers
10	18	Animal Crackers
3	20	Arrowroot
3	35	Graham, 2 1/2" square
1	20	Matzoh, 4" by 6"
5	20	Melba toast, 3 3/4" by 2"
24	20	Oyster
25	20	Pretzels, 3 1/8" long by 1/8" diameter
3	20	Rye wafers, 2" by 3 1/2"
2	20	Rice cakes
6	20	Saltines, 2" square

Measure	Gram Weight	Starchy Vegetables
1/3 cup	70	Beans, peas (dried, cooked)
1/4 cup	50	Baked beans (canned, no pork)
1/2 cup	80	Corn
1 small ear	100	Corn on the cob, 3 to 4" long
1/2 cup	100	Lima beans
2/3 cup	130	Parsnips
1/2 cup	100	Peas, green
1/2 cup	75	Lentils (cooked)
1/2 cup	75	Plantain
1 small	100	Potato, white
1/2 cup	100	Potato, mashed
1 cup	200	Pumpkin
1/2 small	50	Sweet potato, baked
1/3 cup	100	Yam (canned or fresh), sweet potato (canned), plain
3/4 cup	150	Squash, winter (acorn, butternut, buttercup, Hubbard)

Measure	Gram Weight	Prepared Foods (Omit 1 Fat Exchange)
1	35	Biscuit, 2" diameter
¹/₂ cup	30	Chow mein noodles
1	50	Corn bread, 2" cube
1	40	Corn muffin, 2" diameter
6	25	Crackers, round butter type
6	30	Whole-wheat crackers
1 small	40	Muffin, plain
2	45	Pancakes, 4" diameter
10	45	Potatoes, French fried, 2–3¹/₂" long
¹/₄ cup	45	Stuffing, bread (prepared)
2	20	Taco shell, 6" diameter
1	40	Waffle, 5" diameter

Measure	Gram Weight	Special Occasion Foods*
1 slice	25	Angel food cake, plain, ¹/₁₆ of 10" cake (1¹/₂")
1 slice	50	Cake, no icing, ¹/₁₂ cake or 3" square (omit 1 starch and 2 fat)
1 slice	35	Cake, sponge, ¹/₁₆ of 10" cake (1¹/₂")
1 small	30	Croissant, 5" by 2" (omit 2 fat exchanges)
2 small	25	Cookies 1³/₄" (omit 1 fat exchange)
5	20	Gingersnaps, 1³/₄" by ¹/₈"
2 small	20	Shortbread cookies, 1¹/₂" by ¹/₄" (omit 1 fat exchange)
5	20	Vanilla wafers, about 1³/₄" by ¹/₈"
1	30	Doughnut, plain cake (omit 1 fat exchange)
¹/₂ cup	140	Gelatin, sweetened (commercial flavored)
¹/₄ cup	30	Granola (omit 1 fat exchange)
1 small	25	Granola bar (omit 1 fat exchange)
¹/₂ cup	70	Ice cream (omit 2 fat exchanges)
¹/₂ cup	60	Ice milk (omit 1 fat exchange)
2	25	Ice cream cone (cone only)
¹/₄ cup	75	Pudding, sugar sweetened
¹/₃ cup	65	Sherbet
1 oz	30	Snack chips, all varieties (omit 2 fat exchanges)
¹/₃ cup	75	Yogurt, frozen fruit (nonfat)

*Many of these foods contain added sugar and fat. They should be eaten only occasionally, in limited amounts, and with other foods.

Group 4—Vegetable Exchanges

Each serving from the vegetable group contains 2 g of protein, 5 g of carbohydrate, and 25 kcal. One exchange is $^1/_2$ cup (100 g) of vegetable cooked or juice, or $^1/_2$ to 1 cup raw (unless another amount is given).

Artichoke (medium globe)	Jicama (Mexican potato)	Swiss chard
Asparagus (5–7 spears)	Kale	Tomato
Bamboo shoots	Kohlrabi ($^2/_3$ cup)	Raw (1 large)
Bean sprouts	Leeks (2 medium)	Cherry (6)
Beets	Mustard greens	Paste (2 Tbsp)
Beet greens	Okra	Sauce ($^1/_4$ cup)
Broccoli	Onions	Stewed ($^1/_2$ cup)
Brussel sprouts	Pea pods or snow peas	Tomato juice
Carrots	Rutabaga	Turnips
Collard greens	Sauerkraut	Turnip greens
Dandelion greens	Spinach	Vegetable juice cocktail
Eggplant	String beans, green or yellow	Water chestnuts (5)
Green pepper (1 large)		

The following vegetables have little protein, fat, or carbohydrate. One to two cups may be considered "free" and used without substitution in the meal plan.

Alfalfa sprouts	Endive	Rhubarb, artificially sweetened
Cabbage	Escarole	Romaine
Cauliflower	Green onion	Summer squash
Celery	Hot peppers	Watercress
Chicory	Lettuce	Zucchini
Chinese cabbage	Mushrooms	
Cucumber	Radishes	

Group 5—Fruit Exchanges

Each serving from the fruit group contains 15 g carbohydrate and 60 kcal. Fruit may be fresh, unsweetened canned, cooked, frozen, or dried. Juice-packed fruits should be drained; the juice should be counted separately.

Measure	Gram Weight	Fruit	Measure	Gram Weight	Fruit
1 small	100	Apple, 2" diameter	1	130	Orange, 2½" diameter
½ cup	120	Apple juice	½ cup	120	Orange juice
½ cup	120	Apple sauce	¾ cup	165	Orange sections including mandarin
½ cup	120	Apple cider	2½ oz	75	Papaws
4 medium	135	Apricots, fresh	½ medium or 1 cup	150	Papaya
7 halves	25	Apricots, dried	3 medium	60	Passion fruit
½ cup or 4 halves	100	Apricots, canned	1 medium	140	Peach, 2¾" diameter
½ cup	120	Apricot nectar	2 halves	25	Peach, dried
½	60	Banana, 9" long	½ cup	135	Peaches, canned
¾ cup	100	Blackberries	½ cup	120	Peach nectar
¾ cup	100	Blueberries	1 small	100	Pear
¼ or 1 cup chunks	160	Cantaloupe, 6" diameter	2 halves	20	Pear, dried
12 large	80	Cherries, fresh	½ cup	120	Pears, canned
½ cup	120	Cherries, canned	½ cup	120	Pear nectar
⅓ cup	100	Cranberry juice cocktail	2 medium	50	Persimmon, native
1¼ cup	300	Cranberry juice cocktail (low kilocalorie)	¾ cup	120	Pineapple, fresh
2	20	Dates	⅓ cup	100	Pineapple, canned
2	75	Figs, fresh, 2"	½ cup	120	Pineapple juice
1 large	20	Figs, dried	3 or ½ cup	100	Plums, canned
½ cup	125	Fruit cocktail	2	100	Plums, 2" diameter
½ medium	125	Grapefruit	½ medium	80	Pomegranate
½ cup	120	Grapefruit juice	1 medium	150	Prickly pear
¾ cup	155	Grapefruit sections	3 medium	25	Prunes
15 small	90	Grapes	⅓ cup	80	Prune juice
⅓ cup	90	Grape juice	2 Tbsp	20	Raisins
1 medium	100	Guava	1 cup	125	Raspberries
⅛ medium or 1 cup chunks	170	Honeydew	1¼ cup	190	Strawberries
1 large	100	Kiwi	1 medium	175	Tangelo
5 medium	95	Kumquats	2 medium	135	Tangerine, 2½" diameter
½ small	90	Mango	½ cup	120	Tangerine juice
½	120	Nectarine, 3" diameter	1¼ cups	190	Watermelon

Group 6—Fat Exchanges

Each serving from the fat list contains 5 g of fat and 45 kcal.

Measure	Gram Weight	Predominantly Polyunsaturated Fats
1 tsp	5	Margarine: soft, tub (any containing liquid safflower, sunflower, or corn oil as the first ingredient and higher in polyunsaturated than saturated fats)
1 Tbsp	15	Diet margarine (see above)
1 tsp	5	Oil*
2 Tbsp	30	Nondairy cream substitute (liquid)*
1 Tbsp	15	French or Italian-style salad dressing*
2 Tbsp	30	Reduced calorie salad dressing*
1 tsp	5	Mayonnaise*
2 tsp	10	Mayonnaise-type salad dressing*
1 Tbsp	15	Reduced calorie mayonnaise*
1½ tsp	10	Tartar sauce
4 halves	8	Walnuts
4 tsp	5	Pumpkin seeds
1 Tbsp	7	Sunflower seeds (without shells)
		Predominantly Monounsaturated Fats
⅛	30	Avocado, 4" diameter
1 tsp	5	Margarine (any containing soybean, cottonseed, or partially hydrogenated vegetable oil as first ingredient—check label)
1 tsp	5	Oil (Canola, olive, or peanut oil)
9 medium	35	Green olives
5 large	25	Ripe olives
6 whole	8	Almonds
2 medium	10	Brazil nuts
4 large	8	Cashews
5	10	Hazel nuts
3 large	8	Macadamia nuts
10 large	10	Peanuts
5 halves	7	Pecans
20	10	Pistachio nuts
1½ tsp	8	Peanut butter
		Predominantly Saturated Fats
1 tsp	5	Butter, hydrogenated vegetable oil margarine or shortening, palm oil, coconut oil
1 tsp	5	Bacon fat
1 strip	10	Bacon, crisp
2 Tbsp	30	Sour cream
3 Tbsp	45	Half and half (light cream)
1 Tbsp	15	Cream, heavy whipping
2 Tbsp	30	Other nondairy cream substitutes (liquid or powder)
1 Tbsp	15	Cream cheese
2 Tbsp	30	Gravy
1 tsp	5	Lard
¼ oz	7	Salt pork or fat back

*Made with safflower, sunflower, corn, soybean, cottonseed, or sesame oil.

References

1. Abourir NN, Dunn JC. Types of diabetes according to National Diabetes Data Group Classification: limited applicability and need to revisit. Diabetes Care 1990;13:1120–1123.
2. Sims EAH, Callis-Escandon J. Classification of diabetes. A fresh look for the 1990s? Diabetes Care 1990;13:1123–1128.
3. Lillioja S, Mott DM, Howard BV, Bennett PH, Yki-Järvinen H, Freymond D, Nyomba BL, Zurlo F, Swinburn B, Bogardus C. Impaired glucose tolerance as a disorder of insulin action. N Engl J Med 1988;318(19):1217–1225.
4. American Diabetes Association. Position statement: screening for diabetes. Diabetes Care 1991;14(2):7–8.
5. Mykkänen L, Laakso M, Uusitupa M, Pyörälä K. Prevalence of diabetes and impaired glucose tolerance in elderly subjects and their association with obesity and family history of diabetes. Diabetes Care 1990;13(11):1099–1105.
6. Hollander P. Gestational diabetes. Practical Diabetology 1988;7(2):14.
7. Rizza RA, Greene DA. Diabetes mellitus. Med Clin North Am. 1988; 72(6):xi–xii.
8. The Diabetes Control and Complications Trial Research Group. The effect of intensive treatment of diabetes on the development and progression of long-term complications in insulin dependent diabetes mellitus. N Engl J Med 1993;329:977–986.
9. American Diabetes Association. Position statement: nutritional recommendations and principles for individuals with diabetes mellitus. Diabetes Care 1992;15(2):21–28.
10. American Diabetes Association. Position statement: nutritional recommendations and principles for individuals with diabetes mellitus. Diabetes Care 1991;14(2):20–27.
11. Wadden T, Van Itallie TB, Blackburn GL. Responsible and irresponsible use of very-low-calorie diets in the treatment of obesity. JAMA 1990;263(1):83–85.
12. Hansen BC. Dietary considerations for obese diabetic subjects. Diabetes Care 1988;11(2):183–188.
13. Amatruda JM, Richeson JF, Welle SL, Brodows RG, Lockwood DH. The safety and efficacy of a controlled low-energy (very-low-calorie) diet in the treatment of non-insulin-dependent diabetes and obesity. Arch Intern Med 1988;148:873–877.
14. Uusitupa MIJ, Laakso M, Sarlund H, Majander H, Takala J, Pentitilä I. Effects of a very-low-calorie diet on metabolic control and cardiovascular risk factors in the treatment of obese non-insulin-dependent diabetes. Am J Clin Nutr 1990;51:768–773.
15. Brenner BM, Meyer TW, Hostetter TH. Dietary protein intake and the progressive nature of kidney disease. N Engl J Med 1982;307:652–659.
16. Bergstrom J. Discovery and rediscovery of the low protein diet. Clin Nephrol 1984;21(1):29–35.
17. Scott DW, Gorry GA, Gotto AM, Phil D. Diet and coronary heart disease: the statistical analysis of risk. Circulation 1981;63(3):516–518.
18. Nuttall FQ. Diet and the diabetic patient. Diabetes Care 1983;6(2):197–207.
19. Crapo PA. Theory vs fact: the glycemic response to foods. Nutr Today 1984;19:6–11.
20. Diabetes Care and Education Dietetic Practice Group. Diabetes mellitus and glycemic responses to different foods: a summary and annotated bibliography. 1985.
21. Franz M. Glycemic effects of carbohydrates. Diabetes Educator 1985;11:69–70.
22. Hollenbeck CB, Coulston AM, Reaven GM. Comparison of plasma glucose and insulin responses to mixed meals of high-, intermediate-, and low-glycemic potential. Diabetes Care 1988;4(11):323–329.
23. Laine DC, Thomas W, Levitt MD, Bantle JP. Comparison of predictive capabilities of diabetic exchange lists and glycemic index of foods. Diabetes Care 1987;4(10):387–394.
24. Cohen C, Wylie-Rosett J, Shamoon H. Insulin response and glycemic effects of meals in non-insulin-dependent diabetes. Am J Clin Nutr 1990;52:519–523.

25. Hermansen K, Rasmussen O, Arnfred J, Winther E, Schmitz O. Glycemic effect of spaghetti and potato consumed as part of mixed meal on IDDM patients. Diabetes Care 1987;4(10):401–406.

26. American Diabetes Association. Policy statement: glycemic effects of carbohydrates. Diabetes Care 1984;7:607–608.

27. Anderson JW, Gustafson NJ, Bryant CA, Tietyen-Clark J. Dietary fiber and diabetes: a comprehensive review and practical application. J Am Diet Assoc 1987;87:1189–1197.

28. Tietyen J. Dietary fiber in foods: options for diabetes education. Diabetes Educator 1989;15:523–528.

29. Hockaday TDR. Fiber in the management of diabetes. Br Med J 1990;300:1334–1336.

30. Behall KM, Scholfield DJ, McIvor ME, Van Duyn MS, Leo TA, Michnowski JE, Cummings CC, Mendeloff AI. Effect of guar gum on mineral balances in NIDDM adults. Diabetes Care 1989;12:357–363.

31. Rothstein RD. Gastrointestinal motility disorders in diabetes mellitus. Am J Gastroenterol 1990;85(7):782–785.

32. Bertorelli AM, Czarnowski-Hill JV. Review of present and future use of nonnutritive sweeteners. Diabetes Educator 1990;16(5):415–420.

33. Crapo PA. Use of alternative sweeteners in diabetic diet. Diabetes Care 1988;11(2):174–182.

34. Lynch PM. Sugar and fat substitutes: the challenge for today and tomorrow. Diabetes Educator 1990;16(2):101–105.

35. Alfin-Slater RB, Pi-Sunyer FX. Sugar and sugar substitutes: comparisons and indications. Postgrad Med 1987;82(2):46–53.

36. Filer LJ Jr, Stegink LD. Aspartame metabolism in normal adults, phenylketonuric heterozygotes, and diabetic subjects. Diabetes Care 1989;12(1):67–74.

37. Sturtevant FM. Use of aspartame in pregnancy. Int J Fertil 1985;30(1):85–87.

38. Franz M. Is it safe to consume aspartame during pregnancy? A review. Diabetes Educator 1986;12(2):145–147.

39. Franz MJ. Alcohol and diabetes: Part I. Its metabolism and guidelines for the occasional use. Diabetes Spectrum 1990;3(3):136–144.

40. Franz MJ. Alcohol and diabetes: Part II. Its metabolism and guidelines for the occasional use. Diabetes Spectrum 1990;3(4):210–216.

41. Franz MJ. Diabetes mellitus: considerations in the development of guidelines for the occasional use of alcohol. J Am Diet Assoc 1983;83(2):147–152.

42. Kresevic D, McCarthy Slavin S. Incidence of hypoglycemia and nutritional intake in patients on a general medical unit. Nursing Connections 1989;2(4):33–40.

43. Cryer PE, Gerich JE. Glucose counterregulation, hypoglycemia, and intensive insulin therapy in diabetes mellitus. N Engl J Med 1985;313(4):232–241.

44. Schiffrin A, Parikh S. Accommodating planned exercise in type I diabetic patients on intensive treatment. Diabetes Care 1985;8(4):337–342.

45. Maynard T. Exercise: Part I. Physiological response to exercise in diabetes mellitus. Diabetes Educator 1991;17(3):196–204.

46. Jensen MD, Miles JM. The roles of diet and exercise in the management of patients with insulin-dependent diabetes mellitus. Mayo Clinic Proc 1986;61:813–819.

47. Schafer RG. Implementation of low-protein diets for treatment of persons with early diabetic nephropathy. Diabetes Educator 1989;15(3):231–235.

48. Nelson RL. Diabetes and pregnancy. Primary Care 1983;10(2)225–240.

49. American Diabetes Association. Position statement: gestational diabetes mellitus. Diabetes Care 1991;14(2):5–6.

50. Committee on Dietary Allowances Food and Nutrition Board. Recommended dietary allowances, 10th ed. Washington, DC: National Academic Press, 1989:33–34.

51. Magee MS, Knopp RH, Beneditti TJ. Metabolic effects of 1200-kcal diet in obese pregnant women with gestational diabetes. Diabetes 1990;39:234–240.
52. Schrezenmeir J, Stürmer W. Enteral nutrition in diabetes mellitus. Gastroenterology 1989;27:37–41.
53. American Diabetes Association/American Dietetic Association. Exchange lists for meal planning. Alexandria, VA/Chicago, IL: ADA/ADA 1986.

HYPOGLYCEMIA

General Description

For hypoglycemia that results from islet cell tumors and other neoplasms, idiopathic hypoglycemia of childhood, and ketotic hypoglycemia, food is given at frequent intervals in amounts that are necessary to prevent symptoms. Sugars need not be specifically avoided and are particularly useful for the rapid correction of symptoms.

For reactive hypoglycemia, if this is fully documented, the meal plan should avoid large amounts of sucrose and other simple carbohydrates. If 3 regular meals are not well tolerated, smaller feedings at intervals of 2 to 3 hours may, by trial, be recommended.

Nutritional Inadequacy

There are no nutritional inadequacies inherent in the dietary recommendations for hypoglycemia.

Indications and Rationale

Hypoglycemia can result from many causes (mostly from insulin or sulfonylurea treatment of diabetes); classifications have been published.[54,55] Only those categories that involve dietary factors are discussed here.

Hypoglycemia that occurs with islet cell tumors and with some extrapancreatic tumors is elicited by the deprivation of food and tends to become progressively more severe with an increasing duration of fasting. The treatment is surgical. Trials of diet as definitive therapy are inappropriate.

Idiopathic hypoglycemia of infancy and ketotic hypoglycemia occur in infants and in children up to about 5 years of age. Food appropriate for the child's age should be given in frequent feedings. Again, simple sugars need not be specifically avoided. Ketotic hypoglycemia tends to resolve spontaneously, but idiopathic hypoglycemia of infancy may require subtotal pancreatectomy or pharmacologic treatment with diazoxide.

Hypoglycemia that occurs 1 to 3 hours after a meal and resolves spontaneously can be termed "reactive hypoglycemia." Reactive hypoglycemia is a diagnosis often made mistakenly in persons with anxiety or with panic attacks to explain different symptoms that occur throughout the day but have some relation to meals.[56,57] The patient describes partial relief of the symptoms with food, thereby confirming the diagnosis of hypoglycemia, whereas the real cause of the symptoms is anxiety, and the apparent response to the diet may be the result of suggestion. The symptoms of anxiety and of hypoglycemia are qualitatively similar since both are mediated by the release of epinephrine.

The diagnosis of reactive hypoglycemia severe enough to cause significant symptoms can be established if plasma glucose levels of less than 50 mg/dl after ordinary meals are associated with symptoms of epinephrine release, such as tachycardia and feelings of apprehension and anxiety.[58,59] Symptoms should either spontaneously abate in an hour or less or be relieved promptly, consistently, and completely by the ingestion of carbohydrate. However, the glycemic nadir for symptoms is not the same for all people. A rapid decrease in the glucose concentration itself may not provoke epinephrine release and cannot be invoked as a cause for symptoms if the glucose level is well above 50 mg/dl at the time of symptoms. Plasma glucose levels of less than 50 mg/dl may occur in normal, asymptomatic persons during the course of the oral glucose tolerance test. Epinephrine-release symptoms that coincide with the nadir of the plasma glucose concentration in the glucose tolerance test is only suggestive that symptoms occurring after ordinary meals are a hypoglycemic response. The glucose tolerance test should not be used for the diagnosis of hypoglycemia, since it is a challenge to glucose homeostasis in excess of that posed by ordinary meals. Thus, one should not rely on the glucose tolerance test alone for the diagnosis.[60]

A study[58] of patients who regarded themselves as having reactive hypoglycemia showed that there was no significant difference in insulin, glucose, or glucagon levels between those subjects with symptoms and those without.[60] When the subjects were given a standard test meal, no significant hypoglycemia occurred, although some of the subjects had characteristic symptoms. These findings suggest that one should be very skeptical of the diagnosis of reactive hypoglycemia unless one can demonstrate that blood sugar levels are consistently low at the time of symptoms during the course of an ordinary day with ordinary meals.

Documented reactive hypoglycemia with significant symptoms is rare. The disorder sometimes occurs in persons who have had gastric surgery, but the symptoms of "dumping" (see Chapter 9, Postgastrectomy Dumping Syndrome) should be clearly distinguished from those of hypoglycemia. Hypoglycemia that occurs at the fourth hour or later in the glucose tolerance test has been said to predict the later occurrence of diabetes, although this is not clearly established.[61] However, late hypoglycemia may occasionally be found in patients with an insulinoma.

Goals of Dietary Management

The goal of dietary management is to minimize the patient's symptoms or to reduce them to a level that the patient finds tolerable.

Hypoglycemia due to islet cell or extrapancreatic tumors is treated by surgery. While the patient awaits surgery, or if surgery has not succeeded in removing the tumor, frequent feedings are given in order to prevent symptoms. The carbohydrate and protein content of the diet should be emphasized, since fat is largely ineffective in correcting hypoglycemia and would contribute additional kilocalories. Simple sugars rapidly correct symptoms and need not be avoided. Carbohydrates and proteins, which are more slowly absorbed than simple sugar, may be preferable for preventing symptoms since they may extend the intervals between feedings.

The dietary management of reactive hypoglycemia consists of avoiding simple carbohydrates. If several normal-sized mixed meals containing protein, fat, and slowly absorbed carbohydrate are followed by distress, smaller feedings may be tried. The frequency of feedings may need to be increased to provide the necessary caloric intake. The restriction of complex carbohydrates generally does not relieve symptoms and may result in a high fat diet. The meal plans for diabetes offer a reasonable general guide to diet planning in reactive hypoglycemia (see Chapter 8, Diabetes, pp. 158–161).

Physicians: How to Order Diet

The diet order should indicate *diet for reactive hypoglycemia*. If the disorder is indicated, the dietitian determines the appropriate modifications according to the guidelines given and to the tolerances of the patient.

References

54. Service FJ. Hypoglycemias. Compr Ther 1976;2:27–31.
55. Fajans SS, Floyd JC Jr. Fasting hypoglycemia in adults. N Engl J Med 1976;294:766–772.
56. Gastineau CF. Is reactive hypoglycemia a clinical entity? Mayo Clin Proc 1983;58:545–549.
57. Nelson RL. Hypoglycemia: fact or fiction? Mayo Clin Proc 1985;60:844–850.
58. Hofeldt FD. Reactive hypoglycemia. Endocrinol Metab Clin North Am 1989;18(1):185–201.
59. Palardy J, Havrankova J, Lepage R, Matte R, Belanger R, D'Amour P, Ste.-Marie LG. Blood glucose measurements during symptomatic episodes in patients with suspected postprandial hypoglycemia. N Engl J Med 1989;321(2):1421–1425.
60. Hogan MJ, Service FJ, Sharbrough FW, Gerich JE. Oral glucose tolerance test compared with a mixed meal in the diagnosis of reactive hypoglycemia: a caveat on stimulation. Mayo Clin Proc 1983;58:491–496.
61. Felicetta JV. When to worry about hypoglycemia. Postgrad Med 1990;88(1):175–180.

OBESITY

General Description

The management of obesity includes an individualized assessment of the need for weight loss and the determination of appropriate weight and lifestyle goals. The treatment may include dietary, exercise, behaviorial, and/or psychological interventions; emphasis on a particular treatment modality is dependent upon individual circumstances. In general, dietary recommendations include a moderate caloric restriction and modifications in the meal pattern and in the selection of foods.

Nutritional Inadequacy

Weight reduction diets are not inherently inadequate in vitamins or minerals relative to the Recommended Dietary Allowance (RDA). However, diets providing less than 1,200 kcal per day seldom meet the RDA consistently. A daily multiple vitamin supplement is recommended for persons who eat less than 1,200 kcal per day. High potency or "therapeutic" vitamin and mineral supplements are rarely indicated. A multiple vitamin supplement may be appropriate for persons with food aversions or intolerances that greatly limit the variety of food consumed.

Indications and Rationale

Definitions.   Obesity is defined as an excess of body fat relative to lean body mass in comparison to population norms. An ideal medical definition of obesity would be based on the degree of excess body fat at which health risks begin to increase and at which the benefits of treatment outweigh its risks and costs.[62] Because much of the necessary data to make the latter determination is unavailable, and because easy, reliable, and inexpensive means of measuring body fat are not readily available, it is more pragmatic to use the standards for "overweight" instead of those for obesity. Fortunately, being overweight is highly predictive of being overfat, and the exceptions—highly muscular individuals who are overweight but not obese—are relatively easy to identify. For practical purposes, obesity is probably present if body weight is more than 20% above "desirable weight" based upon actuarial height-weight data stratified by age and sex. The benchmark desirable weight currently accepted is the midpoint of the weight range for medium-build individuals from the 1983 Metropolitan Life Insurance Company Tables (see Appendix 4). This is the degree of overweight at which the population risk of adverse health consequences begins to increase.[63] Another standard for "desirable weight" includes a formula based on height, frequently used in the clinical setting (see Table 8-8).[64,65] A more recent height-weight table proposed in the 1990 Dietary Guidelines for Americans, titled "Acceptable Weights for Men and Women," reflects Body Mass Index (BMI) ranges associated with body weight's effect on health and mortality (see Appendix 4).[66] A BMI [weight (kg)/height (m^2)] greater or equal to 27.8 kg/m^2 for men and 27.3 kg/m^2 for women is considered "overweight," whereas "severely overweight" is a BMI greater than or equal to 31.3 kg/m^2 for men and 32.3 kg/m^2 for women.[63]

Some limitations to the use of our current definitions of "overweight" and "obesity" are readily apparent. Individuals who are "metabolically obese, relatively normal weight" do not meet the criteria for the definition of obesity. They may have health problems (hypertension, hypertriglyceridemia, glucose intolerance) that would be expected to improve from weight reduction intervention strategies, however. Conversely, "overweight but healthy adults" (most commonly lower body obese women) may be subjected to repeated weight loss treatments that do not improve their health.

Morbid obesity is arbitrarily defined as being 100 lb or 100% above the "desirable weight" as outlined above. The importance of this definition relates to its

---

TABLE 8-8   Calculation of Desirable Weight*

Women	Allow 100 lb for first 5 ft of height plus 5 lb for each additional inch.
Men	Allow 106 lb for first 5 ft of height plus 6 lb for each additional inch.

*This is for medium frame; subtract or add 10% for small or large frame respectively.

influence on treatment choices. Individuals with long-standing (more than 3 years) morbid obesity complicated by medical problems that could be expected to improve with successful, permanent weight loss may be candidates for bariatric surgery. Nonsurgical approaches to weight control are notoriously unsuccessful in treating morbid obesity.

As can be surmised from the variety of definitions, obesity is not a single disorder, but rather a heterogeneous group of disorders that are associated with varying types and degrees of risk for morbidity and mortality.[67] Management decisions should be based on the evaluation of risk and the consideration of contributing and predisposing factors.[62] The salient questions in the management of obesity are what risks does obesity pose to an individual who has a medical need for weight loss, how much weight should an individual lose, and how should the weight loss be accomplished.

Formulating potentially effective treatment strategies for an individual obese patient requires the collection of a variety of data. These include personal and demographic data, developmental patterns, family history, energy balance, body composition and fat distribution, psychological and behavioral measures, and complications and associated conditions.[67]

Personal and Demographic Data. Personal and demographic data include age, sex, education, occupation, and socioeconomic status. The prevalence of overweight individuals varies with age, sex, race, and socioeconomic status.[63] It has been estimated that as much as one third of the variance in body weight can be accounted for by socioeconomic factors. In the United States, in general, the higher the socioeconomic level, the lower the prevalence of obesity, especially for women. In other societies, particularly in nonindustrialized societies, the pattern is generally reversed. Education and occupation are also important considerations when developing a treatment plan.

Developmental Patterns. Developmental data include the age at onset of obesity, the identifiable circumstances associated with the onset of obesity, and the maximum and minimum adult weight.[67] The individual's personal history of weight changes and the associated events (such as puberty, pregnancy, forced inactivity, and psychological factors) may give some indications of the pathophysiological mechanisms involved and provides information that is important in determining appropriate weight goals. Periods of rapid and substantial weight gain that is then sustained at any age, but particularly during early or late childhood, suggest hyperplasia of fat cells.[68] Individuals with hyperplastic obesity can reduce their fat cell size yet remain overweight because of greater fat cell numbers.[68] This is probably of greater social and psychological consequence than it is a health risk since a reduction in fat cell size tends to correct most metabolic abnormalities.[69] Individuals who have historically been lean and then gain weight with lifestyle and activity changes are probably at a greater risk for health consequences. This is more of a concern if the weight gain is in upper body fat, especially intra-abdominal fat.[70]

Family History. A review of the individual's family background should consider the prevalence of obesity and of medical conditions associated with obesity (diabetes, hyperlipidemia, and hypertension). Recent research suggests that there is a significant genetic component for obesity.[71-73] Severe obesity occurring in individuals who have absolutely no family history of obesity is rare, and its occurrence should prompt a more thorough search for secondary causes of obesity, such as endocrine and central nervous system abnormalities or severe psychiatric disturbances. There is evidence that cardiovascular risks of obesity cluster in families with associated conditions such as hyperlipidemia, NIDDM, and hypertension.[74] A family history of these conditions carries a different prognostic significance than one of family members who tend to live into old age without obesity-related complications in spite of being heavier than average.

Energy Balance. Both caloric expenditure and caloric intake should be considered for their contribution to energy balance. The estimation or measurement of resting energy expenditure (REE) is helpful in allowing one to predict the patient's energy expenditure. Knowledge of daily energy expenditure, in turn, can allow one to provide reasonable goals for daily caloric intake if such goals are needed. REE can be estimated by use of the Mayo Clinic nomogram or the Harris-Benedict equation (see Chapter 3, Nutritional Screening and Assessment). Indirect calorimetry measurements[75] of the resting metabolic rate may be useful for some individuals, particularly those who have severe misconceptions regarding caloric needs.

Only rarely will an individual's measured REE be more than 20% different from that predicted using the above-mentioned methods. Patients in the midst of or just completing a rapid weight loss program (e.g., very low kilocalorie diets [VLCDs] or postbariatric surgery) may have measured REEs 20% below those predicted.[76] Other causes of a markedly subnormal REE include myxedema and prolonged, repeated bouts of food restriction. Occasionally, an obese patient's measured REE will be more than 20% above that predicted. In general, these individuals are likely to be upper body and viscerally obese and admit to consuming large quantities of food.

Most sedentary, nonathletic adults maintain their body weight at a caloric intake approximately 50% above REE.[77] If the individual participates in regular aerobic exercise, it is possible to predict the additional energy expended during exercise. This is most easily done using tables that provide caloric expenditure rates based upon body weight and the type of exercise engaged in.[78]

A precise assessment of the patient's daily caloric intake is virtually impossible using diet history or diet records. Most adults, whether lean or obese, underestimate their true caloric intake. The most helpful information obtained from the diet history includes the meal-snack pattern, the day-to-day variations in intake, the frequency of low calorie diets and binge eating, and the variety of foods eaten. Particular attention should be given to the proportion of calories contributed by fat, sugar, and alcohol, as well as the circumstances associated with adverse changes in eating behavior. VLCDs or the perception of frequent restriction and deprivation increases the likelihood of periods of rebound, uncontrolled overeating, a condition known as "restrained eaters' phenomenon."[79] Frequent snacking and binge eating may be part of an individual's means of dealing with boredom, anxiety, or stress. The role of diet in the development of obesity remains unclear. Reports of eating habits and of food choices of obese and nonobese persons have provided conflicting data but, on the whole, have not substantiated the view that the obese have significantly different food choices or eating patterns[80] or responsiveness to environmental stimuli.[81] Nonetheless, an assessment of dietary intake, of eating patterns, and of influencing factors can guide the recommendations for treatment.

Body Composition and Fat Distribution. Measurements of height and weight are important for obvious reasons. Standard height-weight tables can serve as an initial reference; however, their usefulness is limited. Of greater importance in establishing goals for the individual patient are other assessment data, such as developmental pattern, family history, and complications or associated conditions. An estimation of percent body fat (see Chapter 3, Nutritional Screening and Assessment) may occasionally be useful for determining the degree of obesity and the weight goals for some patients. The concept of body composition also includes a measure of body fat distribution. The distribution of fat that has been described as central, abdominal, truncal, visceral, or upper body obesity is associated with a greater risk of non–insulin dependent diabetes mellitus (NIDDM), glucose intolerance, hyperinsulinemia, hyperlipidemia, and coronary artery disease than lower body, hip and thigh, or gynecoid distribution patterns.[69] A fat distribution pattern can be documented with measurements of the waist and hip circumferences and expressed as the waist-to-hip ratio.[82] Waist-to-hip ratios associated with high risk of obesity-related conditions are approximately 0.95 or above for men and 0.80 or above for women.[66]

Psychological and Behavioral Measures. There is no consistent psychological profile among obese persons,[83] and there is no unanimity of opinion as to the best means of assessing these variables. In the clinical setting, it is often practical only for the physician or the dietitian to make subjective determinations of psychologically related behavior patterns and of the patient's motivation and confidence in having the ability to influence or to improve his or her situation.

Complications and Associated Conditions. Disorders that are clearly associated with obesity and that will usually improve with weight reduction include NIDDM, hypertension, hyperlipidemia, hyperuricemia, and obstructive sleep apnea. Obesity may also be a complicating factor in musculoskeletal impairments, such as degenerative joint disease and chronic low back pain. Complications with general anesthesia and following some types of surgery are more common among very obese persons.

Although rare, a variety of conditions or syndromes are associated with obesity.[67] These include some endocrine disorders, such as Cushing's disease, insulin-producing tumors, and hypogonadal syndromes (Klinefelter's syndrome, Kallman's syndrome), and some chromosomal and congenital anomalies, such as Prader-Labhart-Willi syndrome, Lawrence-Moon-Bardett-Biedel syndrome, and Down's syndrome. Obesity is also associated with central nervous system lesions from trauma or from surgical injury, tumors (such as craniopharyngiomas and metastatic tumors) and infiltrative lesions (such as leukemias, histiocytosis X, and sarcoidosis), and postviral encephalopathies (Kline-Levin syndrome). Syndromes associated with obesity and/or abnormal fat distribution include steatopygia, partial lipoatrophy with secondary lipohypertrophy (Barraquer-Simmons disease), and Madelung's neck or Launois-Bensaude syndromes. The dietary treatment of these unusual syndromes has not proven effective, and one can question whether the major efforts at treatment are appropriate.

Obesity is associated with the use of a number of medications, including corticosteroids (prednisone), the benzodiazapine tranquilizers, tricyclic antidepressants, and lithium.[84] If weight loss is necessary, it may be necessary to change or discontinue psychotherapeutic medications prior to initiating a treatment program.

Determination of Desirable Weight. The term "desirable weight" is used throughout this text to indicate a weight that is likely to be accompanied by benefit to an individual's health. The desirable weight is not necessarily congruent with the ideal weight or the statistical norms that are promulgated by the standard height-weight tables. Rather, the desirable weight is intended to suggest an appropriate or goal weight based on the individual's health status. Both patients and health professionals are attuned to the custom of identifying a particular goal that can be measured in pounds. Although this is an almost universal practice, it is not critical to the achievement of the objectives of weight reduction. In reality, when working with the obese patient in need of weight reduction, more often we are attempting to identify lifestyle goals, which, when accomplished, will result in improved health and weight loss.

The determination of desirable weight should include the consideration of developmental patterns, family history, body composition and fat distribution, and complications and associated conditions. Weight goals may vary substantially among seemingly similar individuals. For example, in a man who weighs 230 lb, the desirable goal weight could justifiably be greater if he had weighed 200 lb during an athletic career or if he had been obese since adolescence and had a healthy, long-lived family background than if he had been 170 lb as a young adult and had gained weight with decreasing physical activity and lifestyle changes, had hypertension, and had a family medical background that included glucose intolerance and premature coronary heart disease. In the former situation, a goal of 200 lb might be appropriate; in the latter situation, a much lower weight goal would be appropriate.

Goals of Dietary Management

The goal of dietary management is to reduce body fat to a level that is accompanied by an improvement in health or is consistent with a reduced risk of complications. Individual goals should be based on functionally important indicators, such as plasma glucose, lipids, and blood pressure, rather than arbitrary weight tables or the rate or degree of weight loss. The treatment should be directed at establishing habits and practices related to food choices, eating behaviors, and physical activity patterns that are conducive to the long-term maintenance of weight loss.

Recommendations

The treatment of obesity includes dietary modifications, physical activity, and behavioral and/or psychological intervention.[85-88] Treatment modalities should be adapted to the circumstances of each patient. No single approach is appropriate for all obese persons. The emphasis that is placed on diet, exercise, and behavioral and/or psychological interventions varies among individuals. Drug therapy for weight reduction, when combined with intensive behavior modification therapy, has been reported to result in greater weight loss than placebo.[89] Unfortunately, weight regain inevitably occurs when the medication is stopped. No anorectic medications are approved for long-term therapy. Surgery for weight reduction is addressed in Chapter 8, Bariatric Surgery.

Dietary Recommendations.   Dietary intervention may include qualitative modifications in food selection, alteration of the meal-snack pattern, and quantitative recommendations for a specific kilocalorie-restricted diet. Emphasis on one or more of these aspects is dependent on individual circumstances and previous dietary patterns.

Relatively high complex carbohydrate, low fat diets, which also tend to be higher in fiber and volume, may be associated with increased satiety and generally form the basis for dietary recommendations. Data support that the nutrient composition of a diet, specifically dietary fat to carbohydrate ratio, may be as important a factor as overall energy intake in weight reduction regimens.[90] In view of the above, the dietary recommendations of the Committee on Diet and Health established by the National Research Council's Food and Nutrition Board appear appropriate to serve as a guide when counseling obese individuals.[91] The dietary recommendations are to reduce fat intake to 30% or less of calories and to increase carbohydrate intake to more than 55% of total calories, primarily by increasing complex carbohydrates (i.e., vegetables, fruits, grains, and legumes), the remaining percentage of calories to come from protein.[91] Although complete restriction of alcohol and of high sugar and/or high fat foods is not necessary, it is generally recommended that they be reduced or used only infrequently. The use of non-nutritive sweeteners and dietetic foods is not universally advocated or prohibited; their utility depends on their caloric content and use in the individual's diet.

For some patients, emphasis should be placed on the redistribution of caloric intake. A structured meal pattern is more conducive to the voluntary control of intake than is an erratic pattern or frequent snacking. Persons who experience episodes of binge eating may benefit from a more equitable distribution of kilocalories throughout the day, especially if deprivation is antecedent to binge eating. For persons with night-eating syndrome and who consume the vast majority of kilocalories in the evening, emphasis should be placed on establishing a 3-meal-per-day pattern and gradually increasing physical activity rather than on further restriction of the caloric intake while maintaining a night-eating pattern.

For most individuals, a moderate caloric restriction that is equal or near to (perhaps approximately 10% above or below) the measured or estimated resting metabolic rate (at present weight) is recommended. This caloric level is sufficient for an average weight loss of 0.5 to 1.0 lb per week, depending on the activity level. Attempts to reduce the proportion of calories from fat are generally warranted. The American Diabetes Association and the American Dietetic Association Food Exchange Lists (see p. 169) with modifications for the occasional use of desserts, sweets, or alcohol can be used to assist with meal planning. Occasional patients consume a large number of calories each day in the form of fruit or vegetable juices or soft drinks. Because the former are considered "healthy," they may not be included by patients in their consideration of total caloric intake. This misconception needs to be addressed.

A moderate caloric restriction is less likely than VLCDs to be associated with undesirable metabolic adaptations, including a reduction in the resting metabolic rate, alterations in appetite control, negative nitrogen balance, electrolyte imbalances, and changes in fluid balance.[92] Furthermore, it appears that repeated caloric deprivation leads to enhanced capacity for physiological adaptation, especially of the metabolic rate, when caloric deprivation (i.e., dieting) is experienced again. Overeating or binge eating following caloric deprivation (i.e., the restrained eaters' phenomenon) compounds the problems posed by the reduction of metabolic rate and may contribute greatly to the cyclically up and down weight pattern that is experienced by many dieters.[93]

The use of VLCDs (diets of 800 kcal or less per day) is not advocated for general use. They should be restricted to extreme circumstances in which rapid weight loss is necessary to ameliorate other life-threatening conditions. Diets that are severely restricted in kilocalories, especially carbohydrates, frequently result in ketosis, diuresis, dehydration, and significant losses in sodium, potassium, calcium, phosphorous, magnesium, and other essential elements.[92] Electrolyte imbalances and cardiac dysrhythmias are a hazard during the use of VLCDs and especially during refeeding. If life-threatening circumstances warrant the use of a VLCD, it should be administered only under the supervision of a physician who is knowledgeable about the regimen's risks and management.[94]

Low kilocalorie diets (diets of 1,200 kcal or less, or less than approximately 50 to 60% of the total calories needed for weight maintenance) do not pose the immediate hazards of very low kilocalorie diets, but they are associated with undesirable metabolic adaptations. And, like very low kilocalorie diets, low kilocalorie diets have not demonstrated convincingly that they result in long-term success.

Weight reduction diets, variously called the Mayo Diet, Mayo Clinic Two-Week Diet, or Mayo Clinic Egg Diet, have had periodic popularity. In general, these diets are relatively low in carbohydrates and high in protein, with varying levels of fat and kilocalories. They advocate the use of a specific combination of foods, such as grapefruit, eggs, and spinach. These diets did not originate at the Mayo Clinic and are neither used nor recommended by the Mayo Clinic.

Physical Activity.   Physical activity has the obvious benefit of increasing the caloric expenditure. Furthermore, increasing physical activity from sedentary to moderate levels is not accompanied by a compensatory increase in the caloric intake and may act to some degree to suppress the appetite.[95,96] The greatest increase in caloric expenditure is with activities that use large muscle groups, that are rhythmic and aerobic in nature, and that can be maintained continuously for a period of time, such as walking, swimming, cycling, running, and endurance game activities. An activity of low to moderate intensity that is maintained for 30 minutes or more, 3 to 5 days per week, is generally recommended for both increased caloric expenditure and improved cardiorespiratory function.[88] For physically deconditioned persons, increases in activity should be made gradually. Substantive, rapid changes from usual activity patterns are discouraged. Those persons who are beginning an exercise program, who are over 35 years of age, and who are deconditioned or who have a major risk factor for cardiovascular disease should consult with their physicians. Persons with restricted mobility, such as might result from a degenerative joint disease or arthritis, should consult with a physician or physical therapist to plan an exercise program. In addition to a formal exercise program, increases in lifestyle activities and the physical actions required for daily living, such as walking and climbing stairs, may contribute to maintaining weight loss.

Behavior Modification and Psychological Intervention. Behavioral approaches are aimed at altering eating, exercise, and lifestyle habits to promote weight control.[86] Techniques and emphasis vary with the individual. Behavioral approaches can take the form of any or all of the following procedures. Records can be kept by the patient of factors that might be related to the urge to eat, such as mood, time of day, varieties of food available, activity, and emotional or situational forces. These records then may enable the identification of situations associated with inappropriate eating. Common examples include watching television, reading a newspaper or book, or seeing or smelling easily available food. Snack type foods in an already opened package might provoke eating, whereas food that requires preparation might be much less tempting.

Once such factors are identified, efforts to control or avoid them can be made. Modifications of eating techniques, such as the cultivation of small bite sizes, the avoidance of rapid eating, or laying down the fork or spoon between bites, might be helpful. A controlled intake of foods that are highly desired by the patient may be more helpful than abstinence, which may ultimately result in binges. A conscious effort can be made by the patient to minimize the discouragement and the guilt that may precede and/or follow binges or that may result from self-perception of appearance or other personal characteristics. Helpful techniques include positive self-statements, imagery, and the establishment of reasonable goals based on consideration of both medical and psychosocial factors.[86]

Physicians: How to Order Diet

The diet order should indicate *weight reduction*. The dietitian makes recommendations according to the preceding guidelines. If a specific treatment approach, caloric level, or weight goal has been previously established in discussions with the patient, the diet order should indicate this information.

References

62. U.S. Department of Health and Human Services. Obesity. In: The surgeon general's report on nutrition and health. Washington, DC: U.S. Government Printing Office, 1988:275–309.

63. National Institutes of Health Consensus Development Conference. Health implications of obesity. Ann Intern Med 1985;103(6 pt 2):983–984,994–995.

64. Hamwi GJ. Therapy: changing dietary concepts. In: Danowski TS, ed. Diabetes mellitus: diagnosis and treatment. New York, Am Diabetes Association, Inc., 1964, vol 1, 73–78.

65. Davidson JK. Controlling diabetes mellitus with diet therapy. Postgrad Med 1976;39(1):114–122.

66. Dietary Guidelines Advisory Committee. Report of the Dietary Guidelines Advisory Committee on the dietary guidelines for Americans, Human Nutrition Information Service U.S.D.A. 1990:7–8,23–24.

67. Callaway CW, Greenwood MRC. Methods for characterizing human obesities: a progress report. In: Hirsch J, Van Itallie TB, eds. Recent advances in obesity research. IV. London: John Libbey, 1985:138–143.

68. Sjöström L. Fat cells and body weight. In: Stunkard AJ, ed. Obesity. Philadelphia: WB Saunders, 1980:72–100.

69. Krotkiewski M, Björntorp P, Sjöström L, Smith U. Impact of obesity on metabolism in men and women. J Clin Invest 1983;72:1150–1162.

70. Anon. The metabolic basis for the "apple" and the "pear" body habitus. Nutr Rev 1991; 49:84–86.

71. Stunkard AJ, Harris JR, Pedersen NL, McClearn GE. The body mass index of twins who have been reared apart. N Engl J Med 1990;322:1483–1487.

72. Bouchard C, Tremblay A, Despres JP, Nadeau A, Lupien PJ, Theriault G, Dussault J, Moorjami S, Pinault S, Fournier G. The response to long–term overfeeding in identical twins. N Engl J Med 1990;322:1477–1482.

73. Sims EAH. Destiny rides again as twins overeat. N Engl J Med 1990;322:1522–1523.

74. Brunzell JD. Are all obese patients at risk for cardiovascular disease? Int J Obes 1984;8: 571–578.

75. Feurer I, Mullen JL. Bedside measurement of resting energy expenditure and respiratory quotient via indirect calorimetry. Nutr Clin Prac 1986;1:43–49.

76. Burgess NS. Effect of a very low calorie diet on body composition and resting metabolic rate in obese men and women. J Am Diet Assoc 1991;91:430–434.

77. Kanaley JA, Andresen-Reid ML, Oenning L, Kottke BA, Jensen MD. Differential health benefits of weight loss in upper-body and lower-body obese women. Am J Clin Nutr 1993;57:20–26.

78. McArdle WD, Katch FI, Katch VL. Exercise physiology: energy, nutrition, and human performance, 3rd ed. Philadelphia: Lea & Febiger, 1991.

79. Polivy J, Herman CP. Dieting and binging: a causal analysis. Am Psychol 1985;40: 193–201.

80. Mahoney MJ. The obese eating style: bites, beliefs, and behavior modification. Addict Behav 1975;1:47–53.

81. Rodin J. Current status of the internal-external hypothesis for obesity.: what went wrong? Am Psychol 1981;36:361–372.

82. Jensen MD. Research techniques for body composition assessment. J Am Diet Assoc 1992;92:454–460.

83. Johnson SF, Swenson WM, Gastineau CF. Personality characteristics in obesity: relation of MMPI profile and age of onset of obesity to success in weight reduction. Am J Clin Nutr 1976;29:626–632.

84. Blundell JE. Pharmacologic adjustment of the mechanisms underlying feeding and obesity. In: Stunkard AJ, ed. Obesity. Philadelphia: WB Saunders, 1980:182–207.

85. Council on Scientific Affairs. Treatment of obesity in adults. JAMA 1988;260:2547–2551.

86. Brownell KD, Wadden TA. The heterogeneity of obesity: fitting treatments to individuals. Behav Ther 1991;22:153–177.

87. Caterson ID. Management strategies for weight control: eating, exercise, and behavior. Drugs 1990;39(Suppl 3):20–32.

88. Pollock ML. The recommended quantity and quality of exercise for developing and maintaining cardiorespiratory and muscular fitness in healthy adults: position statement of the American College of Sports Medicine. Med Sci Sports Exerc 1978;10:8–10.

89. Weintraub M, Sundaresan PR, Madan M, Schuster B, Balder A, Lasagna L, Cox C. Long–term weight control study I (weeks 0 to 34). Clin Pharmacol Ther 1992;51: 586–594.

90. Prewitt TE, Schmeisser D, Bowen PE, Aye P, Dolecek T, Langenberg P, Cole T, Brace L. Changes in body weight, body composition, and energy intake in women fed high- and low-fat diets. Am J Clin Nutr 1991;54:304–310.

91. National Research Council. Diet and health. Washington, DC: National Academy Press, 1989:90,670–672.

92. Davis HJA, Baird IM, Fowler J, Mills IH, Baillie JE, Rattan S, Howard AN. Metabolic response to low and very low calorie diets. Am J Clin Nutr 1989;49:745–751.

93. Jeffery RW, Wing RR, French SA. Weight cycling and cardiovascular risk factors in obese men and women. Am J Clin Nutr 1992;55:641–644.

94. Wadden TA, VonItallie TB, Blackburn GL. Responsible and irresponsible use of very low calorie diets in the treatment of obesity. JAMA 1990;263:83–85.

95. Woo R, Garrow JS, Pi-Sunyer FX. Voluntary food intake during prolonged exercise in obese women. Am J Clin Nutr 1982;36:478–484.

96. Woo R, Garrow JS, Pi-Sunyer FX. Effect of exercise on spontaneous calorie intake in obesity. Am J Clin Nutr 1982;36:470–477.

BARIATRIC SURGERY

General Description

Bariatric surgery was developed in the 1950s as a means of altering the alimentary tract to produce weight loss. Since its introduction, surgery to effect weight loss in obesity has evolved with the goals of optimizing effectiveness and safety. The types of bariatric surgery vary with their approach to caloric restrictions: either complete or selective malabsorption, the anatomical inability to overeat, and induction of early satiety are used either alone or in combination. A cholecystectomy is performed at the time of the bariatric surgery by many surgeons since 80% of patients may develop cholesterol stones. This may be due to a combination of gallbladder bile stasis from lack of cholecystokinin stimulation in the biliopancreatic tract and increased hepatic cholesterol excretion in the bile accompanying mobilization of fat stores with weight loss.

Severe malabsorption, an unexplained cirrhosis, and the development of oxalate nephropathy may result from the jejunoileal bypass procedure. This, as well as serious health complications related to the intestinal "blind loop," prompted most surgeons to abandon this procedure. Patients who have had this procedure in the past may still present with nutritional and metabolic complications.[97]

Gastroplasties (horizontal, vertical, and vertical-banded) attempt to anatomically limit food intake by creating a small upper stomach pouch; malabsorption of ingested nutrients, however, does not occur. The gastric bypass procedure limits intake by creating a small stomach and a "dumping" physiology to inhibit intake of sweets. Less significant nutrient malabsorption develops.[98]

The partial pancreaticobiliary bypass procedure creates a malabsorptive anatomy with many of the attendant nutritional consequences but without leaving a blind intestinal loop or predisposing the patient to cirrhosis.[99] Close nutritional follow-up of all patients undergoing these procedures is essential both to optimize outcome and to prevent nutritional complications.

Indications and Rationale

The surgical treatment of severe obesity may be justified when the risk of remaining overweight exceeds the short- and long-term risks of bariatric surgery. Because the surgical procedures pose significant risks, candidates deserve a careful evaluation.

Criteria for patient selection include (1) a body weight in excess of the average desirable weight by 100 lb or by 100% that has been maintained for 3 to 5 years, (2) the presence of serious health conditions related to obesity that could be expected to improve with successful weight reduction, (3) a history of repeated failure in attempts to lose weight by standard nonsurgical means, and (4) the ability to tolerate surgery and anesthesia. In addition, patients should possess the intellectual capability for complying with the postoperative medical regimen. Because of the risk of growth retardation attributable to prolonged nutritional inadequacies in the child and fetus, bariatric surgery is discouraged in many pediatric patients and women of child-bearing potential.

A preoperative psychiatric evaluation may be helpful to exclude those patients who have a history of substance abuse, unrealistic expectations of the surgery, or who are unlikely to alter their current lifestyle habits.

Goals of Dietary Management

The goals of bariatric surgery diets in the initial postsurgical phase are to (1) facilitate weight loss and (2) prevent the development of nutritional deficiencies as a result of reduced intake and/or malabsorption. Long-term goals are to (1) achieve eating and lifestyle behaviors that are conducive to maintenance of a more desirable weight and (2) detect and treat nutritional deficiencies that develop as a result of reduced intake and/or malabsorption.

VERTICAL BANDED GASTROPLASTY AND GASTRIC BYPASS

Nutritional Inadequacy

In vertical banded gastroplasty and in a gastric bypass, the quantity of food that is consumed is often greatly reduced. There is a potential for nutritional inadequacies. Many patients have difficulty consuming adequate amounts of protein. This problem is particularly pronounced in the first few months that follow surgery but may continue over the long term.[99,100] Such surgery often results in an intolerance to red meats and some meat substitutes. A dislike of or an intolerance to milk, which is a major source of protein for most patients initially following gastroplasty, increases the likelihood of inadequate protein intake. Commercially prepared nutritional supplements (see Appendix 10) may be advisable.

Because the caloric intake is very low and food choices are limited, it is difficult for the individual to be assured of an adequate intake of vitamins and minerals. Clinical signs of deficiencies (such as iron, folate, B_{12}, and in some cases calcium malabsorption in gastric bypass surgery) have been documented in some populations following gastroplasty.[99,101-103] A liquid or chewable multiple vitamin supplement should be taken by these patients daily. Evidence of iron deficiency may require larger amounts of iron in addition to the vitamin. Patients with a gastric bypass may also need monthly vitamin B_{12} injections and may need calcium due to possible inadequate absorption.[101,104]

Dietary Recommendations

Bariatric surgery will necessitate one or more of the following dietary modifications depending upon the procedure: food texture and consistency, volume of solids and liquids, frequency and duration of meals, limited caloric intake, avoidance of foods with a high sugar content, adjustment for food intolerances, and/or malabsorption of nutrients (complete or selective). As with other surgical proce-

TABLE 8-9 Potential Problems Following Gastroplasty and Suggested Dietary Modifications

Potential Problems	Suggestions
Nausea and vomiting	If nausea and vomiting occur after eating a new food, wait several days before trying it again. It may be necessary to eat more liquid or pureed foods temporarily. Eating too fast, eating too much, or insufficient chewing may also cause nausea or vomiting.
Dumping symptoms	Dry solid meals, low in simple sugars but high in complex carbohydrate. Avoidance of simple sugars. Check tolerance to lactose.
Pain in shoulder or upper chest area	The patient should be advised to stop eating if pain occurs during eating and to try to eat later after the pain has resolved.
Dehydration	Dehydration may occur with inadequate fluid intake, especially if there is persistent nausea, vomiting, or diarrhea. At least 6 cups of fluid daily are recommended.
Lactose intolerance	Use lactase-treated milk and lactase enzyme tablets.
Constipation	Constipation may occur temporarily during the first postoperative month but generally resolves with adaptation to changes in the volume of food. The regular use of fruits and fruit juices reduces the risk of recurrent constipation.
Diarrhea	Limit the following foods: high fiber; greasy; milk and milk products, and very hot or cold. Eat small, frequent meals. Drink plenty of fluids.
Blockage of the stoma	The stoma may be temporarily blocked if foods with large particle size are eaten without thorough chewing. If symptoms of pain, nausea, and vomiting persist, a physician should be contacted.
Rupture of the staple line	Rupture of the staple line is unlikely. The patient should be advised to avoid eating an excessive quantity of food at one time.
Stretching of the stomach pouch/stoma dilation	The risk of stretching the stomach pouch can be reduced by avoiding eating large portions of food at one time and by modifying the texture of foods only gradually in the early postoperative weeks. Most surgical techniques now incorporate bands of material that are placed around the stoma to prevent stretching of this opening.
Weight gain or no further weight loss	A careful diet history should be taken. Potential sources of excess kilocalories include the excessive use of high kilocalorie beverages and snacks.

dures that alter the integrity of the stomach, postoperative changes in the texture and volume of food are necessary for all types of bariatric surgeries. More restrictions are necessary in the early postoperative period, with a gradual transition to conventional types of food. When a small pouch is formed, it limits the amount of food or fluid that can be consumed at one time. The diameter of the exit is small, and the consequent slow emptying of the pouch requires the patient to eat 3 to 6 small meals per day and to allow eating intervals of no less than 15 to 30 minutes. The narrow opening from the pouch can be easily blocked with inappropriately sized pieces of food during the early postoperative period; therefore, modification in the consistency of foods and chewing thoroughly are warranted during the first few weeks following surgery, along with following dumping syndrome guidelines (see Chapter 9, Postgastrectomy Dumping Syndrome).

If the type of bariatric surgery involves creation of malabsorption, the dietary recommendations are the same as for other malabsorption procedures (see Chapter 9, Fat Malabsorption).

The patient is encouraged to cultivate and maintain eating habits that limit calorie consumption while maintaining sufficient amounts of essential nutrients, in particular protein.[105] Physical hunger is often minimal, but the psychological urge to eat leads many patients to test the capacity of their gastric pouch with inappropriate amounts and varieties of food.

A rapid weight loss during the early postoperative period may represent considerable loss of lean body muscle mass or so-called fat-free mass. Table 8-9 highlights the potential problems that follow gastroplasty and suggests dietary modifications for their prevention or alleviation.

Modifications in Texture and Consistency.   The diet should progress from liquids to purees, then to soft foods, and finally to a general diet.

A clear liquid diet is the first step of the diet progression and is followed by a full liquid diet according to usual postoperative diet progressions (see Chapter 5, Hospital Diet Progressions). The third step of the progression is pureed foods (blended solid food or prepared baby food), which, like liquids, are thought to cause very little distention of the small stomach pouch. The length of time for advancement to solid foods depends on individual tolerances. Although this varies with each individual, by 12 weeks after surgery most people are eating ordinary solid food, provided they have learned to chew all food to a pureed consistency before swallowing.

Volume of Solids and Liquids.   Patients should be advised to stop eating or drinking when they are full or preferably just before they are full. The subjective feeling of being "full" may change postoperatively compared to the feeling preoperatively. Some patients may never feel full, instead, the feeling of overeating is a distressing epigastric pain that will be relieved only by time (30 to 60 minutes) or by vomiting. Therefore, these patients must learn how much they can eat prior to the onset of epigastric pain. Initially, the small pouch may hold only 2 oz of food at a time. However, the pouch can be stretched by repeatedly challenging it with quantities of food and liquids larger than the pouch can hold, thus defeating the purpose of the surgery. Within the first several months or more after the surgery, the patient is able to gradually eat larger amounts of food.

Liquids create a full feeling but may speed emptying of the pouch and therefore reduce the effectiveness of the surgery. It is important that the patient eat food rather than drink beverages at mealtime. Liquids should be taken between meals.[102] An initial guide is to sip 1 cup over a $1/2$ to 1 hour period. The patient should stop sipping liquids within 45 to 60 minutes of mealtimes. An adequate fluid intake, usually at least 6 cups per day, is encouraged to reduce the risk of dehydration.

Frequency and Duration of Meals. The patient should take small bites of food and eat or drink slowly. Approximately 20 to 30 minutes should be planned initially for each meal. Also, 3 to 6 small meals are better tolerated than 2 or 3 larger meals.

Caloric and Nutrient Intake. The diet is lacking in calories according to what the patient is able to consume. The dietitian monitors the nutrient intake and modifies the diet with supplements if the intake of other nutrients is insufficient.

Food Intolerances. After gastroplasty or gastric bypass, certain foods may be difficult to tolerate because they tend to cause nausea, diarrhea, epigastric or substernal pain or discomfort, vomiting, or blockage of the opening of the stomach.

TABLE 8-10 Foods That May Be Difficult to Tolerate after Gastroplasty/Gastric Bypass

Meats and meat substitutes	Hamburger Tough, gristly meat
Fats	Fried, high fat foods
Starches	Bran Granola Popcorn Whole-grain bread (nontoasted) Whole-grain cereal
Vegetables	Fibrous vegetables (dried beans, peas, celery, corn, cabbage) Raw vegetables Mushrooms
Fruit	Dried fruit Coconut Orange and grapefruit membranes
Miscellaneous	Carbonated beverages Highly seasoned and spicy food Nuts Pickles Seeds Skins
Sweets (postgastric bypass)	Candy Desserts Jam Jelly Sweetened fruit or juice Sweetened beverages Other sweets

Tolerance will vary with each individual.

Generally, foods high in fat, fiber, or sugar and foods that are difficult to chew thoroughly should be avoided. Some people who have had a gastroplasty have found the foods appearing in Table 8-10 difficult to tolerate. After a gastric bypass, sweets may not be tolerated due to the dumping physiology.

Food intolerances vary with the individual. Through trial and error, the patient may demonstrate a tolerance to some of these foods. Any food that causes discomfort should not be eaten.

PANCREATICOBILIARY BYPASS

General Description

In 1975 Scopinaro and colleagues of Italy developed an operation that incorporated a malabsorption syndrome without creating the serious and undesirable side effects of the jejunoileal bypass.[106] The procedure incorporates a subtotal gastrectomy with a long Roux-en-Y limb of the ileum and a distal jejunoileostomy called the "pancreaticobiliary bypass" (PBP). The operation consists of a gastric remnant holding 150 to 400 ml (5 to 10 oz), a gastroenterostomy to an efferent Roux-en-Y limb of the ileum, and a long afferent limb that is anastomosed 50 cm from the ileocecal valve forming a 50 cm common channel for the mixing of food and biliopancreatic secretions. This anatomy effectively bypasses the entire duodenum and jejunum.[107] Unlike the small intestinal bypass, the bypassed segment in this surgery is exposed to the pancreatobiliary secretions. The presence of these secretions prevents the development of both cirrhosis and the "bypass enteritis" seen after small intestine bypass. If the ileal common tract is long enough, it will allow a normal absorption of bile salts, thereby leaving the enterohepatic bile salt circulation undisturbed.

The purpose of a subtotal gastrectomy is to reduce acid production and thereby prevent a stomal ulcer and to increase weight loss during the initial postoperative months due to a decreased gastric reservoir.[107]

Careful preoperative selection of candidates for this procedure is imperative. This operation should be reserved for select patients with "super obesity" (more than 225% above ideal weight) and with the most severe medical problems related to their obesity (e.g., sleep apnea, IDDM, hyperlipidemia with coronary artery disease). The likely level of postoperative compliance should be assessed to ensure long-term health. The same criteria for patient selection involved in the other bariatric surgeries can also be utilized (see p. 196).

Nutritional Inadequacy

The malabsorptive and maldigestive physiology of this procedure results in foul-smelling loose stools that can be offensive and annoying to the patient and family. Diarrhea associated with this procedure is less than with the small intestine bypass so that fluid and electrolyte abnormalities are rarely seen. A two- to three-fold elevated oxalate level in the urine is frequently seen because unabsorbed fatty acids in the colon compete with oxalate for calcium, resulting in free oxalates. In the absence of a dehydrating diarrhea, an increased incidence of renal stones has not been seen. However, encouraging adequate fluid intake is critical.

Reduced serum calcium has occasionally been noted, possibly due to avoidance of milk. Many patients develop a lactose intolerance because the majority of the lactase enzyme is present on the surface of the proximal jejunum. Milk treated with lactase enzyme and milk digestants can be prescribed but have not been proven very effective. The majority of calcium is absorbed in the duodenum, which has been bypassed, and it appears that there is a significant risk for developing metabolic bone disease. Calcium supplementation therefore becomes necessary.

When there is reduced protein digestion and absorption, hypoproteinemia may develop. If detected within the first 6 months, it can be corrected with amino acid supplements and oral pancreatic enzymes. Protein malnutrition may occur in the early stages. The clinical signs consist of asthenia, anemia, alopecia, and edema (with hypoproteinemia and hypoalbuminemia). The cause is usually insufficient food intake. The late onset is most likely related to impaired absorption of protein due to inadequate adaptive changes or to rapid intestinal transit.

The following supplements should be taken daily when needed: a multiple vitamin containing minerals; water soluble forms of vitamins A, D, and K; ferrous fumarate with vitamin C; calcium carbonate; and vitamin B_{12}. In addition, zinc, magnesium, and selenium supplements have been needed in some cases.

Dietary Recommendations

The diet should progress from liquids to mechanical soft and finally to a general diet. A clear liquid diet is the first step of the diet progression and is followed by a full liquid diet according to usual postoperative diet progressions (see Chapter 5, Hospital Diet Progressions). The third step of the diet is mechanical soft foods. The length of time for advancement to solid food depends on individual tolerance. Although this varies with each individual, by 8 weeks after surgery most are eating a regular diet provided they chew food thoroughly to a pureed consistency.

The operation has proven very effective, with a mean weight loss 3 years postoperatively approaching as much as 80% of excess body weight.[106,107] Long-term experience is limited, however. For this reason, close medical supervision is advised.

PATIENT AND FAMILY EDUCATION AFTER BARIATRIC SURGERY

Because of the extent and duration of changes in eating habits that are necessary following bariatric surgery, a detailed explanation of the nature and effects of the surgery is imperative prior to the procedure. Additional education and counseling are suggested during hospitalization to reinforce dietary principles. Because most patients alter their diet according to their tolerances (some of which may have adverse nutritional consequences), diet records should be reviewed periodically.

FOLLOW-UP AFTER BARIATRIC SURGERY

The patient is followed by the surgeon, physician, and dietitian, usually 6 weeks after surgery, then by the physician and dietitian at 3-monthly intervals for 1

TABLE 8-11   Follow-up Care of Patients with Vertical Banded Gastroplasty and Gastric Bypass

	Basal Metabolic Rate	CBC*	Chemistry Group†	Serum Lipids (Total Cholesterol, TG, and HDL)
Preoperative	X	X	X	X
Postoperative hospital care				
6 wk				
3 mo		X	X	
6 mo	X‡	X	X	X§
9 mo		X	X	
12 mo	X‡	X	X	X§
24 mo	X‡	X	X	X§

TG = Triglycerides; HDL = high-density lipoprotein.

*Complete blood count: hemoglobin, hematocrit, erythrocytes, mean corpuscular volume, mean corpuscular hemoglobin, mean corpuscular hemoglobin concentration, red blood cell distribution width, leukocytes, granulocytes, lymphocytes, mononuclear mean platelet volume, platelet count.

†Chemistry group: sodium, potassium, calcium, phosphorus, total protein, glucose, alkaline phosphatase, aspartame aminotransferase, bilirubin—total and direct, uric acid, creatinine, albumin.

‡If weight stabilizes earlier than expected.

§If abnormal preoperatively.

year, then at yearly intervals indefinitely. If problems occur, additional follow-up visits should be scheduled. At each visit, the patient is weighed and specific blood tests are acquired (see Tables 8-11 and 8-12). Also, the health care team questions and discusses with the patient any changes in bowel habit, nausea, vomiting, food intolerance, hydration state, eating and exercise habits, vitamin and mineral supplementation, and any other problems and concerns that develop. When there are difficulties adapting to the required eating and lifestyle changes, a behavioral psychologist can be of assistance in helping patients develop a healthier lifestyle.

Severely overweight females may have fertility problems or irregular menses, which are most likely related to abnormal metabolism of sex steroids by adipose tissue. Weight loss has been found to improve their gynecologic problems and normalize their sex hormones. Patients are encouraged not to get pregnant until after their weight loss has stopped and their weight has stabilized.[98,106]

During the first 3 to 6 months following surgery, nutritional problems may arise due to food intolerances and excessive weight loss (such as a 90 lb weight loss within 3 months). These include protein-calorie malnutrition, dehydration, and specific or general vitamin and/or mineral deficiencies.

The diet assessment should include assessing a 24-hour recall or reviewing a food record or a food frequency questionnaire to determine if the patient is consuming the following:

TABLE 8-12 Follow-up Care of Patients with Pancreaticobiliary Bypass

	Basal Metabolic Rate	CBC*	Chemistry Group†	PT, Vitamin A, E, D, and Trace Element Screen‡	Serum Lipids (Total Cholesterol, TG, and HDL)
Preoperative	X	X	X		X
Postoperative hospital care					
6 wk					
3 mo		X	X	X	
6 mo	X§	X	X	X	X#
9 mo		X	X	X	
12 mo	X§	X	X	X	X#
24 mo	X§	X	X	X	X#

PT = Prothrombin time; TG = triglycerides; HDL = high-density lipoprotein.

*Complete blood count: hemoglobin, hematocrit, erythrocytes, mean corpuscular volume, mean corpuscular hemoglobin, mean corpuscular hemoglobin concentration, red blood cell distribution width, leukocytes, granulocytes, lymphocytes, mononuclear mean platelet volume, platelet count.

†Chemistry group: sodium, potassium, calcium, phosphorus, total protein, glucose, alkaline phosphatase, aspartame aminotransferase, bilirubin—total and direct, uric acid, creatinine, albumin.

‡Such testing may need to be expanded as needed depending on the severity of the malabsorption induced by the surgical procedure. Basic measurements: prothrombin time; vitamin D, A, E; magnesium, zinc, selenium; 24-hr urinary calcium.

§If weight stabilizes earlier than expected.

#If abnormal preoperatively.

- At least 50 g of protein per day
- At least 100 g of carbohydrates per day (preferably complex carbohydrates)
- At least 6 cups of noncaffeinated fluid per day
- The required vitamin and mineral supplement(s)
- Total caloric intake of at least 1,000 to 1,200 per day and gradually up to resting energy caloric requirements for current weight (see Chatper 3, Nutritional Screening and Assessment)
- 3 or more meals daily

In addition, one should check for the following:
- Frequency of nausea and/or vomiting
- Food intolerance(s)
- Chewing food thoroughly
- Changes in bowel habits

Patients should be counseled in an appropriate weight loss diet once they have progressed to and are tolerating a mechanical soft diet. Any other problem areas are addressed as needed (e.g., constipation, lactose intolerance).

Patients that have a vertical banded gastroplasty surgery can ensure failure to lose weight by consuming high caloric density liquids (e.g., ice cream, alcoholic beverages) or semisolid food (e.g., candy, French fries) that can easily pass through the stoma. Weight gain after a gastric bypass can occur from the gradual stretching and enlargement of the stomach pouch and stoma. With most bariatric surgeries, the long-term dietary care is that of maintenance of weight that has been lost. Within 1 year of the surgery, most patients stop losing weight, having achieved a healthier but not "ideal" weight. Careful long-term follow-up is necessary for the maintenance of weight loss and healthy lifestyle habits.[98]

Physicians: How to Order Diet

The diet order should indicate *diet following vertical banded gastroplasty* or *gastric bypass* or *biliopancreatic bypass*. The dietitian makes recommendations according to the preceding guidelines.

References

97. Kirkpatrick JR. Jejunoileal bypass: a legacy of late complications. Arch Surg 1987;122: 610–614.
98. Headley WM, Headley JC. Evolution and current status of surgery for morbid obesity: Part II. J Med Assoc Ga 1989;78:133–140.
99. Diagnostic and Therapeutic Technology Assessment Panel. Gastric restrictive surgery. JAMA 1989;261:1491–1494.
100. Raymond JL, Schipke CA, Becker JM, Lloyd RD, Moody FG. Changes in body composition and dietary intake after gastric partitioning for morbid obesity. Surgery 1986; 99:15–18.
101. Crowley LV, Seay J, Mullin G. Late effects of gastric bypass for obesity. Am J Gastroenterol 1984;79:850–860.
102. Forse RA. Surgical management of obesity. Obesity & Health 1991; March/April: 21–23.
103. Atkinson RL. Massive obesity: complications and treatment. Nutr Rev 1991;49:49–53.
104. Marcuard SP, Sinar DR, Swanson MS, Silverman JF, Levine JS. Absence of luminal intrinsic factor after gastric bypass surgery for moribund obesity. Dig Dis Sci 1989; 34:1238–1242.
105. Kenler HA, Brolin RE, Cody RP. Changes in eating behavior after horizontal gastroplasty and Roux-en-Y gastric bypass. Am J Clin Nutr 1990;52:87–92.
106. Holian DK. Biliopancreatic bypass. In: Dietel M, ed. Surgery for the morbidly obese patient. Philadelphia: Lea and Febiger, 1989:105–111.
107. Scopinaro N, Ginetta E, Friedman D, Adami GF, Traverso E, Bachi V. Evolution of biliopancreatic bypass. Clin Nutr 1986;5:137–146.

OSTEOPOROSIS

General Description

Osteoporosis is a disease characterized by reduced bone mass and impaired skeletal function that results in an increased susceptibility to fractures.[108-110] It is a major skeletal disease in which nutrition may play a role.[109] Dietary recommendations emphasize the maintenance of a nutritionally balanced diet, which includes an adequate calcium intake.

Nutritional Adequacy

Dietary recommendations for osteoporosis fit into any well-balanced diet to meet the Recommended Dietary Allowance (RDA). Calorie-restricted diets, which are often low in calcium, may contribute to an inadequate calcium intake, especially in women.[110] It is difficult to meet RDAs for calcium in diets of 1,200 kcal or less.[111] It is also difficult to meet the RDA for vitamins when caloric intake is under 1,200 per day. A daily multiple vitamin with minerals may be needed to ensure nutritional adequacy.[111]

Indications and Rationale

Osteoporosis afflicts 15 to 20 million Americans each year, causing about 1.3 million fractures in those 45 years of age and older.[108, 109, 112] Often called the "silent disease," osteoporosis may remain unrecognized until the bones become so weak that a strain, bump, or fall causes a fracture or an X-ray reveals a deteriorated vertebra.

It is more common in women than in men for several reasons: (1) they attain less peak bone mass than men; (2) throughout their lives, they tend to consume less calcium than men; and (3) they begin to lose bone density sooner than men and the loss accelerates at menopause due to decreased production of estrogen.[110,113]

Osteoporosis is often divided into two types. Postmenopausal osteoporosis (type I) occurs in women when estrogen levels decline and loss of bone mass accelerates. The loss is most accelerated during the first several years after ovarian function ceases, and may continue up to a decade.[109,112,114,115] Obese women are less prone to type I osteoporosis than thin women, perhaps because of higher production rates of estrone by adipocytes[113] and possibly greater peak bone mass. Age-related osteoporosis (type II) is the inevitable loss of bone with age, which afflicts both men and women. It manifests itself usually after age 70.[109,112] Reduced production of 1,25-dihydroxy vitamin D, higher parathyroid hormone (PTH) activity, and/or impaired bone formation may be contributing factors. A combination of types I and II may occur in individuals aged 66 to 74 years.[112]

TABLE 8-13 Scientific Validity of Osteoporosis Risk Factors[116]

Well Established	Moderate Evidence	Inconclusive or Inadequate Evidence
Obesity (−)	Alcohol (+)	Moderate physical activity
Black ethnicity (−)	Cigarette smoking (+)	Asian ethnicity
Age (+)	Heavy exercise (−)	Parity
Premenopausal oophorectomy (+)	Low dietary calcium (+)	Diabetes
Consumption of corticosteroids (+)		Thiazide diuretic use
Estrogen use (−)		Progestin use
Extreme immobility (+)		Drinking water fluoride
		Caffeine use

+ = Increased risk; − = decreased risk.

With permission from Peck WA, Riggs BL, Bell NH, Wallace RB, Johnson CC, Gordon SL, Shulman LE. Research directions in osteoporosis. Am J Med 1988;84:275–282.

Secondary osteoporosis is bone demineralization that may result from medication use and certain medical conditions.[108,109,112,113] Medications that may result in demineralization of bone include corticosteroids, heparin, or excessive thyroid hormone. Diseases that may result in secondary osteoporosis include hyperthyroidism, hyperparathyroidism, kidney disease, and some forms of cancer (lymphoma, leukemia, multiple myeloma). Diseases of the small intestine, liver, kidney, or pancreas may also result in impaired absorption of calcium and, if chronic, in osteoporosis. Prolonged bed rest and immobilization can also disturb bone homeostasis, leading to bone loss and osteoporosis.

Table 8-13 lists several factors that affect the risk of developing osteoporosis.[116]

Calcium. It is inconclusive whether osteoporotic patients consume less calcium than control subjects.[113] Low dietary calcium may play a permissive, rather than a causative, role in the disorder.[113] It is not yet established whether increased calcium intake prevents osteoporosis; however, insufficient calcium—especially for a prolonged period of time—may reduce peak bone mass, thereby contributing to the development of osteoporosis.[109,110,113] Calcium insufficiency may result from inadequate calcium intake and/or bioavailability (i.e., absorption or utilization by the body).[115] Calcium intake is especially important during the growth years (childhood and adolescence), during pregnancy and lactation, and during the development of peak bone mass (between ages 18 and 30 years).[113,115,117]

The second National Health and Nutrition Examination Survey (NHANES II) indicates that the median daily dietary calcium intake in the United States is 574 mg for females and 826 mg for males.[118] The RDAs for calcium appear in Table 8-14.[119] NHANES II data also revealed that about 50% of all women in North America consume less than 75% of the RDA for calcium and, as postulated, attain a bone mass that is, on average, below their potential peak.[114] Excluding dairy products, the average American diet provides about 300 mg of calcium per day.[120]

Several dietary components (discussed below) have been shown to influence calcium bioavailability and may contribute to an increased risk of osteoporosis.[108,110,113,115,120-123]

Vitamin D. Vitamin D is necessary for efficient absorption of calcium. Its status depends on adequate exposure to sunlight (ultraviolet light forms a precursor to vitamin D in the skin) and to a lesser degree on the dietary intake of this vitamin.

TABLE 8-14 Recommended Dietary Allowance (RDA) for Calcium[116]

Category	Age (yr)	Daily Requirements (mg)
Children	1–10	800
Males	11–24	1,200
	25–51+	800
Females	11–24	1,200
	25–51+	800
Pregnancy/lactation		1,200

Phosphorus. Excessive dietary phosphorus intake has been shown to accelerate bone loss in animal studies, and recent human studies have shown that such increases may also affect calcium balance in humans.

Protein. The effect of protein on absorption of calcium is influenced by the type of protein ingested. Purified protein increases renal excretion of calcium; however, most protein-rich foods contain other nutrients that may reduce the calciuric effect. Increasing the intake of phosphorus, which occurs in high levels in most protein-rich foods (e.g., meat and milk), may counteract the hypercalciuric effect of dietary protein.

Fiber. Fiber and substances found in fibrous foods, such as oxalic acid (see Chapter 14, Urolithiasis, Oxalate) and phytic acid (e.g., wheat bran), may decrease the bioavailability of calcium. The fiber molecules may themselves bind some of the calcium from food and carry it out of the body. Fiber speeds up the movement of intestinal contents through the gastrointestinal tract, allowing less time for calcium absorption. Other influences on calcium bioavailability are the type and size of fiber particles, the level of calcium intake, and length of adaptation to a high fiber diet. There is little evidence that high fiber diets alone induce a mineral deficiency in people who otherwise consume an adequate diet.

Caffeine. Caffeine has been found to increase the loss of calcium through the kidneys and intestine. A moderate amount of caffeine (300 to 400 mg) has a small adverse effect. The effect of caffeine is proportional to intake. An intake of 150 mg of caffeine per day increases urinary excretion of calcium by about 5 mg per day. It is unknown if these calcium losses are due to caffeine or to other compounds in caffeine-containing beverages (e.g., polyphenols, amino acids). (See Appendix 23 for caffeine content of selected foods and beverages.)

Alcohol. People who abuse alcohol are found to have decreased bone mass. Part of this may be related to poor nutrition, although alcohol has been shown to have a direct toxic effect on bone cell formation. More research is needed.

Sugar. Sugars such as sucrose, fructose, xylose, glucose, and lactose have been reported to promote the absorption of calcium in the gastrointestinal tract. The milk sugar lactose can increase serum calcium in some postmenopausal women when calcium solubility or absorption is low.

Lifestyle Habits. Habits that may increase the risk of osteoporosis include smoking and inactivity. The influence of smoking is unclear, although it may be through reduced estrogen levels.[112] Exercise involving weight-bearing activity (because of the gravitational force on bones, joints, and muscles) may reduce bone loss and increase bone mass. Such exercise is particularly important for the elderly, many of whom are sedentary.[124] Studies show that exercise sufficient to produce amenorrhea in young women leads to decreased bone mass.[113]

Goal of Dietary Management

The goal of nutritional management in osteoporosis is to prevent bone loss.

Dietary Recommendations

Persons who have or are at risk of developing osteoporosis should maintain a nutritionally balanced diet that emphasizes adequate calcium intake. Although the role of calcium intake is not entirely clear, current data suggest that it is rational for all people, particularly women, to ingest the RDA for calcium (see Table 8-14).[118] Persons at increased risk of osteoporosis (Table 8-13)—especially postmenopausal women—should ingest calcium levels above the current RDA (i.e., 1,000 to 1,500 mg).[108,109,112,114] During the early postmenopausal period, which may last from several years to about a decade, the dietary increase or supplemental calcium alone may or may not reduce the high rate of bone loss that occurs promptly after ovarian function ceases.[108,112,114,115] An adequate calcium intake throughout life and postmenopausal estrogen therapy maximize bone density and minimize bone loss.[108,112,114,120,125] Calcium intake appears to have a greater influence on improving calcium balance and decreasing bone loss beginning 6 to 10 years after menopause.[120] One study showed that postmenopausal women consuming less than 400 mg of dietary calcium a day had significantly reduced bone loss with supplementation of up to a total intake of 800 mg of calcium per day. Those more than 6 years postmenopausal experienced greater benefit than those less than 5 years.[125]

TABLE 8-15   High Calcium Foods[126]

The following foods contain approximately 300 mg of calcium:

MILK
1/3 cup dry milk powder
1 cup milk (skim, 2%, whole)

CHEESE
1 1/2 oz cheddar type cheese
2 1/2 oz American (processed) cheese
1 3/4 oz Mozzarella (part skim milk) cheese

OTHER DAIRY PRODUCTS
1 3/4 cups ice cream or ice milk
1 cup pudding
6 oz low fat plain yogurt
1 cup low fat fruited yogurt

FISH
5 oz salmon, with bone
7 sardines, with bone

VEGETABLES
2 1/2 cups Great Northern beans (dried, cooked)
1 1/4 cups spinach (fresh, cooked)
2 cups collards (fresh, cooked)

MISCELLANEOUS
1 1/2 cups macaroni and cheese
1 1/4 cups tofu (soybean curd)

Food Sources of Calcium.   Nutrition experts recommend obtaining adequate calcium from food.[115] Table 8-15 shows the calcium content of high calcium foods.[126]

Obtaining an adequate amount of absorbable calcium from food is difficult on a daily basis unless milk or milk products are consumed. In normal healthy individuals, approximately 25 to 35% of the calcium in milk and other dairy products is absorbed.[115] Dark green leafy vegetables (broccoli, kale, collards, mustard, dandelion, turnip greens, and spinach) contain moderate levels of calcium; however, their oxalate and fiber content may reduce the amount available for absorption. The calcium content of grain foods depends on the extent of milling; whole-wheat or graham flours contain more calcium than white flour, which is more highly milled.[110] However, the fiber and phytic acid content of grain products also may interfere with the bioavailability of calcium.[110,115,117] Tofu, processed with calcium sulfate, and fish consumed with bone are good sources of calcium, but are generally eaten too infrequently or sparingly to be major sources. Some of the following foods are being fortified with calcium: orange juice, bread, soft drinks, breakfast cereal, all-purpose flour, milk, and yogurt. However, few of these products have been tested for calcium bioavailability. The product labels should be checked for the amount of calcium in the food.[110]

Persons who have lactose intolerance and who experience bloating, abdominal cramps, flatulence, or diarrhea with the ingestion of milk may have fewer symptoms if milk and milk products are consumed in small amounts at a time and with meals. Lactase enzyme replacement can also be used. (See Chapter 9, Lactose Intolerance, for additional information.)

Calcium Supplements.   Calcium supplements (Table 8-16) may be necessary to achieve an adequate calcium intake. Persons who require calcium supplements should be made aware of the various forms of calcium, their appropriate use, and

---

TABLE 8-16   Calcium Content of Some Commercial Calcium Supplements*

Supplement	Calcium (mg) per tablet
CALCIUM CARBONATE	
Tums™	200
Calcium Rich Rolaids™	220
Tums Ex™	300
Extra Strength Rolaids™	400
Titralac™ (liquid, 1 tsp)	400
Os-Cal 500™	500
Caltrate 600™	600
CALCIUM LACTATE	
Formula 81™	81
CALCIUM CITRATE	
Citracal 200™	200

*This list is not inclusive and does not constitute product endorsement.

the ways of minimizing side effects, such as constipation. More serious side effects from the long-term ingestion of calcium supplements are uncommon, but do occur.[127] These side effects include hypercalcemia, hypercalciuria, urolithiasis, and increased production of gastric acid. Also, the chronic ingestion of large amounts of calcium and of absorbable alkali, such as calcium carbonate, can induce milk-alkali syndrome (subacute or chronic hypercalcemia with fully or partially reversible renal failure). It is unlikely that milk-alkali syndrome will occur with the ingestion of 1 or 2 g of calcium per day. However, the overzealous person who decides "more is better" may be at greater risk.

Several different forms of supplements are available for purchase. Usually calcium carbonate is recommended because it contains the highest percentage of absorbable calcium (40% of the total calcium-salt content). Calcium citrate is 21% calcium, calcium lactate is 13% calcium, and calcium gluconate is only 9% calcium.[110]

Absorption and utilization of calcium supplements appear to be better when supplements are taken with meals and taken throughout the day rather than in a single dose.[128] Calcium carbonate may cause constipation for some people. Calcium-containing antacids are a good source of calcium and have the advantage of being available in chewable or liquid forms, which may be important for those persons who have difficulty swallowing calcium tablets. Calcium citrate supplements, in recent studies, show an efficient calcium bioavailability, reduced risk of renal stone formation, and reduced constipation and gastrointestinal side effects.[129] Also, calcium citrate may be better absorbed than calcium carbonate in individuals in whom gastric acid production may be inefficient (e.g., the elderly).[110]

Bone meal and dolomite are not recommended because they may be contaminated with toxic substances such as lead, mercury, and arsenic. Chelated calcium tablets are not recommended. They are expensive and have no advantage over other types of calcium. Supplemental magnesium is generally not necessary, since magnesium is available in adequate amounts from foods in the diet.

An adequate amount of vitamin D is necessary for bone mineralization. Vitamin D is obtained through regular exposure to sunlight, use of vitamin D–fortified milk, and/or use of a multivitamin supplement. Additional vitamin D, which is present in some calcium supplements, should generally not exceed the adult RDA of 200 IU per day. Larger amounts of vitamin D should not be taken except under supervision of a physician.

Although fluoride increases bone mass, the newly formed bone may have reduced strength, which increases the risk of fractures. It has been found that fluoride supplementation in conjunction with adequate calcium intake is not effective treatment for postmenopausal osteoporosis.[130]

In addition to an overall adequate nutritional intake, the following recommendations may be helpful in reducing a person's risk of osteoporosis.

- Modest caffeine consumption (i.e., no more than 3 cups of coffee per day).[110]
- Avoid diets that exceed 35 g of fiber per day.[115,131]
- Avoid diets excessive in protein. A prudent guide is not to exceed twice the RDA for protein.[119]
- Avoid excess use of alcohol (i.e., no more than 1 to 2 drinks per day). Count as 1 drink: 12 oz of beer, 5 oz of wine, or 1½ oz of distilled spirits, 80 proof.[132]

- Do not smoke.
- Engage in a regular and moderate weight-bearing exercise program.[108,112,123] It is recommended that a physician be consulted for the appropriate exercise recommendations based on the degree of osteoporosis to avoid the risk of fracture. Possibilities for weight-bearing exercises include walking, hiking, jogging, running, aerobic dancing, weight-training, cross-country skiing, and to some extent bicycling.[108] In addition, spine extension and abdominal strengthening exercises have been suggested as part of the treatment plan for osteoporotic patients.[112,133]
- The use of estrogen replacement therapy or other agents such as vitamin D may also be helpful and should be prescribed by a physician.

Physicians: How to Order Diet

The diet order should indicate *diet for osteoporosis*. The specific level of dietary calcium intake recommended should be included in the diet order. If calcium supplements or other therapies are prescribed, they should be documented in the patient's medical record. The physician should inform the dietitian of any other modification or lifestyle habits that need to be addressed.

References

108. Public Health Service, National Institutes of Health, and National Institute of Arthritis and Musculoskeletal and Skin Diseases. Osteoporosis: cause, treatment, and prevention. Bethesda, MD: NIH Publication No. 86-2226:USDHHS, May 1986.
109. U.S. Department of Health and Human Services. Skeletal diseases. In: The Surgeon General's report on nutrition and health. Washington, DC: U.S. Government Printing Office, 1988:311–343.
110. National Dairy Council. Calcium: a summary of current research for the health professional, 2nd ed. Rosemont, IL: National Dairy Council, 1989:1–33.
111. AMA Council on Scientific Affairs. Treatment of obesity in adults. Conn Med 1989; 53(1):21–26.
112. Barth RW, Lane JM. Osteoporosis. Orthop Clin North Am 1988;19(4):845–858.
113. National Research Council. Osteoporesis. In: Diet and health. Washington, DC: National Academy Press, 1989:292–301,352–355,375,615–626.
114. Anderson JJB. Dietary calcium and bone mass through the lifecycle. Nutr Today 1990, 25:9–14.
115. National Dairy Council. Calcium sources: some considerations. Dairy Council Digest 1989;60(3):13–18.
116. Peck WA, Riggs BL, Bell NH, Wallace RB, Johnson CC, Gordon SL, Schulman LE. Research directions in osteoporosis. Am J Med 1988;84:225–282.
117. National Dairy Council. Calcium and osteoporosis: new insights. Dairy Council Digest 1992;63(1):1–6.
118. Walden O. The relationship of dietary and supplementary calcium intake to bone loss and osteoporosis. J Am Diet Assoc 1989; 89(3):397–400.
119. National Research Council. Recommended dietary allowances, 10th ed. Washington, DC: National Academy Press 1989:42,72–73,175–176,179–180.
120. Riggs BL, Melton LG III. The prevention and treatment of osteoporosis. N Engl J Med 1992;327:620–627.
121. Heaney RP, Barger-Lux MJ. Calcium and common sense. New York: Doubleday, 1988: 188–195.

122. Knowles JB, Wood RJ, Rosenberg IH. Response of fractional calcium absorption in women to various coadministered oral glucose dosages. Am J Clin Nutr 1988;48: 1471–1474.

123. Schuette SA, Yasillo NJ, Thompson CM. The effect of carbohydrates in milk on the absorption of calcium by post–menopausal women. J Am Coll Nutr 1991;10(2): 132–139.

124. Halioua L, Anderson JJB. Lifetime calcium intake and physical activity habits: independent and combined effects on the radial bone of healthy menopausal caucasian women. Am J Clin Nutr 1989;49:534–541.

125. Tolstoi LG, Levin RM. Osteoporosis: the treatment controversy. Nutr Today 1992; 27(4):6–12.

126. Pennington JAT. Bowes and Churches' food values of portions commonly used, 15th ed. Philadelphia: JB Lippincott, 1989.

127. Heath H III, Callaway CW. Calcium tablets for hypertension? A consideration of risks and benefits (editorial). Ann Intern Med 1985;103:946–947.

128. Recker RR. Calcium absorption and achlorhydria. N Engl J Med 1985;313:70–73.

129. Pak CYC, Carson JA. Calcium citrate for calcium supplementation. In: Perkin J, ed. Directions in applied nutrition. Frederick, MD: Aspen Publication 1986;1(1):1–4.

130. Riggs BL, Hodgson SF, O'Fallon WM, Chao EYS, Wainer HW, Muhs JM, Cedel SL, Melton LJ III. Effect of fluoride treatment on the fracture rate in postmenopausal women with osteoporosis. N Engl J Med 1990:322(12):802–809,845–846.

131. Schneeman BO. Dietary fiber: comments on interpreting recent research. J Am Diet Assoc 1987;87(9):1163–1164,1166–1168.

132. Dietary Guidelines Advisory Committee. Report of the Dietary Guidelines Advisory Committee on the dietary guidelines for Americans 1990. Human Nutr Info Sx. USDA:1990:12–13,32–33.

133. Sinaki M, Mikkelsen BA. Postmenopausal spinal osteoporosis: flexion versus extension exercises. Arch Phys Med Rehabil 1984;65:593–596.

Gastrointestinal Diseases and Disorders

ABDOMINAL GAS AND FLATULENCE

General Description

Dietary management focuses on the avoidance of foods that are likely to increase intestinal production of gas or foods that the individual finds through trial to increase abdominal gas and flatulence. Behaviors that increase the swallowing of air may also be identified and should be avoided.

Nutritional Inadequacy

The diet is not inherently inadequate in nutrients when compared to the Recommended Dietary Allowance (RDA). However, individual intake should be assessed and supplemented accordingly.

Indications and Rationale

Relief of these symptoms requires an understanding of the possible sources of gas. Five gases (nitrogen, oxygen, hydrogen, carbon monoxide, and methane) make up 99% of bowel gas.[1-3] These gases may either be derived from swallowed air or produced within the intestinal tract. Rapid intestinal transit may also contribute to symptoms by decreasing the time available for the absorption of gases in the intestinal tract.

Nitrogen and oxygen are present in the atmosphere and usually enter the gastrointestinal tract in swallowed air. Ingestion of air is usually responsible for gas in the esophagus and stomach. It is not clear what fraction of swallowed air, if any, passes into the small bowel; however, most swallowed air is regurgitated and usually does not enter the small bowel. A horizontal position may interfere with the normal eructation of stomach gas and increase the likelihood of gas passing into the duodenum.[3]

Hydrogen, carbon dioxide, and methane are produced in the intestine and comprise the bulk of flatus. Hydrogen is formed in the colon by the action of colonic bacteria on fermentable substrate. Carbon dioxide may be produced in the upper intestinal tract when fatty acids, which are released during the digestion of dietary fats, and gastric hydrochloric acid are neutralized by bicarbonate. Like hydrogen, carbon dioxide is also produced in the colon by the action of bacteria on fermentable intestinal contents. Methane is produced in the colon by bacteria, but its production is not related to the ingestion of particular foods. The ability to produce methane appears to be a familial trait.

Normally, gas is reabsorbed through the colonic wall as it passes through the bowel. If colonic motility is disturbed for any reason, bloating and distention may result in abdominal pain.

Complaints of gas usually take one of three forms: (1) excessive belching, (2) abdominal pain or bloating, and (3) excessive passage of flatus.

Excessive Belching. Swallowed air (aerophagia) is usually responsible for belching. Persons with chronic repetitive belching often precede each belch with a swallowing or aspirating maneuver that causes air to enter the esophagus. Aerophagia is usually the result of habit. In some persons, eructation occurs primarily during or immediately after meals.[4] For these persons, habits that are associated with eating and drinking and that result in frequent repetitive swallowing increase the amount of air that is swallowed (Table 9-1). Anxiety may increase

---

TABLE 9-1 Factors That Contribute to Abdominal Gas and Flatulence

Foods That May Contribute to Gas Production (Avoid on a Trial Basis)

Dried beans, dried peas, baked beans, soybeans, lima beans, lentils, cabbage, radishes, onions, broccoli, Brussels sprouts, cauliflower, cucumbers, sauerkraut, kohlrabi, rutabaga

Prunes, apples, raisins, bananas

Bran cereals, excessive amounts of wheat products, excessive amounts of fruit

High lactose foods: milk, ice cream, ice milk, and cream (see p. 266 for additional information on lactose)

The artificial sweeteners sorbitol and mannitol, which are found in some "dietetic" candies and sugar-free gums

High fat foods, such as fried foods, fatty meats, rich cream sauces, gravies, pastries

Sources of Swallowed Air

Frequent, repetitive swallowing that may be caused by ill-fitting dentures, chewing gum or tobacco, sucking on hard candy, or sipping beverages

Eating rapidly and "gulping" food and beverages

"Drawing" on straws, narrow-mouthed bottles, cigars, cigarettes, and pipes

Foods that contain air such as carbonated beverages and whipped cream

Other Factors That May Affect Gas Production or Retention

Reclining after eating

Inactivity

Stress

aerophagia because swallowing is known to increase in response to psychological stress.[5] Foods that include air as part of their natural structure or that have air added in their preparation may also contribute.

Abdominal Discomfort and Bloating.   Abdominal discomfort and bloating, often described by the patient as "gas," are frequently encountered gastrointestinal complaints. Many patients with these complaints show no evidence of excessive gas production, but they appear to have an abnormality of intestinal motility that results in disruption of the passage of gas through the bowel.[2,3] In addition, these patients may sense discomfort with intestinal gas volumes that are well tolerated by most people. Thus, symptoms that are produced by disordered motility and by a heightened pain response to gut distention seem to be misinterpreted as a feeling of increased gas, when in actuality the total intestinal gas volume may be normal.

Excessive Flatus.   Excessive flatus consists of gases that are formed in the colon.[3] Swallowed air does not contribute appreciably to colonic gas. Also, carbon dioxide formed in the duodenum is absorbed as it passes through the small bowel and does not contribute to flatus formation. The excessive production of colonic gas may result from malabsorptive disorders or the ingestion of foods that contain nonabsorbable carbohydrates. In patients with malabsorptive disorders, food constituents such as lactose, which are normally digested and absorbed in the small bowel, are delivered to the colon where they undergo fermentation by the colonic bacteria.

Normal subjects without malabsorptive disorders may also produce large quantities of gas. Certain carbohydrates that cannot be completely digested by enzymes in the small intestine pass unabsorbed into the colon, where bacteria readily ferment them producing hydrogen, carbon dioxide, and methane. Such nonabsorbable carbohydrates are found in legumes and a variety of fruits, vegetables, and grains.[1,6-9] Fructose may be incompletely digested in some persons and therefore could be a cause of symptoms. Fructose is a common constituent of fruits, some sweetened soft drinks, and fruit preserves.[10,11] An often overlooked source of intestinal gas production is the ingestion of sorbitol and mannitol, two artificial sweeteners commonly used in dietetic food products.[10,12-14]

Goals of Dietary Management

The goal of dietary management is to reduce symptoms to a level that the individual finds tolerable.

Dietary Recommendations

A thorough analysis of the patient's dietary intake and eating habits, coupled with restriction or elimination of the likely contributors to gas production, is the most effective approach to treatment. Otherwise healthy persons who complain of gas must be assured that increased gas per se is not harmful. More specific treatment depends on the source of gas (see Table 9-1).

Excessive Belching.   The treatment of chronic repetitive belching should consist of an explanation of the cause and the benign nature of the symptoms.[2-5] Belching can usually be managed by avoiding foods and behaviors that contribute to air swallowing.[2]

Abdominal Discomfort and Bloating.   The treatment of abdominal pain and bloating should include a discussion of the role of emotions in the disturbance of gut motility.[2,3] Since bowel distention from even normal volumes of gas may cause pain in persons with functional abdominal pain, it is often helpful to attempt to reduce the quantity of accumulating gas. Patients should be advised to limit foods that may contribute to gas production, to avoid behaviors that may lead to swallowed air, and to maintain habits that minimize the retention of gas. These measures may relieve the patient's symptoms. The production of carbon dioxide in the stomach may be reduced by using acid neutralizing or acid suppressing agents (i.e., hydrogen ion receptor antagonists).[15] There is limited evidence that activated charcoal may effectively absorb gas in the intestinal tract.[16] Simethicone, by lessening foaming of stomach contents, facilitates belching and may impart some relief.[17]

Excessive Flatus.   If malabsorption has been ruled out, most patients who complain of excess flatus usually benefit by restricting or eliminating gas-producing foods. A diet history will identify those patients who are intolerant to lactose, fructose, sorbitol, or other similar sugars. Patients should be advised to omit foods one at a time on a trial basis until they reach a level of gas that is tolerable. They should also be advised against the unnecessary omission of foods, which may result in nutritional deficiencies. If milk products or other food groups are omitted, foods with similar nutrient content should be substituted. Persons who are trying to increase their fiber intake can minimize gas production by increasing fiber intake gradually over a period of several weeks.[18]

The effect of exercise on flatulence has not been systematically studied. However, the role of exercise in stress management is well documented, and this may help indirectly to prevent distention. Regular exercise is subjectively found to be helpful in relieving or preventing gas and should be encouraged.

Physicians: How to Order Diet

The diet order should indicate: *diet to relieve abdominal gas.*

References

1. Krause MV, Mahan LK. Nutritional care in intestinal diseases. In: Krause MV, Mahan LK, eds. Food, nutrition and diet therapy, 7th ed. Philadelphia: WB Saunders, 1984:439.
2. Levitt MD. Role of gas in functional abdominal pain. South Med J 1984;77:962–963.
3. Levitt MD, Bond JH. Intestinal gas. In: Sleisenger MH, Fordtran JS, eds. Gastrointestinal disease: pathophysiology, diagnosis, management, 4th ed. Philadelphia: WB Saunders, 1989:257–263.
4. Roth JLA. The symptom patterns of gaseousness. Ann N Y Acad Sci 1968;150:108–124.
5. Haderstorfer B, Whitehead WE, Schuster MM. Intestinal gas production from bacterial fermentation of undigested carbohydrate in irritable bowel syndrome. Am J Gastroenterol 1989;84:375–378.
6. Hickey CA, Calloway DH, Murphy EL. Intestinal gas production following ingestion of fruits and fruit juices. Dig Dis 1972;17:383–389.
7. Anderson IH, Levine AS, Levitt MD. Incomplete absorption of the carbohydrate in all-purpose wheat flour. N Engl J Med 1981;309:891–892.

8. Levine AS, Levitt MD. Malabsorption of starch moiety of oats, corn and potatoes. Gastroenterology 1981;80:1209.

9. Stephen AM, Haddad AC, Phillips SF. Passage of carbohydrate into the colon. Gastroenterology 1983;85:589–595.

10. Rumessen JJ, Gudmand-Høyer E. Functional bowel disease: malabsorption and abdominal distress after ingestion of fructose, sorbitol, and fructose-sorbitol mixtures. Gastroenterology 1988;95:694–700.

11. Truswell AS, Seach JM, Thorburn AW. Incomplete absorption of pure fructose in healthy subjects and the facilitating effect of glucose. Am J Clin Nutr 1988;48:1424–1430.

12. Ramry MJR. Dietetic food diarrhea. JAMA 1980;244:270.

13. Hyams JS. Sorbitol intolerance: an unappreciated cause of functional gastrointestinal complaints. Gastroenterology 1983;84:30–33.

14. Jain NK, Rosenberg DB, Ulahannan MJ, Glasser MJ, Pitchumoni CS. Sorbitol intolerance in adults. Am J Gastroenterol 1985;80:678–681.

15. Friedman G. Nutritional therapy of irritable bowel syndrome. Gastroenterol Clin North Am 1989;18:513–524.

16. Jain NK, Patel VP, Pitchumoni CS. Efficacy of activated charcoal in reducing intestinal gas: a double blind clinical trial. Am J Gastroenterol 1985;81:532–535.

17. Jain NK, Patel VP, Pitchumoni CS. Activated charcoal, simethicone, and intestinal gas: a double blind study. Ann Intern Med 1986;105:61–62.

18. Marthinsen D, Fleming SE. Excretion of breath and flatus gases by humans consuming high fiber diets. J Nutr 1982;112:1133–1143.

DELAYED GASTRIC EMPTYING

General Description

The management of delayed gastric emptying is aimed at modifying the composition, consistency, size, and frequency of feedings to a level that the individual can tolerate. This can be accomplished by serving small quantities of liquid to soft foods containing limited amounts of fat and fiber at frequent intervals. The diet should be planned according to individual tolerances. If oral feedings are not tolerated, enteral or parenteral feedings may be necessary.

Nutritional Inadequacy

The nutritional adequacy of the diet depends on the type of diet the patient can tolerate. The full liquid diet may be inadequate in some nutrients. The individual's food intake should be closely assessed. If necessary, the nutritional adequacy of the diet can be improved through the use of liquid dietary supplements. If the diet fails to meet the RDA, it should be supplemented with vitamins and minerals.

Indications and Rationale

Mechanical Obstruction.   Normal gastric emptying may be disrupted by mechanical obstruction. Anatomical obstruction, attributable to pyloric stenosis, peptic ulcer disease, gastric polyps, or gastric carcinoma, causes increased resistance at the gastric outlet. The result is gastric retention, initially of indigestible

TABLE 9-2   Transient and Chronic Conditions That May Be Associated with Impaired Gastric Motility[20-27]

Transient Delayed Gastric Emptying

Postoperative ileus
Acute viral gastroenteritis and other infections
Hyperglycemia
Diabetic ketoacidosis
Hypokalemia and other electrolyte imbalances
Hypothyroidism
Drugs
    Anticholinergics
    Tricyclic antidepressants
    Levodopa
    Opiates (e.g., morphine)
    β-adrenergic agonists
    Alcohol
    Nicotine
    Aluminum hydroxide antacids
    Progesterone

Chronic Gastric Stasis

Diabetes mellitus: autonomic neuropathy
Collagen-vascular diseases
Acid peptic diseases
Achlorhydria and atrophic gastritis (with or without pernicious anemia)
Caloric deprivation (e.g., starvation, anorexia nervosa)
Muscular dystrophies
Central and peripheral neurological disorders
Postgastric surgery (e.g., vagotomy, gastric resection, fundoplication)
Idiopathic pseudo-obstruction
Connective tissue disorders (e.g., lupus erythematosus, scleroderma)

solids, then later of digestible solids and liquids.[19] Mechanical obstruction is almost always managed by surgical intervention. However, when it is inoperable, a feeding tube may be placed beyond the obstruction for the purpose of achieving nutrition and hydration (see the section on Enteral Nutrition Support, Chapter 16).

    Gastric Motility Dysfunction.   Gastric emptying may also be disrupted by alterations in gastric function. Many clinical situations are associated with gastric retention without evidence of structural outlet obstruction (see Table 9-2). All of these conditions appear to be linked by abnormalities of gastric motor function, which present as gastric stasis.[20,21] The term "gastroparesis" has been used to designate this disorder of gastric emptying.

    An understanding of normal gastric physiology and function is helpful in understanding and treating gastric dysmotility. Different mechanisms and regions of the stomach are involved in emptying of the solid and liquid components of gastric contents.[21,28] Gastric emptying of liquids is determined by slow, sustained contractions in the fundus and in the proximal body of the stomach, and gastric emptying of solids by vigorous peristaltic contractions in the antrum or distal part of the stomach. In the process of emptying, the two functions necessary are the antral peristaltic contractions of grinding and mixing (trituration), which reduce solids to the small particle size (less than 2 ml) or near-liquid form that is required for emptying, and the propulsive forces of the fundus, which push the stomach contents into the duodenum. If the stomach has lost its ability to triturate solids into the size necessary for emptying or its ability to generate a gastroduodenal pressure gradient that can push the stomach contents out of the stomach, across the pylorus, and into the duodenum, gastric stasis or gastric retention results.

Motility disorders that are confined to the distal portion of the stomach result in delayed emptying of solids but normal emptying of liquids.[20] Distal gastric dysfunction would preclude the breakdown of solids, but the functioning proximal stomach would retain the capacity to generate the gastroduodenal pressure gradient required for the emptying of liquids. Fundic motility disorders, on the other hand, may delay the emptying of both solids and liquids. Although adequate trituration of solids occurs, the stomach contents do not empty properly because of the impaired gastroduodenal pressure gradient.

Nondigestible solids, such as plant fibers, are resistant to breakdown by antral contractions and, therefore, are not emptied with liquids and digestible solids.[20,28] These solids are retained in the stomach until the rest of the meal is emptied. After the liquids and the digestible solids are digested, powerful contractions sweep the nondigestible solids out of the stomach and down the small intestine to the colon by a special mechanism called the migrating motor complex. Disruption of this motor activity may lead to the retention of indigestible material in the stomach and, occasionally, to the formation of a fibrous bezoar.[22,29,30] A bezoar is a compact mass of fibrous parts of plants that collects in the stomach or small intestine. A loss of normal pyloric function and decreased gastric acidity can cause a predisposition to the formation of bezoars. Thus, patients who have had a vagotomy and pyloroplasty, Billroth I, Billroth II, or Roux-en-Y procedure for peptic ulcer disease may be susceptible to bezoars. Patients with gastroparesis from other causes, such as diabetes mellitus, may also be prone to their development.

The rate at which the stomach empties is influenced by the physical nature and the composition of the gastric contents (i.e., solid or liquid state, original size of the solids, osmolality, and nutrient composition).[20,28,31] Liquids leave the stomach most rapidly. Solids leave the stomach much more slowly in order to allow for the reduction in size to the consistency required for emptying. Fiber is the last dietary constituent to leave the stomach. Osmolality and nutrient composition affect gastric emptying by the action of specific small bowel receptors on neural or hormonal pathways. Fluids of high osmolality have slower emptying rates than do isotonic liquids, which allows for the gradual adjustment of their osmolality to isotonicity in the upper intestine. Although protein, carbohydrate, and fat all slow gastric emptying, fat is the most potent inhibitor. The fatty acid chain length determines the degree of inhibition, with longer chain lengths causing the greatest delay in emptying.

The usual manifestations of gastroparesis may include some combination of nausea, vomiting, early satiety, abdominal pain, postprandial abdominal bloating and distention, anorexia, weight loss, and, at times, bezoar formation.[20,22,23] Symptoms may be of varying degrees of severity.

Some gastroparetic states are acute or transient, such as those associated with certain metabolic abnormalities (which include hyperglycemia, ketoacidosis, and electrolyte imbalances), postoperative ileus, and viral gastroenteritis (see Table 9-2). In these conditions, gastric retention usually resolves or improves as the acute illness abates. Prolonged or chronic gastric retention is often associated with a number of metabolic and endocrine states, some postgastric surgeries, neurological conditions, connective tissue diseases, and such gastric disorders as gastro-esophageal reflux and ulcer disease. In some cases, gastroparesis may be idiopathic. In addition, certain pharmacological agents may cause delayed gastric emptying (see Table 9-2).

The treatment of delayed gastric emptying includes (1) elimination of the cause if possible (e.g., drugs) or treatment of the underlying disorder (e.g., uncontrolled diabetes) if one can be documented, (2) manipulation of the diet, and (3) employment of drugs to improve motility.[20,21] Surgery is rarely indicated in gastroparesis.

Goals of Dietary Management

The dietary management of gastric retention is aimed at planning a diet the individual is capable of digesting, at allowing symptomatic relief, and at assuring adequate nutrition.[20,24] The purpose of the dietary modifications for obstruction is to provide foods that can pass by the partial obstruction. Small feedings are necessary to prevent excessive distention. In delayed gastric motility, the diet is manipulated to find the composition, consistency, and volume of food that the patient's stomach can triturate and empty without nausea, pain, and distention.

Dietary Recommendations

Mechanical Obstruction.   If the obstruction is complete, enteral tube feeding beyond the obstruction or parenteral nutrition may be used. If the obstruction is incomplete, the degree of obstruction determines the type of diet the patient can tolerate. A mechanical soft diet (see Chapter 5) may be tolerated in instances of a lesser obstruction. Emphasis is placed on smaller and more frequent feedings. A full liquid diet (see Chapter 5) can be used if the obstruction is more advanced.

Gastric Motility Dysfunction.   Treatment by dietary manipulation is often helpful. In general, patients with gastric motility disorders tolerate solid foods poorly. Patients with mild disturbances of gastric emptying (as are commonly observed with diabetic, postsurgical, or idiopathic gastroparesis) may tolerate small, frequent meals of soft foods that are lower in fat. Low fiber foods are also advised.[20,29] The dietitian should work with the patient to find the degree of consistency (or particle size) and the level of fat that is tolerated. These patients may also require periodic gastric lavage to remove nondigestible foods.[29] Depending on the patient's tolerance, a variable number of kilocalories may need to be derived from liquids. Table 9-3 summarizes the dietary management for delayed gastric emptying.

TABLE 9-3 Dietary Management for Delayed Gastric Emptying

1. Small, frequent meals
2. Soft to liquid diet as tolerated
3. Reduced fat intake as tolerated
4. Reduced fiber intake as tolerated

Patients with more severe gastroparesis may be unable to triturate and empty solid food but may still be capable of emptying fluids. In these patients, blenderized diets or commercial liquid formula diets may be used. Small amounts of isotonic formula at frequent intervals may be tolerated. Monomeric formulas tend to be poorly tolerated owing to their hyperosmolality.[24]

If the patient is unable to tolerate liquid oral feedings, jejunal feedings may be necessary.[20,24] A continuous infusion by pump is preferable to gravity feeding in order to prevent distention, nausea and vomiting, and dumping syndrome. Feeding into the duodenum may be contraindicated since duodenal contents tend to reflux back into the stomach and duodenal motor abnormalities are commonly associated with gastric motor disorders. In patients unable to tolerate oral or enteral feedings owing to intestinal motility disorders, parenteral nutrition may be necessary.[20,24]

Physicians: How to Order Diet

This diet may be ordered as: *diet for gastroparesis* or *diet for gastric retention*. The dietitian consults with the physician and the patient regarding tolerances and follows the guidelines previously discussed.

References

19. Desai MB, Jeejeebhoy KN. Nutrition and diet in management of diseases of the gastrointestinal tract. In: Shils ME, Young VR, eds. Modern nutrition in health and disease, 7th ed. Philadelphia: Lea & Febiger, 1988:1099–1102.
20. McCallum RW. Motor function of the stomach in health and disease. In: Sleisinger MH, Fordtran JS, eds. Gastrointestinal disease: pathophysiology, diagnosis, management, 4th ed. Philadelphia: WB Saunders, 1989:675–713.
21. Ricci DA, McCallum RW. Diagnosis and treatment of delayed gastric emptying. Adv Intern Med 1988;33:357–384.
22. Gentry P, Miller PF. Nutritional considerations in a patient with gastroparesis. Diabetes Educator 1989;15:374–376.
23. Fich A, Neri M, Camilleri M, Kelly KA, Phillips SF. Stasis syndromes following gastric surgery: clinical and motility features of 60 symptomatic patients. J Clin Gastroenterol 1990;12:505–512.
24. Bistrian BR. Overview of gastrointestinal disorders due to diabetes mellitus: emphasis on nutritional support. JPEN 1989;13:84–91.
25. Camilleri M. Disorders of gastrointestinal motility in neurologic diseases. Mayo Clin Proc 1990;65:825–846.
26. Rigaud D, Bedig G, Merrouche M, Vulpillat M, Bonfils S, Apfelbaum M. Delayed gastric emptying in anorexia nervosa is improved by completion of a renutrition program. Dig Dis Sci 1988;33:919–925.

27. Saltzman MB, McCallum RW. Diabetes and the stomach. Yale J Biol Med 1983;56:179–187.

28. Read NW, Houghton LA. Physiology of gastric emptying and pathophysiology of gastroparesis. Gastroenterol Clin North Am 1989;18:359–373.

29. Emerson AP. Foods high in fiber and phytobezoar formation. JADA 1987;87:1675–1677.

30. Raffin SB. Bezoars. In: Sleisinger MH, Fordtran JS, eds. Gastrointestinal disease: pathophysiology, diagnosis, management, 4th ed. Philadelphia: WB Saunders, 1989:741–745.

31. Meyer B, Beglinger C, Neumayer M, Stolder GA. Physical characteristics of indigestible solids affect emptying from the fasting human stomach. Gut 1989;30:1526–1529.

DIARRHEA

General Description

Diarrhea is generally defined as an increase in the frequency and/or volume of formed or unformed stool.[32,33] Diarrhea is not a disease in itself but a symptom of a variety of diseases or infections. The most common categories of diarrhea are acute (less than 2 weeks duration) and chronic (longer than 2 weeks). Table 9-4 includes examples of the various causes of diarrhea. Treatment depends on the cause of the diarrhea and focuses on four areas: rehydration, medical and/or surgical therapy, nutritional therapy, and prevention of recurrence of the diarrhea.[32,33,39,40]

Nutritional Adequacy

During the acute phase of diarrhea, nutritional intake is often limited. Therefore, the diet is temporarily inadequate in nutrients in comparison with the RDA. However, because of the usually short duration of inadequate intake, a daily multiple vitamin supplement is not indicated.

If diarrhea becomes protracted and chronic in nature or if dietary intake is inadequate because of poor oral intake, therapeutic restrictions (e.g., lactose), or individual food preferences and/or sensitivities, a daily multiple vitamin supplement, that provides nutrients at a level equivalent to the RDA may be recommended. For those who require parenteral administration of fluids for the purpose of maintaining hydration or providing nutritional support, a multiple vitamin supplement can be added to the solution.

Indications and Rationale

Acute.   Acute diarrhea is caused by viral, bacterial, or protozoan infections; by intention or as a side effect of medication; or by altered dietary intake (Table 9-4). Viral-related diarrhea is common and affects all age groups in all parts of the world.[34] Bacterial and protozoan-related diarrheas are also common because of contaminated food and water resources. A cause of diarrhea encountered in the hospital setting is the impairment of intestinal function that results from disuse. When a person has not taken food orally for a week or more, there may be enough decrease in digestive and absorptive functions to produce diarrhea when refeeding is begun. With continued oral feeding of small amounts, intestinal function will gradually be restored and diarrhea will resolve.

TABLE 9-4 Common Causes of Acute and Chronic Diarrhea[32-38]

ACUTE			
Infectious	**Medication/Therapy**	**Dietary Related**	**CHRONIC**
Viral	*Intended effect*	Excessive fruit and	Irritable bowel syndrome
Rotavirus	Laxative	vegetable intake	Inflammatory bowel
Norwalk agent	Lactulose	Lactose intolerance	disease
		Malnutrition resulting	Lactase deficiency/
Bacterial	*Side effect*	in gut atrophy	intolerance
Clostridium	Antibiotics	Enteral feedings	Colon cancer
Staphylococcus	Antacids	Fecal impaction	Carcinoid syndrome
Escherichia coli	Antihypertensives	Heavy metal poisoning	Malabsorption
Campylobacter	Chemotherapy	(mercury, lead,	Celiac sprue
Vibrio species	Colchicine	arsenic)	Pancreatic insufficiency
Shigella	Digoxin	Sorbitol	Surgical
Salmonella	Potassium supplements		Short bowel syndrome
Yersinia	Quinidine		Postgastrectomy
	Radiation therapy		Bacterial overgrowth
Protozoan	Sorbitol		AIDS
Giardia lamblia			Laxative abuse
Entamoeba histolytica			Radiation therapy
Cryptosporidia			Allergy/food sensitivity
Strongyloides stercorali			Motility disorders

Determining the cause of diarrhea is very important because it aids in deciding on the approach to treatment and in preventing recurrence, especially in cases of bacterial and protozoan infections and dietary and medication-related diarrhea. Education regarding the causes of food and water contamination helps minimize the spread of food poisoning and infection. It is also helpful in improving compliance with medical therapy. Adjusting intake of the responsible or offending food item(s) and correcting any malnutrition that may have occurred is necessary to treat dietary-related diarrhea. Diarrhea that develops during a hospitalization may be due to use of antibiotics or other medication. In cases of drug-related diarrhea, the medication may be changed or adjusted to relieve the symptoms.

Diarrhea can be managed by (1) discontinuing intake of the causative food or drug (if possible), (2) providing adequate fluid and electrolyte (e.g., sodium, potassium, chloride) intake to achieve and maintain volume repletion (oral or parenteral), (3) modifying the diet for comfort, and (4) administering antibiotics for protozoan and some bacterial causes.[33,39,40] Commercial or home-made oral rehydration solutions containing glucose, sodium, and other electrolytes have proven very effective in rehydrating pediatric patients and are gaining popularity for use with adults. Glucose facilitates the absorption of sodium and other electrolytes in the small intestine.[33,40] This method has become increasingly helpful for severe cases of diarrhea where parenteral fluids would otherwise be necessary (see Appendix 38, Oral Rehydration Solutions).[32,35,39-41] Fruit juice, Gatorade™ or

TABLE 9-5   Antidiarrheal Medications[33,37,41,42]

Drug	Action	When to Use
Bismuth subsalicylate (Pepto Bismol™)	Inhibits intestinal secretions	Acute diarrhea
Tincture of opium	Antimotility/slows peristalsis	Avoid in infectious diarrhea
Loperamide (Imodium™)	Antimotility/slows peristalsis	Avoid in infectious diarrhea
Diphenoxylate with atropine sulfate (Lomotil™, Lonox™)	Antimotility/slows peristalsis	Avoid in infectious diarrhea
Kaolin- and pectin-containing products	Absorb fluid but do not decrease frequency	Watery diarrhea

other beverages said to correct volume depletion, ginger ale, decaffeinated carbonated beverages, tea, and broth with crackers may be consumed in less severe cases.

Once the diarrhea has begun to abate and the patient is volume repleted, refeeding may begin. Progression from a low fat, low fiber "bland" diet to a usual diet should occur over a 2 to 3 day period as tolerated. Frequent, small meals are generally better tolerated and thus help provide a more adequate nutritional intake. Milk and milk products should be added to the diet cautiously (i.e., limit or avoid full liquid-type diets) in cases of infectious diarrhea, where the small bowel mucosa may have been damaged and a transient decrease in lactase availability occurs.[33,40,41] When diarrhea develops in a patient receiving tube feedings, it is usually not related to the formula, so other causes should be investigated (see Enteral Nutrition Support, Chapter 16).

Medical therapy for acute diarrhea may include parenteral hydration (in severe cases), antibiotics, and over-the-counter antidiarrheal-type medications. Common over-the-counter medications and their mode of action are listed in Table 9-5. Antimotility agents are usually contraindicated in infectious diarrhea because by slowing peristalsis they also cause the toxins to remain in contact with bowel mucosa, hence continuing the disease process. However, they may be helpful in cases of diarrhea from other causes. Further study is needed of the role of kaolin- and pectin-containing products in binding bacteria and toxins to determine their safety and usage.

Chronic.   Diarrhea that lasts longer than 2 weeks requires a physician's evaluation, if not already done, to diagnose the cause and provide effective treatment. Chronic diarrhea may require permanent dietary changes such as a lactose restricted diet for lactase deficiency (Chapter 9, Lactose Intolerance), low fat diet for fat malabsorption (Chapter 9, Fat Malabsorption), high fiber diet for irritable bowel syndrome (Chapter 9, Irritable Bowel, Fiber and Residue Modifications), or gluten-free diet for celiac sprue (Chapter 9, Gluten Sensitivity). In other instances, medical and/or surgical therapy may be necessary for conditions such as inflammatory bowel disease (Chapter 9, Inflammatory Bowel Disease) or cancer (Chapter 12, Cancer).

Goals of Dietary Management

Dietary management is based on an understanding of the cause of the diarrhea. The goals for management are (1) volume repletion, (2) medical and/or surgical therapy, (3) nutritional therapy, and (4) education to prevent recurrence of food poisoning or inappropriate dietary intake. Volume repletion should include extra carbohydrate and electrolyte-containing fluids and/or oral rehydration solutions, often 2 to 3 L/day. Parenteral fluids may be necessary in severe cases. Treatment of the cause as well as the symptoms of diarrhea should begin immediately. Nutritional therapy usually includes 1 to 2 days of a clear liquid diet (Chapter 5, Clear Liquid Diet), which may progress to a diet that is low in fat, low in fiber, "bland," and/or low in lactose. Small, frequent feedings are often better tolerated than 3 meals. Further progression to a general or normal diet occurs as recovery is achieved, usually over 2 to 3 days. Patients should be encouraged to eat a variety of foods, as tolerated, to achieve an adequate and balanced nutritional intake. Patient education regarding the cause and prevention of further episodes should also be included in the plan of care.

Dietary Recommendations

Dietary recommendations are:
1. Initially, encourage patients to consume an adequate amount of fluid to achieve and maintain volume repletion. Appropriate fluids are oral rehydration solutions and clear liquids, especially those that contain sodium and glucose. A clear liquid diet should only be followed for 1 to 2 days due to the inadequacy of most nutrients.
2. When appropriate, advance the diet to include foods that are relatively easy to digest (low fat, low fiber, "bland"). Small, frequent feedings should be provided.
3. Because a temporary lactase deficiency may exist in some instances, milk and milk products should be minimized initially and reintroduced cautiously.
4. After several days and/or abatement of symptoms, further progression to a regular diet is appropriate and necessary to achieve an adequate intake.

Physicians: How to Order Diet

The diet order should indicate the various features necessary, such as: (1) *force oral fluids*, with a goal or minimum amount of fluid indicated in liters, and (2) appropriate dietary modifications (e.g., *clear liquid, low fat, low fiber,* and/or *lactose restricted*). The dietitian determines the appropriate caloric level and other characteristics of the diet based on nutritional assessment, patient tolerance, and discussion with the physician.

References

32. Goldfinger SE. Constipation and diarrhea. In: Wilson JD, Braunwald E, Isselbacker KJ, Petersdorf RG, Martin JB, Fauci AS, Root RK, eds. Harrison's principles of internal medicine, 12th ed. New York: McGraw-Hill, 1991:256–259.
33. Johnson PC, Ericcson CD. Acute diarrhea in developed countries: a rationale for self-treatment. Am J Med 1990;88(6A Suppl):6S–9S.

34. Greenberg NB. Viral gastroenteritis. In: Wilson JD, Braunwald E, Isselbacker KJ, Petersdorf RG, Martin JB, Fauci AS, Root RK, eds. Harrison's principles of internal medicine, 12th ed. New York: McGraw-Hill, 1991:716–717.

35. Wadle KR. Diarrhea. Nurs Clin North Am 1990;25:901–908.

36. Fry RD. Infectious enteritis: a collective review. Dis Colon Rectum 1990;33:520–527.

37. Tabibian N. Diarrhea in critically ill patients. American Family Physician 1989;40:135–140.

38. Greenberger NJ, Isselbacker KJ. Disorders of absorption. In: Wilson JD, Braunwald E, Isselbacker KJ, Petersdorf RG, Martin JB, Fauci AS, Root RK, eds. Harrison's principles of internal medicine, 12th ed. New York: McGraw-Hill, 1991:1252–1268.

39. Taylor CE, Greenough WB. Control of diarrheal diseases. Annu Rev Public Health 1989;10:221–244.

40. Maresca JG, Stringari S. Assessment and management of acute diarrheal illness in adults. Nurse Pract 1986;11:15–28.

41. Brownlee HJ. Family practitioner's guide to patient self-treatment of acute diarrhea. Am J Med 1990;88(6A Suppl):27S–29S.

42. Carpenter CCJ. Acute infectious diarrheal diseases and bacterial food poisoning. In: Wilson JD, Braunwald E, Isselbacker KJ, Petersdorf RG, Martin JB, Fauci AS, Root RK, eds. Harrison's principles of internal medicine, 12th ed. New York: McGraw-Hill, 1991: 519–524.

ESOPHAGEAL REFLUX

General Description

Basic guidelines are given to reduce and/or prevent esophageal reflux symptoms. The use of specific dietary regimens depends on individual patient tolerances to all aspects of medical management.

Nutritional Inadequacy

Dietary modifications for esophageal reflux do not result in a diet that is inherently lacking in nutritional value when compared to the RDA.

Indications and Rationale

Esophageal reflux refers to the regurgitation of gastric contents into the esophagus. The most common symptom is heartburn (substernal pain or discomfort).[43,44] Usually esophageal reflux is a mild condition that can be managed medically. However, chronic reflux may lead to esophagitis, ulceration, hemorrhage, stricture, and/or Barrett's epithelium, which may even necessitate surgical treatment.[43-45] Reflux may occur in patients with or without hiatal hernia, irritable bowel disease, or after gastroesophageal surgery.[45,46]

The esophagus is ordinarily protected from reflux of gastric contents by the contraction of the lower esophageal sphincter. The lower esophageal sphincter is incompetent in persons with chronic esophageal reflux.[43-47] The mean sphincter pressure tends to be lower in these persons so that the likelihood of reflux is increased.[43-46]

Changes in the lower esophageal sphincter pressure normally occur in response to hormonal, mechanical, drug, and dietary factors. Some of the factors that reduce this pressure and therefore increase the chances of reflux include cigarette smoking, alcohol, fatty foods, chocolate, and carminatives (e.g., peppermint and

TABLE 9-6 Pharmaceutical Management of Esophageal Reflux

Action	Examples
Neutralize gastric acid	Antacids (Maalox™)
Neutralize acid and barrier protection	Alginate antacids (Gaviscon™)
Reduce gastric acid secretion	Histamine H_2 receptor blockers (Ranitidine/Zantac™) Proton pump inhibitor (Omeprazole)
Improve lower esophageal sphincter pressure and esophageal acid clearance	Cholinergic agents (Bethanechol™/Urecholine™)
Improve lower esophageal sphincter pressure and gastric emptying	Dopamine antagonists (Metoclopramide/Reglan™)

spearmint oils, garlic, onions, cinnamon).[43,44,46-48] Persons with esophageal inflammation may experience discomfort with the ingestion of citrus and tomato juices. These foods have not been found to consistently decrease lower esophageal sphincter pressure but have a direct irritating effect on inflamed esophageal mucosa.[43,46-48] Some persons associate reflux symptoms with spicy foods. Spices are not believed to affect the esophageal mucosa or the lower esophageal sphincter pressure but are often eaten with high fat or tomato-based foods.

Coffee, decaffeinated coffee, and caffeine have been implicated in esophageal reflux owing to changes in lower esophageal sphincter pressure and increased gastric acid secretion. However, recent studies have shown that coffee produces symptoms primarily through irritation of already damaged esophageal mucosa rather than through these changes in pressure and secretion.[43,47]

Other factors that may predispose to reflux are pregnancy, obesity, and recumbent body position. These tend to increase intra-abdominal pressure.[43,47,48] Nocturnal reflux may be reduced by elevating the head of the bed and by avoiding late evening snacks. Obesity and garments that constrict may increase intra-abdominal pressure. The regression of symptoms is likely to accompany a weight loss. Large meals should be avoided since they may increase gastric pressure on the lower esophageal sphincter.

Table 9-6 summarizes the pharmaceutical management of esophageal reflux. The management may include the use of several medications to treat or to correct reflux.[47,49]

About 5% of individuals with severe reflux require surgery.[50-52] The procedure, called fundoplication, involves creation of a high pressure zone in the lower esophagus that prevents reflux. This is accomplished by wrapping a part of the fundus of the stomach around the lower part of the esophagus.

Goals of Dietary Management

Dietary management is aimed at minimizing symptoms associated with reflux, such as heartburn, and reducing the risk of esophagitis and its sequelae. Dietary recommendations are summarized in Table 9-7.

TABLE 9-7   Recommendations for Esophageal Reflux[43-50]

1. Achieve and maintain a desirable body weight.
2. Avoid large meals. If extra calories are needed, mid-morning and mid-afternoon snacks are permitted.
3. Avoid eating meals or snacks for at least 2 hr before lying down.
4. Avoid or limit foods and beverages that relax the lower esophageal sphincter:
   - Alcohol
   - Carminatives (oils of peppermint or spearmint, garlic, onion)
   - Chocolate
   - High fat foods (fried foods, high fat meats, cream sauces, gravies, margarine/butter, cream, oil, salad dressings)
5. Avoid or limit foods and beverages that can be irritating to damaged esophageal mucosa (according to individual tolerance):
   - Carbonated beverages
   - Citrus fruit and juices
   - Coffee (regular and decaffeinated)
   - Herbs
   - Pepper
   - Spices
   - Tomato products
   - Very hot or very cold foods
6. Encourage the intake of foods that do not affect the lower esophageal sphincter pressure:
   - Protein foods with a low fat content (lean meats, skim or 1% milk, cheeses and yogurt made from skim milk)
   - Carbohydrate foods with a low fat content (breads, cereals, crackers, fruit, noodles, potatoes, rice, vegetables prepared without added fat)

Other Recommendations

Other important antireflux recommendations include elevating the head of the bed, avoiding tight clothing and tight belts, and avoiding smoking.[46-48]

Physicians: How to Order Diet

The diet order should indicate: *antiesophageal reflux diet* or *diet for hiatal hernia*. The dietitian modifies the diet according to the previously identified guidelines and the tolerances of the patient.

References

43. Navab F, Texter EC. Gastroesophageal reflux: pathophysiologic concepts. Arch Intern Med 1985;145:329–333.
44. Gaynor E. Otolaryngologic manifestations of gastroesophageal reflux. Am J Gastroenterol 1991;86(7):801–806.
45. Mann N, Tsai M, Nair PK. Barret's esophagus in patients with symptomatic reflux esophagitis. Am J Gastroenterol 1989;84(12):1494–1496.

46. Friedman G. Nutritional therapy of irritable bowel syndrome. Gastroenterol Clin North Am 1989;18(3):513–523.

47. Kitchin L, Castell DO. Rationale and efficacy of conservative therapy for gastroesophageal reflux disease. Arch Intern Med 1991;151:448–454.

48. Desai MB, Jeejeebhoy KN. Nutrition and diet in management of diseases of the gastrointestinal tract. In: Shils ME, Young VR, eds. Modern nutrition in health and disease, 7th ed. Philadelphia: Lea & Febiger, 1988:1092–1093.

49. Castell DO. Medical therapy for reflux esophagitis: 1986 and beyond (editorial). Ann Intern Med 1986;104:112–114.

50. Larson DE, ed. Mayo Clinic family health book. New York: William Morrow, 1990:593–595.

51. Richter J. Surgery for reflux disease—reflections of a gastroenterologist. N Engl J Med 1992;326(12):825–827.

52. Spechler S. Comparisons of medical and surgical therapy for complicated gastroesophageal reflux disease in veterans: the Department of Veterans Affairs Gastroesophageal Reflux Disease Study Group. N Engl J Med 1992;326(12):786–792.

FAT MALABSORPTION

General Description

The fat restricted diet consists of lowering the individual's usual intake of visible (spreadable and pourable) fat and fat found within food. The level of fat restriction may be adjusted according to the patient's tolerance or according to the physician's order.

Supplementation with medium-chain triglyceride (MCT) fat may be indicated in some situations. The rationale for the use of MCT and guidelines for incorporating them into the diet are given.

Nutritional Inadequacy

This diet is adequate in all nutrients if a proper amount and variety of food are consumed by the patient. One should be alert to the possibility of protein malnutrition since many conditions characterized by fat malabsorption will also show impairment of protein digestion and absorption.

Indications and Rationale

Several disorders can interfere with the normal processes for the utilization of dietary fat. Dietary fats are composed primarily of long-chain triglycerides (LCT), which have a carbon chain length that is greater than 14 carbon atoms. The restriction of fat is likely to be indicated in the treatment of maldigestion, malabsorption, and disorders that involve the transport and the utilization of fat.

Maldigestion.   Maldigestion occurs when there is a defect in the intraluminal breakdown of fat. Causes of maldigestion include disorders that affect gastric, pancreatic, and biliary function.

Pancreatic lipase is responsible for the hydrolysis of most dietary fat. Lipase insufficiency can occur in pancreatitis, cystic fibrosis, pancreatic cancer, and after a resection of the pancreas. It should be noted that pancreatic reserves are large. As much as 90% of pancreatic function can be lost without interfering with fat breakdown and subsequent malabsorption.[53] Oral pancreatic enzyme replacement may partially correct pancreatic insufficiency, so dietary restriction of fat may not be necessary.

Bile acids are responsible for the emulsification of fatty acids into micelles for absorption. Hepatobiliary disease may result in an insufficient production of bile acids or an obstruction to bile flow. Ileal disease or resection decreases the area that is available for the active absorption of bile acids and fat and decreases the bile salt pool. Also, bacterial overgrowth in the small intestine can result in deconjugation of bile salts. A decrease in the amount of bile acids within the intestinal lumen interferes with the emulsification of fatty acids into micelles with a subsequent decrease in the absorption of fat.[53]

Malabsorption.   Malabsorption may occur with conditions that alter the structure and the function of the small bowel mucosa. Celiac sprue or Crohn's disease are examples. The restriction of gluten in sprue and the use of steroids or other drugs in Crohn's disease may be sufficient to correct the malabsorption.

Patients with short bowel syndrome (SBS) have malabsorption that is related to a decrease in the mucosal surface and a decrease in transit time. Recommendations for nutritional therapy depend on the location and extent of the resection and the condition of the remaining bowel. The degree of fat restriction for patients with SBS is currently uncertain. In some studies, fat restriction has failed to benefit patients with less than 150 cm of jejunum that ends in a stoma,[54] whereas other studies substantiate the need for fat restriction to control stomal output and electrolyte losses.[55-57] Patients with a short bowel in continuity with the colon, however, may experience diarrhea because of the cathartic effect of unabsorbed fat and bile salts delivered to the colon. Such patients could benefit from fat restriction to reduce diarrhea and to lessen the likelihood of hyperoxaluria.[58,59]

Transport.   Defects in the lymphatic transport of fat, as found in intestinal lymphangiectasia, chyluria, chylous ascites,[60] and chylothorax, result in the abnormal drainage of lymph into the intestinal lumen, urinary tract, peritoneal space, or a pleural space respectively. There is a loss of chylous lymph, which contains chylomicrons derived from dietary fat. A restriction in LCT aids in the management of these disorders by decreasing chylomicron formation and hence lymph flow. MCTs are rapidly absorbed by the portal route rather than through the lymph system and can be used to supplement the diet.[61]

Utilization.   A diet that is very low in fat is recommended in the management of conditions where the utilization of fat is impaired. One such condition, type I hyperlipoproteinemia, or hyperchylomicronemia, is the result of a defect in the catabolism of chylomicrons by lipoprotein lipase (see Chapter 7, Hyperlipidemia). The clinical features include eruptive xanthomas, hepatosplenomegaly, and pancreatitis. Dietary treatment is directed at alleviating the symptoms and at minimizing chylomicron formation by the restriction of fat to 30 g or less for adults and 15 g or less for children under age 12.

MEDIUM-CHAIN TRIGLYCERIDES

MCT oil is derived from coconut oil through a process of fractionation and of re-esterification of the medium-chain fatty acids with glycerol. MCT oil contains fatty acids primarily of 8 to 10 carbon atoms, whereas usual dietary fats contain fatty acids of 16 to 18 carbon atoms. At room temperature, MCT oil is a thin, clear, light yellow, odorless liquid with a bland taste.[62,63]

MCT are available in two principal forms, MCT oil and formulas that contain MCT oil (see Appendix 10, Enteral Formulas). MCT oil provides 8.3 kcal/g; 1 Tbsp (15 ml) weighs 14 g and provides 116 kcal.

MCT oil is a special purpose food for use as supportive nutritional therapy. It may be used in addition to a fat restricted diet or for nearly total replacement of added dietary fat. The primary purposes for the use of MCT oil are to increase the caloric value and to improve the palatability of a low fat diet.

The rationale for the use of MCT is based on the differences in digestion, absorption, transport, and metabolism between MCT and LCT. Although MCT are rapidly hydrolyzed by pancreatic lipase, absorption can occur before hydrolysis. Bile salts and micelle formation are not required for the dispersion or the absorption of MCT. MCT are transported across the mucosal cell more rapidly than LCT. MCT do not enter the lymph system but are transported through the portal venous system as albumin-bound free fatty acids. They are not incorporated into chylomicrons and therefore do not require lipoprotein lipase for oxidation. MCT may be used as a dietary supplement in most disorders in which a fat restricted diet is indicated.

In addition, the metabolism of MCT under circumstances of carbohydrate restriction produces ketone bodies, which have an anticonvulsant effect. Although many drugs with anticonvulsant actions are now available, a ketogenic diet that incorporates MCT may be used as part of the treatment for seizure disorders.[63] (See also Chapter 25 for a description of Ketogenic Diets.)

MCT should be used cautiously in individuals who are prone to ketoacidosis (such as insulin-dependent diabetic patients) and in patients with cirrhosis. In the former, the ketogenic properties of MCT aggravate any tendency toward metabolic acidosis. In cirrhosis, with or without portacaval shunt, the blood levels of MCT increase owing to the reduced hepatic clearance. Increased levels result in a syndrome that resembles hepatic encephalopathy. This syndrome includes hyperventilation, hyperammonemia, hyperlactacidemia, and disturbed electroencephalogram findings.

The amount of MCT oil used should be small at first and then gradually increased to the desired level. Unpleasant side effects, such as nausea, vomiting, abdominal pain, abdominal distention, and diarrhea, may occur with the rapid introduction of MCT into the diet or the intake of excessively high levels of MCT. Some of the side effects may be related to the hyperosmolar solution that is produced by rapid hydrolysis of MCT. Although the mechanisms are not clearly understood, it may be that the interaction between LCT and MCT or the additive effects cause increased malabsorption and diarrhea when MCT are added to a diet already high in LCT or when excessively large amounts of MCT are incorporated into the diet.

Divided doses of no more than 15 to 20 ml (3 to 4 tsp) at any one time are usually well tolerated. The total daily supplementation should be individualized based on the clinical situation and the therapeutic and nutritional need. Current practice is for the medium- and the long-chain fatty acid content of the diet not to exceed 35 to 40% of the total kilocalories.

The main problems relating to patient compliance are palatability and cost. These can usually be resolved by a variety of methods:

1. Add MCT to beverages by combining 1 tsp (about 5 g) of MCT for each 4 oz of skim milk, juice, or carbonated beverage. Flavoring such as sugar, vanilla, lemon, maple, coffee, or strawberry may be added to milk, if desired.
2. Use MCT in cooking and baking. MCT can be substituted in equal amounts for other fats. Moderately low heat (150–160°C or 300–325°F) should be used when frying foods to prevent the thermal breakdown of MCT. Recipes are available for baked goods.
3. Use MCT in making salad dressings and spreads.
4. Special recipes are available from the manufacturer. Write for "Recipes Using MCT Oil and Portagen," Mead Johnson and Company, Evansville, IN 47721.
5. MCT oil is a very expensive nonprescription item that is available from pharmacies. A physician's prescription along with the HCPC number B4155 can help secure third party reimbursement for MCT.

Goals of Dietary Management

The goals of dietary management are to alleviate the clinical symptoms while providing adequate calories and nutrition.

Dietary Recommendations

Except for the following modifications, the fat restricted diet is patterned after a general well-balanced diet:

- Foods with a high fat content are restricted. The total amount of fat allowed in the daily diet may be determined based on the patient's tolerance or the physician's order.
- No differentiation is made between saturated and unsaturated fat in the diet.
- MCT can be incorporated into the daily diet as needed. Advances in food technology such as the development of fat replacements promise a wider variety of more flavorful food options for patients on fat-restricted diets.[64] See Appendix 22, Fat Substitutes.

Physicians: How to Order Diet

The diet order should indicate: *low fat diet* or *low fat diet with MCT*. If the level of fat is not specified, the dietitian determines the appropriate amounts.

References

53. Friedman HI, Nylund B. Intestinal fat digestion, absorption, and transport. Am J Clin Nutr 1980;33:1108–1139.
54. McIntyre PB, Fitchew M, Lennard-Jones JE. Patients with a high jejunostomy do not need a special diet. Gastroenterology 1986;91:25–33.
55. Higham SE, Read NW. Effect of ingestion of fat on ileostomy effluent. Gut 1990;31:435–438.

56. Mitchell A, Watkins RM, Collin J. Surgical treatment of the short bowel syndrome. Br J Surg 1984;71:329–333.

57. Hessov I, Andersson H, Isaksson B. Effects of a low fat diet on mineral absorption in small-bowel disease. Scand J Gastroenterol 1983;18:551–554.

58. Cummings JH. Short chain fatty acids in the human colon. Gut 1981;22:763–779.

59. Andersson H. Low fat diet in the short-gut syndrome. Lancet Aug 6, 1983;2:347.

60. Ablan CJ, Littooy FN, Freeark RJ. Postoperative chylous ascites: diagnosis and treatment. Arch Surg 1990;125:270–273.

61. Christophe A, Matthys F, Verdonk G. Chylous-fluid triglycerides and lipoproteins in a patient with chylothorax put on a diet of butter or medium-chain triglyceride. Arch Int Physiol Biochem 1980;88:B17–18.

62. Suchev KP. Medium chain triglycerides. Nutr Clin Pract 1986;1:146–150.

63. Bach AC, Babayan VK. Medium-chain triglycerides: an update. Am J Clin Nutr 1982;36: 950–962.

64. Brasitus TA. Advances in food technology provide new options for patients on fat-restricted diets. Resident & Staff Physician 1991;37:63–73.

FIBER AND RESIDUE MODIFICATIONS

HIGH FIBER DIET

General Description

The high fiber diet emphasizes the use of whole-grain bread and cereal products, legumes, vegetables, and fruits in order to increase the intake of dietary fiber. The recommended dietary fiber content of the high fiber diet is 20 to 35 g/day (or approximately 10 to 13 g/1,000 kcal).[65,66] This is about double the amount most Americans consume.

Nutritional Inadequacy

A high fiber diet is nutritionally adequate when compared to the RDA as long as a balanced selection of food items is chosen. High fiber intakes, however, have been associated with a loss of some trace elements in the stool (calcium, iron, and zinc). This has not been found to be of nutritional significance in adults consuming adequate diets.[65] Nevertheless, in populations subsisting on marginal diets, the diet may need to be supplemented.[65]

Indications and Rationale

Dietary fiber is an essential component of a normal diet and appears to be important in both the prevention and treatment of certain diseases. A high fiber diet is now widely accepted as treatment for patients with constipation,[67] and diverticulosis.[67,68] A high fiber diet may also have a role in the management of hypercholesterolemia,[69,70] diabetes,[71,72] and may reduce the risk of developing certain types of cancer.[67,73-77]

Fiber is commonly referred to as roughage, bulk, non-nutritive residue, or unavailable carbohydrate. In the past, many food composition tables have reported fiber content as "crude" rather than "dietary." The term "crude fiber" has no practi-

TABLE 9-8   Food Sources of Various Fiber Components

Insoluble	Soluble
CELLULOSE	**PECTIN**
Whole-wheat flour	Apples
Bran	Citrus fruits
Cabbage family	Strawberries
Dried peas/beans	
Apples	**GUMS**
Root vegetables	Oatmeal
	Dried beans
HEMICELLULOSE	Other legumes
Bran	
Cereals	
Whole grains	
LIGNIN	
Mature vegetables	
Wheat	

From Slavin JL. Dietary fiber: classification, chemical analyses, and food sources. Copyright The American Dietetic Association. Reprinted by permission from J Am Diet Assoc, 1987;87:1164–1168,1171.

cal clinical value since it underestimates the dietary fiber content of foods considerably.[65] The term "dietary fiber" more accurately represents the total fiber content of the food item. Dietary fiber is defined as the portion of plant cells that cannot be digested by human digestive enzymes and therefore cannot be absorbed.[78,79] The principal components of dietary fiber are the major structural components of the plant cell wall: cellulose, hemicellulose, pectins, mucilages, gums, and lignins.[65,78,79]

Dietary fibers are classified by their solubility in water since the solubility of fiber determines, in part, its subsequent physiological effects.[79] In general, soluble fibers (pectin and gums) exert hypolipidemic effects and may lessen postprandial hyperglycemia. Insoluble fibers (cellulose, hemicellulose, and lignin) do not.[65,69-72,79] Insoluble fibers are thought to function mainly as a bulking agent, increasing stool weight and decreasing transit time.[68,79] See Table 9-8 for food sources of various fiber components.

Although the physiological effects of fiber can generally be explained on the basis of their solubility, this does not always hold true. For example, psyllium, which is thought to be highly soluble and has been shown to lower serum cholesterol,[70,80] is also extremely effective in laxation.[79] Thus, it is not always possible to predict the physiological response of a particular fiber based on its solubility. Other physical and chemical characteristics must be considered as well. Particle size of wheat bran can alter its water-holding capacity and, thus, plays an important role in determining transit time and fecal weight.[65,79] Coarse bran is more effective than fine bran in reducing transit time and increasing fecal weight. Other factors such as bacterial degradation and/or adsorption of organic materials may alter the fiber's properties within the colon.

Because of the diverse nature of dietary fiber, it has been difficult to find a method to measure dietary fiber accurately.[78] Currently no ideal method exists. In this text, the most widely accepted and the most complete references for dietary fiber content are used.[80] When available, it is recommended that future literature be used to supplement the tables that are provided.

Bowel Regulation. High fiber diets, especially those high in wheat bran, are useful in the treatment of chronic constipation.[65,67] Fiber increases stool volume, decreases the intracolonic pressure, and decreases intestinal transit time. For most persons with chronic constipation and diverticulosis[68] and for some with irritable bowel syndrome (IBS), an increased intake of fiber may lead to more regular bowel habits and the partial relief of symptoms.[67]

For many years it was believed that a low residue diet was the best treatment for uncomplicated diverticulosis and that the skins and seeds of fruits and vegetables were harmful. These concepts were never validated by controlled studies. In the past decade or two, diets high in fiber, especially whole cereal grains such as bran, have been shown in controlled studies to relieve pain and other associated symptoms of diverticular disease.[68]

Those patients with IBS whose major bowel dysfunction is constipation will be the ones most likely to benefit by increasing their fiber intake.[65] Although the evidence is less conclusive, an increased intake of fiber also appears to benefit some persons with diarrhea. An increased intake of fiber tends to normalize the intestinal transit time. That is, the transit time becomes slower for persons with a rapid transit time. Fiber is also encouraged for those with spinal cord injuries to aid in bowel training.

Diabetes. In diabetes management a high fiber diet improves glycemic control by lessening postprandial hyperglycemia and reducing insulin requirements. High carbohydrate, high fiber diets (55 to 60% carbohydrate, 50 g or more of dietary fiber per day) have been shown to lower insulin levels via increased insulin sensitivity and insulin binding to receptors.[71,72]

Hyperlipidemia. Mechanisms to explain the hypocholesterolemic effect of dietary fiber are less clear. Fiber may exert its lipid-lowering effects by binding bile acids and increasing fecal sterol excretion.[65,70,79,81] However, this probably represents only a small part of the overall mechanism.[65,69,71] Most of its cholesterol-lowering effect is probably indirect, that is, high fiber diets are usually lower in fat and cholesterol. Another indirect benefit of fiber in both diabetes and hyperlipidemia may be its role in weight control. High fiber diets increase satiety, take longer to eat, and are usually lower in calories.[65,69,71,72]

Cancer. Epidemiological and experimental data show a strong relationship between colon cancer and a diet low in fiber.[67,73,74,77] Recent observations suggest that this may also extend to breast cancer.[75,76] At present, the mechanism(s) for cancer inhibition are still not clear. Dietary fiber may play a role in reducing the concentration of fecal carcinogens in the colon, in reducing their contact time through more rapid colonic transit, and perhaps, in reducing their formation through altered bacterial metabolism and lowered pH of colonic contents.[67,73,74,77] In the case of breast cancer, fiber may play a protective role because of its effect on estrogen metabolism and excretion.[75,76] However, the mechanisms clearly involve more than fiber. Diets high in fiber-dense foods are often higher in other nutrients and lower in fat and calories. Thus, the effects of fiber must be considered in the context of the entire diet and the interactions of dietary components. The role of dietary fiber in health and disease management is discussed further in other sections of this manual. Refer to: Chapter 2, Diet and Cancer Risk; Chapter 7, Hyperlipidemia; Chapter 8, Diabetes Mellitus; and Chapter 9, Irritable Bowel Syndrome.

Goals of Dietary Management

Nutritional therapy is generally directed toward increasing the consumption of unrefined breads and cereals, legumes, vegetables, and fruits. The diet plan seeks to increase the intake of fiber over the amount that was usual for the individual.

Dietary Recommendations

A high fiber intake is generally considered to consist of 20 to 35 g of dietary fiber per day (or 10 to 13 g per 1,000 kcal). The consumption of more than 50 g of dietary fiber has no additional benefit and may cause intolerance (fullness, flatulence) and/or problems with absorption of trace elements.

Table 9-9 presents the dietary fiber content of selected foods. It can be helpful for evaluating current dietary fiber intake as well as for planning a high fiber diet. In most cases, food preparation techniques may change the fiber structure but do not significantly change the fiber content.

Initially, a high fiber diet may produce some unpleasant effects, such as increased flatulence and borborygmus. These symptoms are likely to be less of a problem with gradual increases in intake of high fiber foods and often resolve with time as the person becomes accustomed to the diet. Patients should be advised to increase their intake of high fiber foods gradually in order to minimize these gastrointestinal discomforts. If intolerance occurs, the individual should also be advised to try various sources of fiber in order to identify foods that are best tolerated. Patients with IBS may be more prone to developing these symptoms. Better tolerance and improved symptoms can be expected if the total fiber intake is distributed throughout the day. Adequate fluid intake (8 or more cups each day) is important in establishing good utilization of increased fiber consumption. A regular exercise program is also helpful in promoting bowel regularity and general good health.

Fiber supplements ranging from bran tablets to cellulose powders have been proven effective in treating constipation and may also have an adjunctive role in the management of hypercholesterolemia[69,70,81] and diabetes.[72] They may play an important part in the management of some patients. However, many of the commercially available highly purified soluble fiber supplements may produce side effects such as nausea, flatulence, fullness, and abdominal discomfort in some individuals.[65,69,72] Also, supplementation with a concentrated or purified dietary fiber source lacks the nutritional balance provided by a diet containing a variety of foods. Additionally, data on the effect of fiber supplements on nutrient absorption are limited.[78] For these reasons, fiber supplements should only be used for a specific therapeutic purpose in selected patients as prescribed by a physician.

TABLE 9-9 Dietary Fiber Content of Selected Foods

Food Groups	Grams per Serving (per exchange-sized, edible portion*)[80]				
	≤ 0.5	0.6–1.0	1.1–2.0	2.1–3.0	≥ 3.1§
FRUIT†‡	Apples (cooked, canned)	Apples (peeled, dried*)	Apples (skin on)	Boysenberries	Blackberries (4)
	Apricots (cooked, canned)	Applesauce	Cranberries (raw, 1 cup)	Gooseberries	Elderberries (5)
	Banana	Apricots (raw, dried)	Figs (raw)	Kumquats	Guava (5)
	Cherries	Blueberries (canned)	Papaya	Pear	Raspberries (4)
	Coconut (dried, shredded, 1/4 cup)*	Cantaloupe	Prunes (dried)		
	Cranberry sauce (strained, 1/2 cup)	Cranberry relish (1/2 cup)			
	Currants (dried)*	Coconut (raw, 1/4 cup)*			
	Dates*	Figs (canned, dried)*			
	Fruit juice	Fruit cocktail (canned)			
	Grapefruit	Honeydew			
	Grapes	Kiwi fruit			
	Mandarin oranges	Mango			
	Peaches (cooked, canned)	Nectarine			
	Pineapple (canned)	Orange			
	Plums (cooked, canned)	Peach (raw, dried*)			
	Pomegranate	Pears (canned, dried*)			
	Raisins*	Pineapple (raw)			
	Tangerine	Plums (raw)			
		Prunes (canned, cooked)			
		Rhubarb (cooked 1/2 cup, raw 1 cup)			
		Strawberries			
		Watermelon			

*Food may be a significant source of fiber in larger quantities.

†Includes all forms (raw, dried, cooked) for fruits and vegetables except where noted.

‡All raw fruits, raw vegetables, and nuts (including those with 0.5 g of fiber or less) may be contraindicated for some disease states.

§Actual dietary fiber content listed in parentheses.

Continued.

TABLE 9-9   Dietary Fiber Content of Selected Foods—cont'd

Food Groups	≤ 0.5	0.6–1.0	1.1–2.0	2.1–3.0	≥ 3.1§
			Grams per Serving **(per exchange-sized, edible portion*)[80]**		
VEGETABLES†‡	Bamboo shoots	Asparagus	Artichoke, globe or		
	Bean sprouts (cooked,	Beans (string)	French		
	canned)	Bean sprouts (raw)	Broccoli (cooked)		
	Cabbage (cooked)	Beets	Brussels sprouts		
	Celery	Broccoli (raw)	Carrots (raw)		
	Eggplant	Cabbage (raw)	Chicory		
	Endive	Carrots (cooked)	Kohlrabi (raw)		
	Lettuce	Cauliflower	Mushrooms, Shitake		
	Onions (cooked)	Cucumber	Rutabagas		
	Radishes	Greens	Soybean sprouts (raw)		
	Summer squash	beet	Turnips (raw)		
	(cooked)	collard			
	Tomato paste	dandelion			
	Tomato puree	kale			
	Vegetable juice	mustard			
	Water chestnuts	spinach			
	Watercress	Swiss chard			
		turnip			
		Green pepper			
		Kohlrabi (cooked)			
		Mushrooms			
		Okra			
		Onions (raw)			
		Parsley			
		Soybean sprouts			
		(cooked)			
		Summer squash (raw)			
		Tomato			
		Spaghetti/tomato			
		sauce			
		Turnips (cooked)			

STARCHES

Bagel, white	Cheerios™	Artichoke, Jerusalem	Beans (dried, cooked)	Barley (3.5)
Bread, white	Corn	Beans, baked	40% branflakes	All-Bran™ (9)
Cornflakes	Cream of Wheat™	Beans, garbanzo	Flour, whole-wheat	Bran Buds™ (8)
Corn Chex™	Oatmeal	Beans, lima	Parsnips	100% Bran™ (6)
Corn grits	Puffed wheat	Bread, whole-wheat	Peas (dried, cooked)	Bran muffin (3.5)
Cream of Rice™	Soybeans (cooked)	Farina	Pumpkin	Bulgur (3.5)
Flour, white	Sweet potato or yam	Granola	Raisin bran	Lentils (4)
Graham crackers		Grapenuts™	Rykrisp™	Wheat bran (9)
Maltomeal™		Peas, blackeyed	Shredded Wheat™	
Plantain		Peas, green	Spaghetti, macaroni, noodles (whole-wheat)	
Potato chips		Popcorn (1½ cup)	Squash, winter	
Potatoes (no skin)		Ralston™	Wheat germ	
Puffed rice		Rice (brown, wild)		
Rice Chex™		Roll or bun, whole-wheat		
Rice Krispies™		Wheat flakes		
Rice, white		Wheaties™		
Roll or bun, white				
Saltines				
Spaghetti, macaroni, noodles (refined)				

MEAT SUBSTITUTES

		Peanut butter

FATS AND OILS‡

Avocado*
Nuts*
  Almonds
  Brazil
  Cashews
  Hazelnuts
  Macadamia
  Peanuts
  Pecans
  Pistachios
  Walnuts
Seeds*
  Pumpkin
  Sunflower
Soybean nuts*

Physicians: How to Order Diet

The diet order should indicate: *high fiber diet*.

RESTRICTED FIBER DIET

General Description

The restricted fiber diet limits the intake of high fiber foods such as whole-grain bread and cereal products, nuts, seeds, legumes, and certain fruits and vegetables. It is more liberal than the low residue diet. The degree of fiber restriction will depend on the patient's condition and the goals of management.

Nutritional Inadequacy

The diet is not inherently lacking in nutrients when compared to the RDA. However, the individual's food intake should be assessed and supplemented as needed.

TABLE 9-10   Fiber Restricted Diets for Disease States[68,82-85]

Disease or Condition	Degree of Restriction	Comments
Diverticulitis	Acute: low residue Resolving: restricted fiber	Gradual progression to high fiber diet
Gastroparesis	Severe: low residue Mild to moderate: restricted fiber	Severity of the condition will determine the patient's tolerance. Small, frequent meals. Avoid all *raw* fruits and vegetables since they can cause bezoars. High fat diet may further decrease gastric emptying (see also Chapter 9, Delayed Gastric Emptying)
Small bowel obstruction or stricture	Intermittent and/or partial: restricted fiber High likelihood of recurrent obstruction: low residue	Small, frequent meals Site of stricture or obstruction will also be a factor in determining degree of residue restriction
Bowel fistula (i.e., rectovaginal or enterocutaneous)	Low residue	May need elemental diet or parenteral nutrition
Inflammatory bowel disease	See above for small bowel obstruction, stricture, and fistula	Also see Chapter 9, Inflammatory Bowel Disease
Radiation enteritis	See above for small bowel obstruction, stricture, and fistula	
Bowel preparation for surgery	Low residue	Use a milk-free formula if a supplement is indicated

Indications and Rationale

The degree of fiber restriction will depend on the severity of the patient's disease and on the goals for management. A more restrictive diet may be needed during acute exacerbations of gastrointestinal diseases and a less restrictive diet during the resolution of such exacerbations. The fiber restriction may be temporary (e.g., as a transition to a general diet after intestinal surgery) or it may be used for long-term management of chronic conditions such as motility disorders or intermittent or recurrent small bowel obstructions. The severity of these conditions will also help to determine the degree of fiber restriction. Table 9-10 lists various disease states and the degree of fiber restriction indicated.

TABLE 9-11   Restricted Fiber Diet

Food Groups	Allow	Avoid
Meat, and meat substitutes	Tender meat, poultry, fish, seafood, and eggs	Tough or coarse meats, peanut butter
Milk	All dairy products with allowed ingredients	Dairy products containing more than 0.5 g of fiber per serving
Starches*	Most refined breads, cereals, rice and pasta (check label for fiber content), white potatoes without skins	Whole-grain breads, cereals, rice and pasta; starchy vegetables, legumes, popcorn with more than 0.5 g of fiber per serving (see Table 9-9)
Vegetables*	Those with 0.5 g or less of fiber per serving: bamboo shoots, bean sprouts (cooked and canned), cabbage (cooked), celery, eggplant, endive, lettuce, onions (cooked), radishes, summer squash (cooked), tomato paste, tomato puree, vegetable juice, water chestnuts, watercress	All others with more than 0.5 g of fiber per serving (see Table 9-9)
Fruits*	Those with 0.5 g or less of fiber per serving: apples (cooked, canned), apricots (cooked, canned), banana, cherries, coconut (dried, shredded, $1/4$ cup), cranberry sauce (strained, $1/2$ cup), currants (dried), dates, fruit juice, grapefruit, grapes, mandarin oranges, peaches (cooked, canned), pineapple (canned), plums (cooked, canned) pomegranate, raisins, tangerine	All others with more than 0.5 g of fiber per serving (see Table 9-9)
Fats and oils*	Avocado, nuts (almonds, Brazil, cashews, hazelnuts, macadamia, peanuts, pecans, pistachios, walnuts), seeds (pumpkin, sunflower), soybean nuts	

*Contains ≤ 0.5 g of fiber per exchange-size portion. May provide a significant amount of fiber in larger quantities.

Goals of Dietary Management

The goal of this diet is to reduce the fiber intake to a level that minimizes the amount of indigestible solids while providing adequate nutrition.

Dietary Recommendations

A restricted fiber diet can be accomplished by avoiding whole-grain products, legumes, and fibrous fruits and vegetables (Table 9-11). All foods with more than 0.5 g of dietary fiber per serving should be avoided (Table 9-9). In some less severe conditions, foods with 0.5 to 1 g of fiber per serving may be allowed based on the dietitian's discretion and the patient's tolerance. These foods should always be introduced cautiously. Patients should also be advised to chew foods thoroughly, eat slowly, and avoid large meals because these measures may improve tolerance.

Physicians: How to Order Diet

The diet order should indicate: *restricted fiber diet*. The dietitian assists the patient in establishing food tolerances, liberalizing the diet if indicated, and ensuring a nutritionally adequate diet.

LOW RESIDUE DIET

General Description

The low residue diet consists of foods that are very low in dietary fiber. Foods that increase the fecal residue despite the low content of fiber may also be excluded. This diet is used primarily as a pre- or postsurgical diet but may be necessary in cases of partial intestinal obstructions and severe disorders of motility.

Nutritional Inadequacy

The diet may be low in a number of nutrients. It is intended to be used for a short time only. If long-term use is necessary, supplementation with a liquid or chewable multiple vitamin and mineral supplement is indicated. An elemental or polymeric formula may be used if additional calories and protein are needed.

Indications and Rationale

The low residue diet may be used pre- and postoperatively for intestinal surgery. It may also be used during acute exacerbations of inflammatory bowel disease or diverticulitis and when there is bowel stricture or partial obstruction. The low residue diet may also be used for palliative purposes in patients with advanced cancer. Usually the diet is to be used for a short time only or as a transition from a liquid diet to one that is more moderate in fiber content.

The term "residue" refers to unabsorbed dietary constituents, sloughed cells from the gastrointestinal tract, and intestinal bacteria found in feces after digestion.[86-88] Some foods, such as milk and the connective tissue of meats, are low in dietary fiber but may contribute to stool volume,[89-90] particularly in individuals with altered gastrointestinal capabilities. The restriction of these residue-producing foods is based on tradition and is not well documented in the literature.[87,88,90] The need for restriction of these foods should be examined on an individual basis.

TABLE 9-12 Low Residue Diet

Food Groups	Allow	Avoid
Starches	Most refined breads, cereals, rice and pasta, and other products made from refined grains	Whole- grain breads, cereals, rice, pasta, and other products made from whole grains, starchy vegetables, legumes, popcorn
Fruits	Fruit juices except prune	All fruits, including canned
Vegetables	Vegetable juices	All vegetables, including potatoes
Milk	Milk and foods made from milk (pudding, ice cream, cheeses, strained creamed soups) up to 2 cups per day	Milk and foods made from milk (pudding, ice cream, cheeses, strained creamed soups) in excess of 2 cups per day
Meat and Meat Substitutes	Tender meat, poultry, fish, and eggs	Tough or coarse meats, peanut butter
Miscellaneous		Seeds, nuts

Goals of Dietary Management

The goal of the low residue diet is to minimize fecal volume. Nutritional therapy is generally directed toward establishing a tolerance to food.

Dietary Recommendations

Table 9-12 summarizes the dietary recommendations for a low residue diet. Patients should be offered smaller, more frequent meals. They should also be encouraged to eat slowly and to chew foods thoroughly.

Physicians: How to Order Diet

The diet order should indicate: *low residue diet.* The dietitian will clarify the degree of restriction with the physician. If a more restrictive diet is preferred, one should order a commercial formula with elemental or polymeric nutrient sources (see Chapter 16, Enteral Nutritional Support, and Appendix 10, Enteral Nutritional Formulas). A milk-free formula is required in instances where a minimal stool volume is desired.

The dietitian assists the patient in establishing food tolerances, adjusting the diet as indicated, and ensuring a nutritionally adequate diet.

References

65. Kritchevsky D. Dietary fiber. Annu Rev Nutr 1988;8:301–328.
66. U.S. Department of Health and Human Services, Public Health Service. 1990. Healthy people 2000: national health promotion and disease prevention objectives. DHHS Publication No. (PHS) 91–50212:118–119.
67. Klurfeld DM. The role of dietary fiber in gastrointestinal disease. JADA 1987;87:1972–1977.

68. Naitove A, Almy TP. Diverticular disease of the colon. In: Sleisinger MH, Fordtran JS, eds. Gastrointestinal disease: pathophysiology, diagnosis, management, 4th ed. Philadelphia: WB Saunders, 1989:1419–1433.

69. Todd PA, Benfield P, Goa KL. Guar gum: a review of its pharmacological properties, and use as a dietary adjunct in hypercholesterolemia. Drugs 1990;39:917–928.

70. Miettinen TA. Dietary fiber and lipids. Am J Clin Nutr 1987;45:1237–1242.

71. Smith U. Dietary fibre, diabetes and obesity. Int J Obes 1987;11 (Suppl 1):27–31.

72. Anderson JW, Gustafson NJ, Bryant CA, Tietyen-Clark J. Dietary fiber and diabetes: a comprehensive review and practical application. JADA 1987;87:1189–1197.

73. Trock BJ, Lanza E, Greenwald P. High fiber diet and colon cancer: a critical review. Recent Prog Res Nutr Cancer 1990;145–157.

74. Kritchevsky D. Fiber and cancer. Med Oncol Tumor Pharmacother 1990;7:137–141.

75. Rose DP. Dietary fiber in breast cancer. Nutr Cancer 1990;13:1–8.

76. Rose DP, Goldman M, Connolly JM, Strong LE. High-fiber diet reduces serum estrogen concentrations in premenopausal women. Am J Clin Nutr 1991;54:520–525.

77. Greenwald P, Lanza E, Eddy GA. Dietary fiber in the reduction of colon cancer. JADA 1987;87:1178–1188.

78. Slavin JL. Dietary fiber: classification, chemical analyses, and food sources. JADA 1987;87:1164–1171.

79. Slavin JL. Dietary fiber: mechanisms or magic on disease prevention? Nutr Today 1990;6–10.

80. Human Nutrition Information Service, U.S. Department of Agriculture. Government Printing Office, Composition of foods. Washington, DC: 1982–1990.

81. Bell LP, Hectorne K, Reynolds H, Balm TK, Hunninghake DB. Cholesterol-lowering effects of psyllium hydrophilic mucilloid. JAMA 1989;261:3419–3423.

82. Alpers DH. Dietary management and vitamin-mineral replacement therapy. In: Sleisenger MH, Fordtran JS, eds. Gastrointestinal disease: pathophysiology, diagnosis, management, 4th ed. Philadelphia: WB Saunders, 1989:1994–2006.

83. Donaldson RM. Crohn's disease. In: Sleisenger MH, Fordtran JS, eds. Gastrointestinal disease: pathophysiology, diagnosis, management, 4th ed. Philadelphia: WB Saunders, 1989;1327–1358.

84. Earnest DL, Trier JS. Radiation enteritis and colitis. In: Sleisenger MH, Fordtran JS, eds. Gastrointestinal disease: pathophysiology, diagnosis, management, 4th ed. Philadelphia: WB Saunders, 1989;1369–1382.

85. Emerson AP. Foods high in fiber and phytobezoar formation. JADA 1987;87:1675–1677.

86. Beyer PL, Flynn MA. Effects of high- and low-fiber diets on human feces. JADA 1978; 72:271–277.

87. Kramer P. The meaning of high- and low-residue diets (editorial). Gastroenterology 1964;6:649–652.

88. Weinstein L, Olson RE, Van Itallie TB, Caso E, Johnson D, Inglefinger FJ. Diet as related to gastrointestinal function. JAMA 1961;11:935–941.

89. Christian GM, Alford B, Shanklin CW, DiMarco N. Milk and milk products in low residue diets: current hospital practices do not match dietitians' beliefs. JADA 1991;91:341–342.

90. Watts JH, Graham DCW, Jones F, Adams FJ, Thompson DJ. Fecal solids excreted by young men following the ingestion of dairy foods. Am J Dig Dis 1963;4:364–375.

GLUTEN SENSITIVITY: CELIAC SPRUE AND DERMATITIS HERPETIFORMIS

General Description

The diet eliminates gluten, which is the protein found in wheat, oats, rye, and barley. The widespread use of gluten-containing grain products in restaurant and commercially processed foods, and difficulty in recognizing the presence of gluten in many other foods can make strict adherence difficult. This makes thorough nutritional counseling of utmost importance. Secondary malabsorption of fat and lactose may necessitate initial restriction of fat and milk-containing foods until the bowel has regained its digestive and absorptive ability.

Nutritional Inadequacy

A gluten-free diet is not nutritionally inadequate; however, when malabsorption is present, appropriate vitamin and/or mineral supplements should be prescribed at least until the disorder is corrected. If the patient is also lactose intolerant and is not able to consume or tolerate adequate amounts of lactase-treated dairy products, calcium supplementation to meet requirements may be indicated (see Chapter 9, Lactose Intolerance). Vitamin D supplementation may also be needed initially for patients with metabolic bone disease. Iron, folate, or vitamin B_{12} supplementation may be necessary for patients with anemia.

Indications and Rationale

Celiac Sprue. Celiac sprue can be defined as a chronic disease in which the gliadin protein fraction of gluten causes a mucosal lesion of the small intestine that impairs nutrient absorption.[91] Celiac sprue is also termed gluten-sensitive enteropathy, nontropical sprue, and gluten-induced enteropathy. In children it is termed celiac disease (see Chapter 24, Gluten Sensitive Enteropathy: Celiac Disease). Several mechanisms, which include a disorder of immunological function or a direct toxic effect, have been postulated to explain the detrimental effects of gluten. The disease damages primarily the mucosa of the small intestine, especially the duodenum and proximal jejunum. Biopsy reveals a flat mucosal surface with absence or severe blunting of normal intestinal villi. Histologic examination confirms loss of normal villous structure. The result of these changes is usually diarrhea and steatorrhea. (Although diarrhea is the most common complaint, it is not always present.) Flatulence, abdominal distention, weight loss, and weakness also occur.[92]

Extraintestinal symptoms may result from anemia and metabolic bone disease such as osteomalacia. Anemia is usually a result of iron deficiency and hence tends to be microcytic, while folate and, to a lesser extent, vitamin B_{12} deficiencies contribute. Osteomalacia may be prominent, with manifestations of bone pain and tenderness.[91]

The clinical presentation of celiac disease is highly variable and exemplifies the subtleties involved in malabsorption syndromes. Malabsorption of protein, fat and fat soluble vitamins, vitamin B_{12}, folate, iron, calcium, and other nutrients can occur. The degree is dependent upon the location, extent, and duration of the disease.

The diagnosis is confirmed by evidence of malabsorption, a small bowel biopsy demonstrating the characteristic although not diagnostic lesion of a flat jejunal mucosa with the loss or severe blunting of normal villi, and by the subsequent improvement of biochemical findings and clinical symptoms following institution of a gluten-free diet.

Once gluten is removed from the diet, there is a gradual improvement in symptoms over a period of weeks to months. Initially there is a relief of symptoms and later the return of intestinal mucosa to near normal condition.

Gluten-sensitive enteropathy should be considered a chronic disease that is controlled by diet. An asymptomatic state depends on the lifelong maintenance of a gluten-free diet. Patients should be cautioned against ingesting gluten once they start to gain weight and to feel better. The ingestion of gluten damages the mucosa and causes recurrent symptoms, although several weeks or more may elapse before the symptoms are observed. An assessment of dietary adherence is critical in determining whether the recurrent symptoms are related to sprue or to another unrelated problem.

Failure to respond to a gluten-free diet is not common, but it may occur. The most common reasons for lack of response are the wrong diagnosis or failure to strictly adhere to the diet. Other possible reasons include secondary lactase deficiency, concurrent disease, such as pancreatic insufficiency, jejunal or ileal ulceration, or, rarely, intestinal lymphoma.[92,93] Collagenous sprue is an extremely rare entity and is characterized by a lack of response to dietary therapy.[94]

Dermatitis Herpetiformis.   Dermatitis herpetiformis is a chronic inflammatory disease of the skin. It is usually diagnosed in young or middle-aged adults and is characterized by an itching, blistering rash. It is also accompanied in the majority of patients by a jejunal lesion similar to that of sprue. Gastrointestinal symptoms may be present, but more often are not. The histologic appearance of both the jejunum and the skin lesions may respond to gluten withdrawal and relapse with a challenge of gluten. Therefore, long-term adherence to a gluten-free diet is recommended.[92]

Goals of Dietary Management

The goals of dietary management are the remission of clinical symptoms, the normalization of absorptive function, and the regeneration of mucosal villi.

Dietary Recommendations

The strict, lifelong avoidance of gluten is paramount. Gluten is a protein found only in the grains of wheat, oats, rye, and barley (Table 9-13). Although abstaining from these grains appears to be direct and simple, strict dietary adherence is difficult for most patients. Gluten-containing grains and products that are made from them are a staple in the American diet. The widespread use of emulsifiers, thickeners, and other additives derived from gluten-containing grains in commercially processed foods further complicates the strict adherence to a gluten-free diet. It is necessary for patients to read food labels carefully and to avoid products that list ingredients that cannot be verified as gluten-free by the manufacturer. The unintentional consumption of gluten is the most common cause of recurrence of symptoms. Other reasons patients may fail to maintain a strict gluten-free diet are boredom with the taste of alternatives to wheat breads, crackers, and pasta and the limited availability of appropriate foods when eating away from home. Patients should be encouraged to use gluten-free bread replacements to maintain adequate carbohydrate and kilocalorie intake.

Initially, a high kilocalorie and high protein diet should be recommended, especially if weight loss and specific deficiencies owing to malabsorption are pronounced. The kilocalorie and protein recommendations may be normalized as absorption improves. Supplemental vitamins and minerals may also be indicated initially but may not continue to be necessary as absorption improves.

TABLE 9-13   Sources of Gluten*

Foods That Contain Gluten	Foods That May Contain Gluten	Foods That Do Not Contain Gluten
Beverages		
Cereal beverages (e.g., Postum™), malt, Ovaltine™, beer and ale	Commercial chocolate milk; cocoa mixes; other beverage mixes; dietary supplements	Coffee; tea; decaffeinated coffee; carbonated beverages; chocolate drinks made with pure cocoa powder; wine; distilled liquor
Meat and Meat Substitutes		
Commercially breaded meats	Meat loaf and patties, cold cuts and prepared meats, stuffing, cheese foods and spreads; commercial soufflés, omelets, and fondue; soy protein meat substitutes	Pure meat, fish, fowl, egg, cottage cheese, and peanut butter
Fat and Oil		
Commercial gravies, white and cream sauces	Commercial salad dressing and mayonnaise, nondairy creamer	Butter, margarine, vegetable oil
Milk		
Milk beverages that contain malt	Commercial chocolate milk	Whole, low-fat, and skim milk; buttermilk
Grains and Grain Products		
Bread, crackers, cereal, and pasta that contain wheat, oats, rye, malt, malt flavoring, graham flour, durum flour, pastry flour, bran, or wheat germ; barley; millet; pretzels; communion wafers[96]	Commercial seasoned rice and potato mixes	Specially prepared breads made with wheat starch†, rice, potato, or soybean flour or cornmeal; pure corn or rice cereals; hominy grits; white, brown, and wild rice; popcorn; low protein pasta made from wheat starch
Vegetables		
Commercially breaded vegetables or vegetables with a cream or cheese sauce	Commercial seasoned vegetable mixes; canned baked beans	All fresh vegetables; plain commercially frozen or canned vegetables
Fruit		
	Commercial pie fillings	All plain or sweetened fruits; fruit thickened with tapioca or cornstarch
Soup		
Most commercial soup and soup mixes; soup that contains barley, wheat pasta; soup thickened with wheat flour or other gluten-containing grains	Broth	Soup thickened with cornstarch, wheat starch, or potato, rice, or soybean flour; pure broth

Continued.

TABLE 9-13 Sources of Gluten*—cont'd

FoodsThat Contain Gluten	Foods That May Contain Gluten	Foods That Do Not Contain Gluten
Desserts		
Commercial cakes, cookies, and pastries; commercial dessert mixes	Commercial ice cream and sherbet, puddings	Gelatin; custard; fruit ice; specially prepared cakes, cookies, and pastries made with gluten-free flour or starch; pudding and fruit filling thickened with tapioca, cornstarch, or arrowroot flour
Sweets		
	Commercial candies, especially chocolates	
Miscellaneous‡		
	Ketchup; prepared mustard; soy sauce; commercially prepared meat sauces and pickles; white vinegar; flavoring syrups (syrups for pancakes or ice cream)	Monosodium glutamate; salt; pepper; pure spices and herbs; yeast; pure baking chocolate or cocoa powder; carob; flavoring extracts; artificial flavoring; cider and wine vinegar

*The terms "commercially prepared" and "commercial" are used to refer to partially prepared foods purchased from a grocery or food market and to prepared foods purchased from a restaurant.

†Wheat starch may contain trace amounts of gluten. Avoid if not tolerated.

‡Medications may contain trace amounts of gluten.[95] A pharmacist may be able to provide information on the gluten content of medications.

For some patients, lactose and fat may need to be restricted initially because of secondary lactase deficiency and fat malabsorption. Dairy products and fats should be reintroduced into the diet gradually since a degree of lactose intolerance and fat malabsorption may continue indefinitely for some patients. (See Chapter 9, Lactose Intolerance, and Chapter 9, Fat Malabsorption.)

Physicians: How to Order Diet

The diet order should indicate: *gluten-free diet.* The need for secondary restrictions, such as lactose and fat, should also be indicated according to individual patient tolerance.

Food Labeling

Gluten-containing grains are widely used in the preparation of foods. A thorough review of the list of ingredients on the label reveals obvious sources of gluten, but the patient should also be alert to less obvious food sources of gluten such as pasta products, cold cuts, commercial soups and salad dressings, sauces, and instant cereal beverage mixes. The labels on commercial breads should also be reviewed since some products include wheat flour. The following ingredients when listed on food labels may or may not contain gluten:

cereal	hydrolyzed vegetable protein
cereal additive	modified food starch
emulsifier	stabilizer
flavoring	starch
hydrolyzed plant protein	vegetable protein

If one of these ingredients is listed on the label, the absence of gluten should be verified by calling or writing to the manufacturer to request information on the gluten content. When the ingredients are not listed on the label, the manufacturer should also be contacted for complete ingredient information.

Substitutions for Wheat Flour

Most patients find special cookbooks helpful. Recipes can be modified by the following substitutions.

For baking, 1 cup of wheat flour may be replaced by:

1 cup of wheat starch

1 cup of corn flour

1 scant cup of fine cornmeal

$^3/_4$ cup of coarse cornmeal

$^5/_8$ cup (10 Tbsp) of potato flour

$^7/_8$ cup (14 Tbsp) of rice flour, white or brown

1 cup of soy flour plus $^1/_4$ cup of potato starch flour

$^1/_2$ cup of soy flour plus $^1/_2$ cup of potato starch flour

For thickening, 1 Tbsp of wheat flour may be replaced by:

$1^1/_2$ Tbsp of cornstarch, potato starch flour, rice flour, or arrowroot starch

2 tsp of quick-cooking tapioca

Patient Support Groups

At the time of publication, these patient support groups are active.

American Celiac Society
45 Gifford Avenue
Jersey City, NJ 07304
(201) 432-2986

Gluten-Intolerance Group
PO Box 23053
Seattle, WA 98102
(201) 325-6980

Celiac Sprue Association/United States of America, Inc.
PO Box 31700
Omaha, NE 68131
(402) 558-0600

References

91. Trier JS. Celiac Sprue. N Engl J Med 1991;325(24):1709–1719.
92. Kelly CP, Feighery CF, Gallagher RB, Weir DG. Diagnosis and treatment of gluten-sensitive enteropathy. Adv Intern Med 1990;35:341–363.
93. Holmes GKT, Prior P, Lane MR, Pope D, Allan RN. Malignancy in coeliac disease: effect of a gluten-free diet. Gut 1989;30:333–338.
94. Greenberger NJ. Gastrointestinal disorders: a pathophysiologic approach, 4th ed. Chicago: Mosby–Year Book, 1989:147.
95. Patel DG, Krough CME, Thompson WG. Gluten in pills: a hazard for patients with celiac disease. Can Med Assoc J 1985;133:114–115.
96. Bentley AC. A survey of celiac-sprue patients: effect of dietary restrictions on religious practices. The J Gen Psychol 1988;115(1):7–14.

INFLAMMATORY BOWEL DISEASE

General Description

Recommendations for inflammatory bowel disease (IBD) are variable and depend on the nutritional status of the individual, the location and extent of the disease, and the nature of the surgical or medical management.

Nutritional Inadequacy

Dietary modifications for IBD are based on individual food tolerances. Each person's diet should be assessed for nutritional adequacy and supplemented to provide the RDA for nutrients. Extra supplementation may be necessary to correct additional needs that are attributable to malabsorption and to increased requirements. Pharmacotherapy may also contribute to nutrient deficiencies. Examples include sulfasalazine (interferes with folate absorption), corticosteroids (suppress calcium absorption), and cholestyramine (impairs absorption of fat and fat-soluble vitamins).

Indications and Rationale

IBD is a general term that refers primarily to two related but clinically and pathologically distinct disease processes—chronic ulcerative colitis (CUC) and Crohn's disease. CUC is an idiopathic inflammatory disorder that is confined to the mucosa of the large intestine. The extent of the process may vary from the rectum alone (ulcerative proctitis) to the entire large intestine (pancolitis). Involvement is generally uniform; it begins in the rectum and spreads proximally in a continuous fashion. Crohn's disease, or regional enteritis, on the other hand, may involve the small or the large intestine or both, and its distribution may be interspersed with areas of healthy bowel. As opposed to CUC, Crohn's disease involves all layers of the intestinal wall and is more commonly associated with stricture formation, with fistulous tracts, and with abscesses. The pathology of the two diseases may be indistinguishable. In approximately 10% of cases of IBD, the pathology of even a resected specimen may have features of both CUC and Crohn's and be designated "indeterminate."

The major symptoms and signs of IBD include abdominal pain, diarrhea, intestinal bleeding, protein loss, and fever. These symptoms result in nutritional wasting owing to a decreased intake from anorexia, an increased loss of nutrients from maldigestion and malabsorption, loss of nutrients across the diseased gastrointestinal tract (i.e., protein), drug-nutrient interactions, and an increase in requirements due to abscess, infection, and fever. Malnutrition occurs with sustained and unsupported chronic disease.[97,98] Fluid and electrolyte imbalances may occur with acute exacerbations or in patients with Crohn's disease and short bowel syndrome (SBS).

Management is directed toward the control of symptoms and treatment of complications. This may include pharmacotherapy, surgery, and nutritional support. Pharmacotherapy may involve anti-inflammatory agents such as corticosteroids and antibacterials such as metronidazole for abscesses and fistulas. The judicious use of anticholinergics and antidiarrheal agents (Lomotil™ or loperamide) may also have a role in symptomatic care. Other drug therapies being explored include immunomodulators (e.g., cyclosporine, 6-MP, methotrexate), omega-3 fatty acids in fish oil (inflammatory inhibitors), short-chain fatty acid enemas to enhance mucosal growth and repair in diversion colitis, and control of free radical damage with copper and zinc dependent superoxide dismutase.[99]

Medications most commonly used for the treatment of IBD may also result in nutrient malabsorption: sulfasalazine inhibits folate absorption; cholestyramine, a bile acid–binding resin used to treat diarrhea for patients with ileal resection, may result in fat and fat-soluble vitamin malabsorption; and corticosteroids decrease intestinal calcium absorption and may contribute to steroid-induced osteoporosis (see Appendix 2, Drug-Nutrient Interactions).

Surgery is curative in CUC, and newer ileostomy alternatives (see p. 256) make this approach more acceptable to the younger population. Crohn's disease, however, tends to recur following surgical resection of the affected segments in the majority of patients. For this reason, one is more conservative in the treatment of Crohn's disease, reserving surgery for truly refractory disease or for significant complications such as obstruction, abscess, fistulae, or bleeding. Patient education and psychological support are important aspects of the management for patients with IBD.

Goals of Dietary Management

The nutritional goals are to replace the nutrient losses that are associated with the inflammatory process, to correct the body deficits, and to provide sufficient nutrients to achieve energy, nitrogen, fluid, and electrolyte balance. Dietary recommendations should also be designed to avoid aggravating symptoms.

Dietary Recommendations

A nutritional assessment should be performed to determine the patient's nutritional status and to estimate the patient's needs (see Chapter 3, Nutritional Screening and Assessment). The approach to nutritional therapy must take into account the intestinal function, including previous intestinal resections, the site and the extent of the disease process (Fig. 9-1), and the anticipated medical and surgical treatment.

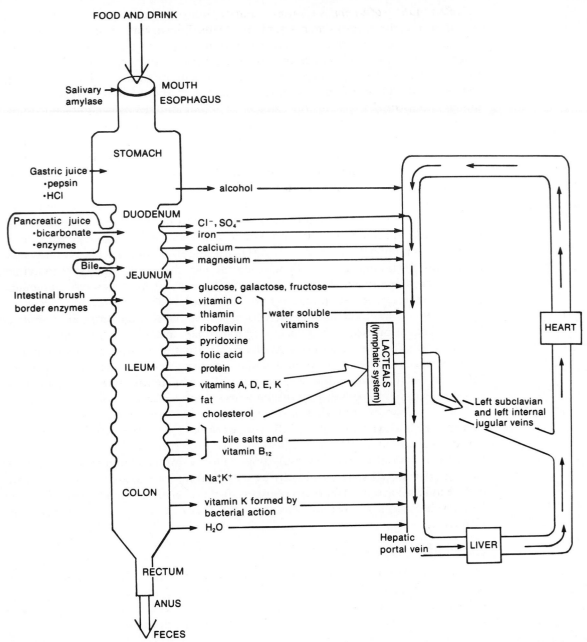

FIGURE 9-1 The site and the extent of the disease process and the effect on nutrient absorption. (Reprinted with permission from Mahan LK, Arlin M. Krause's food, nutrition and diet therapy, 8th ed. Philadelphia: WB Saunders, 1992:13.)

Inflammation of the Large Bowel.   During the acute phase, diarrhea, tenesmus, and frequent bowel movements are a problem. Pharmacological agents are used to control symptoms. The extent of diet control depends on the severity of symptoms. The patient who suffers from severe abdominal cramps and diarrhea and who is rapidly becoming dehydrated needs hospitalization. Oral intake may increase the amount of liquid that is presented by the small intestine to the colon and may consequently aggravate diarrhea. Oral intake of both food and fluid is restricted, although one can expect only diminution, not abolition, of peristaltic and secretory activity. Parenteral nutritional support is used to provide the nutritional and fluid needs of these patients. This support can be administered peripherally for short-term management or centrally if the course is fulminating and the therapy is likely to be more extended.

As the patient improves and the number of bowel movements decrease, oral intake can be initiated. Transitional feedings may commence according to patient tolerance. Monomeric or polymeric enteral formulas can be provided via tube or, with a well-motivated patient, taken orally. A minimal residue diet, a low fiber diet, or a regular diet that includes fiber may be provided to the degree that the patient feels is tolerable. The restriction of fiber for chronic colitis is based on anecdotal experience, and there are no good studies to demonstrate that fiber has a deleterious effect. For the patient with chronic colitis who is asymptomatic, the intake of fiber should not be limited if fiber does not induce symptoms. It has been shown that soluble fiber is broken down by colonic bacteria into short-chain fatty acids, primarily butyric, which promotes colonic mucosal growth and repair and decreases inflammation.[100] It has recently been shown that marine fish-oil supplements (rich in n-3 fatty acids) may also reduce the inflammation associated with ulcerative colitis.[101-103] It is postulated that fish oils may exert their beneficial effects by shifting their eicosanoid synthesis to less inflammatory processes or by modulating levels of certain cytokines.

Because lactase deficiency may be present, tolerance for lactose-containing foods can be established by either laboratory testing or subjective trial. If intolerance exists, lactase enzyme may be added to the milk. Although it seems prudent to limit the intake of spices, their exact effect on the colon has not been studied. The patient's food preferences should be encouraged and not limited because of the spice content. Unless marked improvement in symptoms is experienced when lactose and spices are limited, restriction of dietary choices is discouraged.[98-104]

Inflammation of the Small Bowel.   Acute and chronic Crohn's disease is similar to acute and CUC, with some exceptions. For acute flares with evidence of severe obstruction, all oral feeding is stopped and nasogastric suction and intravenous nutritional support are initiated. If the complete or partial obstruction does not respond to medical management, surgical resection of the stenotic segment is indicated.

Pharmacological treatment of Crohn's disease will usually induce remission.[105,106] However, treatment without consideration of nutritional status can result in critical loss of visceral protein, limit the body's immune response, limit the ability for tissue repair, and ultimately result in medical and surgical treatment failure.[107] Patients with Crohn's disease, in the absence of infection and fever, do not have increased energy expenditure.[108] Significant losses of fat as well as visceral and somatic proteins frequently occur, and the change in body composition may be associated with poor response to medical and surgical management.[109] Nutritional support via enteral or parenteral routes can allow for maintenance of nutritional status (if the patient cannot fulfill nutritional needs orally) while the disease is being treated.[110]

Several investigations have tried to determine whether nutritional therapy might be effective as primary treatment for Crohn's disease. These studies have included bowel rest with complete restriction of oral intake and with total parenteral nutrition in order to eliminate luminal irritation and potential dietary antigens. Although remission was achieved in two-thirds of hospitalized patients in a 3 week hospitalization, over half the patients had recurrences of symptoms in a 1 year follow-up.[107] It is known that this form of bowel rest may result in "bowel starvation" and promotion of gut atrophy,[111] possibly due to the absence of glutamine, a preferred metabolic substrate for the small intestine that is absent in standard parenteral nutrition.[112]

Elemental diets provide nitrogen as individual amino acids. These and peptide-based enteral formulas, by removing whole proteins that could serve as antigenic stimulants, have also been tested as a primary form of therapy for Crohn's disease.[112] Glutamine is present in enteral formulas and has been found to maintain gut mucosa and prevent translocation of bacteria in rats.[114] Enteral formulas have also been shown to decrease intestinal protein losses[115] and to decrease intestinal permeability.[116]

There is also growing evidence that other enteral nutrients may be efficacious in the treatment of Crohn's disease, including short-chain fatty acids (from colonic conversion of fiber) to decrease inflammation and provide gut-specific fuels for distal small bowel and colonic mucosal growth and repair.[100] Further, it has been shown that clinical remission may be achieved with enteral nutrition without the need for achieving repletion of nutritional status.[117] For these reasons, except in the presence of acute exacerbations, abscess, or fistulas proximal in the gut, the enteral route (tube or oral) is preferred over parenteral nutrition.

In general, no specific oral diet is recommended for patients with Crohn's disease. Instead, emphasis is on maintaining overall nutrition with food within the patient's tolerance. However, patients with Crohn's disease may experience selective malabsorption of nutrients that is directly proportional to the site and to the extent of small bowel involvement or resection. Therefore, the diet should be planned with this in mind. (See the section on short bowel, p. 258.)

Intolerance to specific food items has been cited as a source of symptoms by patients. Individualized diet counseling aimed at eliminating offending foods while optimizing the patient's nutritional status has been found to be beneficial. In one prospective study, individual counseling over a 6 month period was associated with a significant decrease in the Crohn's disease activity index, increased incidence of remission, decreased need for medication therapy, a reduction in the number of days spent in the hospital, and a reduction in the amount of time lost from work in comparison to control patients who did not receive dietary counseling.[118]

Lactose maldigestion is increased in some individuals with Crohn's disease, especially those with extensive small bowel disease or resection. However, intolerance is variable, and small amounts (up to 250 ml) of milk may be consumed according to individual preference since milk is the major dietary source of calcium and protein.[119] (See Chapter 9, Lactose Intolerance).

Varying the amount of dietary fiber in management of IBD is controversial. A low fiber diet may be necessary for patients at risk for intestinal obstruction or stricture of the small bowel. Clinical studies, however, have failed to show that prolonged use of a low fiber diet has significant therapeutic effect on patient outcome when compared with a normal diet.[120,121] Lifting of this dietary restriction resulted in a more appealing and nutritious diet without causing symptomatic deterioration or precipitation of intestinal obstruction.[120]

Steatorrhea may occur with small bowel involvement. Malabsorption of fat and increased excretion of calcium, magnesium, and zinc may result from excessive bowel movements. For patients with colonic continuity and steatorrhea, the risks of hyperoxaluria and kidney stone formation are increased.[122] Increased urinary oxalate excretion occurs because of increased colonic absorption of dietary oxalate, which results because calcium, in the presence of steatorrhea, preferentially complexes with fatty acids and is no longer available to bind with oxalate. This leads to increased availability of soluble oxalate for absorption by the colon and excretion by the kidneys. Stool losses of magnesium indirectly facilitate calcium oxalate stones. Bicarbonate losses with diarrhea contribute to systemic acidosis, which coupled with dehydration, contributes to uric acid kidney stones. Patients may benefit from a decreased fat and oxalate intake and calcium supplementation.

Anemia is also common and may be caused by iron, folate, vitamin B_{12}, or copper deficiencies, or it may occur as a result of chronic inflammation and hemorrhage (e.g., anemia of chronic disease). Other deficiencies include electrolytes, minerals (calcium and magnesium), vitamin C (due to increased demand), vitamins D and K (disrupted enterohepatic circulation), and trace metals (in particular zinc and selenium).[123] Additional vitamin and mineral supplementation may be necessary for these nutrients because of increased losses that are attributable to malabsorption, increased needs due to infection and/or pharmacotherapy, or decreased intake.

Patients with Crohn's disease lose protein from their gastrointestinal tract in amounts that correlate well with the severity of their disease.[124] Anorexia and malabsorption are also contributing factors for hypoalbuminemia. Hypoalbuminemia can also result from cytokine-induced reduction in albumin synthesis in the acutely ill patient with IBD. Serum albumin level is more a marker of disease activity than of nutritional status.

Colostomy.   A colostomy may be constructed when a segment of colon or rectum (or both) is removed because of disease or obstruction. Dietary management depends on the colostomy site because the output from the stoma is proportional to the length of the remaining bowel (Fig. 9-2). Patients with colostomies in the transverse or the descending colon often achieve control of colonic function so that they have relatively little loss of fluid secretions from the stoma and can control evacuation by daily irrigation. Cecostomies or colostomies in the ascending colon have a more liquid stool output and therefore a greater loss of fluid and electrolytes. Most patients with colostomies can return to a normal diet after surgery. Dietary modification is based solely on individual tolerance. Restriction

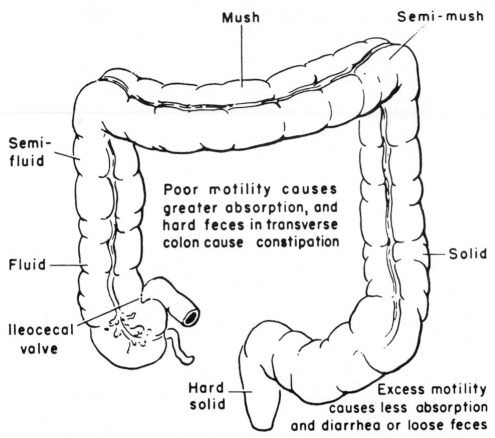

FIGURE 9-2 The colostomy site and its effect on output. (Reprinted with permission from Guyton AC. Textbook of medical physiology, 8th ed. Philadelphia: WB Saunders, 1991:706.)

should be limited to only those foods that produce annoying side effects for the individual, such as gas or loose stools.[125] The patient may feel greater comfort and may find caring for the ostomy easier by following the guidelines in Table 9-14.

Ileostomy.   An ileostomy is usually fashioned when the entire colon and rectum is removed. The consistency of output is more liquid than that from a colostomy. Although more water, sodium, and other minerals are lost, fluid and electrolyte balance may eventually be achieved, depending upon the length of remaining gut and upon the adaptation that results with increased absorption. After a conventional ileostomy, the effluent will usually plateau at approximately 500 ml per day. As with patients with colostomies, dietary restrictions should be based solely on the individual's intolerances.[125] The patient with an ileostomy may also benefit from the general guidelines in Table 9-14.

Ileal Pouch/Anal Anastomosis.   The ileal pouch/anal anastomosis is an alternative to an ileostomy. This surgical procedure removes the diseased colon and rectal mucosa while preserving the anal sphincter. A pouch is made from terminal ileum

TABLE 9-14   Dietary Guidelines for Colostomy and Ileostomy

Guidelines	Reasons
1. Eat meals at regular times—three or more times daily.	1. Bowel pattern may be more regular.
2. Chew all foods thoroughly.	2. Chewing well assists the digestive process and reduces the chance of stomal blockages.
3. Drink adequate fluids, 8 to 10 glasses per day.	3. Increased fluids are recommended to prevent constipation and dehydration.
4. Avoid gaining excessive weight.	4. Excess weight may affect stomal function.
5. Limit foods that may produce excessive gas, or loose stools or that may not be completely digested.	5. Colostomy: foods that have caused problems prior to surgery may continue to do so as they are digested before they reach the colon. Ileostomy: during the first 4 to 6 weeks, limit foods that have caused problems prior to surgery in order to decrease the chance for stomal blockage and to reduce the amount of gas and stool.
6. Eat a smaller evening meal.	6. This will reduce nocturnal stool output.
7. Try new foods one at a time.	7. This will help determine food tolerance.

The following list has been developed from anecdotal accounts and should be regarded as only an initial guideline. Because of the nature of the ostomy and of the remaining gastrointestinal tract, the foods that alter function may not be the same as those that produce the same effect in the unaltered gastrointestinal tract.

GAS FORMING FOODS

Asparagus
Beans
Broccoli
Brussels sprouts
Cabbage
Carbonated beverages
Cauliflower
Onions

INCOMPLETELY DIGESTED FOODS

Cabbage	Mushrooms	Spinach
Celery	Nuts	Tough skins
Coconut	Olives	from fruits
Corn	Peas	and
Cucumbers	Pickles	vegetables
Dried fruit	Pineapple	
Green peppers	Popcorn	
Lettuce	Seeds	

THICKENING FOODS

Applesauce
Bananas
Breads
Cheeses
Pasta
Peanut butter (creamy)
Starchy foods

THINNING FOODS

Apple juice
Grape juice
Prune Juice
Highly seasoned food

ODOR REDUCING FOODS

Buttermilk
Cranberry juice
Parsley
Yogurt

ODOR PRODUCING FOODS

Asparagus
Eggs
Fish
Garlic
Onions

Reminders:
- Eating more than one food from within a list may intensify the effect.
- Do not eliminate a food from the diet without trying it several times.
- The stool may appear red after eating beets. Do not mistake it for blood. Broccoli, asparagus and spinach may darken the stool.

and is pulled through the rectal muscular tube and attached to the anus. This preserves anal continence and allows for a more normal pattern of evacuation. A temporary ileostomy is usually made at the time of surgery to protect the pouch and to allow time for healing. After 2 to 3 months, the ileostomy is closed and bowel continuity is established. The dietary management for patients with ileal pouch/anal anastomosis is directed toward managing the temporary ileostomy and achieving bowel control. The consistency and the frequency of bowel movements vary from patient to patient. To increase the consistency of the stool, patients may wish to avoid those foods that tended to loosen the stool during the temporary ileostomy. Fresh fruits and vegetables and their juices may also have a laxative effect. Patients may find that eating the main meal at mid-day and avoiding large quantities of fluids in the evening result in fewer bowel movements during the night.

Short Bowel Syndrome.   Patients sometimes have many operations to resect areas of inflamed or strictured intestine. Even though surgery for Crohn's disease has become more conservative, it is now one of the most common causes of SBS.[126] The symptoms and the consequences of SBS depend on the site and the extent of the small bowel that is removed, on the time that has lapsed since resection, on the presence of the ileocecal valve, on the condition of the remaining gut, and on whether or not there is colon continuity.[127]

Ileal resections of less than 100 cm are frequently associated with bile salt malabsorption. The malabsorbed dihydroxy bile salts cause a secretory diarrhea by stimulating cyclic adenosine monophosphate in the colonic mucosa. In this setting, resins such as cholestyramine that are capable of binding bile salts may be given to help control diarrhea. Yet these may further aggravate fat malabsorption.

Resections of more than 100 cm are more problematic because the malabsorbed fatty acids also contribute to secretory diarrhea. With the more extensive resections, carbohydrate malabsorption further contributes to an osmotic diarrhea.[128]

Proximal bowel resections are better tolerated than distal resections since the ileum can compensate for most of the absorptive functions of the jejunum.[128,129] Extensive ileal resection, however, can result in more severe diarrhea and steatorrhea.

Calcium and magnesium deficiency can occur due to the binding of calcium and of magnesium in malabsorbed stool fat,[130] to inadequate dietary intake, or to both. One frequent complication is calcium-oxalate nephrolithiasis in patients with colonic continuity.[131] Because the small bowel is the site of vitamin and mineral absorption, nutritional deficiencies are likely. The steatorrhea of SBS may result in the malabsorption of fat-soluble vitamins. Vitamin B_{12} deficiency may occur if the site for absorption, the terminal ileum, is impaired or resected. The dietary intake of vitamins, such as vitamins C and folate, may be reduced due to the restriction of fruit and vegetable intake. Supplemental calcium, in amounts of 500 mg or more per day of elemental calcium, may help prevent both oxalate nephrolithiasis and calcium deficiency. Magnesium deficiency is common, but oral magnesium preparations contribute to diarrhea. Iron therapy given orally (or by injection if not tolerated orally) is helpful to correct iron deficiency anemia. Hence, routine multiple vitamin-mineral supplementation is indicated.

Nutritional support may influence bowel function significantly. Parenteral support is indicated if the patient cannot take adequate nutrients or if the oral diet aggravates symptoms (see Chapter 16, Parenteral Nutrition). The ability to secrete normal concentrations of digestive enzymes decreases when patients are not allowed oral intake and are given only total parenteral nutrition for prolonged periods.[111,112] Villous growth is stimulated by the presence of food. Therefore, it is preferable to return to oral feedings as soon as possible, even in small amounts, rather than to depend on prolonged parenteral feeding. Enteral nutritional support may be helpful as either a sole source of nutrition or as a supplement to the food intake (see Chapter 16, Enteral Nutrition). Selection of the appropriate formula is based on the individual's digestive and absorptive capabilities.

The dietary management for patients with SBS should take all of the aforementioned factors into account.

Patients with small bowel to colon continuity may initially require fat restriction, and depending on the severity of malabsorption, the patient may also benefit from the use of MCT fat (see Chapter 9, Fat Malabsorption). In the presence of colonic continuity, dietary sources of oxalate should also be limited for the prevention of urolithiasis. Modifications in lactose and in fiber can be made according to individual tolerance. There is current evidence that fiber may enhance gut function by promoting mucosal growth.[100] Vitamins and minerals should be supplemented according to the intake and to the capability of absorption.

The management of fluid and electrolyte deficits may be difficult for patients with SBS. Pharmacotherapy is of paramount importance in the management of fluid and electrolyte balance due to excessive gastrointestinal losses. Intravenous hydrogen-ion blockers help decrease gastric secretions. Cholestyramine is helpful in controlling bile salt malabsorption for patients with less than 100 cm of ileal resection and with a colon. Antimotility agents may be initiated to control diarrhea. The synthetic analog of Sandostatin, octreotide, has been used effectively in reducing by 50% the large volume fluid and electrolyte losses in the end-jejunostomy patient.[131]

Oral rehydration solutions have been used successfully to manage high output diarrhea.[132] The mechanism is based on the coupled absorption of glucose and sodium. If glucose absorption is not damaged in the small intestine, the intake of glucose activates the mechanisms for absorption of sodium and water with the glucose, which results in the reversal of net water secretion and in the correction of diarrhea. (See Appendix 38 for examples of oral rehydration solutions.) The amounts and the rate of oral intake depend on the degree of dehydration and of diarrhea. In general, the intake should match the output.

Physicians: How to Order Diet

The diet order should reflect the underlying disorders: *diet for chronic ulcerative colitis, Crohn's disease, colostomy, ileostomy, ileal pouch/anal anastomosis,* or *short bowel syndrome.* The dietitian plans the nutritional program according to the preceding guidelines.

References

97. Alfonso JJ, Rombeau JL. Nutritional care for patients with Crohn's disease. Hepatogastroenterology 1990;37(1):32–41.
98. Seidman EG. Nutritional management of inflammatory bowel disease. Gastroenterol Clin North Am 1989;18(1):129–155.

99. Cole AT, Hawkey CJ. New treatments in inflammatory bowel disease. Br J Hosp Med 1992;47(8):581–587.

100. Goodlad RA, Lenton W, Ghatei MA, Adrian TE, Bloom SR, Wright NA. Effects of an elemental diet, inert bulk and different types of dietary fibre on the response of the intestinal epithelium to refeeding in the rat and relationship to plasma gastrin, enteroglucagon and PYY concentrations. Gut 1987;28:171–180.

101. Salomon P, Kornbluth AA, Janowitz HD. Treatment of ulcerative colitis with fish oil n-3 omega fatty acid: an open trial. J Clin Gastroenterol 1990;12(2):157–161.

102. Ross E. The role of marine fish oils in the treatment of ulcerative colitis. Nutr Rev 1993;51(2):47–49.

103. Stenson WF, Cort D, Rodgers J, Burakoff R, De Schryver-Kecskemeti K, Gramlich TL, Becker W. Dietary supplementation with fish oils in ulcerative colitis. Ann Intern Med 1992;116:609–614.

104. Culpepper-Morgan JA, Floch MH. Bowel rest or bowel starvation: defining the role of nutritional support in the treatment of inflammatory bowel diseases. Am J Gastroenterol 1991;86(3):269–271.

105. Summers RW, Switz DM, Sessions JT, Becktell JM, Best WR, Kern F, Singleton JW. National cooperative Crohn's disease study: results of drug treatment. Gastroenterology 1979;77:847–869.

106. Malchow H, Ewe K, Brandes JW, Goebell H, Ehms H, Sommer H, Jesidinski H. European cooperative Crohn's disease study (ECCDS): results of drug treatment. Gastroenterology 1984;86:249–266.

107. Greenberg GR, Fleming CR, Jeejeebhoy KN, Rosenberg IH, Sales D, Tremaine WJ. Controlled trial of bowel rest and nutritional support in the management of Crohn's disease. Gut 1988;29:1309–1315.

108. Chan AT, Fleming CR, O'Fallon WM, Huizenga KA. Estimated versus measured basal energy requirements in patients with Crohn's disease. Gastroenterology 1986;91:75–78.

109. Fischer JE, Foster GS, Abel RM, Abbott WM, Ryan JA. Hyperalimentation as primary therapy for inflammatory bowel disease. Am J Surg 1973;125:165–175.

110. Christie PM, Hill GL. Effect of intravenous nutrition on nutrition and function in acute attacks of inflammatory bowel disease. Gastroenterology 1990;99:730–736.

111. Johnson LR, Copeland EM, Dudrick SJ, Lichtenberger LM, Castro GA. Structural and hormonal alterations in the gastrointestinal tract of parenterally fed rats. Gastroenterology 1975;68:1177–1183.

112. O'Dwyer ST, Smith RJ, Hwang TL, Wilmore DW. Maintenance of small bowel mucosa with glutamine-enriched parenteral nutrition. JPEN 1989;13:579–585.

113. O'Morain CA. Nutritional therapy in ambulatory patients. Dig Dis Sci 1987;32:95s–99s.

114. Smith JL, Arteaga C, Heymsfield SB. Increased ureagenesis and impaired nitrogen use during infusion of a synthetic amino acid formula: a controlled trial. N Engl J Med 1982;306:1013–1018.

115. Logan RF, Gillon J, Ferrington Ferguson A. Reduction of gastrointestinal protein loss by elemental diet in Crohn's disease of the small bowel. Gut 1981;22:383–387.

116. Sanderson IR, Boulton P, Menzies I, Walker-Smith JA. Improvement of abnormal lactulose/rhamnose permeability in active Crohn's disease of the small bowel by an elemental diet. Gut 1987;28:1073–1076.

117. Giaffer MN, North G, Holdsworth CD. Controlled trial of polymeric versus elemental diet in treatment of active Crohn's disease. Lancet 1990:335;816–819.

118. Imes S, Pinchbeck B, Thomson ABR. Diet counselling improves the clinical course of patients with Crohn's disease. Digestion 1988;39:7–19.

119. Pironi L, Callegari C, Cornia GL, Lami F, Miglioli M, Barbara L. Lactose malabsorption in adult patients with Crohn's disease. Am J Gastroenterol 1988;83(11): 1267–1271.

120. Levenstein S, Prantera C, Luzi C, D'Ubaldi A. Low residue or normal diet in Crohn's disease: a prospective controlled study in Italian patients. Gut 1985;26(10):989–993.

121. Ritchie JK, Wadsworth J, Lennard-Jones JE. Controlled multicentre therapeutic trial of unrefined carbohydrate, fibre rich diet in Crohn's disease. BMJ 1979;2:764–766.

122. Mandell I, Krauss E, Millan JC. Oxalate induced acute renal failure in Crohn's disease. Am J Med 1980;69:628–632.

123. Stokes MA. Crohn's disease and nutrition. Br J Surg 1992;79:391–394.

124. van Hees PAM. An index of inflammatory activity in patients with Crohn's disease. Acta Gastroenterol Belg 1984;47:282–288.

125. National Foundation for Ileitis and Colitis. Questions and answers about diet and nutrition. New York: NFIC, 1985.

126. Stokes MA, Hill GL. The short gut. Curr Pract Surg 1990;2:139–145.

127. Purdum PP, Kirby DF. Short bowel syndrome: a review of the role of nutritional support. JPEN 1991;15:93–101.

128. McClenahan JE, Fisher B. Physiological effects of massive small intestinal resection and colectomy. Am J Surg 1950;79:684–688.

129. Bristol JB, Williamson RCN, Chir M. Nutrition, operations and intestinal adaptation. JPEN 1988;12(3):299–309.

130. Hessov I, Hasselblad C, Fasth S, Hult_n L. Magnesium deficiency after ileal resections for Crohn's disease. Scand J Gastroenterol 1983;18:643–649.

131. Rosen GH. Somatostatin and its analogs in short bowel syndrome. Nutr Clin Pract 1992;7:81–84.

132. Newton CR, McIntyre PB, Lennard-Jones JE, Gonvers JJ, Preston DM. Effect of different drinks or fluid and electrolyte losses from a jejunostomy. J R Soc Med 1985;78:27–34.

IRRITABLE BOWEL SYNDROME

The diet emphasizes identification and elimination of individual food intolerances (e.g., lactose intolerance), appropriate fiber consumption, and elimination of foods identified as contributing to flatulence. The diet should also be low in fat, especially for patients with symptoms of diarrhea.[133,134] Regular meals and exercise are often helpful. Adequate protein and calories should be provided to maintain a desirable weight and good nutrition.

Nutritional Inadequacy

The potential for vitamin and mineral deficiencies exists. These depend on the patient's food intolerances and choices. A calcium supplement may be needed for patients following a lactose restricted diet. (See Chapter 8, Table 8-16, Calcium Content of Commercial Calcium Supplements.) A multiple vitamin and mineral supplement that meets the RDA is recommended for diets with significant food exclusion.

Indications and Rationale

IBS is characterized by abdominal pain and a change in bowel habits.[135] Persons frequently complain of abdominal pain, excessive gas and bloating, and indigestion. Constipation, diarrhea, and alternation between the two often occur. Typically, symptoms appear after a meal and are temporarily relieved by evacuating the bowels. Other symptoms such as nausea, dysmenorrhea, lower abdominal cramping, and fatigue may also exist. Abdominal bloating and flatulence are also very common complaints.

IBS is a chronic disorder that may be prevalent in as many as 22 million people.[136] IBS is reported twice as often by women as by men and is found primarily in Caucasians.[133] IBS is often considered a functional disorder since there are no signs of disease upon physical examination or objective testing. The causes of IBS are unknown but may include diet (e.g., food intolerance, low fiber), significant gut motility disorders involving small and/or large intestines, psychiatric disorders, and stress. Generally, prior to treatment, organic disease is excluded by a medical evaluation. Subsequently the possible aspects of stress and diet are investigated. Much of the current research regarding IBS has involved evaluation of possible intestinal motility disorders. There is evidence that the bowel is more sensitive to normal stimuli in IBS than in healthy individuals, and some patients have abnormal small bowel, or colonic motility.[135,137] New techniques involving smooth muscle myoelectric frequency or pressure recordings of contractions have been used.[133] Currently, possible hypotheses for causes of motility disorders are (1) size and content of meals, (2) medications, (3) hormonal fluctuations at menses, and (4) psychological stress.

Stress and other psychological factors need to be considered and discussed by the physician. Stress tends to increase colonic spasms in patients with IBS. This may be mediated by the central nervous system. Many stressors have been identified as potential factors: marital, business or career problems, family concerns, sexual difficulties, abuse, and fear of diseases. Patients with IBS may have more symptoms of anxiety and depression than other individuals with gastrointestinal disorders.[136] Although there appears to be a link between psychological symptoms and IBS, it has yet to be determined whether it is a cause or effect relationship. Stress may be decreased with simple forms of relaxation training and/or exercise.

Diet also affects gastrointestinal motility. An increase in myoelectric activity and motility in the colon is associated with high caloric and fat content of ingested food. Fatty foods and meals have been shown to induce a gastrocolic response, which may exacerbate irritable bowel syndrome[133] (see Chapter 9, Diarrhea). This activity may be reduced by consuming smaller, more frequent meals that are low in fat. Timing of meals should also be addressed because this may regulate bowel function.

A decrease in gas-producing foods and beverages may help alleviate IBS symptoms. Flatulence is most often a result of bacterial fermentation of unabsorbed carbohydrate. Normally, 10 to 20% of ingested carbohydrate may be maldigested.[134] Recent research has implicated the ingestion of fructose with or without sorbitol in IBS symptoms. This could explain why apple, grape, and pear juice may be associated with diarrhea and abdominal distress.[134] Additional gas-producing items include carbonated beverages, beans, legumes, and cabbage. Also, air swallowing associated with sucking candy, chewing gum, and smoking may cause problems (see Chapter 9, Abdominal Gas and Flatulence).

Recent studies confirm that food intolerances and allergies are not a major factor in the pathogenesis of IBS. However, identification of a possible food intolerance is essential.[138,139] Commonly, patients with diarrhea and/or gas exhibit food intolerances. Lactose is especially troublesome. Thus, lactose-containing products should be reduced or eliminated according to individual intolerance (see Chapter 9, Lactose Intolerance). Additional evidence suggests possible individual intolerance to citrus fruits, onions, gluten, potatoes, chocolate, eggs, caffeine, alcohol, and nuts.[140]

Another major area of research is in the use of fiber and bulking agents to regulate bowel function. In general, a high fiber diet is recommended to increase residue that reaches the distal colon, to normalize gastrointestinal motor function, and to decrease intraluminal colonic pressures.[134] Much discussion has occurred regarding which type and quantity of dietary fiber is most effective. The types of fiber studied include wheat, vegetable, and fruit fibers. Wheat bran is considered to be most effective, especially for patients with constipation (see Chapter 9, Fiber and Residue Modifications), although controlled studies do not exist.[141] It is interesting to note that some controlled studies using placebos demonstrated the same efficacy rate as wheat bran.[140,142] Other fiber supplements such as psyllium, ispaghula, and methylcellulose also provide relief from constipation. Unfortunately, high fiber diets may also increase gas and bloating; thus dietary fiber should be increased gradually. Over time, these symptoms may dissipate as the gastrointestinal tract adjusts.[142]

Adjunctive medication therapy may be necessary as well.[136] Antidiarrheal medications may be appropriate for some patients. Cathartics are usually discouraged because they may cause smooth muscle damage with long-term use.

Goals of Dietary Management

The goals of dietary management appear in Table 9-15.

Dietary Recommendations

Meals are planned to be well balanced, high in fiber, and low in fat. Timing of meals should be addressed because this may help regulate bowel function. A lactose restriction may be added (see section for lactose restricted diets). Additional food intolerances will be addressed according to the individual patient's symptoms.

TABLE 9-15 Dietary Recommendations for Irritable Bowel Syndrome

1. Identify food intolerance(s).
2. Avoid offending foods as needed:
   - Milk and daily products (see Chapter 9, Lactose Intolerance)
   - Gas forming foods and beverages (see Chapter 9, Abdominal Gas)
   - Foods containing high amounts of fructose and raffinose
   - Dietetic foods containing sorbitol
3. Encourage regular, small, frequent, and low fat meals (see Chapter 9, Fat Malabsorption).
4. Gradually increase dietary fiber to approximately 15 to 25 g/day. Discuss use of bulking agents with the physician.
5. Limit caffeine and alcohol intake.
6. Exercise regularly and practice stress reduction techniques.
7. Drink 8 or more cups of water or fluid per day.

Physicians: How to Order Diet

The diet order should specify: *diet for irritable bowel syndrome*. The dietitian will individualize a meal schedule per patient's needs.

References

133. Friedman G. Nutritional therapy of irritable bowel syndrome. Gastroenterol Clin North Am 1989;18(3):513–524.

134. Kellow JE, Langeluddecke PM. Advances in the understanding and management of the irritable bowel syndrome. Med J Aust 1989;151(2):92,95–99.

135. Camilleri M, Prather CM. The irritable bowel syndrome: mechanisms and a practical approach to management. Ann Intern Med 1992;116(12):1001–1008.

136. Drossman DA. Irritable bowel syndrome. American Family Physician 1989;36(6):159–164.

137. Drossman DA, Thompson WG. The irritable bowel syndrome: review and a graduated multicomponent treatment approach. Ann Intern Med 1992;116(12):1009–1016.

138. McKee AM, Prior A, Whorwell PJ. Exclusion diets in irritable bowel syndrome: are they worthwhile? J Clin Gastroenterol 1987;9(5):526–528.

139. Floch MH. The irritable bowel syndrome: the possible link between dietary fiber deficiency and disturbed intestinal motility. Am J Gastroenterol 1988;83(9):963–964.

140. Johnsen R, Jacobsen BK, Forde OH. Associates between symptoms of irritable colon and psychological and social conditions and lifestyle. BMJ 1986;292:1633–1635.

141. Odes HS. Wheat and nonwheat dietary fibers—is there a choice? J Clin Gastroenterol 1987;9(2):131–134.

142. Thompson WG. A strategy for management of the irritable bowel. Am J Gastroenterol 1986;81(2):95–100.

LACTOSE INTOLERANCE

General Description

Lactose, a disaccharide, is the primary carbohydrate in milk. Lactose restriction limits milk and milk products according to individual tolerance. Most individuals with lactose intolerance are able to tolerate small amounts of lactose containing foods.

Nutritional Inadequacy

The diet may be low in calcium, riboflavin, and vitamin D, depending upon the extent of lactose restriction and of age-related nutrient requirements. The RDA for all these nutrients can be met through the use of lactase enzyme–treated milk and milk products. If these products are not used, supplementation may be indicated. In particular, the need for calcium supplementation should be considered for children, adolescents, postmenopausal women,[143] pregnant and lactating women, and women who are at risk for developing osteoporosis. Calcium supplementation is generally contraindicated for individuals with hypercalcemia, hypercalciuria, or a history of calcium-containing urolithiasis. The current practice is to recommend calcium supplements, usually calcium carbonate, to meet or slightly exceed the RDA. (See Chapter 8, Table 8-15, for the calcium content of foods, and Table 8-16, for the calcium content of supplements.) Vitamin D supplementation is necessary only if the individual has inadequate exposure to sunlight. Vitamin D supplements should not exceed the RDA. Supplementary riboflavin is rarely indicated because of its availability from other foods.

Indications and Rationale

Lactase deficiency can be defined as a lowered level of intestinal lactase activity. Lactose intolerance is the condition of intestinal symptoms that follows the ingestion of lactose in a subject with lactase deficiency. It should be noted that a lactase deficient subject may tolerate small amounts of milk without symptoms; thus, the person is somewhat lactose tolerant. This same person may develop symptoms following an intake of greater quantities of lactose, and at that level of intake the person is considered lactose intolerant.[144] Lactase deficiency is not a debilitating disorder, but it can cause uncomfortable and unpleasant symptoms. It is, in fact, a "normal" condition, as the majority of people in the world have lactase deficiency. Lactose intolerance varies in degree among individuals who are affected, rarely appearing as complete or total intolerance.

In the individual with sufficient lactase, lactose is hydrolyzed by the intestinal enzyme lactase into glucose and galactose. If the amount of the enzyme is insufficient to hydrolyze the lactose ingested, some undigested lactose remains in the intestine. Through osmotic effect, the undigested lactose causes water to be drawn into the digestive tract, which results in intestinal symptoms. The undigested lactose passes into the large bowel where it is fermented by normal colonic bacteria to form fatty acids, carbon dioxide, and hydrogen. Symptoms of lactose intolerance include abdominal cramping, flatulence, and diarrhea and may occur shortly after the ingestion of lactose or a few hours later. The severity of symptoms depends upon the amount of lactose that is ingested and the degree of intolerance to lactose.

Secondary lactase deficiency can occur in those with acute or chronic diseases that involve damage to the intestine, such as tropical or celiac sprue, or Crohn's disease[145] or in those who have had small bowel or gastric surgery. Periods of disuse of the intestinal tract, as are encountered with the extended use of central parenteral nutrition, may cause atrophy of the small intestine and hence lactase deficiency. The recovery from such functional impairment can usually be accomplished through the gradual resumption of dietary intake over a period of several weeks.

The diagnosis of lactase deficiency can be determined by (1) a diet history that relates the intake of milk and of milk products to the symptoms, (2) trial of a lactose restricted diet and observation of the elimination of symptoms, (3) a hydrogen breath test to measure the hydrogen in expired air following the ingestion and colonic metabolism of lactose (see Chapter 17 for a discussion of diet in the preparation for a hydrogen breath test), (4) a small bowel biopsy to measure lactase activity, and (5) a lactose tolerance test. The lactose tolerance test is performed by measuring plasma glucose levels following the ingestion of a lactose load. In the adult, an increase in plasma glucose that is less than 20 mg/dl in any

TABLE 9-16 Lactose Content of Foods

LACTOSE-FREE FOODS

Broth-based soups
Plain meat, fish, poultry, peanut butter
Breads that do not contain milk, dry milk solids, or whey
Cereal, crackers
Fruit, plain vegetables
Desserts made without milk, dry milk solids, or whey
Tofu and tofu products, such as tofu-based ice cream substitute
Nondairy creamers

LOW LACTOSE FOODS (0–2 g/SERVING)

¹/₂ cup	Milk treated with lactase enzyme
¹/₂ cup	Sherbet
1-2 oz	Aged cheese
1 oz	Processed cheese
	Butter or margarine
	Commercially-prepared foods containing dry milk solids or whey

Some medications and vitamin preparations may contain a small amount of lactose. Generally, the amount is very small and is tolerated well.

HIGH LACTOSE FOODS (5–8 g/SERVING)

¹/₂ cup	Milk (whole, skim, 1%, 2%, buttermilk, sweet acidophilus)
¹/₈ cup	Powdered dry milk (whole, nonfat, buttermilk—before reconstituting)
¹/₄ cup	Evaporated milk
3 Tbsp	Sweetened condensed milk
³/₄ cup	Heavy cream
¹/₂ cup	Half and Half
¹/₂ cup	Sour cream
¹/₂ cup	White sauce
¹/₂ cup	Party chip dip or potato topping
³/₄ cup	Creamed or low fat cottage cheese
1 cup	Dry cottage cheese
³/₄ cup	Ricotta cheese
2 oz	Cheese food or cheese spread*
³/₄ cup	Ice cream or ice milk
¹/₂ cup	Yogurt†

*Lactose content is higher than that of aged cheese and of processed cheese because of the addition of whey powder and of dry milk solids.

†Yogurt may be tolerated better than foods with similar lactose content because of hydrolysis of lactose by bacterial lactase found in the culture. Tolerance may vary with the brand and the processing method.

of the samples, taken 30, 60, 90, and 120 minutes after a 50 g lactose load, is strongly suggestive of lactase deficiency.[146]

The prevalence of lactase deficiency is high in many populations not of northern European origin. These include persons of Mediterranean origin, blacks, Asians, Greeks, Jews, Mexicans, American Indians, and Aborigines. This is a primary intolerance with no history or signs of underlying intestinal disease.

Goals of Dietary Management

The goals of dietary management are to provide a nutritionally adequate diet and to minimize or reduce symptoms to a level that the patient finds tolerable.

Dietary Recommendations

Tolerance for lactose varies among individuals. The following guidelines may be helpful for individuals who are suspected of or diagnosed as having lactase deficiency.

1. Establish the individual's tolerance level by gradually adding small amounts of lactose-containing foods to a lactose-free diet.
2. Most people can tolerate 5 to 8 g of lactose at a given time, which is the amount in $^1/_2$ cup of milk or the equivalent (see Table 9-16).
3. Small amounts of lactose that are within the individual's tolerance level can generally be taken on several occasions throughout the day.
4. Lactose is generally tolerated if it is taken along with other foods rather than taken alone as a beverage or as a snack.[147]
5. Yogurt may be better tolerated than milk since the bacterial lactase that is found in the yogurt culture hydrolyzes lactose, in addition to the hydrolysis that occurs in the intestinal tract.[148,149] However, tolerance to yogurt may vary with different brands and processing methods.
6. Lactase enzyme is available as Lactaid™, Lactrase™, or Dairy Ease™ and may be added to milk 24 hours in advance of ingestion. In addition, a tablet form is available that can be ingested just before eating a meal that contains lactose. Depending on the degree of intolerance, $^1/_2$ to 3 tablets may be used.[150]
7. Special commercially prepared low lactose foods, including milk, ice cream, and cottage cheese, are available in some supermarkets and in some areas.
8. Lactobacillus acidophilus milk is probably not better tolerated than regular milk.[151,152]
9. Cocoa and chocolate milk may be better tolerated than milk, although there is individual variation.[153]

Table 9-16 presents the lactose content of foods.

Appendix 10 presents lactose-free enteral formulas.

Physicians: How to Order Diet

The diet order should indicate: *lactose restricted diet*. The dietitian plans the diet according to the preceding guidelines and modifies the diet according to the needs and tolerances of the patient.

References

143. Anon. Metabolic bone disease as a result of lactase deficiency. Nutr Rev 1979;37:72–73.
144. Newcomer AD, McGill DB. Clinical importance of lactase deficiency. N Engl J Med 1984;310:42–43.
145. Pironi L, Callegari C, Cornia GL, Lami F, Miglioli M, Barbara L. Lactose malabsorption in adult patients with Crohn's disease. Am J Gastroenterol 1988;83:1267–1271.
146. Skinner S, Martins R, eds. The milk sugar dilemma: living with lactose intolerance. Michigan: Medi-Ed Press, 1985:15.
147. Martini M, Savaiano D. Reduced intolerance symptoms from lactose consumed during a meal. Am J Clin Nutr 1988;47:57–60.

148. Kolars JC, Levitt MD, Mostafa Aouji DAG, Savaiano DA. Yogurt—an autodigesting source of lactose. N Engl J Med 1984;310:1–3.

149. Anon. In vivo digestion of yogurt lactose by yogurt lactase. Nutr Rev 1984;42:216–217.

150. Kligerman AE. Relative efficiency of a commercial lactase tablet. Am J Clin Nutr 1990;51:890–893.

151. Newcomer AD, Park P, O'Brien PC, McGill DB. Response of patients with irritable bowel syndrome and lactase deficiency using unfermented acidophilus milk. Am J Clin Nutr 1983;38:257–263.

152. Savaiano DA, Abdelhak Abou El Anouar DAG, Smith DE, Levitt MD. Lactose malabsorption from yogurt, pasteurized yogurt, sweet acidophilus milk, and cultured milk in lactase-deficient individuals. Am J Clin Nutr 1984;40:1219–1223.

153. Lee C, Hardy C. Cocoa feeding and human lactose intolerance. Am J Clin Nutr 1989;49:840–844.

PEPTIC ULCER DISEASE

General Description

Dietary guidelines are given that help avoid extreme stimulation of gastric acid secretion and may reduce the symptoms of peptic ulcer disease. Slight modifications in the patient's usual diet may be recommended and are based on the individual's food intolerances. However, diet plays a minor role in the cause of ulcers, with medications being the mainstay of treatment.

Nutritional Inadequacy

Dietary modifications for peptic ulcer disease do not result in a diet inadequate in nutrients when compared to the RDA.

Indications and Rationale

A peptic ulcer is an erosion or disintegration in the mucosal lining of the esophagus, stomach, or duodenum. It typically occurs in the lower part of the stomach (gastric ulcer) or in the initial portion of the duodenum (duodenal ulcer). The cause is not fully known.[154] Normally the linings of the esophagus, stomach, and duodenum are kept intact by a balance between the acid produced in the stomach and the resistance of these linings to breakdown. When the balance is disrupted, the result may be an ulcer. It is estimated that peptic ulcers occur in 1 of every 10 individuals. The occurrence of duodenal ulcers peaks between ages 40 and 50 years; gastric ulcers peak between ages 60 and 70 years.[154]

The goals of ulcer treatment are to relieve symptoms, heal the ulcer, prevent reoccurrence, and avoid complications. Medication acts to decrease the acidity of stomach secretions (antacids) or to decrease acid production (H_2 blockers) or as protection for the lining of the esophagus, stomach, or duodenum (sucralfate). The vast majority of patients with peptic ulcer disease respond well to medication.[154] In some instances, the rationale for diet has been physiologically inappropriate and the food restrictions have been unwarranted. A bland or what may be referred to as an "ulcer diet" is no more effective than a general diet in speeding the rate of ulcer healing and in reducing gastric acid secretion. Controlled trials in patients with a duodenal ulcer have shown that these diets do not hasten the remission of symptoms or prevent recurrences.[155-158] However, bland diets probably are not detrimental to most persons if they are used for a short time and may be of psychological benefit to some. Prolonged adherence to these regimens is not necessary.

Current dietary therapy consists largely of eliminating foods that (1) increase secretion of stomach acid, (2) worsen symptoms, and (3) damage the lining of the esophagus, stomach, or duodenum. Such diets may hasten healing to some extent. However, the beneficial effect is not perceptible statistically because of the difficulties in evaluating degrees of healing and the variability of response among subjects. The approach to diet for peptic ulcer disease must be individualized. Following are various dietary features that have been studied for effects on peptic ulcer disease and that should be considered when developing dietary guidelines for each patient.

Rough or Coarse Food. Rough or coarse food has previously been excluded from bland diets on the presumption that it irritates the gastric mucosa. This presumption has not been found to be true. In fact, clinical studies are showing that a high fiber diet may have a prophylactic effect in the prevention of duodenal ulcer relapse.[158,159]

Milk. In the past, milk was an important part of ulcer diets because it was believed to buffer gastric contents. While it is true that milk, in addition to many other foods, has a transient buffering effect, it tends to be a strong secretagogue for acid production, owing largely to its calcium and protein content. It has been found that whole, low fat, and nonfat milk each produce a significant increase in mean gastric acid secretion 2 to 3 hours after ingestion.[157,160] Since milk has only a transient buffering effect on gastric acid that is followed by a sustained rise in acid secretion, frequent milk ingestion is not recommended for ulcer treatment.[156-158,160]

Spices, Condiments, and Acidic Foods. Spices, condiments, and fruit juices, although frequently producing dyspepsia, have not been shown to cause ulcer disease or impair ulcer healing.[156,158,161] The spices most often implicated are black pepper, chili powder, and red pepper.[155] The restriction of spices and other foods should be determined by individual tolerances.

Caffeine and Decaffeinated Beverages. It is rational to recommend a restriction of stimulators of gastric acid secretion, which include regular coffee and tea, other sources of caffeine, and decaffeinated coffee and tea.[155,156] These foods may worsen dyspeptic symptoms. Appendix 23 presents the caffeine content of beverages and some medications. Also presented are beverages without caffeine.

Alcohol. Alcohol is thought to directly damage the gastric mucosa. During treatment for gastric ulcers, patients should be advised to minimize their alcoholic intake.[156,157]

Small Volume, Frequent Feedings. Small volume, frequent feedings have not been found to be more effective than 3 meals per day in the long-term treatment of peptic ulcer disease. In fact, some authorities advise against extra feedings because they increase acid secretion and may unduly complicate the patient's eating pattern. However, some patients claim relief of symptoms with frequent feedings, especially during the acute stages.[156]

Smoking.   Smoking has been associated with the occurrence of ulcers and with the prevention of ulcer healing. Avoidance of smoking is advised.[155,156]

Goals of Dietary Management

The goals of dietary management are to avoid the stimulation of gastric acid secretion and the direct irritation of gastric mucosa, which may delay the healing of the ulcer and the resolution of symptoms.

Dietary Recommendations

Limit or avoid coffee, decaffeinated coffee, caffeine-containing beverages, and alcoholic beverages. Meal size and other specific food selections should be individually determined by the patient. Gradual increase in the intake of fiber may be helpful. Cigarette smoking should be stopped.

Physicians: How to Order Diet

The diet order should indicate: *diet for peptic ulcer.*

References

154. Larson DE, ed. Mayo Clinic family health book. New York: William Morrow, 1990:603–607.
155. Marotta RB, Floch MH. Diet and nutrition in ulcer disease. Med Clin North Am 1991; 75(4):967–977.
156. Gaska JA, Tietze KJ. Current concepts in the treatment of peptic ulcer disease: a case oriented approach. Am Pharmac 1989;NS29(11):48–53.
157. Desai MB, Jeejeebhoy KN. Nutrition and diet in the management of diseases of the gastrointestinal tract. In: Shils ME, Young VR, eds. Modern nutrition in health and disease. Philadelphia: Lea & Febiger, 1988:1099–1102.
158. Berstad A. Dietary treatment of peptic ulcer. Scand J Gastroenterol 1987;129(Suppl): 228–231.
159. Rydning A. Dietary fibre and peptic ulcer. Scand J Gastroenterol 1987;129(Suppl):232–240.
160. Ippoliti AF, Maxwell V, Isenberg JI. The effect of various forms of milk on gastric acid secretion. Ann Intern Med 1976;84:286–289.
161. Graham DY, Lacey-Smith J, Opekun AR. Spicy food and the stomach—evaluation by videoendoscopy. JAMA 1988;260(23):3473–3475.

POSTGASTRECTOMY DUMPING SYNDROME

General Description

The dietary management of dumping syndrome is aimed at reducing the volume and the osmotic effect of food that enters the proximal small bowel, thereby preventing small bowel distention and late hypoglycemia. This can be achieved by (1) limiting the intake of simple sugars (mono- and disaccharides), (2) consuming small, frequent meals, and (3) limiting fluids with meals. Because symptoms vary greatly in severity and duration, the diet should be individualized and modified according to the patient's symptoms.

Nutritional Inadequacy

The modifications for dumping syndrome do not result in a diet that is inherently inadequate in nutrients when compared to the RDA. However, each individual's diet should be assessed for nutritional adequacy because of the variation in food tolerances. The long-term restriction of important nutrients may warrant supplementation (e.g., calcium supplementation for the restriction of milk because of lactose intolerance).

Indications and Rationale

Dumping syndrome may develop as a complication of a total or subtotal gastrectomy or of any surgical procedure that removes, disrupts, or bypasses the pyloric sphincter, such as vagotomy and pyloroplasty, and including some surgical procedures for morbid obesity (see Chapter 8 for dietary management after bariatric surgeries).[162,163] As many as 20 to 40% of patients experience an element of dumping symptoms immediately after surgery, but symptoms usually decrease with time; only 5% or less of patients suffer chronic disability because of dumping. Occasionally, symptoms of dumping may appear for the first time several months or years after surgery.

Dumping syndrome can be divided into early and late phases.[162-165] The intensity and duration of symptoms vary considerably with the individual, but there are common characteristics. The early phase occurs 15 to 30 minutes postprandially and is characterized by gastrointestinal symptoms of epigastric fullness, abdominal cramps, nausea, and/or diarrhea and vasomotor symptoms of tachycardia, postural hypotension, sweating, weakness, flushing, and/or syncope. However, some patients may experience the intestinal symptoms without the associated vasomotor phenomena or vice versa.

Most of the early phase symptoms are related to rapid gastric emptying with consequent distention of the upper small intestine. The hypertonicity of the "dumped" intestinal contents produces a rapid influx of fluid as the hyperosmolar content is diluted. The syndrome may be aggravated by consumption of meals that are high in simple carbohydrate, which increases the osmolality of the gastric contents, and/or meals with large volumes of liquids, which enhances the rate of emptying of food from the stomach.[164] Fullness, cramps, and nausea can be attributed to rapid jejunal filling. Diarrhea is due to the rapid entry of hypertonic liquids into the small intestine, thereby overwhelming its absorptive capacity and resulting in the passage of large volumes of unabsorbed material into the colon.[164] Reflex mechanisms initiated by jejunal distention and the release of hormones may also increase colonic motility, which further decreases intestinal transit time.

Like the gastrointestinal symptoms, the vasomotor abnormalities can be evoked by the rapid filling of the jejunum with hypertonic material. This can cause a combination of autonomic reflexes, hemoconcentration that is secondary to a rapid osmotic shift of plasma fluid into the bowel lumen with a subsequent fall in the blood volume, and an excessive release of vasoactive hormones, all of which may account for many of the vasomotor symptoms.

The late phase occurs about 2 to 4 hours postprandially and is associated with symptoms that have been attributed to hypoglycemia; that is, perspiration, hunger, nausea, anxiety, tremors, and/or weakness.[164] The late phase is seen much less frequently than the symptoms of early dumping.

The medical treatment of dumping syndrome consists almost entirely of dietary management.[163-165] Most drug therapy is usually not effective. Octreotide, a long-lasting somatostatin analog, has recently been found to be helpful in many disabled patients.[166] Surgical revision may be necessary in severe cases, but in itself may not always be successful in alleviating the problem.

Goals of Dietary Management

The goals of dietary management are to provide a nutritionally adequate diet and to reduce symptoms to a level that the patient finds tolerable. This can be achieved through manipulations and restrictions that are designed to normalize or at least slow gastric emptying, thereby controlling the volume and the osmolality of food that enters the jejunum.[164,167-169] Sometimes the dumping symptoms may be of such severity that the person exists in a state of semistarvation with protein-calorie malnutrition. Although inadequate intake appears to be the main cause for malnutrition after gastrectomy, steatorrhea and enteric protein losses must also be considered.[164,170] Regular screening is emphasized to detect early iron, vitamin B_{12}, protein, and vitamin D deficiencies.

Dietary Recommendations

Early satiety and the desire to ameliorate symptoms frequently result in decreased food intake and subsequent weight loss after gastric surgery.[164] The diet should be adjusted to meet the patient's needs with an increase in complex carbohydrate, protein, and fat (if tolerated) to provide sufficient kilocalories. Table 9-17 presents the dietary recommendations for postgastrectomy dumping syndrome.

Following gastrectomy, the patient's nutritional status should be assessed to determine whether or not malabsorption and/or dietary restriction are having

---

TABLE 9-17   Dietary Recommendations for Postgastrectomy Dumping Syndrome

1. Small, frequent meals are recommended to decrease intestinal distention caused by the rapid emptying of a large meal.
2. Mono- and disaccharides should be kept to a minimum to prevent the formation of hyperosmolar intestinal contents. Sugar, honey, syrup, and other foods high in sugar should be avoided initially and may need long-term limitation.
3. Tolerance to milk and to other lactose-containing products should be established by a gradual introduction into the diet. Lactose reduced milk is usually not tolerated, because lactase enzymes simply reduce disaccharides to monosaccharides, which are just as likely to promote dumping.
4. Fluids should not be taken with meals but may be taken 45 to 60 minutes before or after meals. Initially, it may be helpful to limit the volume of fluids to 4 oz per serving. The restriction of fluids retards gastric emptying of solids. Hypertonic liquids are emptied rapidly and should be avoided. Adequate fluids between meals should be encouraged to prevent dehydration.
5. Lying down for 15 to 30 minutes after meals may help to decrease the symptoms of dumping. If the patient is also bothered by reflux, lying flat after eating is not recommended.

adverse effects. Mild anemia is a common finding, generally developing several years after a partial or total gastrectomy.[164,168,171,172] The cause may be multifactorial, and its presence should be assessed by monitoring serum iron, B_{12}, and folate levels. An inadequate nutritional intake as well as gastrointestinal blood loss may be contributing factors. Most patients with dumping have had an antiulcer operation (antrectomy, vagotomy) performed to decrease acid production by the stomach. This interferes with iron conversion and its subsequent absorption, which may lead to iron deficiency. Serum albumin and dietary protein intake should be monitored to determine whether maldigestion-malabsorption of protein and/or inadequate protein intake are causing protein malnutrition. Mild steatorrhea of 10 to 15 g/day of fecal fat is a common finding. However, its contribution to malnutrition is usually not significant.[164,171,173] An uncommon and late complication is metabolic bone disease (osteomalacia), which appears to involve alterations in vitamin D metabolism.[164,171,172,174]

The vast majority of symptoms resolve or improve with time.[163,168] As foods are better tolerated, patients are more willing and able to liberalize the diet. Only a minority of patients need to maintain the restrictions for extended periods of time. Most are able to identify their own levels of tolerance with guidance from a dietitian. Additional dietary modifications may be necessary for those with malabsorption.

Physicians: How to Order Diet

The diet order should indicate: *diet for postgastrectomy dumping syndrome*. The dietitian plans the diet according to the guidelines previously mentioned and modifies the diet according to the needs and tolerances of the patient.

References

162. Herrington JL. Postgastrectomy syndromes. In: Bayless TM, ed. Current therapy in gastroenterology and liver disease, 1984–1985. Philadelphia: BC Decker, 1984:69–76.
163. Cooperman AM. Postgastrectomy syndromes. Surg Annu 1981;13:139–161.
164. Meyer JH. Chronic morbidity after ulcer surgery. In: Sleisenger MH, Fordtran JS, eds. Gastrointestinal disease: pathophysiology, diagnosis, management, 4th ed. Philadelphia: WB Saunders, 1989:962–987.
165. Spiro HM. Postgastrectomy and post-vagotomy syndrome. In: Clinical gastroenterology, 3rd ed. New York: MacMillan, 1983:434–455.
166. Geer RJ, Richards WO, O'Dorisio TM, Woltering EO, Williams S, Rice D, Abumrad NN. Efficacy of ocreotide in treatment of severe postgastrectomy dumping syndrome. Ann Surg 1990;212:678–687.
167. Williamson J. Physiological stress: nutritional care for patients having surgery, trauma or burns. In: Krause MV, Mahan LK, eds. Food, nutrition, and diet therapy, 7th ed. Philadelphia: WB Saunders, 1984:689–706.
168. Alpers DH, Clouse RE, Stenson WF. Restrictive diets. In: Alpers DH, Clouse RE, Stenson WF, eds. Manual of nutritional therapeutics, 2nd ed. Boston: Little, Brown, 1988:277–332.
169. Shils ME, Young VR. Appendix A-31. In: Shils ME, Young VR, eds. Modern nutrition in health and disease, 7th ed. Philadelphia: Lea & Febiger, 1988:1583–1585.
170. Sategna-Guidetti C, Bianco L. Malnutrition and malabsorption after total gastrectomy. J Clin Gastroenterol 1989;11:518–524.

171. Desai MB, Jeejeebhoy KN. Nutrition and diet in management of diseases of the gastrointestinal tract. In: Shils ME, Young VR, eds. Modern nutrition in health and disease, 7th ed. Philadelphia: Lea & Febiger, 1988:1103–1107.
172. Tovey FI, Godfrey JE, Lewin MR. A gastrectomy population: 25–30 years on. Postgrad Med J 1990;66:450–456.
173. Cristallo M, Braga M, Agape D, Primiguani M, Zuliani W, Vecchi M, Murone M, Sironi M, DiCarlo V, DeFranchis R. Nutritional status, function of the small intestine and jejunal morphology after total gastrectomy for carcinoma of the stomach. Surg Gynecol Obstet 1986;163:225–230.
174. Klein KB, Orwoll ES, Lieberman DA, Meier DE, McClung MR, Parfitt AM. Metabolic bone disease in asymptomatic men after partial gastrectomy with Billroth II anastomosis. Gastroenterology 1987;92:608–616.

10 / *Hepatobiliary Diseases*

HEPATOBILIARY DISEASES

General Description

Patients with liver disease are frequently malnourished for a variety of reasons (Table 10-1).[1] Dietary restrictions of sodium and fluid are commonly required to manage ascites and pedal edema. Protein restrictions are necessary in some cases of hepatic encephalopathy. Some patients may become glucose intolerant in the later stages of their disease. Others may require frequent high carbohydrate feedings to compensate for decreased capacity to store glycogen and lessened capacity for gluconeogenesis. Patients with chronic cholestatic liver diseases (primary biliary cirrhosis, primary sclerosing cholangitis, choledocholithiasis, secondary biliary stricture, and biliary atresia) commonly have steatorrhea, which may respond to a modification of dietary fat (i.e., restriction of ordinary dietary fats and possibly the addition of medium chain triglycerides). In all cases of liver disease, attention should be given to the patient's electrolyte, fluid, vitamin, and mineral status, with appropriate dietary modification and/or supplementation as needed.

Nutritional Inadequacy

The goal of dietary management in liver disease is to promote nutritional adequacy within necessary dietary guidelines. The diet is not inherently lacking in nutrients as compared to the Recommended Dietary Allowance (RDA) unless severe protein, sodium, and/or fluid restrictions are required. Potential amino acid deficiencies exist in diets that provide less total protein than the RDA of 0.8 g of protein per kilogram of dry body weight. To counter this risk, approximately 75% of the total protein intake should be high biological value protein or complementary vegetable proteins. Diets of 50 g of protein or less per day provide inadequate calcium, iron, phosphorus, thiamine, riboflavin, niacin, and folic acid by RDA criteria. Therefore, a daily multiple vitamin that includes approximately 1mg of folic acid is recommended.

TABLE 10-1   Potential Causes of Malnutrition in Liver Disease[1]

1. Decreased intake of food
    (i.) Decreased quantity of food
        (a.) Anorexia, nausea and vomiting, early satiety
        (b.) Hospitalization related
    (ii.) Decreased quality of food
        (a.) Unpalatable diets
        (b.) Hospitalization related
2. Impaired digestion and absorption
    (i.) Impaired digestion
        (a.) Pancreatic deficiency
        (b.) Bile salt deficiency
    (ii.) Impaired absorption
        (a.) Mucosal defect (portal hypertensive enteropathy)
3. Increased energy requirements
4. Inefficient protein synthesis
5. Accelerated protein breakdown
6. Increased protein oxidation*

*Protein oxidation is a term used to describe irreversible amino-nitrogen loss occurring at the amino acid level but extrapolated to precursor tissue protein.

Reprinted with permission: McCullough AJ, Tabill AS. Disordered energy and protein metabolism in liver disease. Semin Liver Dis 1991;11:265–277, Thieme Medical Publishers.

Indications and Rationale

Energy.   An adequate supply of kilocalories is necessary to allow protein synthesis and prevent the use of amino acids for energy. Several studies suggest that when metabolic parameters are corrected for decreased lean body mass and fluid overload, patients with chronic liver disease (cirrhosis) may be hypermetabolic.[2-4] If alterations in protein, carbohydrate, and/or fat metabolism exist, the standard proportion of kilocalories that each nutrient usually provides will need to be adjusted. In addition, distributing kilocalories in a meal plan which includes at least an evening snack has been shown to maintain a more positive nitrogen balance in patients with cirrhosis than in similar patients receiving the same amount of kilocalories distributed as three meals per day, as a means of decreasing the accelerated starvation rate, which can occur in the fasting state.[5]

Protein.   Usual protein requirements in stable liver disease have been determined to be 0.7 to 1.0 g/kg of dry or desirable body weight per day,[6-8] while others have suggested that up to 1.5 g/kg per day may be required in stressed patients to achieve anabolism.[9] It has been determined that approximately 1.0 g/kg of ideal body weight per day was required to reach nitrogen balance in patients being prepared for orthotopic liver transplantation.[10]

Hepatic encephalopathy or coma is a potential and serious complication of liver disease. Hepatic encephalopathy is associated with changes in consciousness, behavior, and neurologic status (see Table 10-2).[11] In chronic encephalopathy,

TABLE 10-2 Clinical Stages of Hepatic Encephalopathy[11]

Stage	Mental State
I	Mild confusion, euphoria or depression, decreased attention, slowing of ability to perform mental tasks, irritability, disorder of sleep pattern
II	Drowsiness, lethargy, gross deficits, inability to perform mental tasks, obvious personality changes, inappropriate behavior, intermittent disorientation (usually for a time)
III	Somnolent but rousable, unable to perform mental tasks, disorientation with respect to time and/or place, marked confusion, amnesia, occasional fits of rage, speech present but incomprehensible
IV	Coma

Reprinted with permission: Gammel SH, Jones EA. Hepatic encephalopathy. Med Clin North Am 1989;73:793-813.

symptoms may be subclinical and detected only by special testing, vary in severity, and be worsened rapidly by gastrointestinal bleeding, sedatives, renal failure, infection, or severe constipation.

The cause of hepatic encephalopathy is unknown, but precipitating factors that are coupled with chronic liver disease have been identified. The three proposed general mechanisms that lead to hepatic coma are (1) an accumulation of various toxins owing to impaired hepatic function (ammonia appears to be a marker of impaired clearance of toxins associated with encephalopathy), (2) false neurotransmitters (altered plasma amino acid composition; decreased ratio of branched chain amino acids [BCAA] to aromatic amino acids), and (3) an increase in serum and brain neuroinhibitory substances (increased gamma-aminobutyric acid [GABA] levels and augmented density of cerebral GABA receptors).[11-14]

A widely accepted concept is that hepatic encephalopathy is closely associated with increased levels of blood ammonia. This increase can be caused by decreased production of urea, which results from impaired liver function, by increased bacterial production of ammonia in the intestine from available nitrogenous substrates (dietary protein, gastrointestinal hemorrhage), by enterohepatic circulation of urea, by renal failure (increased availability of urea for enterohepatic circulation), and by constipation (increased ammonia production and prolonged transit time, which allows increased absorption).[11,14] Other proposed causes contributing to hepatic encephalopathy include infection (increased catabolism of body protein coupled with abnormal ammonia metabolism), sedative abuse, excessive diuretics, which cause fluid and electrolyte imbalances, anesthesia and surgery, elevated levels of blood mercaptans (methionine metabolites), and altered BCAA to aromatic amino acid ratio and its effect on neurotransmitter synthesis.[14] Acute hepatic encephalopathy in the absence of pre-existing liver disease is usually seen in conjunction with acute viral hepatitis or with toxin/drug-induced liver damage. The medical management of hepatic encephalopathy is aimed at the identification and treatment of precipitating factors.[15]

Since ammonia is a product of protein metabolism, dietary protein has often been restricted. However, sufficient protein and caloric intake to maintain nitrogen balance must be provided. Severe protein restriction is usually not necessary unless a documented protein intolerance exists, and may actually be harmful by promoting the catabolism of lean body tissue.[6,16,17] Metabolic abnormalities that are associated with liver disease (hyperglucagonemia and hyperinsulinemia) coupled with the needs for tissue repair or other stress situations may actually increase protein requirements for cirrhotic and encephalopathic individuals.[1,9,17]

Several studies have explored the advantages of using nonmeat sources of dietary protein in the treatment of hepatic encephalopathy.[18,20] Nonmeat sources of dietary protein, such as vegetable and dairy products, contain lower amounts of ammonia-producing substrates, methionine, and aromatic amino acids, and have a higher BCAA content than meat protein. Vegetable proteins also contain lower amounts of ammonia and mercaptans. However, compliance with vegetable protein diets may be difficult. Because of the bulkiness of vegetable protein diets, some patients with various eating problems (e.g.. early satiety or bloating) may not be able to eat enough food to assure nutritional adequacy of the diet. Furthermore, research has not found significant differences in mental status, nitrogen balance, and plasma amino acids when a diet of vegetable protein is ingested versus a diet of animal protein.[11] Although dairy protein sources have not been shown conclusively to be more advantageous than meat protein, it seems reasonable to use dairy protein sources to the extent that they are accepted by the patient. The role of enteral and parenteral BCAA in supplying either supplementary or total protein nutrition in the protein intolerant patient is controversial at best. Two reviews of the literature (meta-analysis) reached different conclusions on its appropriate use for treatment of encephalopathy.[22,23] While definitive studies still need to be completed to determine the true level of benefit versus cost of high BCAA supplements, their use to increase the total intake of nitrogen in the traditionally protein intolerant patient or to provide total nutrition for a patient with severe encephalopathy may be appropriate and beneficial.

Fat.   Most patients with liver disease continue to tolerate dietary and intravenous forms of fat, so it should be used as an integral form of kilocalories in the diet.[3,6,15] In some cases of severe steatorrhea (stool fat greater than 25 g per 24 hours), a diet restricted in ordinary dietary fat, perhaps with the addition of medium chain triglycerides, may be beneficial in reducing the degree of stool fat (kilocalorie) and vitamin and mineral losses. These measures may also improve the patient's general well-being due to relief from diarrheal symptoms (see Chapter 9, Fat Malabsorption).

Electrolytes and Fluid

Sodium.   Sodium restriction (90 mEq or 2 g) is often necessary when edema and/or ascites are present. Balancing adequate kilocalorie and protein intake, diuretic therapy, and fluid restriction (if necessary) can help prevent further sodium restrictions. Lower levels of sodium intake may be necessary to maintain sodium balance; however, dietary compliance decreases due to a lack of palatability and decreased variety. Special food items and preparations are also required. Special attention is necessary for diets less than 45 mEq of sodium per day because it is difficult to maintain a relatively high kilocalorie and protein intake at that level of sodium intake.

Potassium. It is usually not necessary to restrict potassium in liver disease unless serum levels rise as a result of impaired renal function or from diuretic usage (e.g., spironolactone). In some cases, a high potassium diet and/or supplements may be necessary when using potassium-wasting diuretics (e.g., Lasix™).

Magnesium. Mild to moderate decreases in serum magnesium levels may occur because of increased urinary losses due to chronic alcohol ingestion or malabsorption or from enteropathy or pancreatic insufficiency. Attempts should be made to supplement with oral magnesium preparations (magnesium oxide), but these may cause diarrhea and are usually not totally successful in replacing body stores. Parenteral (I.M.) magnesium is sometimes required.

Fluid. Fluid restrictions are often used to assist with the correction of ascites and edema especially when serum sodium levels drop below 128 mEq/L. Fluid allowances such as 1,500 ml per day or the equivalent of the previous day's fluid losses may be specified.

Vitamins

Water-soluble. A multiple vitamin supplement that provides the RDA amounts of B vitamins is usually adequate to meet deficiencies. Supplemental thiamine and vitamin C may also be necessary.[24]

Fat-soluble. Deficiencies of fat-soluble vitamins are very common in chronic liver disease (especially the cholestatic diseases) and contribute to the osteoporosis often seen in such diseases.[16,24,25] Water-miscible forms of the vitamins (e.g., Aquasol A™, and Aquasol E™) should be used to supplement along with regular monitoring of serum levels to ensure adequacy of the supplementation.

Minerals

Zinc. Zinc deficiency is common in many types of liver disease. It may be due to a combination of decreased intake, decreased absorption, increased urinary excretion, and altered metabolism.[24-26]

Iron. Supplementation of iron in cases of anemia is indicated, but, care must be taken to avoid iron overload because of the hepatotoxic nature of excessive iron.[24,26]

Copper. Dietary copper intake should be restricted in cases of Wilson's disease along with proper chelation therapy (e.g., D-penicillamine) (see Chapter 10, Copper Metabolism).

Calcium. Interpretation of serum calcium levels requires consideration of frequent hypoalbuminemia in liver disease. Adequate dietary and/or supplemental calcium intake (up to 1,500 mg per day) should be encouraged, especially in those patients at risk for or who have osteoporosis (patients with cholestatic liver disease or steroid-treated autoimmune chronic active hepatitis).[26,27]

Goals of Dietary Management

Nutritional therapy is generally directed at clinical manifestations of the disease rather than at the cause. The goals of dietary management are to maintain adequate nutrition, to prevent the catabolism of body protein tissue, to control edema and ascites, and to prevent or to ameliorate the symptoms of hepatic encephalopathy to the greatest possible extent.

Dietary Recommendations

The diet should be individualized according to the needs of each patient. If protein intake needs to be restricted due to hepatic encephalopathy, the highest amount that will not provoke encephalopathy should be used, with a goal of 1.0 g/kg of dry (or desirable) body weight (for 0 or stage 1 encephalopathy). If this level is not tolerated, further restriction to 0.75 or 0.5 g/kg of dry (desirable) weight may be used (stage 2 encephalopathy). To avoid muscle catabolism, the long-term total protein content of the diet should not be less than 35 to 50 g per day. Once the encephalopathy is resolved or controlled, the patient's tolerance may be challenged with increases of 10 to 20 g of dietary protein every 3 to 5 days until the highest amount tolerated is reached. Some patients may tolerate larger total amounts of protein if the majority comes from dairy, starch, and vegetable sources while limiting meat type (animal) sources to 20 to 40 g per day (≤ 0.5 g/kg).

For patients whose symptoms require ongoing treatment with conventional low protein diets or who are receiving no protein due to stage 3 or 4 encephalopathy, supplementation with a high BCAA and low aromatic amino acid formula may be indicated. The formula should be decreased as the oral intake of protein increases. There is a limited benefit to oral supplementation with the formula for patients who are able to take more than 50 g per day of protein from food.

Caloric intake should be sufficient to prevent the catabolism of body protein for energy. Kilocalories equal to Harris-Benedict (basal plus 20% or 30 kcal/kg of dry or desirable weight) should be adequate to meet most patients' requirements. However, 150 to 170% of Harris-Benedict (basal) may be needed in some patients who are extremely catabolic, stressed, restless, or who require weight gain.[9] In this type of patient and in the fluid overloaded patient when it is difficult to estimate dry weight, indirect calorimetry may be helpful to better define actual caloric requirements. Since many patients are anorexic, drowsy, and have early satiety, they may have difficulty consuming enough kilocalories at mealtime, so supplements and/or between meal feedings (especially at bedtime) may be necessary to increase caloric intake and to help maintain muscle mass.

A sodium intake of 90 mEq or less is appropriate if ascites and edema are present and if the patient is in a positive sodium balance. A rapid gain in weight may indicate that some fluid is being retained and that the sodium level may need to be reduced to 60 mEq or less. Diets that contain as little as 20 to 45 mEq of sodium per day may be necessary for patients whose edema and ascites are resistant to diuretic therapy. However, these diets are very restrictive, unpalatable, and difficult to comply with.

The fluid intake is variable and must be controlled in relation to the urinary output, changes in weight, and serum electrolyte values. After vigorous diuretic therapy and resulting losses of sodium, there is the possibility of significant dilutional hyponatremia if the patient is allowed to drink water to fully satisfy thirst. Fluid restrictions usually begin at 1,500 ml per day and may decrease to 1,200 or 1,000 ml depending on response and urinary losses. Suggestions on how to cope with thirst are necessary to improve compliance with fluid restriction.

The diet for hepatic diseases or hepatic encephalopathy can be planned with the use of the exchange lists for protein, sodium, fluid, and potassium control (see Chapter 14, Renal Exchange Lists, for Protein, Sodium, and Potassium Control).

Physicians: How to Order Diet

The diet order should indicate (1) the *specific level of protein*. The most common levels are 1.0, 0.75, and 0.5 g/kg of dry (or desirable) body weight or a minimum of 40 g per day; (2) the *specific level of sodium*. The most common levels are 90, 60, 45 and 20 mEq. If there is a positive sodium balance, the level given should be able to put the patient into a negative sodium balance; and (3) the *specific level of fluid*. The most common levels are 1,500, 1,200, and 1,000 ml per day. The dietitian determines the appropriate caloric level and other characteristics of the diet based on nutrition assessment, patient tolerance, and discussion with the physician.

References

1. McCullough AJ, Tabill AS. Disordered energy and protein metabolism in liver disease. Semin Liver Dis 1991;11:265–277.
2. Shanbhogue RLK, Bistrian BR, Jenkins RL, Jones C, Benotti P, Blackburn GL. Resting energy expenditure in patients with end-stage liver disease and in normal population. JPEN 1987;11:305–308.
3. Dolz C, Raurich JM, Ibanez J, Obrador A, Marse P, Gaya J. Ascites increases the resting energy expenditure in liver cirrhosis. Gastroenterology 1991;100:738–744.
4. Schneeweiss B, Graninger W, Ferenci P, Eichinger S, Grimm G, Schneider B, Laggner AN, Lenz K, Kleinberger G. Energy metabolism in patients with acute and chronic liver disease. Hepatology 1990;11:387–393.
5. Swart GR, Zillinkens MC, Van Vuvre JK, van den Berg JWO. Effect of a late evening meal on nitrogen balance in patients with cirrhosis of the liver. Br Med J 1989; 299:1202–1203.
6. Munoz SJ. Nutritional therapies in liver disease. Semin Liver Dis 1991;11:278–291.
7. O'Keefe SJD, Abraham RR, Davis M, Williams R. Protein turnover in acute and chronic liver disease. Acta Chir Scand 1980;507(suppl):91–101.
8. Morgan MY, Levine JA. Nutritional management of patients with liver disease. J Clin Nutr Gastroenterol 1986;1:303–314.
9. Shronts EP, Teasley KM, Thoele SL, Cerra FB. Nutrition support of the adult liver transplant candidate. J Am Diet Assoc 1987;87:441–451.
10. Plevak DJ, DiCecco SR, Wiesner RH, Porayko MK, Janzow DJ, Hammel K. Nutritional support in liver transplantation: identifying calorie and protein requirements. Mayo Clin Proc (at press, March 1994).
11. Gammel SH, Jones EA. Hepatic encephalopathy. Med Clin North Am 1989;73:793–813.
12. Fischer JE, Baldessarini RJ. False neurotransmitters and hepatic failure. Lancet 1971; 2:75–80.
13. Schafer DF, Jones EA. Hepatic encephalopathy and the gamma-aminobutyric acid neurotransmitter system. Lancet 1982;1:18–20.
14. Butterworth RF. Pathogenesis and treatment of portal-systemic encephalopathy: an update. Dig Dis Sci 1992;37:321–327.
15. Mullen KD, Weber FL. Role of nutrition in hepatic encephalopathy. Semin Liver Dis 1991;11:292–304.
16. Talbot JM. Guidelines for the scientific review of enteral food products for special medical purposes. JPEN 1991;15(suppl):122S–129S.
17. Silk DBA, O'Keefe SJD, Wicks C. Nutritional support in liver disease. Gut 1991;(suppl): S29–S33.
18. Uribe M, Marquez MA, Ramos GG, Ramos-Uribe MH, Vargas F, Villalobas A, Ramos C. Treatment of chronic portal-systemic encephalopathy with vegetable and animal protein diets: a controlled crossover study. Dig Dis Sci 1982;27:1109–1116.

19. De Bruijn KM, Blendis LM, Zilm DH, Carlen PL, Anderson GH. Effect of dietary protein manipulations in subclinical portal-systemic encephalopathy. Gut 1983;24:53–60.

20. Greenberger NJ, Carley J, Schenker S, Bettinger I, Stamnes C, Beyer P. Effect of vegetable and animal protein diets in chronic hepatic encephalopathy. Dig Dis 1977; 22:845–855.

21. Shaw S, Warner TM, Lieber CS. Comparison of animal and vegetable protein sources in the dietary management of hepatic encephalopathy. Am J Clin Nutr 1983;38:59–63.

22. Naylor CD, O'Rourke K, Detsky AS, Baker JP. Parenteral nutrition with branched-chain amino acids in hepatic encephalopathy: a meta-analysis. Gastroenterology 1989;97: 1033–1042.

23. Ericksson LS, Conn HO. Branched-chain amino acids in the management of hepatic encephalopathy: an analysis of variants. Hepatology 1989;10:228–246.

24. Mezitis NHE. Nutritional management in liver disease. Nutr Clin Prac 1988;3:108–112.

25. DiCecco SR, Wieners EJ, Wiesner RH, Southorn PA, Plevak DJ, Krom RAF. Assessment of nutritional status of patients with end-stage liver disease undergoing liver transplantation. Mayo Clin Proc 1989;64:95–102.

26. McClain CJ, Marsano L, Burk RF, Bacon B. Trace metals in liver disease. Semin Liver Dis 1991;11:321–339.

27. Hay JE. Nutritional aspects of chronic cholestatic liver disease. Support Line (Dietitians in Nutrition Support) Newsletter 1991;13:15–17.

COPPER METABOLISM

General Description

The medical management of Wilson's disease aims at preventing copper from accumulating to toxic levels. Prevention of copper accumulation cannot be achieved by diet alone, but with the use of copper-depleting medications such as D-penicillamine or trientine, some of the excess copper in the body can be eliminated through the kidney and further accumulations prevented. Copper is widely distributed in foods and does not occur exclusively in particular food groups. For patients with Wilson's disease it is recommended that dietary intake not exceed 1.5 mg of copper per day.

Nutritional Inadequacy

The low copper diet is not so restrictive that it imposes the danger of nutritional inadequacy. However, patients who are taking D-penicillamine may be at risk for a vitamin B_6 deficiency because of the possible antipyridoxine effect of the drug. It is standard practice to administer 25 mg daily of vitamin B_6 to patients who are on D-penicillamine therapy.[28]

Indications and Rationale

A copper-restricted diet may be appropriate in the treatment of Wilson's disease as a supplement to drug therapy.

Wilson's disease (hepatolenticular degeneration) is an inherited disorder of copper metabolism characterized by the abnormal transport and storage of copper.[29] Copper accumulates primarily in the liver, brain, kidney, and cornea and may have a toxic effect on these tissues. The primary metabolic defect is in the

TABLE 10-3   Copper Content of Foods*[33-35]

Food Groups	High (>0.2 mg/Portions Commonly Used†) (Avoid)	Moderate (0.1 to 0.2 mg/Portion) (No More Than 6 Servings/Day)	Low (0.1 mg/Portions Commonly Used†) (May Be Eaten as Desired)
Meat and Meat Substitutes			
	Lamb; pork; pheasant; quail; duck; goose; squid; salmon; all organ meats including liver, heart, kidney, brain; all shellfish, including oysters, scallops, shrimp, lobster, clams, and crab; meat gelatin; soy protein meat substitutes; tofu; all nuts and seeds	All other fish (3 oz); dark-meat turkey (3 oz); peanut butter (2 Tbsp)	Beef; cheese; cottage cheese; eggs; light meat turkey, cold cuts and frankfurters that do not contain pork, dark turkey, or organ meats; all others not listed on high or moderate list
Fats and Oils			
	Avocado	Olives (2 med); cream (½ cup)	Butter; cream; margarine; mayonnaise; nondairy cream substitutes; oils; sour cream; salad dressings (made from allowed ingredients); all others not listed on high or moderate list
Milk			
	Chocolate; cocoa; soy milk		All other dairy products; milk flavored with carob
Starch			
	Dried beans including soybeans, lima beans, baked beans, garbanzo beans, pinto beans; dried peas; lentils; millet; barley; wheat germ; bran breads and cereals; cereals with > 0.2 mg of copper per serving (check label); soy flour; soy grits; sweet potatoes (fresh)	Whole-wheat bread (1 slice); potatoes in any form (½ cup or 1 small); pumpkin (¾ cup); melba toast (4); whole-wheat crackers (6); parsnips (⅔ cup); winter squash (½ cup; green peas (½ cup); instant oatmeal (½ cup); instant Ralston™ (½ cup); cereals with 0.1 to 0.2 mg of copper per serving (check labels); dehydrated and canned soups (1 cup)	Breads and pasta from refined flour; canned sweet potatoes; rice; regular oatmeal; cereals with < 0.1 mg of copper per serving (check label); all others not listed on high or moderate list

*Data available on the average copper content of foods varies greatly. There is disagreement on the copper content of the usual American diet, with estimates that range from 1 mg of copper a day to 5 mg a day. The concentration of copper in foods is affected by many factors, including soil conditions, geographic location, species, diet, processing method, and contamination in processing. The exact copper content of the foods is difficult to verify. It is estimated that avoidance of high copper foods and restriction of moderate copper foods results in a diet of approximately 1 mg/day. For practical purposes, diets are designed to limit foods that tend to have a higher copper content than other foods, and not to achieve a specific level of copper in the diet.

†Portions commonly used are those generally accepted as typical portion sizes in various nutrient data source manuals.

Continued.

TABLE 10-3   Copper Content of Foods—cont'd

Food Groups	High (>0.2 mg/Portions Commonly Used†) (Avoid)	Moderate (0.1 to 0.2mg/Portion) (No More Than 6 Servings/Day)	Low (0.1 mg/Portions Commonly Used†) (May Be Eaten as Desired)
Vegetables			
	Mushrooms; vegetable juice cocktail	Bean sprouts (1 cup); beets (¹/₂ cup); spinach (¹/₂ cup cooked, 1 cup raw); tomato juice and other tomato products (¹/₂ cup); broccoli (¹/₂ cup); asparagus (¹/₂ cup)	All others, including fresh tomatoes
Fruits			
	Nectarines; dried fruits including raisins, dates, and prunes (dried fruits are permitted if dried at home)	Mango (¹/₂ cup); pears (1 medium); pineapple (¹/₂ cup); papaya (¹/₄ average)	All others
Desserts			
	Desserts that contain significant amounts of any foods high in copper		All others
Sugar and Sweets			
	Chocolate; cocoa	Licorice (1 oz); syrups (1 oz)	All others including jams, jellies, and candies made with allowed ingredients; carob; flavoring extracts
Miscellaneous			
	Brewers yeast; copper-containing vitamin supplements	Ketchup (2 Tbsp); dehydrated and canned soups	Homemade soups from allowed ingredients
Beverages‡			
	Instant breakfast beverages; mineral water; alcohol§; soy-based beverages; copper fortified formulas	Postum™ and other cereal beverages (1 cup); carbonated beverages (12 oz)	All others including fruit flavored beverages; lemonade

‡A water sample from the patient's home water supply should be analyzed for copper content. Demineralized water should be used if the water contains more than 100 μg/L.

§Although not necessarily high in copper, alcoholic beverages are discouraged because of their action as a hepatotoxin.

liver, where a block of biliary copper excretion causes accumulation of copper.[30] There is also a decrease in the incorporation of copper into ceruloplasmin, the main copper-containing protein exported from the liver. Symptoms of Wilson's disease may include hepatic, neurological, and psychiatric dysfunctions.

Long-term therapy consists primarily of the use of a copper removal agent such as D-penicillamine or trientine to keep the patient in a satisfactory copper balance.[31] Some patients have been treated successfully with pharmacological doses of zinc, which promotes copper binding to intestinal cells and subsequent excretion in the stool.[32] A low or very low copper diet may be an appropriate adjunct. Treatment usually improves neurological and hepatic symptoms. Lifelong treatment of asymptomatic patients with the Wilson's metabolic defect prevents the disease.

Goals of Dietary Management

The restriction of copper may be advised for patients with Wilson's disease. The diet is considered adjunctive to copper removal therapy.

Dietary Recommendations

A diet that is very low in copper (≤ 1.0 mg per day) allows foods of low copper content and limits servings from the moderate copper content group. Foods of high copper content should be avoided. A low copper diet (≤ 1.5 mg per day) restricts only those foods high in copper content. Table 10-3 presents the copper content of foods.

A water sample from the patient's home water supply should be analyzed for copper content. Demineralized water should be used if the water contains more than 100 µg/L.

Although not necessarily high in copper, alcoholic beverages are discouraged because of their action as an hepatotoxin.

Physicians: How to Order Diet

The diet order should indicate *low copper diet* (avoidance of high copper foods) or *very low copper diet* (avoidance of high and limited moderate copper content foods).

References

28. Smithgall JM. The copper controlled diet: current aspects of dietary copper restriction in management of copper metabolism disorders. J Am Diet Assoc 1985;35:609–611.
29. Dobyns WB, Goldstein NP, Gordon H. Clinical spectrum of Wilson's disease (hepatolenticular degeneration). Mayo Clin Proc 1979;54:35–42.
30. Frommer DJ. Defective biliary excretion of copper in Wilson's disease. Gut 1974;15:125–129.
31. Scheinberg IH, Sternlieb I. Wilson disease. Philadelphia: WB Saunders, 1984.
32. Brewer GJ, Hill GM, Prasud AS, Cossack ZT, Rabbani P. Oral zinc therapy for Wilson's disease. Ann Intern Med 1983;99:314–320.
33. Leveille GA, Zabik ME, Morgan KJ. Nutrients in foods. Cambridge, MA: The Nutrition Guild, 1983.
34. Hook L, Brandt IK. Copper content of some low-copper food. J Am Diet Assoc 1966;49:202–203.
35. Pennington JAT, Church HN. Bowes and Church's food values of portions commonly used, 15th ed. Philadelphia: JB Lippincott, 1989.

SCLEROTHERAPY

General Description

Sclerotherapy is currently the primary treatment of choice for the majority of patients who present with esophageal variceal bleeding.[36-38] Esophageal varices are enlarged or protruding veins that anastomose with tributaries of the portal vein of the lower esophagus. The cause of esophageal variceal bleeding is generally thought to be portal hypertension. Causes of portal hypertension include alcoholic liver disease, portal vein thrombosis, schistosomiasis, and inferior vena caval obstruction by tumor or thrombus.

Sclerotherapy is performed using an endoscope, which injects sclerosants such as sodium tetradecyl sulfate into a varix. The procedure provides hemostasis in patients who are actively bleeding and may be useful for long-term treatment to prevent recurrent hemorrhage.

Dietary Recommendations

Usually, clear liquids of room temperature are recommended for the first 24 hours following the procedure. Soft foods may be tolerated thereafter with a gradual progression to a general diet. Other dietary restrictions may need to be included according to the patient's underlying medical condition (e.g., sodium control).

References

36. Thatcher BS. Therapeutic endoscopy for gastrointestinal bleeding. AFP 1986;34(4): 139–43.
37. Sarin SK, Kumar A. Sclerosants for variceal sclerotherapy: a critical appraisal. Am J Gastroenterol 1990;85(6):641–649.
38. Rice TL. Treatment of esophageal varices. Clin Pharm 1989;8(2):122–131.

11 / *Neurologic Diseases*

PARKINSON'S DISEASE

General Description

Diet therapy alone is not an effective treatment for Parkinson's disease. However, in certain patients, dietary modification may help potentiate and stabilize the response to levodopa therapy. Levodopa is the foundation of medical treatment for Parkinson's disease and is typically formulated with a dopa decarboxylase inhibitor, which dramatically reduces the dosage requirement and minimizes side effects. The dopa decarboxylase inhibitor employed in this country is carbidopa and is a component of the drug named Sinemet™. Dietary amino acids can inhibit the transport of levodopa into the circulation and, hence into the brain.[1] Thus, protein redistribution diets have a place in selected Parkinson patients. However, the vast majority of Parkinson patients do not require a special diet.

Modifications of dietary protein in Parkinson patients should be made with attention to adequate nutrition and to satisfying the patient's minimum protein requirements. The consistency of the diet may need to be modified depending upon impairment of chewing or swallowing. Parkinson patients' diets should also be modified to contain adequate fiber to reduce constipation and to avoid gas-forming foods.

Nutritional Inadequacy

Diets recommended for Parkinson's disease patients are not inherently lacking in nutrients, vitamins, and minerals. However, certain patients do not consume balanced diets for a variety of reasons. In those patients, a multiple vitamin that meets 100% of the Recommended Dietary Allowance (RDA) is advised.

Prior to the advent of the dopa decarboxylase inhibitor carbidopa, which is part of the Sinemet™ formulation, avoidance of supplementary vitamin B$_6$ (pyridoxine) was advised. This vitamin can facilitate the premature conversion of levodopa to dopamine, reducing potency. This is not a problem when levodopa is formulated with carbidopa, hence special multivitamins devoid of supplementary B_6 are not necessary.

A study has shown that severe restriction of daytime dietary protein (10 g or less) allowed mean intake of most nutrients to remain above RDA levels.[2] However, significant decreases occurred in protein, calcium, iron, phosphorus, riboflavin, and niacin intakes. Healthy and highly motivated patients may maintain adequate intake of most nutrients while restricting daytime dietary protein. However, nutrient intakes may be compromised in patients whose regular diets are marginally adequate.

It has been suggested that other dietary amino acids, such as L-tryptophan, may effectively treat certain aspects of Parkinson's disease. L-Tryptophan is a precursor of serotonin, a neurotransmitter chemically similar to levodopa. Large doses of l-tryptophan are not particularly useful in the treatment aspect of Parkinson's disease and may actually lead to clinical deterioration by antagonizing levodopa absorption. Therefore, L-tryptophan has no place in Parkinson's disease treatment. Furthermore, L-tryptophan preparations have been associated with the serious illness eosinophilic myalgia.

Indications and Rationale

Idiopathic Parkinson's disease is a degenerative central nervous system condition characterized by the progressive loss of cells within the substantia nigra.[3,4] These cells release the neurotransmitter dopamine, and it is the loss of dopamine that is primarily responsible for the motor deficits. Common characteristics include (1) slowness of movement, (2) muscular rigidity, (3) resting tremor, and (4) postural instability. This disease is much more common in senior citizens, and it is slightly more prevalent in men than women.[4]

The cause of Parkinson's disease is unknown. The primary medical treatment is directed at replenishing cerebral dopaminergic tone. Although there are synthetic dopamine agonists, such as pergolide or bromocriptine, the most effective treatment is administration of the dopamine precursor levodopa. Direct administration of dopamine is ineffective because of failure to cross the blood brain-barrier into the brain. The naturally occurring, large, neutral amino acid levodopa does enter the brain, carried by a specific transport system. Once levodopa has entered the brain, it can be decarboxylated to dopamine, potentially replenishing this depleted neurotransmitter.

Premature conversion of levodopa to dopamine outside the brain is undesirable for two reasons. First, circulating dopamine is trapped outside the blood-brain barrier. Secondly, circulating dopamine can induce a variety of side effects. The most prominent is nausea. The nausea is due to passage of circulating dopamine into the brain's chemoreceptive trigger zone; this is one of the few areas of the brain where the blood-brain barrier is patent. Formulation of levodopa with the dopa decarboxylase inhibitor carbidopa is fairly effective in preventing most of the premature conversion of levodopa to dopamine prior to brain entry. Nonetheless, occasional patients do experience nausea. For many, this is mild, and tolerance to the nausea rapidly develops. In others, this is more troublesome. It is worth emphasizing that the nausea is primarily cerebrally mediated rather than due to a direct gastric irritant effect upon the stomach.

The large, neutral amino acids generated from the metabolic breakdown of dietary protein can inhibit the absorption of levodopa.[1] Thus, administering levodopa/carbidopa with meals may result in suboptimal absorption. Most patients do not require a special diet; rather, administering doses on an empty stomach, such as 1 hour before each meal, is adequate. Occasional patients who find they tolerate levodopa/carbidopa better with food might try consuming several soda crackers at the time of levodopa/carbidopa administration rather than a larger meal containing protein.

Patients with longer standing Parkinson's disease frequently experience short-duration responses to levodopa/carbidopa, with the beneficial effect lasting for only a few hours (or less) after each dose. In some, the response to medication is erratic and fluctuating, with doses that occasionally do not "kick in." It is these patients that may benefit from manipulation of dietary protein. Numerous articles have been written in the recent past outlining therapeutic strategies.[5-9]

Patients wishing to remain in their optimum state during the daytime can sometimes benefit from redistribution of dietary protein. Daytime restriction of dietary protein to 10 g or less before 5 P.M. has been shown to improve efficacy of levodopa and reduce response fluctuations for some Parkinson's disease patients. (The remaining day's requirement for dietary protein is consumed after 5 P.M.[5,7-9]) However, patients should be aware of the consequence of consuming a larger protein meal in the evening, which can result in a suboptimal levodopa effect following that meal with consequent rigidity, slowness, and tremor. For some patients, the tendency to confine these symptoms to the evening allows adequate performance of daytime activities, both occupational and social.

Meals containing great amounts of protein, such as large steaks, may also effectively turn off the levodopa response in many Parkinson patients. Patients should be aware of this relationship and in many cases will do best by keeping the protein content of their meals more moderate. Patients also benefit from instruction in protein content of the diet. Occasional patients consume frequent snacks of protein-containing substances such as ice cream, with deleterious effects upon their Parkinson control.

Weight loss is an occasional problem in patients with Parkinson's disease. This can be due to one or more of a variety of factors. Causes include increased energy expenditure related to medication-induced involuntary movements (dyskinesia) or severe tremor. Patients may experience difficulty feeding themselves due to Parkinson symptoms or the medication-related dyskinesias. Depression, dementia, dysphagia might also be factors. (See Chapter 5, Dysphagia.) Weight loss might also be due to nausea secondary to dopamine-active medications. Finally, self-imposed protein restriction in hopes of potentiating Sinemet™ can be associated with weight loss.

Constipation is also a common problem in Parkinson's disease patients. The cause is typically twofold. First, Parkinson's disease is frequently associated with at least low grade autonomic dysfunction. Secondly, the anti-Parkinson medications may also contribute to constipation. The worst offenders are the anticholinergic drugs.

TABLE 11-1   Dietary Goals in Parkinson's Disease

Maintain desirable weight.

Prevent lessening of therapeutic effect of anti–Parkinson drugs.

Lessen swallowing difficulties resulting from disease and/or medication–induced dry mouth.

Regulate bowel function through provision of adequate sources of fiber and fluid.

Maintain optimal hydration.

However, dopamine-active medications can also contribute to constipation. Inadequate fluid and fiber intake in patients experiencing difficulties with swallowing or holding a glass or cup might also contribute.

Symptomatic postural hypotension is also occasionally seen in patients with Parkinson's disease. Again, the causes are predominantly twofold. First, Parkinson's disease-related autonomic dysfunction may predispose to orthostatic hypotension. Secondly, the anti-Parkinson medications may result in an exacerbation of this problem. The condition may be further exacerbated by patients' inappropriate restriction of their sodium intake, as is common practice by many senior citizens. For many such patients, simply normalizing or increasing dietary sodium is adequate to treat symptomatic orthostatic hypotension.

Goals of Dietary Management

The goals of the diet for individuals with Parkinson's disease appear in Table 11-1.

Dietary Recommendations

Intervention is individualized according to each patient's needs. Instruction to optimize kilocalorie and nutrient intake within the individual's ability to prepare food, chew, and swallow it should be based upon a complete diet history. Dietary protein redistribution may prove beneficial and could be considered on a trial basis. Therapeutic modifications to optimize dietary sodium, fluid, and fiber intake in order to normalize orthostatic hypotension, hydration, and bowel function may be indicated. Food texture and consistency can be altered for those with impaired chewing and swallowing. Supplemental vitamins and minerals that meet 100% of the RDA may be needed if the diet is inadequate.

Physicians: How to Order Diet

The diet order should indicate *diet for Parkinson's disease.* Nutritional needs will be determined by the dietitian and individualized according to the patient's symptoms (e.g., dysphagia, constipation, hypotension, weight loss). The physician should indicate if a protein redistribution diet is to be tried.

References

1. Carter JH, Nutt JG, Woodward WR, Hatcher LF, Trotman TL. Amount and distribution of dietary protein affects clinical response to levodopa in Parkinson's disease. Neurology 1989;39(4):552–556.

2. Paré S, Barr SI, Ross SE. Effect of daytime protein restriction on nutrient intakes of free-living Parkinson's disease patients. Am J Clin Nutr 1992;55:701–707.

3. Duvoisin RC. Parkinson's disease: a guide for patient and family, 2nd ed. New York: Raven Press, 1984.

4. Muenter MD. Movement disorders. In: *Clinical medicine.* Philadelphia: Harper & Row, 1985;11(6):1–46.

5. Pincus JH, Barry K. Influence of dietary protein on motor fluctuations in Parkinson's disease. Arch Neurol 1987;44(3):270–272.

6. Kurlan R. Editorial. Arch Neurol 1987;44(11):1119–1121.

7. Riley D, Lang AE. Practical application of a low–protein diet for Parkinson's disease. Neurology 1988;38(7):1026–1031.

8. Tsui JK, Ross S, Poulin K, Douglas J, Postnikoff D, Calne S, Woodward W, Calne DB. The effect of dietary protein on the efficacy of L-dopa: a double-blind study. Neurology 1989; 39(4):592–594.

9. Yen PK. Does a low–protein diet help with Parkinson's? Geriatr Nurs 1990;11(1):48.

12 / *Oncologic Diseases*

CANCER

General Description

Anorexia, maldigestion, malabsorption, and difficulties in mastication and swallowing are common factors that make protein-calorie malnutrition a common problem in patients with advancing cancer. The dietitian should seek to provide foods that can be consumed in quantities that are sufficient to meet protein and kilocalorie needs, to correct nutritional deficits, and to minimize weight loss. Suggestions on how this may be accomplished are given.

Indications and Rationale

The maintenance of an adequate nutritional status may reduce the complications from oncologic therapy and should contribute to the patient's sense of well-being. For these reasons, nutritional care is an important part of supportive management for the patient with cancer.

Nutritional Effects of Cancer

Protein-calorie malnutrition is the single most common secondary diagnosis in patients with cancer. It tends to be severe in patients with tumors of the head and neck, stomach, pancreas, lung, colon, and ovary but less pronounced in patients with breast cancer.[1,2] Clearly the presence of malnutrition with cancer is a poor prognostic sign.[3-5] Malnutrition adversely affects not only tissue function and repair but also humoral and cellular immunocompetence. Changes in drug metabolism through alterations in liver function may also occur. Thus, malnutrition can interfere with the delivery of oncologic therapy and enhance the severity of side effects of treatment. Malnourished patients do not tolerate surgery, chemotherapy, or radiation therapy as well as those in a better nutritional state.[5,6] Thus, the cachexia may become more immediately threatening to life than the local effects of the cancer.

293

Cancer cachexia presents clinically with anorexia, alterations in taste sensation, weight loss, muscle wasting, and malnutrition, which results in a decline in general physical and mental functions. The pathogenesis of the anorexia-cachexia syndrome is incompletely understood. Metabolic by-products of tumor metabolism or the host response to cancer may directly cause anorexia or early satiety or may do so secondarily by an effect on hypothalamic function.[7-9] In some cases, the anorexia may be more likely the result of early satiety than of impaired perception of hunger.[9] Both interleukin-1 and tumor necrosis factor (cachectin), products of activated macrophages, enhance triglyceride release from adipose cells and amino acids from muscle cells. These cytokines may be important factors in cancer cachexia, but the precise manner by which they accomplish this is not clear. Tumor metabolites may also be responsible for the abnormalities of sensations of taste and smell that have been observed in persons with cancer.[7,8,10-12]

Patients may have a heightened or decreased sensitivity to sweet taste. The taste thresholds for salty and sour foods are often increased, while they are decreased for bitter foods. The decreased threshold for bitter taste (urea as a test substance) is often responsible for the aversion to meat that is frequently experienced by patients with cancer.

Psychological stresses that are associated with cancer may contribute to anorexia.[7,13,14] Even in the absence of true depression, the presence of pain, lack of sense of well-being, discouragement, and anxiety about the treatment of the disease or its prognosis may cause emotional stress, which diminishes the enjoyment of eating.[15] A conditioned aversion to eating certain foods may develop if patients experience nausea or other discomforts, perhaps as a consequence of radiation therapy or chemotherapy, during or after eating these foods.[15] Such aversions may persist long after the therapy has been completed. Nutritional deficiencies or excesses may result if patients avoid foods they consider as contributing to the genesis of the cancer or if they consume larger quantities of allegedly beneficial foods.

Although a decreased intake of nutrients appears to be the dominant cause of wasting, it cannot entirely explain the progressive weight loss that often occurs despite an apparently adequate intake. Other mechanisms that have been suggested include an abnormal adaptation to starvation with an increased rather than a decreased metabolic rate, parasitization of the host tissues by the growing tumor, and derangements in intermediary metabolism.[1,5,16,17] In general, a tumor burden is usually thought to be too small to act as a metabolic drain of sufficient magnitude to produce host wasting. However, the presence of a tumor could induce derangements in the metabolism of carbohydrate, fat, and protein, which may cause an increase in energy requirements.

Nutritional Effects of Cancer Therapies

Besides the effects of the tumor itself, various modalities used in the treatment of cancer may have an adverse effect on nutritional status.[18] The malnutrition that results from treatment assumes even more importance when one realizes that many cancer patients are already debilitated from their disease. Antitumor therapies may produce only mild, transient nutritional disturbances, such as mucositis from chemotherapy; however, cancer therapies may lead to severe, permanent nutritional problems, as in small bowel resection or as in disabilities of chewing and swallowing after head and neck surgery.

Surgical Therapy

Radical surgery of the head and neck region may lead to significant malnutrition by altering the normal route of nutritional intake. Although some of these changes are temporary, many patients have permanent difficulty with chewing, swallowing, and risk of aspiration. Resection of the esophagus or the stomach can cause postprandial symptoms such as gastric stasis or dumping syndrome, which may lead to inadequate caloric intake (see Chapter 8, Delayed Gastric Emptying and Postgastrectomy Dumping Syndrome).

The nutritional sequelae of intestinal resection are directly related to the site and extent of resection and to the individual functions of the various segments.[19] The ability of various segments of the small intestine to increase their absorptive capabilities over a period of several months prevents major clinical problems after small bowel resection unless the bowel resection is massive, in which case malabsorption becomes the primary problem of nutritional management. Colon surgery is usually well tolerated from a nutritional standpoint. The large water and electrolyte losses in the early postoperative period decrease rapidly soon after surgery.

Weight loss that is secondary to anorexia and malabsorption is common in patients with pancreatic cancer. Some degree of nutritional repletion prior to surgery is desirable but not always feasible. Pancreatectomy may lead to pancreatic endocrine and/or exocrine insufficiency, which may result in diabetes and significant malabsorption. The administration of pancreatic enzymes, histamine H_2 receptor blockers, and insulin may lessen but not entirely correct the trends toward malnutrition that result from malabsorption and insulin-dependent diabetes.[20] Conventional dietary restrictions for diabetes may need to be liberalized by the inclusion of sugar-containing foods to achieve adequate caloric intake.

Chemotherapy

Chemotherapeutic agents may contribute to malnutrition through a variety of direct and indirect mechanisms, including anorexia, nausea, vomiting, mucositis, organ injury (toxicity), and learned food aversions.[1,21,22] These agents affect normal cells as well as malignant tissues and are most active on rapidly proliferating cells such as the epithelial cells of the alimentary tract. The degree to which gastrointestinal functions are affected depends on the particular chemotherapy agent, drug dosage, duration of the treatment, rates of metabolism, and the individual's susceptibility. Mucositis is a major gastrointestinal toxicity and may be greatly intensified when radiation therapy is given concurrently with chemotherapy. Mucositis can affect any part of the alimentary tract and may lead to ulceration, bleeding, and malabsorption. The renewal rate of the alimentary tract mucosa is rapid so that the mucositis from chemotherapy is usually short-lived.

Nausea and vomiting commonly accompany the administration of many antitumor drugs and may even occur in anticipation of chemotherapy.[23,24] Indirect effects of chemotherapy that may contribute to malnutrition include fungal infections of the gastrointestinal tract and learned food aversions.[25] Candidiasis of the gastrointestinal tract is not an uncommon occurrence during chemotherapy, especially in patients with leukemias and lymphomas. Candidiasis in the oral cavity, pharynx, or esophagus can produce oral discomfort and dysphagia.

Weight gain is common in women who undergo adjuvant chemotherapy for breast cancer. It is not clear, however, whether the weight gain is a direct effect of chemotherapy.[26,27]

Radiation Therapy

The complications of radiation vary according to the region of the body radiated, dose, fractionation, and associated antitumor therapy such as surgery or chemotherapy. The patient's nutritional status at the initiation of radiation is also important.[19] Complications may develop acutely during radiation or become chronic and progress even after radiation has been completed. For example, when the salivary glands are in the field of radiation, saliva production decreases in conjunction with an increase in viscosity. In addition to causing mouth dryness and impaired swallowing, the decrease in salivation causes an alteration in the composition of the oral bacterial flora, which in turn promotes caries formation. Secondary infection, such as candidiasis, may also develop. For some, the thick, scant secretions may create a feeling of nausea.[28]

The mucosa of the alimentary tract is sensitive to radiation, which can produce a sore mouth or throat, painful ulcerations, bleeding, or even chronic radiation ulcer. Radionecrosis of oral tissue may result from the combination of trauma and infection superimposed on highly radiated tissues. Trismus can occur from tumor infiltration or postradiation fibrosis.

Damage of the microvilli of the taste cells often results in altered, suppressed, or heightened taste sensation or in complete loss of taste sensation, which is described as "mouth blindness." Bitter and acid tastes are most often impaired; salty and sweet tastes are less influenced. In most patients, taste returns gradually within 2 to 4 months of completion of therapy but may take up to 1 year. These symptoms have a profound effect on the desire and ability to eat and may combine to create a potentially serious situation since patients are often already anorectic and undernourished. Unless nutritional intervention is provided, many patients lose weight during radiation therapy. If oral feeding becomes impossible, enteral feedings may be indicated (see Chapter 16, Enteral Nutrition).

Patients with tumors of the esophagus, like those with cancer of the oral cavity, are often in a marginal nutritional state at the start of radiation therapy because of impaired swallowing and perhaps because of habits of tobacco and alcohol use. Fatigue during eating, attributable to shortness of breath and anorexia, often contributes to weight loss in patients with cancer of the lung. Radiation to the thoracic area induces esophagitis with its accompanying sore throat and dysphagia. This usually disappears following the cessation of therapy. Tumor necrosis, however, may result in delayed complications such as sinus tract formation, ulceration with possible fistula, or obstruction from fibrosis and stricture.

Abdominal or pelvic radiation may result in altered intestinal function. Patients who receive upper abdominal radiation often experience nausea and vomiting, and those who receive radiation to the lower abdomen often experience diarrhea. Damage to the intestinal mucosa can produce malabsorption as well as fluid and electrolyte deficiencies. Acute radiation enteritis usually disappears following therapy. However, late effects of abdominopelvic radiation occur in a small percentage of patients. The effects may occur months to years after the completion of radiation therapy and may be manifested as intestinal obstruction, fistula formation, or chronic enteritis.[29]

Goals of Dietary Management

Nutritional support of the cancer patient must be individualized. Nutritional therapy should be undertaken with the overall prognosis of the patient clearly in mind so that the aggressiveness of dietary intervention (supportive, adjunctive, definitive) can be appropriately adjusted. All patients with nutritional problems should have frequent dietary consultation and should be helped to understand that nutrition is an integral part of the total management of their disease. Dietary modifications depend on the extent of anorexia, taste alterations, early satiety, nausea, weight loss, and consequences of treatment.

Dietary Recommendations

Some general considerations in designing a diet for the cancer patient follow.

1. A detailed history should be obtained to determine past weight changes, food preferences and eating habits, use of food/nutritional supplements, present kilocalorie and protein intake, food intolerances, taste abnormalities, distribution of meals throughout the day, who does the cooking, and whether the patient eats alone. Consideration should be given to nutritional side effects from past or current treatment.

2. Information obtained in the diet history should be carefully considered in the formulation of the nutritional care plan. Table 12-1 outlines the potential nutritional problems of cancer therapy with suggested dietary approaches to help meet nutritional needs.[30,31,32]

3. The effect of cancer on metabolism is only partially understood, and it is not possible to be precise about the minimum intake of kilocalories and protein that would be sufficient to meet the needs of cancer patients.[33,34] Furthermore, the energy sources (carbohydrate and fat) and the quantity and quality of protein that would promote nitrogen balance cannot yet be stated. For these reasons, the recommendations for daily kilocalorie and protein intake should be monitored and adjusted according to individual patient response.

4. If the patient has been losing weight, the first realistic goal of nutritional intervention may be to prevent a further loss of weight. Multiple studies have now demonstrated that megestrol acetate can result in appetite stimulation in patients with advanced cancer.[35,36] This therapy may be of note for patients suffering from anorexia/cachexia.

5. If the patient is nauseated from the underlying cancer, radiation, or chemotherapy, the use of an antiemetic drug, such as prochlorperazine (Compazine™) may be helpful. The drug should be given 30 to 60 minutes before planned meals. Likewise, if pain hinders eating, the systematic administration of analgesics may enhance the patient's willingness and desire to eat.

TABLE 12-1   Potential Nutrition Problems of Cancer and Cancer Therapy with Suggested Nutritional Approaches

Problem	Frequent Small Meals	Increase Kcal/ Protein Content of Foods	High Protein High Kcal Supplement	Avoid Strong Odors	Cool or Room Temperature Foods	Increase Fluid Intake	Increase Fiber Intake	Eat and Drink Slowly
Loss of appetite and early satiety	X	X	X		±			
Diarrhea*	X				X	X		X
Nausea and vomiting	X			X	X	X		X
Chewing and swallowing difficulties (sore mouth or throat)	X	X	X		X	X		X
Constipation						X	X	
Abdominal gas/bloating								X
Dry mouth						X		
Taste/smell alterations				±	±			

*Diarrhea secondary to malabsorption, dumping syndrome, or other causes may require different treatment modalities (see Chapter 9, Diarrhea).

6. The necessity of changing lifetime meal and snack patterns should be frankly explained to the patient. For example, the patient who was conditioned to omitting snacks or desserts to avoid gaining weight before the diagnosis of cancer should be told that this routine is no longer appropriate. Previous dietary restrictions may need to be liberalized (e.g., cholesterol, fat, and total calorie control).

TABLE 12-1   Potential Nutrition Problems of Cancer and Cancer Therapy with Suggested Nutritional Approaches—cont'd

Decrease Fiber Intake	Avoid Excessive Fat	Avoid Gas-Forming Foods	Regular Exercise if Tolerated	Limit Liquids at Mealtime	Select Soft, Moist Foods; Add Sauce, Gravy	Avoid Highly Seasoned Foods	Comments
	±		X	X			Pleasant mealtime atmosphere. Appetite may be best in the morning.
X	X	X		X		X	Clear liquids helpful initially. Limit beverages containing caffeine and alcohol. Trial avoidance of lactose. Antidiarrheal medication per physician.
	X			X		X	Clear, cool beverages. Rest after meals with head elevated. Antiemetic per physician.
					X	X	Coarse-textured and acidic foods may aggravate. Avoid alcohol, tobacco, and commercial mouthwashes.
			X				Stool softener and/or laxative may be necessary.
X	X	X	X				Limit high lactose foods if not tolerated. See Chapter 9, Abdominal Gas and Flatulence.
					X		Tart foods or hard candy (preferably sugar-free) may be used to stimulate saliva. Avoid alcohol, tobacco, and commercial mouthwashes.
							Use seasonings to enhance food flavors. Avoid cooking odors. For meat aversion, try alternative protein sources.

7. Recommendations should take into account the patient's strength and ability to prepare food. If the patient is alone part of the day, suggestions to make food easily obtainable should be given.

8. The patient should be given dietary guidelines in writing and should be gently encouraged to eat the suggested foods in the recommended amounts. However, the patient should not be excessively pressured by friends or relatives

concerning poor nutritional intake. Such action may increase anxiety and become counterproductive.

9. Food should fill the diet prescription whenever possible. Sometimes supplementation with high kilocalorie, high protein liquid feedings is necessary. Predigested formulas should be used only if specifically indicated, as in situations of malabsorption (see Chapter 9, Fat Malabsorption).

10. A multiple vitamin/mineral supplement should be given to patients who are not able to ingest a well-balanced diet or who have specific deficiencies.

The patient's progress should be evaluated at regular intervals to determine whether the nutritional state is improving. Follow-up also offers a means of support and reinforcement so that the diet prescription can be advanced or modified in response to treatment.

If efforts at oral feeding fail or are impossible, the use of alternative feeding methods such as tube feeding or central parenteral nutrition may be necessary. The use of aggressive nutritional support is beneficial for many patients who undergo therapy and who have a high probability of positive response to therapy. However, the use of nutritional support for terminal cancer patients is of questionable benefit. More appropriate are suggestions for oral feedings as tolerated and the provision of emotional support. For the end-stage patient, the pleasurable aspects of eating should be emphasized, with less concern for quantity and nutrient content.

Weight gain and obesity are common in patients with breast cancer. Skeletal metastasis may cause more problems, such as pathologic fractures, in the overweight person. Some evidence suggests that the cancer recurrence rate may be adversely affected by the patient being overweight.[37,38] Therefore, obesity should be treated by gradual weight reduction through moderate calorie control and, if appropriate, exercise.

Nutrition and Its Role in Cancer Protection

Epidemiologic and animal studies over a period of years indicate that patterns of food consumption and some dietary components may increase the risk of cancer. The speculation that types of diets and individual food components offer protection against cancer risk is unproven. However, the National Cancer Institute and the American Cancer Society have established prudent dietary guidelines for food selection. The reader is referred to Chapter 2, Diet and Cancer Risk, for this information.

References

1. Costa G, Donaldson S. The nutritional effects of cancer and its therapy. Nutr Cancer 1980;2:22–29.
2. Wood RM, Lander VL, Mosby EL, Hiatt WR. Nutrition and the head and neck cancer patient. Oral Surg Oral Med Oral Pathol 1989;68:391–395.
3. Balducci L, Hardy C. Cancer and malnutrition—a critical interaction: a review. Am J Hematol 1985;18:91–103.
4. Copeland EM III, Souba WW. Nutritional considerations in treatment of the cancer patient. Nutr Clin Pract 1988;3:173–174.
5. DeWys WD, Begg C, Lavin PT, Band PR, Bennett JM, Bertino JR, Cohen MH, Douglass HO, Engstrom PF, Ezdinli EZ, Horton J, Johnson GJ, Moertel CG, Oken MM, Perlia C,

Rosenbaum C, Silverstein MN, Skeel RT, Sponzo RW, Tormey DC. Prognostic effect of weight loss prior to chemotherapy in cancer patients. Am J Med 1980;69:491–497.

6. Dreizen S, McCredie KB, Keating MJ, Andersson BS. Nutritional deficiencies in patients receiving cancer chemotherapy. Postgrad Med 1990;87:163–167.

7. DeWys WD. Anorexia in cancer patients. Cancer Res 1977;37:2354–2358.

8. DeWys WD. Anorexia as a general effect of cancer. Cancer 1979;43:2013–2019.

9. Theologides A. Pathogenesis of anorexia and cachexia in cancer. Cancer Bull 1982;34: 140–149.

10. Fearson KCH, Carter DC. Cancer cachexia. Ann Surg 1988;208:1–5.

11. Vickers ZM, Nielsen SS, Theologides A. Food preferences of patients with cancer. J Am Diet Assoc 1981;79:441–445.

12. Nielsen SS, Theologides A, Vickers ZM. Influence of food odors on food aversions and preferences in patients with cancer. Am J Clin Nutr 1980;33:2253–2261.

13. Sutton A. Cancer cachexia. Nursing Times 1988;84:65–66.

14. Bernstein I. Physiological and psychological mechanisms of cancer anorexia. Cancer Res 1982;42(suppl):715s–720s.

15. vanEyes J. Nutrition and cancer: physiological interrelationships. Ann Rev Nutr 1985;5: 435–461.

16. DeWys WD. Pathophysiology of cancer cachexia: current understanding and areas for future research. Cancer Res 1982;42(suppl):721s–726s.

17. Wachman BA, Hardin TC. Cancer cachexia: the metabolic alterations. Nutr Clin Pract 1988;3:191–197.

18. Shils ME. Nutrition and diet in cancer. In: Shils ME, Young VR, eds. Modern nutrition in health and disease, 7th ed. Philadelphia: Lea & Febiger, 1988:1380–1422.

19. Lawrence W. Nutritional consequences of surgical resection of the gastrointestinal tract for cancer. Cancer Res 1977;37:2379–2386.

20. Perez MM, Newcomer AD, Moertel CG, Go VLW, DiMagno EP. Assessment of weight loss, food intake, fat metabolism, malabsorption, and treatment of pancreatic insufficiency in pancreatic cancer. Cancer 1983;52:346–352.

21. McAnena OJ, Daly JM. Impact of antitumor therapy on nutrition. Surg Clin North Am 1986;66:1213–1228.

22. Morrow GR. Chemotherapy-related nausea and vomiting: etiology and management. Cancer 1989;39:89–104.

23. Zook DJ, Yasho JM. Psychologic factors: their effect on nausea and vomiting experienced by clients receiving chemotherapy. Oncol Nurs Forum 1983;10:76–81.

24. Laszlo J, Lucas VS, Stevenson D. Chemotherapy. In: Laszlo J, ed. Physician's guide to cancer care complications: prevention and management. New York: Marcel Dekker, 1986:61–145.

25. Holland JCB, Rowland J, Plumb M. Psychological aspects of anorexia in cancer patients. Cancer Res 1977;37:2425–2428.

26. See JS. Nutrition management of the patient with breast cancer. In: Bloch AS, ed. Nutrition management of the cancer patient. Rockville, MD: Aspen Publishers, 1990: 149–158.

27. Heasman KZ, Sutherland HJ, Campbell JA, Elhakim T, Boyd NF. Weight gain during adjuvant chemotherapy for breast cancer. Breast Cancer Res Treat 1985;5:195–200.

28. Ross BT. The impact of radiation therapy on the nutrition status of the cancer patient: an overview. In: Bloch AS, ed. Nutrition management of the cancer patient. Rockville, MD: Aspen Publishers, 1990:173–180.

29. Kokal WA. The impact of antitumor therapy on nutrition. Cancer 1985;55:273–278.

30. Kouba J. Nutritional care of the individual with cancer. Nutr Clin Pract 1988;3:175–182.

31. Kelly K. An overview of how to nourish the cancer patient by mouth. Cancer 1986;58: 1897–1901.
32. Levy MH, Catalano RB. Control of common physical symptoms other than pain in patients with terminal disease. Semin Oncol 1985;12:411–430.
33. Kern KA, Norton JA. Cancer cachexia. JPEN 1988;12:286–297.
34. DeWys WD. Management of cancer cachexia. Semin Oncol 1985;12:452–460.
35. Loprinzi CL, Ellison NM, Schaid DJ, Krook JE, Athmann LM, Dose AM, Mailliard JA, Johnson PS, Ebbert LP, Geeraerts LH. Controlled trial of megestrol acetate for the treatment of cancer anorexia and cachexia. J Nat Cancer Inst 1990;82:1127–1132.
36. Loprinzi CL, Goldberg RM, Burnham NL. Cancer-associated anorexia and cachexia. Drugs 1992;43(4):499–506.
37. Ahmann DL, O'Fallon JR, Scanlon PW, Payne WS, Bisel HF, Edmonson JH. A preliminary assessment of factors associated with recurrent disease in a surgical adjuvant clinical trial for patients with breast cancer with special emphasis on the aggressiveness of therapy. Am J Clin Oncol (CCT) 1982;5:371–381.
38. Camoriano JK, Loprinzi CL, Ingle JN, Therneau TM, Krook JE, Veeder MH. Weight change in women treated with adjuvant therapy or observed following mastectomy for node-positive breast cancer. J Clin Oncol 1990;8:1327–1334.

13 / *Psychological Disorders*

ANOREXIA NERVOSA AND BULIMIA NERVOSA

General Description

The dietary recommendations for patients with eating disorders include a meal plan designed to meet current energy and nutrient needs. For the patient with anorexia nervosa, the initial meal plan reflects nutrient needs and identifies energy allowances that consider the degree of starvation. For these patients, relatively small, gradual increases are made in the kilocalorie level of the diet during treatment. For patients with bulimia nervosa, the recommended kilocalorie level may be constant through the course of the treatment. For both anorexia nervosa and bulimia nervosa, it is essential that a meal plan consider individual needs. Education about normal nutritional needs and the physiologic effects of starvation and refeeding is also an important component of the treatment plan. Management often requires long-term nutritional counseling and ongoing patient support.

Nutritional Inadequacy

The initial kilocalorie recommendations in anorexia nervosa may be low, which may result in all the nutrients being less than the Recommended Dietary Allowance (RDA). As the kilocalorie level is increased during treatment, the diet will meet the RDA for all nutrients. A vitamin/mineral supplement is usually not needed.

The dietary recommendations in bulimia nervosa are designed to meet the RDA for all nutrients.

Indication and Rationale

Anorexia Nervosa. Anorexia nervosa is characterized by self-imposed weight loss, endocrine dysfunction, and a misperception of body image. The illness occurs most often in females shortly after puberty or later in adolescence, but onset can be premenarchal or later in life. Less commonly the illness occurs in males. Psychological characteristics include misperception of the body image with

303

the patient seeing herself as being fatter than she is, fear of becoming fat, and denial of fatigue. The physiological accompaniments consist of the somatic changes associated with semistarvation, notably lowered basal metabolic rate and reduced gonadotropin production, which results in the cessation of menses in females. Specific dietary inadequacies can lead to nutritional deficiencies and osteoporosis.[1,2]

Among females, more than half the cases begin before the age of 20 years. Fewer than 10% have premenarchal onset. Late onset, after the age of 25 years, occurs in about a quarter of cases. Lifetime prevalence is about 0.3% in females and 0.02% in males. Among 15 to 19 year old females the prevalence is 0.5%. Incidence of the disorder in the young female population has been increasing in Western countries since the 1930s. Among women older than 25 years, and among males, the rates have remained constant.[3]

Nutritional intervention should be undertaken when significant weight has been lost and when eating patterns are severely distorted. Hospitalization becomes necessary when an inordinate amount of weight, generally more than 25% of body weight, has been lost; when eating patterns are severely out of control; and when there is little motivation by the patient to change. Treatment of the patient may involve care by a pediatrician, an internist, a psychiatrist, or a general physician and collaboration with a dietitian. Communication among the practitioners and a coordinated approach to treatment are essential. The family may also benefit from therapy and/or from support groups. In the hospital setting, teamwork is especially important to assure consistency in treatment.[4,5]

Requirements for medical treatment vary greatly and depend on the age of the patient, the duration and severity of the starvation, and the degree of dehydration or of other complications. The diet history, the presence of binge-eating and of vomiting, and the abuse of laxatives and diuretics influence the approach to treatment. Restoring normal physiological function by the correction of changes that are associated with starvation is the initial aim of the treatment. Too rapid a reversal of the hypometabolic state by rapid refeeding may cause excessive peripheral edema. Some edema is to be expected during refeeding and should not be cause for alarm. Nearly all patients should be able to resume an oral intake of small amounts of regular food. This approach is much preferable to liquid food substitutes given orally or as tube feeding, because the aim is for the patient to resume normal eating habits.

Patients often react to the changes associated with refeeding with the fear that they are becoming fat. An explanation of the physiologic changes that are associated with starvation[2,6] and a careful explanation of the treatment are essential before treatment is begun. The long-term goal, beyond restoring normal eating patterns, is for the patient to become an effective, independently functioning individual.

The treatment of patients with anorexia nervosa can be exceedingly difficult and time-consuming. Hospitalization, which includes long-term intensive psychotherapy coordinated with nutritional rehabilitation, is often necessary.[5] Some patients require only a brief hospitalization while others can be managed entirely as outpatients. The treatment principles are no different for hospitalized patients than for outpatients. Hospitalization is required when medical complications warrant it or when eating behaviors are severely out of control. Principles involve the restoration of a satisfactory nutritional state, preferably through the patient's own efforts, and the restoration of an adequate weight and normal eating patterns.

During the initial phase of hospitalization, the intravenous restoration of fluids and electrolytes may be required. Oral intake may need to be supported by peripheral parenteral nutrition if the nutritional status is precarious. Central parenteral nutrition and tube feedings are generally not needed.

The treatment goals are set with the patient, and there should be flexibility in implementing the program. The setting of a series of goal weights that are acceptable to the patient is often useful. These weights should be individualized based on an understanding of the patient's growth patterns as demonstrated by the standard growth charts. At first, dependence on the therapist and on the program is fostered; in time there is a gradual movement toward greater responsibility and autonomy for the patient.

Clinical judgment dictates whether dietary instruction should be avoided entirely. Some patients, especially children, respond best when the external pressure to eat is removed and the normal drive to eat is allowed to reassert itself. In other instances, specific advice about meal plans and food choices is helpful in initially structuring the dietary guidelines and in resolving decisions about eating. Care must be taken not to reinforce the compulsive rituals and the preoccupation with food that exist in many patients. Principles, rather than rigid plans, should be conveyed.[7]

Bulimia Nervosa. Bulimia nervosa is a disorder characterized by frequent binge-eating and purging associated with loss of control over eating and a persistent overconcern about body shape and weight. The disorder occurs predominantly in adolescent girls and young adult women. It is often associated with normal weight, but it also occurs as a sequel to anorexia nervosa and may be present in emaciated individuals. Milder forms of the disorder are common, being seen in young women who use purging as a means of weight control and in those who induce vomiting occasionally after eating excessively. To the extent that semistarvation is a feature in bulimic syndromes, physiologic changes similar to those seen in anorexia nervosa occur. The diversity of eating patterns makes it impossible to generalize, however. Reduced basal metabolic rate is a common feature, even among patients whose weight is within the normal range. Daily variations in caloric intake lead to nonpainful enlargement of the salivary glands. Habitual vomiting causes erosion of the dental enamel. Vomiting and laxative abuse may cause metabolic alkalosis and hypokalemia leading to muscular weakness, cardiac arrhythmias, renal impairment, and even death.[1,8]

Bulimia nervosa and its variants are now more frequently seen than anorexia nervosa. When strict criteria for diagnosing bulimia nervosa are used, the prevalence rate for adolescent and young adult women is 1 to 2% of the population. It is rare among males. When broader criteria for binge-eating and purging are used, the prevalence rates are from 3 to 9% and more males are included.

Most patients with bulimic behaviors can benefit from nutritional counseling when they are motivated to change their behaviors. Willingness by the patient to acknowledge the aberrant behaviors and to make changes increases the likelihood that nutritional intervention will be effective. Many treatment approaches have been advocated, including individual and group psychotherapy and psychopharmacologic treatment. There is a great diversity among patients with bulimic syndromes. Therefore, treatment requires individualization. Nonetheless, several principles are basic to the treatment. The principles include education about the physiologic changes that result from fasting and refeeding and about the nutritional and health consequences of harmful behaviors. Periods of food deprivation should be avoided. Guidelines about kilocalorie needs and food choices are often helpful. The undesirable behaviors are often minimized by regulating eating habits and by structuring daily routines. When the binge-purge pattern is severely out of control and the complications, such as hypokalemia from vomiting and laxative abuse, have ensued, hospitalization may be needed. Metabolic derangements are corrected in the hospital. Psychiatric hospitalization can provide a structured environment to interrupt and prevent the harmful eating and purging behaviors.

Goals of Dietary Management

The goal of dietary treatment in anorexia nervosa is to aid the patient in reestablishing a normal eating pattern.[7] While this is also the ultimate goal in bulimia nervosa, the initial goal is for the patient to gain control of the bulimic behaviors. The diet helps in achieving the goals initially by resolving decisions about eating and later by providing guidelines for appropriate food choices.

The following dietary recommendations and the techniques for their implementation were developed for outpatient treatment; however, the same principles apply to hospitalized individuals.

Experience has suggested that there are a variety of eating patterns among patients with anorexia nervosa or bulimic syndromes. This variability in the dietary patterns makes it essential to tailor the diet to each patient's specific needs.[9]

Several specific areas need to be included in the formulation of a dietary treatment plan that reflects the needs of each patient with anorexia nervosa or bulimia nervosa. The first is a detailed diet history, which helps to identify the particular areas that will require the greatest amount of attention during the treatment. It also provides an opportunity for the dietitian to become acquainted with the patient and to begin developing the rapport that is necessary for working together successfully. The history taking is followed by determining the kilocalorie content of the initial diet, designing a diet plan, gradually increasing the kilocalorie content of the diet, identifying weight gain expectations, and formulating a maintenance diet plan.

Dietary Recommendations: Anorexia Nervosa

Diet History.   The initial diet history forms the basis for the dietary management of the patient with anorexia nervosa, from the design of the initial dietary guidelines to those of the weight maintenance diet. It should identify, as accurately as possible, the patient's eating pattern before the reduction of food intake and evolution of the present practices. The current kilocalorie and protein intake should be estimated along with the current eating pattern, which includes meal and snack frequency and content. Family eating patterns, which include where and with whom the patient eats, should be determined. Food likes, dislikes, preferences, and aversions need to be identified; true food dislikes must be differentiated from aversions (and "fear" foods) that have resulted from recent dietary manipulations. The occurrence of fasting, binge-eating, vomiting, and laxative/diuretic abuse should be determined and documented. The kind, frequency, and duration of physical activity also need identification.

Kilocalorie Content of Initial Diet. When a patient's food supply has been insufficient to meet energy needs for some time, the body adjusts to a lower level of metabolism in order to conserve energy. As a result, the basal or resting energy expenditure is reduced.

Generally, the basal energy requirement can be estimated by using the Nomogram for present weight (see Appendix 6). However, because of the lowered basal metabolic rate that results from starvation, the calculated basal kilocalorie requirement overestimates actual basal kilocalorie needs. Therefore, a diet planned at the calculated basal level usually results in stopping or at least slowing weight loss.

In severely malnourished patients, it may be helpful to determine the actual kilocalorie expenditure by measuring oxygen consumption. Such measurements can be used to guide planning of the initial diet. Occasionally, a series of oxygen consumption measurements can be made, and increasing metabolic rates can be regarded as an indicator of improvement in the physiological function. However, this degree of precision is usually not essential in formulating an initial kilocalorie prescription or for follow-up.

To determine the kilocalorie content of the initial diet, the calculated basal kilocalorie requirement is compared with the estimated kilocalories of the current diet, as obtained in the initial diet history. If the basal kilocalories are 200 to 250 kcal more than the current kilocalorie intake obtained from the history, the patient probably will not accept more than the estimate of basal kilocalories. If the discrepancy is less, an addition of 200 to 250 kcal to the basal kilocalories may be appropriate. If an estimate of the current kilocalorie intake cannot be made, an initial prescription that is equal to the basal kilocalorie requirement is appropriate. If the kilocalorie content of the initial diet is set too high, the patient may feel overwhelmed rather than challenged; consideration of motivation and of readiness to accept diet instructions is essential. Usually, the initial goal is to stop the weight loss while beginning to establish regularity in the eating pattern.

Often the patient is reluctant to start following the diet because he or she fears that eating and weight gain will become uncontrollable and excessive. Providing an explanation of the energy relationship using the individual's own kilocalorie needs, as well as reassuring the patient that the kilocalorie level of the diet will be monitored, may help to give the individual the confidence to try what is suggested.

Diet Plan Design. The priority in designing the diet plan is that the diet be of an appropriate nutrient composition and kilocalorie content. The dietitian should discuss with the patient the body's nutrient needs for growth, development, and maintenance and how these needs can be met by food. The initial and progressive diets are designed to include foods from each of the basic food groups, with portions being increased as kilocalorie increases are made. Supplementary vitamins are rarely necessary since vitamin deficiencies are infrequent among patients with anorexia nervosa and since the prescribed maintenance diet contains sufficient vitamins. In most cases, the need for eating a varied diet must be emphasized frequently. The diet plan should respect and reflect the patient's likes and dislikes.

Initially, weighing meats and measuring the other foods in the diet is recommended to ensure that adequate portions are being taken. If the portion sizes are determined in relation to the patient's present desire for food, adequate intake usually will not be achieved. In the initial stages of treatment, measuring portions also gives the patient greater confidence that overeating will not occur than if the portion sizes were estimated. As eating becomes more comfortable for the individual, estimating the food portions is encouraged.

The individualized meal plan should ensure that a wide variety of foods are included in 3 meals, with or without snacks. Abdominal distention, which is attributable to the presence of increased bulk in the gastrointestinal tract, and slowed gastric emptying often result in the feeling of fullness. The patient recognizes that more has been eaten than in the past. This contributes to the initial discomfort that is felt after eating the prescribed diet. The reasons for this discomfort should be discussed with the patient so that it is understood that such initial discomfort is normal and that over time the capacity for food will increase, and less discomfort will be experienced, as the diet is consistently eaten. In contrast to low kilocalorie weight reduction diets, the bulk content of meals should not be excessive in the initial stages because of the easy filling and the discomfort that is experienced.

The dietary plan is presented as a minimum guideline, and it is emphasized that the patient may eat more of any of the foods, or eat foods that are not on the diet, as long as the prescribed diet is eaten. Yet most patients are not comfortable in modifying the prescribed diet until they have gained confidence in using it and feel assured that they are not gaining too rapidly.

It is helpful to provide specific written dietary guidelines based on the six food exchange lists. Also, for many patients it is useful to expand the food exchange lists to include desserts, sweets, and a "favorite foods list" that includes special recipes, fast foods, and convenience foods, with an indication of the food exchange value of these foods. Written instructions should contain a daily meal plan and a sample menu, which can be completed by the patient and the dietitian at the initial consultation. This approach allows the diet to be viewed by the patient as guidelines for normal nutritional needs.

Keeping a food record is useful for most patients. Records can include a hunger rating as well as where meals are eaten, with whom, feelings and symptoms felt, and kinds and amounts of foods eaten. Record keeping can be discontinued as soon as eating becomes comfortable and spontaneous. In the hospital, food intake should be monitored through kilocalorie counts or through close observation of the food intake in the context of a well-supervised environment.

While constipation is a frequent concern, it is usually not a problem once the quantity of food that is eaten increases and a more regular pattern of eating is established. Diarrhea may occur during the initial stages as the kilocalorie intake increases.

Diet Progression.   The progression of the kilocalorie content of the diet is highly individual. The increases should present a challenge while being realistic.

In general, increments of 200 kcal per week can be made during the early stages of treatment, with greater increases as the patient becomes more comfortable with eating. Increase in the number of kilocalories should be made slowly. This allows time for the psychological changes that are needed for acceptance of the weight gain. With some patients, the kilocalorie content of the diet may not be changed for several weeks if efforts need to be directed toward difficult changes in other areas, such as eating patterns or expanding the variety of foods eaten.

Weight Gain Expectations.   In general, as long as progress continues to be made (initially by stopping the weight loss, followed by consistent increases in the weight), dietary treatment is considered to be satisfactory. Usually, one cannot expect the patient to gain a specific number of pounds each week. The patient must be reassured that the weight gain that results from the rehydration of refeeding does not represent a rapid accumulation of body fat and will resolve spontaneously if the prescribed diet is continued. A long-term goal weight should be set considering the previous weight history or growth pattern and the weight the patient will accept. The goal weight can be renegotiated as the treatment progresses.

Diet Plan for Weight Maintenance.   Dietary guidelines should be designed for weight maintenance when the patient reaches her goal weight. The goal weight is determined individually based on knowledge of the previous growth history. It is the weight at which normal physiological functions are presumed to occur. Menstruation often returns at this weight. However, there can be a delay of months or years after the goal weight is attained before this function is resumed. Sometimes a lower weight is selected as an initial goal, with re-evaluation when the initial goal is reached.

Food records during this phase are again useful because they offer reassurance to the patient that the food intake is appropriate. Also, such records, along with the patient's weight response, enable the dietitian to evaluate the appropriateness of the kilocalorie level of the maintenance diet. Because of variations in activity, the level for weight maintenance may require adjustment.

Dietary Recommendations: Bulimia Nervosa

The principles of dietary treatment used for patients with anorexia nervosa can be adapted for patients with bulimia nervosa. The specific areas that need consideration in the bulimia nervosa treatment program are similar to those in the anorexia nervosa program with the following additional considerations.

Diet History.   During the initial diet history, the factors that trigger the bulimic behaviors should be identified, as well as when and how frequently they occur. Also, the occurrence of fasting should be noted along with its frequency and duration. It is useful to determine what foods are usually eaten during an eating binge and what a patient identifies as an eating binge. Purging methods used, whether vomiting, laxative/diuretic abuse, and/or exercise, should be identified.

Information in these areas is helpful in acquainting the dietitian with the patient and in defining the areas that will need the greatest attention during the coming weeks of nutrition education.

Kilocalorie Content of Initial Diet.   The kilocalorie content of the initial diet should be set at a level that the patient can accept and that results in weight stabilization. It is important not to set the kilocalorie level of the initial diet too high so that the patient is fearful that weight gain will result and may be tempted to purge or fast. Likewise, the kilocalorie level should not be to low so as to impose too great a restriction on food intake and result in further binge-eating. It should be a compromise that the patient can accept and that results in weight stabilization. Emphasis during the initial stages is usually not on changing weight but on establishing more acceptable eating patterns.

The kilocalorie level of the initial diet can be set by determining the basal kilocalories by means of the Harris-Benedict equation or the Mayo Clinic Nomogram for present weight (see Appendix 6). A diet planned at this level usually results in weight stabilization. If the patient is very active, a kilocalorie allowance for activity should be added. The addition of kilocalories for activity equal to 10 to 15% of the basal kilocalories is generally sufficient. Usually this kilocalorie level is also acceptable to the patient.

Diet Plan Design.   In designing the diet, the priorities are similar to those in anorexia nervosa. Eating 3 meals each day at regular times is important. Uncontrolled eating binges are often minimized by maintaining a regular mealtime pattern and eating adequately at meals. Planning a wide variety of foods, including "fear" foods, is essential. Overeating on previously forbidden foods is frequently experienced by patients who limit or avoid the use of specific ("fear") foods. Also, the use of snacks needs to be carefully considered. Some patients feel that snacks may trigger a binge; others feel that they need snacks to help prevent the overwhelming hunger that they perceive as occurring between meals and that results in triggering a binge. Fasting, skipping meals, and eating inadequate amounts at meals may contribute to the occurrence of binges.

Food records are helpful and should include a notation of the times of the binges, the kinds of foods eaten, and the occurrence of vomiting and laxative and/or diuretic abuse.

Weight Gain or Loss.   Generally the kilocalorie level of the diet does not change during treatment. When the patient has regulated the dietary intake and begins to feel more confident with the ability to control eating behaviors while keeping weight relatively stable, the kilocalorie level of the diet and the need for a gradual weight loss program can be reassessed. If body weight is inappropriate, a realistic goal may be set. A daily kilocalorie level of less than 1,400 kcal or one that results in more than a 1 lb loss per week is perhaps too restrictive and may reinitiate binge-eating, fasting, and purging.

Diet Plan for Weight Maintenance.   A weight maintenance diet should be designed at a suitable time. The kilocalorie level of this diet can be determined by the basal kilocalories for the height, age, sex, and goal weight, with the addition of an appropriate increment for activity. A goal weight that is physiologically appropriate should be set. Previous growth history is a useful guide. Setting a goal weight that is too low may result in a less than comfortable intake of kilocalories for weight maintenance, which may again initiate a binging, purging, and/or fasting cycle.

Follow-up support and nutrition counseling should continue even after weight has been stabilized and eating behaviors regulated.

Physicians: How to Order Diet

The diet order should indicate diet for *anorexia nervosa* or *bulimia nervosa*. The dietitian determines the variety of foods and the kilocalorie level according to the previously outlined principles.

References

1. Lucas AR, Huse DM. Behavioral disorders affecting food intake: anorexia nervosa and bulimia nervosa. In: Shils ME, Young VR, eds. Modern nutrition in health and disease, 8th ed. Philadelphia: Lea & Febiger, 1994:977–983.
2. Lucas AR, Callaway CW. Anorexia nervosa and bulimia. In: Berk JE, ed. Bockus gastro-enterology, 4th ed. Philadelphia: WB Saunders, 1985:4416–4434.
3. Lucas AR, Beard CM, O'Fallon WM, Kurland LT. 50-year trends in the incidence of anorexia nervosa in Rochester, Minnesota: a population-based study. Am J Psychiatry 1991;148:917–922.
4. Bruch H. Eating disorders: obesity and anorexia nervosa. New York: Basic Books, 1973.
5. Andersen AE. Practical comprehensive treatment of anorexia nervosa and bulimia. Baltimore: Johns Hopkins Press, 1985.
6. Keys A, Brožek J, Henschel A, Mickelsen O, Taylor HL. The biology of human starvation. Vol. 1 and 2. Minneapolis: University of Minnesota Press, 1950.
7. Huse DM, Lucas AR. Dietary treatment of anorexia nervosa. J Am Diet Assoc 1983;83: 687–690.
8. Kirkley BG. Bulimia: clinical characteristics, development and etiology. J Am Diet Assoc 1986;86:468–475.
9. Huse DM, Lucas AR. Dietary patterns in anorexia nervosa. Am J Clin Nutr 1984;40: 251–254.

TYRAMINE CONTROLLED DIET

General Description

This diet restricts foods that contain large amounts of tyramine either naturally or through aging. Aging is a process that increases tyramine content by protein breakdown. Foods that have high levels of other pressor amines and foods that have been implicated in hypertensive reactions during monoamine oxidase therapy are also restricted.

Nutritional Inadequacy

The tyramine-controlled diet is not inherently lacking in nutrients when compared to the RDA. However, for those diets restricted to 1,200 kcal or less, it is difficult to meet the RDA consistently. A multiple vitamin supplement that provides nutrients at a level equivalent to the RDA is recommended for persons who consume 1,200 kcal or less. A multiple vitamin supplement may also be warranted for persons who have food aversions or intolerances that greatly limit the variety of food choices.

Indications and Rationale

The diet should be used as a precautionary measure for all patients who take monoamine oxidase (MAO) inhibitor drugs. These drugs, such as tranylcypromine

(Parnate™), phenelzine (Nardil™), and isocarboxazid (Marplan™), are utilized in the treatment of depression and anxiety disorders.

The concomitant ingestion of foods that have a high concentration of tyramine may precipitate a hypertensive crisis characterized by headaches and nausea. Tyramine and other pressor amines (catecholamines) are normally degraded in the body by the enzyme monoamine oxidase. MAO inhibitors interfere with this process, and the result is the accumulation of unmetabolized tyramine and a variety of pressor amine substances in the adrenergic nerve terminals. The ingestion of tyramine may trigger the sudden release of large quantities of pressor amines from their nerve terminal storage sites. Some of the released catecholamines are strongly active vasopressor materials; therefore, a hypertensive crisis may occur.

Goals of Dietary Management

In patients who take MAO inhibitors, it has been reported that as little as 6 mg of tyramine may cause increased blood pressure and that 25 mg may induce a hypertensive crisis. Thus the intake should be kept below 5 mg per day.[10]

TABLE 13-1   Food Sources of Tyramine*[10-13]

Food Group	Types of Food
Beverages	Red wines including Chianti Sherry Vermouth Beer: limit to 12–24 oz per day if approved by physician White wine: limit to 4–8 oz per day if approved by physician
Meat and meat substitutes	Caviar Cheese, aged and processed Herring, pickled or dried Liver Sausage: dry, summer, pepperoni, hard salami, bologna
Vegetables	Snow pea pods Italian green beans Fava beans Sauerkraut
Soups	Soups packaged with yeast products: miso (a soup stock commonly used in Oriental cooking)
Miscellaneous	Concentrated yeast extract: brewer's yeast, yeast supplements, Marmite (an English beverage and sandwich spread) Salad dressings containing cheese Soy sauce in large amounts

*Data available on the content of tyramine and other pressor amines show a great deal of variation. The tyramine content is likely to vary among different brands of a particular food, since several factors related to the preparation, processing, and storing of foods may contribute to their tyramine content. Various methods of analysis also present different results. The tyramine content may also vary with the time the food is left unrefrigerated: the longer the time, the greater the protein degradation. For practical purposes, the diet is intended to prohibit or limit foods that tend to be high in tyramine or other pressor amines and foods that have been implicated in the development of a hypertensive crisis in patients who take monoamine oxidase inhibitors.

Dietary Recommendations

In general, only fresh foods or freshly prepared frozen or canned foods should be eaten. Avoid any protein food that has been aged, stored, or refrigerated.

1. Cottage cheese, cream cheese, farmer's cheese, and ricotta cheese may be used.
2. Yeast leavened products made with baker's yeast are allowed.
3. Check labels of canned and packaged foods carefully.
4. Remember tyramine restriction when selecting foods in a restaurant.

Table 13-1 presents foods that are high in tyramine.

In addition to the aforementioned dietary restrictions, certain medications should be avoided while receiving an MAO inhibitor. These include many cold tablets and decongestants, most allergy and asthma medications, some high blood pressure pills, all antidepressants, the anti-obsessional drug Anafranil™, and the pain medication Demerol™. Prior to beginning an MAO inhibitor, the physician should evaluate all the medications taken, including over-the-counter preparations. The patient should be reminded to consult a physician or pharmacist prior to taking any new medication.[11]

Physicians: How to Order Diet

The diet order should indicate *tyramine control* or request dietary precautions during the use of MAO inhibitors.

References

10. McCabe BJ. Dietary tyramine and other pressor amines in MAOI regimens: review. J Am Diet Assoc 1986;86:1059–1064.
11. Lippmann S. Monoamine oxidase inhibitors. Am Fam Physician 1986;34:113–119.
12. Shulman KI, Walker SE, MacKenzie S, Knowles S. Dietary restriction, tyramine, and the use of monoamine oxidase inhibitors. J Clin Pharmacol 1989;9:397–402.
13. Brown C, Taniguchi G. The monoamine oxidase inhibitor-tyramine interaction. J Clin Pharmacol 1989;29:529–532.

Indications and Rationale

Table 14-2 summarizes the dietary guidelines for chronic renal failure.

Protein.   Animal research and preliminary human research suggest that early intervention with protein restriction not only prevents the symptoms of chronic renal failure (CRF) but *may* preserve kidney function.[8,9] Conclusive evidence that dietary protein intake influences the progression of renal failure is not yet available. However, based upon research thus far, protein restriction in these patients seems prudent.

The appropriate time to initiate a protein restricted diet continues to be debated. There have been studies that demonstrate the benefit of early protein restriction when the creatinine clearance drops below 70 ml/min/1.73 m^2,[10] while others are hesitant to specify a level of function because the safety of long-term use and the absolute benefit of a low protein diet are yet to be determined.[11] Without a consensus regarding the opportune time to initiate such a regimen, the exact protein determination and the timing of its implementation should be based on the protocol of the individual nephrologist.[6]

At the Mayo Clinic, a lower protein diet is implemented when deemed appropriate based on the patient's rate of disease progression and ensuing symptoms. Typically, a restriction in the range of 0.6 to 0.8 g/kg of body weight is initiated when the patient's creatinine clearance approaches 30 ml/min/1.73 m^2.

It should be noted that the suggested protein intake is based on actual body weight (corrected for edema), not ideal or desired weight. However, for the obese patient (more than 125% of ideal body weight), it is suggested that an adjusted body weight be used to determine protein needs. To calculate the patient's adjusted body weight, the following formula is used.[6]

TABLE 14-2   Dietary Guidelines in Chronic Renal Failure

Component	Comments
Sodium	Generally 60–90 mEq Calculate sodium level ± 10% of diet order
Kilocalories	Sufficient for weight maintenance, weight gain, or slow weight loss (0.2–0.4 kg or ½–1 lb/wk) Encourage nonprotein calories (unsaturated fat, carbohydrate)
Protein	0.6–0.8 g/kg of body weight + 24 hr urinary protein loss Approximately 60–70% of protein from high biological value sources (meat, poultry, fish, egg, milk); high protein foods should be distributed throughout the day
Potassium	Generally no restriction of food sources Avoid potassium chloride (salt substitutes)
Phosphorus	Reduced intake is inherent in low protein diet Further restriction only if serum phosphorus level elevated
Calcium	Calcium carbonate supplements if ordered by physician

$$[(ABW - IBW) \times 0.25] + IBW = \text{Adjusted Weight in Kg}$$

Where: ABW = actual body weight in kg
IBW = ideal body weight in kg
0.25 = 25% of body fat tissue that is considered to be metabolically active

If proteinuria is present, an amount of protein equal to that lost in the urine, as determined by a 24 hr urine collection, should be added to the calculated daily protein allowance (see Chapter 14, Nephrotic Syndrome). Approximately 60 to 70% of the total protein should be of high biological value (eggs, milk, and meat) to assure an adequate intake of essential amino acids.[6] It is recommended that high protein foods be distributed throughout the day and not saved for consumption in a single meal in order to optimize protein utilization.

Metabolic acidosis can occur in CRF patients due to reduced capacity of the diseased kidneys to excrete hydrogen ions. Studies indicate that this acidosis accelerates protein degradation and that correction of this condition may, to a degree, prevent the catabolic state of uremia. Metabolic acidosis can be corrected with use of a supplemental alkali agent such as calcium carbonate.[12]

Close follow-up of patients by the use of 7 day food records is advised so that protein intake can be modified according to the patient's medical and nutritional status.

Kilocalories. Utilization of dietary protein is directly influenced by total caloric intake. Therefore, adequate caloric intake is of vital importance to the patient with renal disease in order to (1) prevent catabolism of body protein, (2) ensure that dietary protein is not used as an energy source, (3) maintain a constant body weight, and (4) favor the preservation of normal vigor and feelings of well-being. Patients need to be reminded to maintain an adequate caloric intake since they often adhere more closely to the protein restriction and neglect their caloric needs. Patients should be encouraged to consume adequate kilocalories from nonprotein sources. Because CRF appears to increase the risk for coronary heart disease, it may be prudent to substitute carbohydrates and unsaturated fats for saturated fats.[13]

Consumption of these nonprotein kilocalories, along with the dietary protein, may spare endogenous tissue protein from use as an energy source. Caloric needs can be determined according to the guidelines described in Chapter 3, Nutritional Screening and Assessment.

Weight reduction should be approached cautiously because of the risk of catabolism of lean body tissue in addition to the catabolism of body fat. Unless the need for immediate weight loss is compelling, stringent caloric restriction is not recommended, since it may be hazardous, especially if renal function is less than 15% of normal. A moderate caloric deficit, no more than 250 to 500 kcal/day, is recommended.

Sodium. The level of sodium intake should be specific to the patient's needs. The goal is to adjust sodium intake to just below the level that results in edema or hypertension (or both). This will achieve maximum renal function compatible with control of these symptoms.[14] If edema or hypertension is present, a sodium intake of 60 to 90 mEq/day is often indicated. In the extremely edematous patient, more strict control (less than 60 mEq of sodium per day) and diuretics may be needed initially. The diet should be planned to provide within 10% of the prescribed level of sodium.* A measured amount of added salt is necessary only in rare instances. Most CRF patients can conserve sodium reasonably well. If the patient's adherence to this dietary recommendation is in question, a 24 hour urinary sodium study could be performed to determine the patient's level of compliance.

Potassium. The serum potassium level usually remains within the normal range when urinary volume is normal. Dietary potassium control becomes more important when urine volume decreases to below normal.[15] However, as a precaution, patients should be advised to avoid potassium chloride (salt substitute) unless the physician prescribes it as a medication to correct hypokalemia. With normal urine output, hypokalemia usually does not occur unless excess sodium intake necessitates increased use of diuretics, thereby resulting in a corresponding loss of potassium.

Calcium and Phosphorus. As the glomerular filtration rate declines to 30% of normal or less, the dietary phosphate load is greater than the kidney can excrete.[16] Consequently the serum phosphorus concentration rises and may in turn cause the serum calcium level to decrease. Also, the impaired production of 1,25-dihydroxyvitamin D_3 by diseased kidneys decreases the intestinal absorption of dietary calcium. These factors lead to a lowered serum calcium concentration, which stimulates increased secretion of parathyroid hormone. Renal osteodystrophy and metastatic calcification are two of the demonstrable complications that may result from the body's adjustments to normalize serum calcium and phosphorus levels.

Some degree of restriction of phosphorus and calcium is inherent in a low protein diet. On a low protein diet the daily phosphorus intake is already well below the usual American intake (1,500 mg/day).[17] Phosphorus intake should not exceed 800 to 900 mg/day. Generally the phosphorus intake can be controlled by using limited quantities of dairy products and whole-grain breads and cereals (see Appendix 24 for the phosphorus content of foods). For patients with severe hyperphosphatemia it may be necessary to use a phosphate binder to decrease serum phosphorus. It is current practice to use an aluminum-containing phosphate binder initially and then switch to an aluminum-free phosphate binder for long-term use since aluminum toxicity is a potential problem. Calcium salts, such as calcium carbonate and calcium acetate, are the preferred binding agents because they can also help meet the increased calcium needs of the CRF patient.[10]

Goals of Dietary Management

The goals of dietary management are (1) to control sodium intake, thereby maximizing renal function, preventing edema, and controlling blood pressure; (2) to provide adequate nonprotein calories, thereby preventing muscle catabolism; (3) to limit protein intake, thereby preventing excessive accumulation of nitrogenous waste products and preventing uremic toxicity; and (4) to aid in controlling serum potassium, calcium, and phosphorus levels.

---

*In other situations, such as management of hypertension, the diet prescription is interpreted to mean less than or equal to the desired sodium level. The diet may actually provide considerably less than the prescribed level. However, in renal disease, the diet should be planned to provide the prescribed level ± 10%.

Dietary Recommendations

The food exchange list for protein, sodium, and potassium control is used for meal planning (see pp. 348–356). Unless serum potassium is elevated, the potassium subgroupings are not necessary.

Chronic Renal Failure and Diabetes

Some compromises must be made in the usual diabetic diet when diabetes mellitus is complicated by renal failure. The requirements of the protein controlled diet generally take priority.

The decrease in protein intake requires a corresponding increase in intake of fat and carbohydrate. Low protein products can be used as a source of kilocalories. To assure adequate kilocalories, one also may have to include simple carbohydrates, such as sugar, jellies, and sugar-sweetened fruit. If simple carbohydrates are consumed, they should be measured carefully and distributed evenly throughout the day to minimize fluctuation in blood sugar levels. Patients are often reluctant to eat simple sugars; thus the rationale behind their incorporation must be clearly stated to ensure compliance.

The food exchange list for protein, sodium, and potassium control, rather than the diabetic exchange list, is used for meal planning. Consistency in timing and in composition of meals and the use of additional food for increased exercise and to prevent hypoglycemic reactions are still appropriate.

Physicians: How to Order Diet

The diet order should indicate: the *specific level of protein* (the most common levels are 40 and 50 g) and the *specific level of sodium* (the most common levels are 60 and 90 mEq).

The dietitian will calculate caloric needs. The diet order should indicate if weight loss is desired. Restriction of potassium, other than to caution against use of potassium chloride, is not included unless specifically requested. Restriction of phosphorus beyond that inherent in the diet is not included unless specifically requested.

References

6. Renal Dietitians Dietetic Practice Group of the American Dietetic Association. Guideline for nutrition care of patients receiving conservative treatment for end-stage renal disease. In: Wilkins KG, Brouns Schiro K, eds. Suggested guidelines for nutrition care of renal patients, 2nd ed. Chicago: ADA, 1992:10–12.
7. Carron D. A review of vitamin supplements for adults undergoing hemodialysis. CRN Quarterly 1985;9:7–8.
8. Liddle VR. Nutrition for the patient with end-stage renal disease. In: Lancaster LE, ed. The patient with end-stage renal disease. New York: John Wiley & Sons, 1984: 92.
9. Hartnett MN. Low-protein diets in chronic renal insufficiency: a meta-analysis. Therapeutico: ACP Journal Club 1992(July/Aug):11.
10. Massry SG, Kopple JD. Requirements for calcium, phosphorus and vitamin D. In: Mitch W, Klahr S, eds. Nutrition and the kidney. Boston: Little, Brown, 1993:96–113.
11. Hunsicker LG. Studies of therapy of progressive renal failure in humans. Semin Nephrol 1989;9(4):380–394.

12. Sugino N, Ando A, Arai J. Chronic renal failure: the Japanese experience. In: Mitch WE, Stein JH, eds. The progressive nature of renal disease, contemporary issues in nephrology, 2nd ed. New York: Churchill-Livingstone, 1992;26:183–202.
13. Grundy SM. Management of hyperlipidemia of kidney disease. Kidney Int 1990;37:847–853.
14. Kopple JD. Nutritional management of chronic renal failure. Postgrad Med 1978;64(5):135–144.
15. Bansal VK. Potassium metabolism in renal failure: nondietary rationale for hyperkalemia. J Renal Nutr 1992;2(3):8–12.
16. Delmez JA, Slatopolsky E. Hyperphosphatemia: its consequences and treatment in patients with chronic renal disease. Am J Kidney Dis 1992;19(4):303–317.
17. Subcommittee on the tenth edition of the RDAs. Food and Nutrition Board, Committee on Life Sciences, National Research Council. Recommended dietary allowances, 10th ed. Washington, DC: National Academy Press, 1989.

HEMODIALYSIS

General Description

The diet emphasizes controlled intake of protein, kilocalories, sodium, potassium, fluid, calcium, and phosphorus. Recommended levels are dependent on the frequency of dialysis and on the individual's medical situation.

Nutritional Inadequacy

The dialysis patient is at risk for deficiencies of water-soluble vitamins, particularly vitamin B_6 and folic acid, due to poor intake or loss of these nutrients during the dialysis procedure.[18]

The fat-soluble vitamins A, E, and K usually do not require supplementation. In fact, cases of vitamin A toxicity have been reported in renal failure patients. A daily supplement of water-soluble vitamins that includes 0.8 to 1.0 mg of folic acid is recommended. (Examples of such preparations include Nephrovite™ and Nephrocaps™. Other preparations may also be available.) Vitamin D (usually in the form of 1,25-dihydroxyvitamin D_3) may be supplemented for those individuals in need.

Trace minerals also may be lost in the dialysate, but the extent of the losses is unknown. Therefore, daily supplementation is not recommended unless a specific deficiency is suspected or documented.

The risk of nutrient deficiencies is greater when the patient has poor dietary intake. Poor intake may be the result of poor appetite, of nausea and vomiting, or of limitations on food choices imposed by therapeutic dietary restrictions.

Indications and Rationale

Although the dialysis machine is capable of duplicating much of the kidney's function, it does not have the flexibility of the normal kidney. Without nutritional intervention, dangerous levels of waste products can accumulate between dialysis treatments.[19] Dietary recommendations should be based upon the frequency of dialysis, the level of residual intrinsic renal function, and the size of the patient. In patients with significant residual renal function, more stringent dietary restrictions

TABLE 14-3 Dietary Guidelines for Hemodialysis

Component	Comments
Protein	1–1.2 g/kg of body weight, adjusted according to individual dialysis characteristics
Kilocalories	Sufficient for weight maintenance, weight gain, or slow weight loss ($^1/_2$–1 lb/wk) Encourage nonprotein kcal from fats, oils, and simple carbohydrate
Sodium	60–120 mEq, generally 90 mEq Calculate the sodium level ± 10% of the diet order
Potassium	60–70 mEq
Fluid	Limit beverages and foods that are liquid at room temperature to an amount equal to urine volume plus 1,000 ml
Phosphorus	Restrict dietary phosphorus
Calcium	Calcium carbonate supplements if ordered by the physician

may permit some lengthening of the interval between dialysis sessions. Table 14-3 summarizes the dietary guidelines for patients receiving hemodialysis.

Protein. The protein intake of the patient must be sufficient to maintain nitrogen balance and to replace amino acids lost during dialysis. However, the protein intake must be low enough to prevent excessive interdialytic accumulation of waste products. From 10 to 13 g of amino acids are thought to be lost per dialysis treatment.[18]

At the Mayo Clinic, dietary protein prescription and dialysis therapy are individually tailored according to the patient's desired postdialysis body weight ("dry weight") and residual kidney function via a test method called urea kinetic modeling.[20]

The overall goals of urea kinetic modeling are (1) to individualize the length of dialysis necessary to maintain blood urea nitrogen (BUN) or urea within a target range and (2) to identify those patients who require more intensive nutritional therapy.

Urea kinetic modeling is a computerized clinical tool for assessing protein metabolism and for monitoring the efficacy of diet and of the patient's compliance. Urea kinetic modeling utilizes the net protein catabolic rate (PCR) which reflects the amount of protein that is catabolized per kilogram of body weight per 24 hours. This provides useful information for the determination of nitrogen balance. Urea kinetic analysis uses the patient's PCR, the residual renal function, and the dialyzer characteristics to forecast the length of treatment time necessary to maintain a plasma urea or BUN level within a designated target range (plasma or blood urea × 0.47 = BUN).

Catabolized protein can be either endogenous (muscle catabolism) or exogenous (dietary) in origin. To determine the source of catabolized protein, the patient's reported protein intake from a 3 day food record is compared to the PCR. This comparison indicates if the patient's protein intake is inadequate or excessive. Nutritionally stable patients have a PCR equivalent to the reported dietary protein intake. Correlation of dietary protein intake, the PCR, changes in weight, and changes in serum albumin can assist in the identification and prevention of catabolism and in the maintenance of optimum nutritional status.

In general, the protein requirements of the average adult with minimal residual renal function who requires dialysis 3 times a week can usually be supplied by a diet that provides 1.0 to 1.2 g of protein per kilogram of body weight. Current research recommends that approximately 50% of the total protein intake should be of high biological value (eggs, meats, and milk). However, in our practice, a higher level of high biological value of protein is encouraged whenever possible. Some research suggests that up to 1.4 g of dietary protein per kilogram of body weight is desirable, especially for those patients who are initially malnourished or who develop signs of protein-energy malnutrition.[18]

Kilocalories.   Adequate caloric intake is necessary to prevent catabolism of lean body tissue. Caloric needs generally remain the same as they were before dialysis and can be determined according to the guidelines described in Chapter 3, Nutritional Screening and Assessment.

Adequate intake of nonprotein kilocalories is encouraged to prevent the use of dietary protein for energy. The primary sources of nonprotein kilocalories are fats, oils, simple carbohydrates, and low protein products.[19] However, one must remember that hemodialysis patients can often undergo repeated stresses, which call upon their body's nutritional stores. These stressors include various injuries, infections, and repeated dialysis vascular access surgery. During these metabolic insults, energy requirements go up and dietary intake typically declines. Therefore, frequent assessment of each patient's nutritional requirements is necessary to maintain optimum nutritional status.[21]

If weight reduction is necessary, it should be approached cautiously because of the risk of catabolism of lean body tissue. Only slow weight loss, no more than $1/2$ to 1 lb/week, should be attempted. Correspondingly, the recommended caloric deficit should be no more than 250 to 500 kcal/day.

Sodium.   Control of sodium intake to 60 to 120 mEq/day is usually necessary to control hypertension and edema. Restriction of sodium is extremely helpful in blunting thirst and thus preventing excessive fluid intake and weight gain.[19]

Potassium.   Potassium restriction is essential. Hyperkalemia and rapid changes in serum potassium can result in cardiac dysrhythmia and death.[19] Dietary potassium intake determines the amount of potassium removed during dialysis. Using a dialysate with a low potassium concentration removes more potassium and allows liberalization of dietary potassium (up to 100 mEq/day). However, this method leads to interdialytic hyperkalemia and large changes in serum potassium during each dialysis session.

Fluid.   Limitation of fluid is often the most difficult aspect of the diet for the dialysis patient. If the body retains excess water but sodium intake is restricted, a state of hyponatremia and "water intoxication" may occur. This state is characterized by tremulousness and disorientation, but not necessarily edema.

Fluid sources are (1) beverages and foods that are liquid at room temperature, such as ice cream and gelatin, (2) water content of nonliquid foods, and (3) water formed from the oxidation of food. For practical purposes, the water content of nonliquid foods and the water formed from oxidation of food can be disregarded since they are approximately equal to insensible water loss (respiration, perspiration, and fecal losses) in the stable dialysis patient.[18] Insensible loss may be elevated in states of fever or extensive burns or in a warm dry environment. Water of metabolism may be substantially increased in catabolic states or with a large oral or parenteral intake of calories. It is reasonable to consider as dietary fluid sources only beverages and foods that melt at room temperature. To achieve the optimal interdialytic weight gain of less than 1 kg per day, the total dietary fluid allowance can be calculated by adding urine volume and 1,000 ml.

Calcium and Phosphorus. Hypocalcemia and hyperphosphatemia must be controlled in the uremic state to avoid hyperparathyroidism and to minimize skeletal changes and soft-tissue calcification.[19] The kidney is the site of conversion of 1-hydroxyvitamin D_3 to 1,25-dihydroxyvitamin D_3, the most active form of vitamin D. Deficiencies of 1,25-dihyroxyvitamin D_3 may contribute to renal bone disease. Serum calcium and phosphorus levels are difficult to manage by dietary means alone. Therefore, calcium supplements and phosphate binders are necessary to ensure adequate control.

Methods for controlling phosphorus have been modified because of the potential for aluminum toxicity with prolonged use of aluminum-containing phosphorus binders. Currently, the preferred therapy is a strict dietary phosphorus limitation in conjunction with the use of calcium carbonate or calcium acetate as phosphate binders. It is essential that the phosphate binders be taken at mealtime.[22,23]

Usual phosphorus intake can be determined from 3 or 4 day food records. A specific level of phosphorus intake is not recommended. High phosphorus foods are proscribed, and lower phosphorus alternatives are recommended. (See Appendix 24 for phosphorus content of foods.)

Hypercalcemia and an increase in serum phosphorus levels sometimes occur on this program. Therefore, calcium and phosphorus must be closely monitored. Persistent elevations in phosphorus, especially when coupled with hypercalcemia, may necessitate use of aluminum-containing phosphate binders, which are currently the most effective means of reducing serum phosphorus.

Other Nutritional Problems

Patients on chronic maintenance dialysis commonly develop hypertriglyceridemia and/or hypercholesterolemia.[24] Dietary efforts to regulate hypertriglyceridemia consist of weight control and avoidance of alcohol. Simple carbohydrates are an important calorie source, and it is often not feasible to restrict them. Usual recommendations for control of hypercholesterolemia are often not practical. Total fat intake is generally high since fat is a major nonprotein calorie source. However, the use of mono- and polyunsaturated fat is recommended. In actual practice, high cholesterol- and saturated fat-containing foods, such as eggs and cheese, are not limited because of their importance as protein sources. Exercise is encouraged to control weight and to promote an increase in high-density lipoprotein.

Another common nutritional concern is poor appetite, partly owing to changes in taste acuity and in food preferences, especially for red meat and sweets. Changes in gut motility may also affect appetite.[19] Enteral supplements of high protein and/or high caloric content are frequently needed by the dialysis patient to maintain adequate nutrition. In an attempt to increase protein intake, increased use of dairy products may be encouraged and the serum phosphorus may be allowed to rise slightly above 5.5 mg/dl, provided the product of serum calcium concentration (mg/dl) multiplied by serum phosphorus concentration (mg/dl) is less than 60.

If, despite aggressive dietary counseling and oral nutritional supplements, patients continue to lose weight and/or their albumin levels decline, an intradialytic parenteral nutrition (IDPN) program may be necessary to restore proper nutritional status. Advantages of IDPN therapy include reduced catabolic stress from dialysis because dialysate losses are replaced, and the dialysis treatment offers convenient access to the circulation so that costly hospital administration of parenteral nutrition can be avoided and infused fluids can be removed as the solution is given, thus minimizing the possibility of fluid overload. Concerns regarding IDPN include hyperglycemia during infusion of highly concentrated dextrose and possible reactive hypoglycemia after infusion is completed, azotemia, electrolyte imbalance, and hyperlipidemia as a result of infused lipids. All of these possible effects can be minimized or avoided with close follow-up and prompt treatment should they occur.

It remains unclear if IDPN is an effective temporary treatment for malnourished patients. However, it is a fairly new and very costly treatment regimen, and ongoing research is necessary to fully understand its implications.[25]

Drug Therapy

Human recombinant erythropoietin (EPO) has recently been introduced for the treatment of anemia in end-stage renal disease. The kidney is the source of EPO synthesis, which is therefore lacking in the person who has severe renal disease. Recombinant human EPO is given intravenously after each dialysis treatment. Long-term therapy can restore the hematocrit to normal levels, practically eliminating the need for transfusions, and thus decreasing the risks of immunological sensitization, infection, and iron overload. Treatment of anemia with EPO has been reported to increase predialysis urea and potassium values. These increases have been attributed to an increase in appetite due to an overall improved sense of well-being, as well as a decrease in dialyzer clearance if the hematocrit is increased above 36%. With the risk of elevated urea and potassium, it is important that the dietitian educate the patient regarding the possible effects of EPO therapy, closely monitor laboratory values, and adjust the dietary prescription as needed.[26]

Goals of Dietary Management

The goals of dietary management are (1) to provide sufficient protein to compensate for essential amino acids and nitrogen lost in the dialysate, to maintain nitrogen balance, and yet to prevent excessive accumulation of waste products; (2) to provide adequate kilocalories to prevent catabolism of lean body tissue; (3) to limit sodium intake to control blood pressure and thirst and prevent edema; (4) to control potassium to prevent hyperkalemia and cardiac arrhythmia; (5) to control fluid intake to prevent hyponatremia and excess interdialytic weight gain; and (6) to limit phosphorus to control hyperphosphatemia and minimize renal osteodystrophy.

To ensure that these goals are achieved, the nutritional status and overall nutrient intake of all patients should be regularly evaluated.

Dietary Recommendations

The food exchange list for protein, sodium, and potassium control is used for meal planning (see pp. 348-356). Additional modifications of the list may be necessary for restriction of phosphorus (see Appendix 24) and saturated fat.

Physicians: How to Order Diet

The diet order should indicate: the *specific level of protein* (generally the initial order is 1 to 1.2 g of protein per kg of body weight), the *specific level of sodium* (generally the initial order is 90 mEq of sodium; the usual range is 60 to 120 mEq of sodium), the *specific level of potassium* (the most common level is 60 to 70 mEq or less daily), and the *specific amount of fluid.*

The dietitian will calculate caloric needs. The diet order should indicate if weight loss is desired. Restriction of phosphorus is routinely included. Dietary modifications for hyperlipidemia are included if the patient has hyperlipidemia.

References

18. Bergstrom J. Nutritional requirements of hemodialysis patients. In: Mitch WE, Klahr S, eds. Nutrition and the kidney. Boston: Little, Brown, 1993:263–289.
19. Harum P. Renal nutrition for the renal nurse. Am Nephrol Nurs Assoc J 1984;11(5): 38–43.
20. Sargent J, Gotch F. Urea kinetics: a guide to nutritional management of renal failure. Am J Clin Nutr 1978;31:1696–1702.
21. Allman MA, Stewart PM, Tiller DJ, Horvath JS, Duggin GG, Truswell AS. Energy supplementation and the nutritional status of hemodialysis patients. Am J Clin Nutr 1990;51:558–562.
22. Slatopolsky E, Weerts C, Lopez-Hilker S, Norwood K, Zink M, Windus D, Delmez J. Calcium carbonate as a phosphate binder in patients with chronic renal failure undergoing dialysis. N Engl J Med 1986;315:157–161.
23. Schiller LR, Santa Ana CA, Sheikh MS, Emmett M, Fordtran JS. Effect of the time administration of calcium acetate on phosphorus binding. N Engl J Med 1989;320:1100–1113.
24. Lindner A, Charra B, Sherrard DJ, Scribner BH. Accelerated atherosclerosis in prolonged maintenance hemodialysis. N Engl J Med 1974;290:697–701.
25. Cano N, Labastie-Coeyrehourg J, Lacombe P, Stroumza P, diCostanzo-Dufetel J, Durbec JP, Coudray-Lucas C, Cynober L. Peridialytic parenteral nutrition with lipids and amino acids in malnourished hemodialysis patients. Am J Clin Nutr 1990;726–730.
26. Eschbach JW, Egrie JC, Downing MR, Browne JK, Adamson JW. Correction of the anemia of end-stage renal disease with recombinant human erythropoietin. N Engl J Med 1987;316:73–78.

PERITONEAL DIALYSIS

CONTINUOUS AMBULATORY PERITONEAL DIALYSIS AND CONTINUOUS CYCLIC PERITONEAL DIALYSIS

General Description

The diet emphasizes high protein intake to offset the loss of protein in the dialysate, adequate calories to maintain a desirable weight, and moderate sodium restriction.

Nutritional Inadequacy

As in hemodialysis, the patient undergoing peritoneal dialysis is at risk for deficiencies of water-soluble vitamins and minerals. The extent of losses is unknown. A daily multiple vitamin that includes water-soluble vitamins, particularly folic acid, is recommended. For patients receiving human recombinant EPO for correction of anemia, supplementation with iron may be necessary to maintain adequate iron stores to maximize the effectiveness of the drug.

Indications and Rationale

Currently, two types of peritoneal dialysis are utilized at the Mayo Clinic—continuous ambulatory peritoneal dialysis (CAPD) and continuous cyclic peritoneal dialysis (CCPD). Table 14-4 summarizes the dietary guidelines for CAPD and CCPD.

Continuous Ambulatory Peritoneal Dialysis. CAPD is a self-dialysis technique that does not require a machine, unlike other dialysis techniques. This self-dialysis technique is accomplished by having the patient perform exchanges of dialysate into the peritoneal cavity 4 to 5 times daily. Since dialysis is continuous, a steady state of metabolic end products, electrolytes, and fluid can be achieved.[27] Dialysis exchanges vary in volume and in concentration. Currently, each exchange is a volume of 1.0, 1.5, 2.0, or 3.0 L with a dextrose concentration of 1.5, 2.5, or 4.25%. The percentage is defined in grams of dextrose per deciliter.

TABLE 14-4 Dietary Recommendations for Peritoneal Dialysis

Component	CAPD	CCPD
Protein	1.2–1.5 g/kg of body weight	Same
Kilocalories	Dietary kcal = Total kcal Requirement − kcal from Dialysate kcal from Dialysate = Glucose Concentration (g/L) × 3.7 kcal/g × 0.8 × Volume (L)	Same
Sodium	90–120 mEq	Generally not restricted
Potassium	Use high potassium foods in moderation If serum potassium is elevated, restrict to 60–70 mEq	Generally not restricted
Fluid	Generally not restricted	Same
Phosphorus	Avoid very high phosphorus foods, except meat; limit milk to ½ cup/day	Same
Calcium	Calcium carbonate supplements as ordered by the physician	Same
Simple carbohydrates	If hypertriglyceridemia exists, or if above desired weight, limit intake	Same
Alcohol	If hypertriglyceridemia exists, avoid unless prescribed by physician to increase appetite	Same
Saturated fat	If hypercholesterolemia exists, use unsaturated fats rather than saturated fats	Same
Cholesterol	If hypercholesterolemia exists, restrict only if able to consume adequate protein from low cholesterol sources	Same

Perceived benefits of CAPD by the patient include freedom from in-center dialysis, liberalization of diet, and an increased sense of well-being. The major disadvantage of CAPD is the risk of peritonitis with the potential need for hospitalization.

Diabetic patients are frequently chosen to receive CAPD in the hope of better blood glucose control and lower morbidity.[28] The patient has the option of administering insulin directly into the dialysate bag, thus avoiding subcutaneous injections. When insulin is added to the dialysate, rather than being injected subcutaneously, less fluctuation of plasma glucose levels occurs. In general, the dose of insulin delivered in this manner is 3 to 4 times that required subcutaneously.

Continuous Cyclic Peritoneal Dialysis. CCPD is a home dialysis technique that utilizes an automated device to provide nocturnal exchanges. During each night there are five to six 2 L exchanges of approximately 1½ hours in duration. During each day there is a single 1 L exchange that dwells within the peritoneal cavity for approximately 12 hours or until initiation of dialysis that evening. There appears to be less risk of peritonitis with CCPD than with CAPD because the patient has fewer line connections to make (i.e., one connection at night and a disconnection in the morning as opposed to multiple daily connections with CAPD).[29]

Calories. Dietary caloric needs of the peritoneal dialysis patient are generally lower than for the hemodialysis patient because of the significant calorie contribution from the peritoneal dialysis exchanges. The literature[27] frequently cites the kilocalorie contribution of the dialysate as 400 to 800 kcal. However, the volumes of the exchanges vary greatly and thus affect this rough estimate. Dietary caloric needs can be calculated by determining total caloric needs (see Chapter 3, Nutritional Screening and Assessment) and subtracting the kilocalories provided by the dialysate.

Generally, it is assumed that 80% of the glucose in the dialysate is absorbed. The kilocalories contributed by the dialysate can be estimated by multiplying the grams of glucose (expressed as the monohydrate) by the number of liters, then by 3.7 kcal/g and then by 80%.[30] The following equations can be used:

Kcal From Dialysate = Glucose Concentration (g/L) × Volume (L) × 3.7 (kcal/g) × 0.8
For example, 2,000 ml of 4.25% glucose would provide approximately 231 kcal
(42.5 g/L × 2.0 L × 3.7 kcal/g × 0.8)

Protein. As in hemodialysis, peritoneal dialysis removes needed nutrients as well as unwanted waste products. Protein losses, primarily albumin, may be 9 g or more per day.[31] A protein intake of 1.2 to 1.5 g/kg/day is recommended to replace protein losses. Hemoglobin, serum albumin, urea, and total serum protein are used as the key indicators of adequacy of protein intake. Sudden decreases in these values are seen in patients with inadequate oral intake or with excessive losses accompanying peritonitis.

It has been suggested that appetite improves in patients receiving peritoneal dialysis so that increasing protein intake is easier.[31,32] However, this depends upon the individual. Many patients are unable to achieve the 1.2 to 1.5 g of protein range.[33] If the patient exhibits evidence of protein malnutrition, protein supplementation and/or maintenance hemodialysis may become necessary.[34]

Sodium.   Restriction of sodium is generally more liberal than in other treatment modalities for chronic renal failure. Current practice for CAPD is to recommend 90 to 120 mEq of sodium. Sodium restriction helps prevent fluid retention. If fluid retention were to occur, higher concentrations of dextrose in the dialysis exchanges would be required to remove edema fluid. Restriction of sodium is less necessary with CCPD than with CAPD because of greater losses in the dialysate during the 12 hour exchange. Unfortunately, chronic use of high dextrose concentrations in the dialysate promotes adipose tissue weight gain because of the added caloric intake. More rigorous sodium restriction may be necessary for patients with diabetes mellitus so that lower dextrose concentrations can be used in dialysis. Patients with hypertension, excess fluid weight gain, or congestive heart failure may also benefit from further reduction of sodium intake.

Potassium.   Serum potassium is usually kept within normal limits with CAPD because of the frequency of dialysis, so a potassium restriction is not always needed. However, hypokalemia can occur in patients on 5 exchanges per day.[32] Hyperkalemia can also occur owing to higher protein requirements and the corresponding higher potassium content of the diet. Dietary potassium should be limited to 60 to 70 mEq/day if the serum potassium is elevated. Otherwise, high potassium foods may be used in moderation. Restriction of potassium is less necessary with CCPD than with CAPD because the 12 hour exchange removes more of this mineral.

Fluid.   Restriction of fluid intake is usually not necessary. Up to 2 L/day may be tolerated and removed by using higher concentrations of dextrose in the dialysate. However, for some patients it may be preferable to restrict fluid and sodium intake to prevent edema rather than try to mobilize fluid by using a higher glucose concentration in the dialysate because the latter approach may result in excessive weight gain.

Phosphorus.   The need for phosphorus control with peritoneal dialysis is similar to that in hemodialysis patients. The goal is to normalize serum calcium and phosphorus levels to avoid hyperparathyroidism, thus minimizing skeletal changes and soft-tissue calcification. There is no evidence that the need for phosphate binders is reduced.[33] Dietary control of phosphorus is difficult due to recommendations for a higher meat intake, which is necessary to obtain adequate protein. Therefore, high phosphorus foods should be restricted when possible and lower phosphorus foods substituted. Food records can be used to assess current intake of phosphorus. (See Appendix 24 for phosphorus content of foods.)

Calcium.   Increased calcium intake is desirable. However, dairy products are generally limited in an effort to control serum phosphorus. Milk intake is limited to 1/2 cup per day unless the patient has difficulty consuming adequate protein. Milk may be an alternative for those who cannot obtain sufficient protein from meat because acceptance of milk is often better than for meat. An increase in the serum phosphorus level slightly above 5 mg/dl may be accepted in an attempt to achieve adequate protein intake. Milk intake is limited for the patient who is able to consume adequate protein from meat. Calcium supplements may be used in an effort to maintain serum calcium levels.

In most regards, the nutritional considerations for CCPD are similar to those for CAPD. In peritoneal dialysis substantial loss of protein in the dialysate means that the patient must maintain a high protein intake. Determination of caloric needs in CAPD and CCPD are similar, including calculations of the kilocalorie contribution of the dialysate. Given the previously mentioned need for a higher protein intake, phosphorus control can be difficult to achieve. Restriction of sodium, potassium, and fluid is less often necessary with CCPD than with CAPD because of the greater loss of these nutrients from the body to the dialysate during the 12 hour exchange. However, restriction of sodium and fluid are necessary if hypertension or fluid overload is present.

Other Nutritional Problems

Serum cholesterol and triglycerides increase with the length of peritoneal dialysis therapy. Kurtz et al[33] reported an increase in the very low-density lipoproteins and a low, but stable, high-density lipoprotein cholesterol fraction. Low-density lipoprotein (LDL) remained normal throughout therapy.

The reasons for the lipid changes are not known. It has been theorized that triglycerides become elevated because of the higher calorie intake and possible glucose absorption from the dialysate. The increase in triglycerides may also be related to an increase in weight, to changes in fatty acid oxidation, or to a decrease in lipoprotein lipase activity, which results in reduced peripheral triglyceride clearing.[35]

Weight control measures and restriction of cholesterol, saturated fat, simple carbohydrate, and alcohol are recommended to manage hyperlipidemia. These dietary modifications are recommended only to the degree that they are possible without compromising adequacy of protein and nonprotein caloric intake. Cholesterol intake usually cannot be greatly decreased because of the need for adequate protein. In fact, patients who have nausea or taste acuity changes are often advised to consume high quality protein in the form of eggs in an attempt to meet their needs. Generally, unsaturated fats can be substituted for saturated fats, and it may be possible to reduce total fat intake slightly. However, since high protein foods are often sources of fat, it may not be possible to greatly reduce total fat intake. Simple carbohydrates and alcohol are restricted as a means of controlling hypertriglyceridemia but also to control weight gain, which may have a greater effect on the hyperlipidemia.

Weight gain is commonly seen with peritoneal dialysis.[36] The dialysate contributes a significant caloric load. It appears that the weight gain is the result of fat deposition and correction of protein deficits, with an associated increase in the mass of muscle since hypertension and edema are generally not seen with such weight gains. Avoidance of excessive weight gain is an important aspect of nutritional care, especially for those patients who use higher concentrations of dextrose.

Dehydration may occur with peritoneal dialysis and should be anticipated when a change is made from hemodialysis to peritoneal dialysis. Dehydration is characterized by excessive fluid removal and extracellular fluid volume deficits, manifested by weight loss and low blood pressure, especially drops in orthostatic blood pressure. A lower concentration of dextrose in the dialysate may be effective in correcting dehydration. Dehydration may also occur in people who are extremely weight conscious and who restrict their calorie and/or sodium intake excessively.

Another common nutritional problem is early satiety. The intra-abdominal volume of the dialysate may cause the patient to feel full and to have difficulty consuming adequate nutrients, particularly protein. It may be helpful for the patient to drain the dialysate prior to meal time and to reinfuse with the fresh exchange at the end of the meal. Small, frequent meals also may help to relieve the sense of fullness.

Goals of Dietary Management

The goals of dietary management are (1) to provide sufficient protein to compensate for large losses of protein and essential amino acids in the dialysate and to maintain nitrogen balance; (2) to limit sodium intake if necessary to control blood pressure and thirst and to prevent excess edema; (3) to prevent excessive weight gain; (4) to limit phosphorus to control hyperphosphatemia and renal osteodystrophy; and (5) to control hyperlipidemia.

Dietary Recommendations

The food exchange list for protein, sodium, and potassium control can be used for meal planning (see pp. 348–356). Modifications can be made to liberalize sodium and potassium restrictions. Additional modifications may be necessary for restriction of saturated fat or phosphorus (see Appendix 24).

Physicians: How to Order Diet

The diet order should indicate: *diet for CAPD or CCPD.*

The dietitian will calculate caloric needs based on the concentration of the dialysate and on the number of exchanges made each day. The diet order should also indicate if weight loss is desired. The dietitian will follow the preceding guidelines for modification of other dietary constituents.

References

27. Nolph KD, Lindblad AS, Novak JW. Current concepts: continuous ambulatory peritoneal dialysis. New Engl J Med 1988;318:1595–1600.
28. Senekjian H, Koerpel BJ. CAPD in the diabetic patient. Dialysis Transplant 1984;13: 780–783, 812.
29. Diamond SM, Henrich WL. Nutrition and peritoneal dialysis. In: Mitch W, Klahr S, eds. Nutrition and the kidney. Boston: Little, Brown, 1988:198–223.
30. McCann L. Peritoneal dialysis and nutritional considerations. In: Gillit D, Stover J, Spinozzi NS, eds. A clinical guide to nutrition care in end-stage renal disease. Chicago: The American Dietetic Association, 1987:43–51.
31. Bouma S, Dwyer JT. Glucose absorption and weight change in 18 months of CAPD. JADA 1984;84:194–197.
32. Moncrief JW. Continuous ambulatory peritoneal dialysis: impact on management of patients with end-stage renal disease. Nephron 1981;27:226–268.
33. Kurtz SB, Wong VH, Anderson CF, Vogel JP, McCarthy JT, Mitchell JC, Kumar R, Johnson WJ. Continuous ambulatory peritoneal dialysis: three-years' experience at the Mayo Clinic. Mayo Clin Proc 1983;54:633–639.
34. Smathers JS, Moles K, Sandroni S. Strategies to improve protein intake in peritoneal dialysis patients. J Renal Nutr 1992;2:33–36.

35. Easter G. Guidelines for nutritional intervention of the adult CAPD patient. Contemp Dial Nephrol 1989;July:20–27.

36 Baig F, Brubaker KA, Ali AS. Nutritional implications in CAPD. Contemp Dial 1982;Mar: 37–41.

NEPHROTIC SYNDROME

General Description

The diet emphasizes controlled intake of sodium, protein, and kilocalories.

Nutritional Inadequacy

The diet is not inherently lacking in nutrients as compared to the RDA.

Indications and Rationale

Nephrotic syndrome arises from the abnormal passage of plasma proteins into the urine as a result of increased glomerular capillary membrane permeability. A number of pathological processes result in glomerular capillary wall injury, including immune complex diseases affecting the kidney (e.g., lupus nephritis) and diabetic renal disease. A 24-hour urinary protein excretion greater than 3.0 g is indicative of nephrotic range proteinuria.[37]

The nephrotic syndrome is characterized by increased urinary excretion of albumin and other serum proteins, accompanied by hypoalbuminemia and edema formation. A sodium intake range of 60 to 90 mEq is usually quite helpful in the control of hypertension (often in conjunction with blood pressure medications) and edema. (See Chapter 7, Hypertension.)

Increased dietary protein does stimulate albumin synthesis but it may also increase glomerular permeability. The result is that the albumin synthesized is lost in the urine. In addition, excessive protein may be responsible for an increased glomerular filtration rate and renal blood flow, which may accelerate the progression of glomerular sclerosis.[37]

Therefore, according to current research, a dietary protein intake of 0.8 to 1 g/kg/day is generally recommended for patients with normal serum creatinine and urea levels.[38-40] However, if a patient with reasonably good renal function develops protein calorie malnutrition, has proteinuria greater than 15 g of protein per day, is receiving high dose corticosteroid therapy, or has other conditions that may require a higher protein intake to avoid malnutrition, a trial period of moderately increased dietary protein intake is recommended. There is no certainty that this increase will maintain or restore optimal nutritional status, but it should be attempted under close medical supervision.[40] In cases where the glomerular filtration rate is decreased, the amount of protein allowed should be determined in the same way as for patients with chronic renal failure, with an additional amount of protein equivalent to the 24 hour urinary protein loss.

Caloric intake for patients with nephrotic syndrome should be calculated according to individual needs (see Chapter 3, Nutritional Screening and Assessment).

TABLE 14-5 Dietary Guidelines in Nephrotic Syndrome

Components	Comments
Kilocalories	Sufficient for weight maintenance, weight gain, or slow weight loss ($1/2$ to 1 lb/week)
Protein	Generally 0.8–1.0 g of dietary protein per kg of body weight in patients with normal creatinine and urea levels
	If protein needs are high because of malnutrition or other concurrent conditions, and if renal function is good, a moderately increased protein intake may be warranted
	If the glomerular filtration rate is reduced, less than 0.8 g of dietary protein per kg of body weight plus 24 hr urinary protein loss
Sodium	60–90 mEq of sodium
	Calculate the sodium level to ± 10% of the diet order
Cholesterol and fat	Stringent dietary restrictions not necessary

Care should be taken to avoid insufficient caloric intake since this results in catabolism of lean body tissue.[41] Weight reduction should be approached cautiously because of the risk of catabolism of lean body tissue (i.e., proteins) in addition to fat. Stringent caloric restriction is not recommended unless immediate weight loss is compelling. A slow to moderate weight loss of no more than $1/2$ to 1 lb/week is recommended. Table 14-5 summarizes the dietary guidelines for nephrotic syndrome.

Other Nutritional Problems

Hyperlipidemia is a common manifestation of nephrotic syndrome. Increased serum concentration of total cholesterol and LDL cholesterol have been the most frequently reported abnormalities in patients with nephrotic syndrome. In addition, increases in triglycerides and very low-density lipoproteins have been found, especially in patients with massive proteinuria.[42] It is felt that these elevated serum lipid concentrations are due to increases in lipoprotein production. Typically, serum albumin concentrations are inversely related to serum lipid concentrations.

The extent to which hyperlipidemia contributes to the development and progression of atherosclerosis in patients with nephrotic syndrome is unclear.[40,42] Until conclusive studies are available, and in light of other dietary restrictions, dietary treatment of hyperlipidemia remains a secondary goal. However, when possible, patients will be advised to follow a lipid lowering regimen (see Chapter 7, Hyperlipidemia). Treatment directed toward inhibiting cholesterol and LDL synthesis with the hydroxymethylglutanyl-coenzyme A reductase inhibitors has been suggested and is currently under investigation.[43,44]

Goals of Dietary Management

The primary goals of dietary management are to control hypertension, minimize edema, decrease urinary albumin loss, offset protein malnutrition, slow progression of renal disease, prevent muscle catabolism, and supply adequate energy. Control of hyperlipidemia, which is a common manifestation, is not a primary dietary concern at this time, but current research indicates a need for further evaluation.

Dietary Recommendations

The food exchange list for protein and sodium control can be used for meal planning. This list appears on pages 348 through 356.

Physicians: How to Order Diet

The diet order should indicate: the *specific level of protein* (see preceding guidelines) and the *specific level of sodium* (the usual range is 60 to 90 mEq). The dietitian will calculate caloric needs.

References

37. Mansy H, Goodship THJ, Tapson JS, Hartley GH, Keavfy P, Wilkinson R. Effect of a high protein diet in patients with the nephrotic syndrome. Clin Sci 1989;77:445–451.
38. Olmer M, Pain C, Dussol B, Berland Y. Protein diet and nephrotic syndrome. Kidney Int 1989;36(27):S152–S153.
39. Kaysen GA. Nutritional management of nephrotic syndrome. J Renal Nutr 1992;2(2):50–58.
40. Kaysen GA. The nephrotic syndrome: nutritional consequences and dietary management. In: Mitch WE, Klahr S, eds. Nutrition and the kidney. Boston: Little, Brown, 1993:213–242.
41. Guarnieri GF, Toigo G, Situlin R, Carraro M, Tamaro G, Lucchesli A, Oldrizzi L, Rugiu C, Maschio G. Nutritional state in patients on long-term low-protein diet or with nephrotic syndrome. Kidney Int 1989;36(27):S195–S200.
42. Keane WF, Kasiske BL. Hyperlipidemia in the nephrotic syndrome. N Engl J Med 1990; 323(9):603–604.
43. Joven J, Villabona C, Vilella E, Masana L, Alberti R, Valles M. Abnormalities of lipoprotein metabolism in patients with the nephrotic syndrome. N Engl J Med 1990;323(9):579–584.
44. Rabelink AJ, Hene RJ, Erkelens DW, Joles JA, Koomans HA. Effect of simvastatin and cholestyramine on lipoprotein profile in hyperlipidemia of nephrotic syndrome. Lancet 1988;2(8624):1335–1338.

UROLITHIASIS

General Description

Generous fluid intake is recommended in the management of all types of kidney stone disease. Other diet modifications are based on the type of stone formed and are generally directed at reduction of excessive intake of a particular dietary constituent.[45]

Indications and Rationale

The major components of urinary stones are calcium, oxalate, uric acid, phosphate, and cystine. Chemical analysis of stones can determine the predominant components. Recommendations for or contraindications to dietary modification are discussed for each of these constituents and for other nutritional factors affecting urolithiasis.[46-49]

Dilution of the urine is of primary importance.[48,50,51] The goal is to minimize precipitation of the offending substance into urinary stones. Fluid intake should be distributed throughout the day to assure a constantly high urine output. In general, the patient should be advised to drink 240 to 300 ml (8 to 10 oz) of fluid per hour while awake and on one occasion during the night if arising to void. Fluid must be consumed to maintain a recommended urine volume of 2 L/day for women and 2.5 L/day for men. More fluid intake is recommended in warm climates and for physically active people.

At least half of the fluid ingested should be water. Other beverages may contain large amounts of potentially lithogenic substances and may need to be restricted. See the following individual sections for beverages that may require restriction.

References

45. Wendland BE. Nutritional management of patients with kidney stones. Nephrol News Issues 1991;Oct:32–43.

46. Smith LH, Van Den Berg CJ, Wilson DM. Nutrition and urolithiasis. N Engl J Med 1978; 298:87.

47. Benson EA, Brannen GE, Bush WH. Urinary tract stones: medical management. Postgrad Med J 1985;77:193–198, 201.

48. Lingeman JE, Preminger GM, Wilson DM. Kidney stones: medical management. Patient Care 1990;Oct 15:85–105.

49. Coe FL, Parks JH, Asplin JR. The pathogenesis and treatment of kidney stones. N Engl J Med 1992;327:1141–1152.

50. Vahlensieck W. The importance of diet in urinary stones. Urol Res 1986;14:283–288.

51. Consensus Conference. Prevention and treatment of kidney stones. JAMA 1988;260(7): 977–981.

CALCIUM CONTROL

General Description

Calcium intake can be controlled by restricting milk and foods made from milk.

Nutritional Inadequacy

Diets for the management of hypercalciuria are not inherently lacking in nutrients for adults age 25 to 50 as compared to the RDA. Recommendations of 800 mg of calcium for men and 1000 mg for women will not meet the RDA for individuals under 25 years of age or for pregnant and breast-feeding women. However, calcium supplements are not advised.

Indications and Rationale

In normal persons, urinary calcium excretion has little correlation with calcium consumption since intestinal absorption of calcium decreases when dietary intake is excessive.

Half of the patients with idiopathic calcium urolithiasis (ICU) have normal urinary calcium levels. The other half have elevated urinary calcium, which can be due to three causes: 10% of these patients have renal hypercalciuria due to a renal "leak" of calcium; the remaining 90% are equally divided between those who have absorptive hypercalciuria, diet independent (type I), in which urinary calcium is elevated irrespective of dietary calcium intake, and those who have absorptive hypercalciuria, diet dependent (type II), in which urinary calcium is elevated only with high dietary calcium intake (Fig. 14-1).

It is recommended that patients with absorptive hypercalciuria, diet dependent (type II) follow a calcium controlled diet. However, the recommended level of calcium intake depends upon the sex of the individual. Men are advised to limit their calcium intake to 800 mg/day. Prior to the onset of menopause, women are advised to consume 1,000 mg of calcium per day, while it is recommended that postmenopausal women consume 1,200 mg/day. Restriction of daily calcium intake to less than these levels yields no additional clinical benefit and is usually not recommended, since it may result in a negative calcium balance. Also, a low calcium intake tends to increase oxalate absorption from the diet due to its decreased availability in the gastrointestinal tract to bind with the oxalate, thus potentially increasing the risk of stone formation.[52] In addition to a controlled calcium intake, these patients are advised to decrease their oxalate intake (see Oxalate Restriction, p. 339).

An excessive calcium intake should be avoided because it may produce hypercalciuria significant enough to promote stone formation, even when intestinal calcium absorption is normal.[53] Patients with absorptive hypercalciuria, diet independent (type I) and renal hypercalciuria should limit their calcium intake to approximately 800 to 1,000 mg/day.

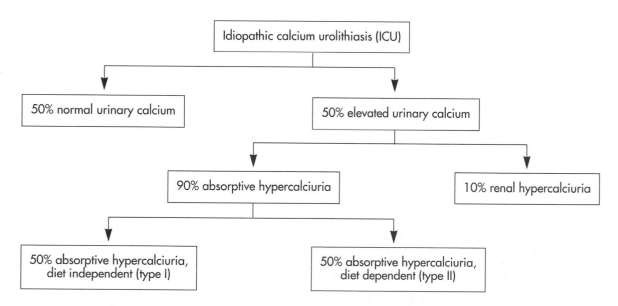

FIGURE 14-1 Occurrence of idiopathic calcium urolithiasis.

Excessive amounts of dietary sodium, animal protein, and sugars can aggravate hypercalciuria. Therefore, excesses of these dietary constituents should be avoided in patients with hypercalciuria. Patients should be encouraged to be prudent with their intake of these constituents.

A moderate sodium restriction (90 to 150 mEq/day) may be beneficial to patients with hypercalciuria by reducing the amount of calcium excreted in the urine.[53,54] When thiazide diuretics are used to reduce the urinary excretion of calcium, high sodium intake can overcome the response. Therefore, a 90 mEq sodium restriction should be followed in conjunction with thiazide medication (see Chapter 7, Hypertension).

A high insoluble fiber diet has been shown to increase fecal calcium excretion by binding calcium and preventing its absorption.[55] Bran fiber provides phytic acid, which combines with dietary calcium in the intestine to form calcium phytate, which is excreted in the stool, thus lessening the excretion of calcium via the kidney. Fiber also decreases gut transit time, thus reducing time for calcium absorption.[56]

Hypercalciuria is a common complication of spinal cord injury (SCI) and non-weight-bearing immobilization. It is also associated with a high incidence of urolithiasis in SCI patients. However, bladder stones in SCI patients are frequently the consequence of indwelling Foley catheters and bladder infections.[57]

Calcium is not routinely restricted for SCI patients. Adequate calcium is recommended to prevent negative calcium balance and its long-term consequences. Hypercalciuria may lead to negative calcium balance and osteoporosis, thus resulting in fractures of the long bones in the lower extremities. Lack of weight bearing leads to calcium loss from bone and, in turn, hypercalciuria.

Goals of Dietary Management

The goals of dietary management are to reduce the level of calcium in the urine and to maintain a dilute urine.

Dietary Recommendations

Sufficient control of calcium can generally be accomplished by limiting milk and foods made from large amounts of milk. However, other foods such as sardines, fish canned with bones, quick-cooking cereals, quick breads, sweet potato, beet greens, Swiss chard, collards, dandelion greens, kale, mustard greens, okra, spinach, turnip greens, endive, escarole, rhubarb, and dried fruits may contribute a substantial amount of calcium to the diet if used frequently and in large amounts. It is not necessary to restrict these foods unless a diet history reveals a high frequency of use and the situation warrants their exclusion.

The calcium content of a diet that includes a variety of foods but no milk products can be estimated to provide approximately 200 mg of calcium per 1,000 kcal/day. For most persons this is equivalent to 300 to 500 mg of calcium per day. The amounts of milk and milk products permitted in the diet must be carefully planned to achieve the desired level of calcium[58] (Table 14-6).

Physicians: How to Order Diet

The diet order should indicate: the *specific level of calcium* desired, such as 800 mg to 1,000 mg.

TABLE 14-6   Calcium Control

General Recommendations

Fluid: 250–300 ml/hr while awake and on one occasion at night if patient arises; at least 50% as water
Sodium: Moderate restriction, 90–150 mEq/day, or avoidance of excessive sodium intake
Fiber: High fiber diet

Disorder	Specific Recommendations

Absorptive Hypercalciuria, Diet Dependent (type II)	Calcium controlled diet
	Men: 800 mg/day
	Women:
	   Premenopause—1,000 mg/day
	   Postmenopause—1,200 mg/day
	Oxalate controlled diet (see Tables 14-7 and 14-8)

Renal Hypercalciuria and Absorptive Hypercalciuria, Diet Independent (type I)	Encourage adequate, but not excessive calcium intake
Hypercalciuria resulting from immobilization (e.g., spinal cord injury)	Encourage adequate calcium intake

The dietitian will make additional recommendations according to the preceding guidelines.

References

52. Curhan GC, Willett WC, Rimm EB, Stampfer MJ. A prospective study of dietary calcium and other nutrients and the risk of symptomatic kidney stones. N Engl J Med 1993;328: 833–838.
53. Pak CYC, Smith LH, Resnick MI, Weinerth JL. Dietary management of idiopathic calcium urolithiasis. J Urol 1984;131:850–852.
54. Muldowney FP, Freaney R, Moloney MF. Importance of dietary sodium in the hypercalciuria syndrome. Kidney Int 1982;22:292–296.
55. Vahlensieck W. The importance of diet in urinary stones. Urol Res 1986;14:283–288.
56. Shah PJR, Williams G, Green NA. Idiopathic hypercalciuria: its control with unprocessed bran. Br J Urol 1980;52:426–429.
57. Lamid S, El Ghatit AZ, Melvin JL. Relationship of hypercalciuria to diet and bladder stone formation in spinal cord injury patients. Am J Phys Med 1984;63:182–187.
58. Pennington JAT. Bowes and Church's food values of portions commonly used, 16th ed. Philadelphia: JB Lippincott, 1994.

OXALATE RESTRICTION

General Description

Oxalic acid occurs primarily in food of plant origin. The diet excludes foods that are high in oxalates and is intended to provide less than 50 mg of oxalate per day.

Nutritional Inadequacy

There are no nutritional inadequacies inherent in an oxalate restricted diet.

Indications and Rationale

Oxalic acid, or oxalate, is the end product of both glyoxylic acid and ascorbic acid metabolism. Normal urinary excretion of oxalate is less than 0.48 mM per 24 hours, of which approximately 10% comes from oxalate in the diet. However, large fluctuations in urinary oxalate may be attributable to variations in diet.[59]

Dietary calcium and oxalate absorption are inversely related. Calcium normally combines with oxalate in the intestinal lumen and makes it less available for absorption. Therefore, a diet extremely low in calcium will increase urinary oxalate excretion.

Urine is commonly supersaturated with calcium oxalate since this compound is poorly soluble. Small increases in urinary oxalate concentration greatly increase the potential for crystal formation. Control of dietary oxalate may be of benefit to those who are susceptible to calcium oxalate urolithiasis since increased urinary excretion of oxalate is likely after ingestion of high oxalate foods.

Restriction of oxalate, in addition to a calcium controlled diet, is recommended for absorptive hypercalciuria type II. A low calcium diet tends to increase oxalate absorption from the diet because of decreased availability of calcium to bind oxalate.[60] Once absorbed into the body, the oxalate is not metabolized, but excreted into the urine. An oxalate and calcium controlled diet effectively reduces the rate of stone formation. However, many persons find strict long-term adherence to this type of diet difficult[61] (Tables 14-7 and 14-8).

Enteric hyperoxaluria is a consequence of intestinal malabsorption.[66] The increase in urinary oxalate excretion is attributable to enhanced absorption of dietary oxalate. Oxalate is normally sequestered by calcium in the intestinal lumen and is poorly absorbed. In malabsorptive states, fatty acids bind with calcium so that oxalate is more available for absorption. The malabsorbed fatty acids and bile salts also increase colonic permeability to oxalate. A low fat diet may be warranted

---

TABLE 14-7   Oxalate Restriction

General Recommendations

Diet: Low oxalate
Fluid: 240 to 300 ml/hr while awake and on one occasion at night if patient arises; 50% as water
Ascorbic acid: No more than 1 g/day

Additional Recommendations

Idiopathic hyperoxaluria: adequate calcium intake
Absorptive hypercalciuria, type II: calcium controlled diet (see pp. 336–339)
Enteric hyperoxaluria: high calcium intake (supplement with 1 g of calcium carbonate); low fat diet if
   there is significant steatorrhea

TABLE 14-8 Approximate Oxalate Content of Selected Foods*[62-65]

Little or No Oxalate (<2 mg/serving)	Moderate Oxalate (2–10 mg/serving)	High Oxalate (>10 mg/serving)
BEVERAGES		
Beer, bottled (light, mild flavor)	Coffee (limit to 8 oz/day)	Beer, 4 oz/day (dark, robust)
Carbonated cola (limit to 12 oz/day)		Ovaltine and other beverage mixes
Distilled alcohol		Tea
Lemonade or limeade without added		Chocolate milk
vitamin C		Cocoa
Wine: red, rosé, white (3–4 oz)		
MILK		
Buttermilk		
Whole, low fat, or skim milk		
Yogurt with allowed fruit		
MEAT AND MEAT SUBSTITUTES		
Eggs	Sardines	Baked beans canned in tomato sauce
Cheese		($^1/_3$ cup)
Beef, lamb, or pork		Tofu ($^1/_2$ cup)
Poultry		
Fish and shellfish		
VEGETABLES ($^1/_2$ cup cooked, 1 cup raw)		
Avocado	Asparagus	Beans: green, wax, dried
Cauliflower	Broccoli	Beets: root, greens
Cabbage	Brussels sprouts	Celery
Mushrooms	Carrots	Chives
Onions	Corn: sweet white or yellow	Collards
Peas, green (fresh or frozen)	Green peas, canned	Cucumbers
Potatoes, white	Lettuce	Dandelion greens
Radishes	Lima beans	Eggplant
	Parsnips	Escarole
	Tomato, 1 small or juice (4 oz)	Kale
	Turnips	Leeks
		Mustard greens
		Okra
		Parsley
		Peppers, green
		Pokeweed
		Potatoes, sweet
		Rutabagas
		Spinach
		Summer squash
		Swiss Chard
		Watercress
FRUITS/JUICES ($^1/_2$ cup canned or juice, 1 medium fruit)		
Apple and apple juice	Apricots	Blackberries
Avocado	Black currants	Blueberries
Banana	Cherries, red sour	Currants, red
Cherries, Bing	Cranberry juice (4 oz)	Dewberries

Continued.

TABLE 14-8 Approximate Oxalate Content of Selected Foods*[62-65]—cont'd

Little or No Oxalate (<2 mg/serving)	Moderate Oxalate (2–10 mg/serving)	High Oxalate (>10 mg/serving)
FRUITS/JUICES—cont'd		
Grapefruit, fruit and juice	Grape juice (4 oz)	Fruit cocktail
Grapes, green	Orange, fruit and juice (4 oz)	Grapes, purple
Mangoes	Peaches	Gooseberries
Melons: cantaloupe, casaba, honeydew, watermelon	Pears	Lemon peel
	Pineapple	Lime peel
Nectarines	Plums, purple	Orange peel
Pineapple juice	Prunes	Raspberries
Plums, green or yellow		Rhubarb
		Strawberries
		Tangerine
		Juices made from the above fruits
BREAD/STARCHES		
Bread	Cornbread (2" square)	Amaranth (½ cup)
Breakfast cereals	Sponge cake (1" slice)	Fruit cake
Macaroni	Spaghetti, canned in tomato sauce (½ cup)	Grits, white corn
Noodles		Soybean crackers
Rice		Wheat germ and bran (1 cup)
Spaghetti		
FATS/OILS		
Bacon		Nuts: peanuts, almonds, pecans, cashews, walnuts (⅓ cup)
Mayonnaise		
Salad dressing		Nut butters (6 Tbsp)
Vegetable oils		Sesame seeds (1 cup)
Butter, margarine		
MISCELLANEOUS		
Coconut	Chicken noodle soup, dehydrated	Carob or tahini (¾ cup)
Jelly or preserves (made with allowed fruits)		Chocolate, cocoa (3–4 oz)
		Vegetable soup (½ cup)
Lemon, lime juice		Tomato soup (½ cup)
Salt, pepper (limit to 1 tsp/day)		Marmalade (5 Tbsp)
Soups with allowed ingredients		
Sugar		

*Considerable variation exists in the oxalate content of a single type of food. Factors such as growing conditions, age of the plant, bioavailability, and the patient's gastrointestinal abnormalities all affect individual absorption of oxalate.[65] Therefore, the foods have been categorized into low, moderate, and high oxalate groups rather than giving exact values. The data available on the oxalate content of foods are limited and variable. Many foods have been analyzed for oxalate content using specific name brands or varieties. Data have been extrapolated to include the broader category of food for which analysis of oxalate content is available. The diet is intended to limit oxalate intake to less than 50 mg/day. Therefore, foods high in oxalate should be restricted and food with moderate oxalate should be limited. Little or no oxalate containing foods may be consumed as desired unless a portion size is indicated.

if steatorrhea is significant. Calcium restriction is contraindicated because of the mechanisms of increased oxalate absorption. In fact, calcium supplements up to 1 g/day may be recommended.[67] The poor calcium absorption in these patients usually protects against hypercalciuria, which should be watched for as a potential hazard.

Oxalate is an end product of ascorbic acid metabolism; therefore, ascorbic acid supplementation may increase urinary oxalate excretion. If supplementation with ascorbic acid is warranted, limit the level to 1 g/day. Patients should be cautioned not to exceed this amount.

Goals of Dietary Management

The goals of dietary management are to reduce the level of oxalate in the urine and to maintain a dilute urine.

Dietary Recommendations

The dietary recommendations for an oxalate reduced diet are given in Table 14-7.

Physicians: How to Order Diet

The diet order should indicate: *low oxalate diet.*

The dietitian will make additional recommendations according to the preceding guidelines.

References

59. Finch AM, Kasidas GP, Rose GA. Urine composition in normal subjects after oral ingestion of oxalate-rich foods. Clin Sci 1981;60:411–418.
60. Massey LK, Sutton RAL. Modification of dietary oxalate and calcium reduces urinary oxalate in hyperoxaluric patients with kidney stones. JADA 1993;93(11):1305–1307.
61. Hodgkinson A. Comment: Is there a place for a low-oxalate diet? J Hum Nutr 1981;35:136.
62. Massey LK, Roman-Smith H, Sutton RAL. Effect of dietary oxalate and calcium on urinary oxalate and risk of formation of calcium oxalate kidney stones. JADA 1993;93(8)901–906.
63. Ney DM, Hofmann AF, Fischer C, Stubblefield N. The low oxalate diet book for the prevention of oxalate kidney stones. San Diego: University of California Press, 1981.
64. Krause M, Mahan L. Food nutrition and diet therapy, 7th ed. Philadelphia: WB Saunders, 1984:944–945.
65. Brinkley L, McGuire J, Gregory J, Pak CYC. Bioavailability of oxalate in foods. Urology 1981;17:534–538.
66. Stauffer JQ. Hyperoxaluria and calcium oxalate nephrolithiasis after jejunoileal bypass. Am J Clin Nutr 1977;30:64–71.
67. Lingeman JE, Preminger GM, Wilson DM. Kidney stones: medical management. Patient Care 1990;Oct 15:85–105.

PHOSPHATE RESTRICTION

Attempts to control the formation of phosphate-containing stones through the use of a low phosphate diet and phosphate binding agents have been largely unsuccessful and are no longer used in the management of stone disease.

LOW METHIONINE DIET

Cystinuria is an inherited disorder that involves decreased gastrointestinal and renal transport of the amino acids cystine, lysine, arginine, and ornithine. The only major complication in this disorder is the tendency to form cystine stones because of the low urinary solubility of cystine. Cystine is the end product of methionine metabolism. Urinary excretion of cystine can be lowered by reducing dietary intake of methionine, and this can be accomplished by decreasing the total protein content of the diet. Stringent restriction of protein is rarely recommended; however, excessive dietary protein (more than 100 g/day) should be avoided.[68] Alkalinization of the urine increases solubility of cystine; thus, avoidance of acid-ash foods increases the effectiveness of alkalizing agents. A low sodium diet may be beneficial because a high sodium intake increases urinary excretion of cystine.[69]

References

68. Vahlensieck W. The importance of diet in urinary stones. Urol Res 1986;14:283–288.
69. Jaeger P, Portmann L, Saunders A, Rosenberg L, Thier S. Anticystinuric effects of glutamine and of dietary sodium restriction. N Engl J Med 1986;315:1120–1123.

PURINE RESTRICTION

General Description

Specific kinds of meats and meat extracts are high in purines.

Nutritional Inadequacy

There are no nutritional inadequacies inherent in a purine restricted diet.

Indications and Rationale

Persons with disorders affecting purine metabolism, such as gout and urinary uric acid lithiasis, may be advised to reduce their intake of purine.

Uric acid stones may develop as a result of hyperuricuria, dehydration, or excessive acidity of the urine. Uric acid is the end product of purine metabolism. Foods high in purines generally have a high acid-ash content and tend to acidify the urine and increase urinary excretion of uric acid. Exclusion of foods extremely high in purines may be helpful.[70]

Goals of Dietary Management

The goals of purine restriction are to supplement the effect of medication by decreasing plasma and urine levels of uric acid.

Dietary Recommendations

Historically, dietary efforts to reduce purine intake have been relatively comprehensive. All meats, fish, and poultry contain moderate to high amounts of purine. Some vegetables contain low to moderate amounts of purine. Efforts to greatly restrict these foods are generally unnecessary because of their relatively insignificant effect compared to that of medications aimed at reducing uric acid excretion.

TABLE 14-9 Dietary Recommendations for Gout and Hyperuricemia[72-74]

Purines are normally formed in the body during the metabolic breakdown of nucleoproteins. In certain genetic disorders, including gout, the relatively insoluble purine, *uric acid,* tends to accumulate and deposit in the toes and other joints. Drug treatment is generally prescribed for patients with gout; however, dietary restriction of purine yielding foods may also be advised.

- *Avoid Foods Highest in Purines (150–825 mg/100 g)*
  Anchovies (363 mg/100 g)
  Brains
  Kidney (beef—200 mg/100 g)
  Game meats
  Gravies
  Herring
  Liver (calf, beef—233 mg/100 g)
  Sardines (295 mg/100 g)
  Scallops
  Sweetbreads (825 mg/100 g)

- *Limit Foods High in Purines (50–150 mg/100 g)*
  Asparagus
  Breads and cereals, whole grain
  Cauliflower
  Eel
  Fish, fresh and saltwater
  Legumes, beans, lentils, peas
  Meat—beef, lamb, pork, veal
  Meat soups and broths
  Mushrooms
  Oatmeal
  Peas, green
  Poultry—chicken, duck, turkey
  Shellfish—crab, lobster, oysters
  Spinach
  Wheat germ and bran

- *Consume Foods Lowest in Purines (0–50 mg/100 g)*
  Beverages—coffee, tea, sodas
  Breads and cereals except whole grain
  Cheese
  Eggs
  Fats
  Fish roe
  Fruits and fruit juices
  Gelatin
  Milk
  Nuts
  Sugars, syrups, sweets
  Vegetables (except those listed above)
  Vegetable and cream soups

- *Reduce Weight if Overweight*

- *Avoid Alcohol*

It is generally sufficient to simply avoid an excessive intake of purines since the diet is considered an auxiliary measure to medications.

Specific Dietary Recommendations

Avoid excessive intake of meat, fish, and poultry. Intake of dietary protein should not exceed 100 g daily,[71] since excessive animal protein may increase urinary uric acid from purine load and lower urine pH. Avoid extremely high purine foods, and limit the intake of high purine foods (see Table 14-9).[72] Those with gout should reduce weight if overweight. Weight loss should be gradual because rapid weight loss can aggravate hyperuricuria and decrease urine pH. Excessive alcohol intake should also be avoided.[73,74]

Physicians: How to Order Diet

The diet order should indicate: *purine control.*

References

70. Lingeman JE, Preminger GM, Wilson DM. Kidney stones: medical management. Patient Care 1990;Oct 15:85–105.
71. Vahlensieck W. The importance of diet in urinary stones. Urol Res 1986;14:283–288.
72. Pennington JAT. Bowes and Church's food values of portions commonly used, 16th ed. Philadelphia: JB Lippincott, 1994:387.
73. Faller J, Fox IH. Ethanol-induced hyperuricemia. N Engl J Med 1982;307:1598–1602.
74. Roubenoff R. Gout and hyperuricemia. Rheum Dis Clin North Am 1990;16(3):539–550.

OTHER DIETARY CONSIDERATIONS: ACID-ASH AND ALKALINE-ASH DIETS

General Description

Foods that render the urine acid are spoken of as "acid-ash" foods since the ash remaining after their metabolism is acid in reaction. Foods that leave alkaline ash after metabolism cause the urine to become alkaline.

Indications and Rationale

Dietary manipulations that decrease the pH of the urine may be useful in the management of infection-type urinary stones and, together with methenamine mandelate, some urinary tract infections. Alkalinization of the urine may retard formation of uric acid, cystine, and calcium oxalate calculi.[75,76]

Description of foods as either acid-ash or alkaline-ash is based on the reaction of the ash that remains after the combustion of foods under laboratory conditions. Acid-ash foods tend to promote a more acidic urine. Conversely, alkaline-ash foods tend to promote a more alkaline urine. Tables are available that list amounts of acid or alkali to be derived from the metabolism of various foods, but there are enough uncertainties in the application of these data that planning diets to manipulate the pH of the urine should be regarded as qualitative rather than quantitative.[77] An acid-ash or alkaline-ash diet is generally considered to be supplemental to acidifying or alkalinizing medications.

Catabolic states tend to favor an acid urine. Even such a minor process of catabolism as overnight fasting results in an acid urine. In addition, the average diet is somewhat acid-ash.

The use of cranberry juice has gained popular appeal and may be self-prescribed by some persons. Normal amounts of cranberry juice may be consumed, if desired, since it is a liquid; however, it contains oxalate and provides no apparent benefits other than the fluid it provides.[78]

Goals of Dietary Management

The goal of acid- and alkaline-ash diets is to supplement the effect of medications in altering the pH of the urine.

Dietary Recommendations

Both acid-ash and alkaline-ash diets tend to become monotonous so that compliance by the patient is often poor. Since diet is generally considered an auxiliary measure to acidifying or alkalinizing medications, it may be sufficient to simply avoid excessive use of particular foods. For example, if medical treatment is directed at acidifying the urine, the diet should not contain large amounts of alkaline-ash foods; complete avoidance of all alkaline-ash foods, however, probably would not yield any further benefit and is unwarranted. A strict dietary regimen is rarely necessary.

Potentially Acid or Acid-Ash Foods	
Meat	Meat, fish, fowl, shellfish, eggs, all types of cheese, peanut butter, peanuts
Fat	Bacon, nuts (Brazil nuts, filberts, walnuts)
Starch	All types of bread (especially whole-wheat), cereal, crackers, macaroni, spaghetti, noodles, rice
Vegetables	Corn, lentils
Fruit	Cranberries, plums, prunes
Desserts	Plain cakes, cookies

Potentially Basic or Alkaline-Ash Foods	
Milk	Milk and milk products, cream, buttermilk
Fat	Nuts (almonds, chestnuts, coconut)
Vegetables	All types (except corn, lentils), especially beets, beet greens, Swiss chard, dandelion greens, kale, mustard greens, spinach, turnip greens
Fruit	All types (except cranberries, prunes, plums)
Sweets	Molasses

Neutral Foods	
Fats	Butter, margarine, cooking fats, oils
Sweets	Plain candies, sugar, syrup, honey
Starch	Arrowroot, corn, tapioca
Beverages	Coffee, tea

Physicians: How to Order Diet

The diet order should indicate: *acid-ash* or *alkaline-ash diet.*

References

75. Fellström B, Danielson BG, Karlström B, Lithell H, Ljunghall S, Wide L. Effects of high intake of dietary animal protein on mineral metabolism and urinary supersaturation of calcium oxalate in renal stone formers. Br J Urol 1984;56:263–269.
76. Simpson DP. Citrate excretion: a window on renal metabolism. Am J Physiol 1983;244: 223–234.
77. Dwyer J, Foulkes E, Evans M, Ausman L. Acid/alkaline ash diets: time for assessment and change. JADA 1985;85:841–845.
78. Kahn DH, Panariello VA, Saeli J, Sampson JR, Schwartz E. Effect of cranberry juice on urine. JADA 1967;51:251–254.

FOOD EXCHANGE LISTS FOR PROTEIN, SODIUM, AND POTASSIUM CONTROL

The following list is adapted from the 1986 American Diabetes Association and American Dietetics Association exchange lists for meal planning.[79] Modifications to the lists were made considering protein, sodium, and potassium control.

For patient education, this list has been simplified in respect to potassium content of foods. Fruits and vegetables which are available in different forms (i.e., juice, dried, fresh, canned) are all grouped together and assigned to reflect the average potassium content of all forms.

The average protein content of the starch group is 2 g instead of 3 g due to omission of dried beans, legumes, bran and whole grain items, necessary for optimal mineral control. Based on current nutrient content data,[80] the average protein content of the vegetable group in the renal exchange diet is 1 g of protein instead of 2 g.

TABLE 14-10   Summary of Nutrients in One Serving From Each Exchange Group

Exchange Group	Kcal*	Protein (g)	Fat (g)	Carbohydrate (g)	Sodium (mEq)	Potassium (mEq)	Phosphorus (mg)
Meat	75	7	5	Trace	1–3–8	2.5	70
Milk	Varies	4	0–2.5–5	6	2.5	4	115
Dessert (made with milk)	150	4	Varies	18	2.5	4	115
Starch	70	2	Trace	15	0.5–8	1.5–4–7–12†	45
Vegetable	25	1	Trace	5	0.5–12	4–7	30
Fruit	60	0.5	Trace	15	Trace	2–4–7	15
Low Protein product	100	0.2	2	20	0.5	Trace	Trace
Fat	45	Trace	5	Trace	0–2	Trace	1
Calorie supplement	100	Trace	Trace	25	Trace	Trace	Trace
Beverage	Varies	Varies	Varies	Varies	Varies	Trace–2–4	Varies

*Average calories per serving noted.

†Potassium content of most starch servings is approximately 1.5 mEq. The higher levels of potassium reflect the potassium content of starchy vegetables within the starch group.

The National Renal Diet food lists for planning renal diets[81] have been reviewed, however, we have not adopted those guidelines at this time as our current exchange lists better satisfy the educational needs of our patient population.

Table 14-10 summarizes the average nutrient contents of foods from each exchange group.

Meat and Meat Substitute

Each exchange contains approximately 7 g of protein and 2.5 mEq of potassium. The sodium content varies. Portion sizes refer to cooked weights.

Unsalted: 1 mEq of Sodium	
1 oz	Beef, lamb, pork, or veal
1 oz	Poultry
1 oz	Fish; any fresh or frozen
¼ cup	Salmon or tuna, fresh or unsalted, waterpacked
1 oz	Unsalted cheese
2 Tbsp	Unsalted peanut butter* (limit to 1 serving daily)

Salted: 3 mEq of Sodium	
1	Egg (no salt added)
¼ cup	Egg substitute (no salt added)
1 oz	Lightly salted meat, fish, poultry (¼ tsp of salt per lb)
1 oz	Liver, heart, kidneys
1 oz	Clams, crab, lobster
2 oz (1 med)	Oysters
1 oz (2 med)	Shrimp
1 oz	Swiss cheese†

High Sodium: 8 mEq of Sodium	
¼ cup	Cottage cheese†
1 oz	Cheese†: brick, cheddar, Colby, mozzarella
2 Tbsp	Regular peanut butter* (limit to 1 serving/day)

*These foods contain 6 mEq of potassium and are low biological value protein.
†These foods contain 1 mEq of potassium.

Milk and Milk Products

Each exchange contains approximately 4 g of protein, 2.5 mEq of sodium, and 4 mEq of potassium.

½ cup	Skim, 2%, or whole milk*
½ cup	Half and half*
¼ cup	Evaporated milk*
2 Tbsp	Nonfat dry milk (before adding liquid)
⅔ cup	Whipping cream, light*
¾ cup	Whipping cream, heavy*
½ cup	Yogurt (plain)

*These foods are to be included in fluid allowance.

Desserts Made with Milk

The following milk products contain additional carbohydrate. Omit one-half serving of carbohydrate supplement in addition to one serving of milk for diabetic patients.

1/3 cup	Bread pudding	3/4 cup	Ice cream*
1/2 cup	Chocolate milk*	2/3 cup	Ice milk*
1/3 cup	Custard	1/2 cup	Pudding
1/2 cup	Frozen yogurt dessert*	1/2 cup	Yogurt (flavored)

---

* These foods are to be included in fluid allowance.

Starch

Each exchange contains approximately 2 g of protein and 1.5 mEq of potassium unless otherwise specified. Sodium content is indicated. Unsalted cooked cereal, rice, pasta, and starchy vegetables are prepared without salt and contain less than 1 mEq of sodium. Salted cooked cereal, rice, pasta, and starchy vegetables are prepared with 1/8 tsp of salt per serving and contain approximately 10 mEq of sodium per serving.

Unsalted: Less Than 1 mEq of Sodium (Average, 0.5 mEq)

Bread

1 slice	Unsalted bread
1	Tortilla, 6-in diameter

Crackers

6	Saltines, unsalted, 2 1/2-in square

Cereal

1/2 cup	Barley
1/2 cup	Cooked cereal (no salt)
3/4 cup	Corn flakes, unsalted
1/4 cup	Granola
1/2 cup	Grits (cooked, no salt)
1 1/2 cups	Puffed wheat or rice, unsalted
1 biscuit	Shredded wheat, unsalted
1 Tbsp	Wheat germ (2 mEq of potassium)

Rice and Pasta

1/3 cup	Rice (cooked, no salt)
1/2 cup	Pasta, spaghetti, noodles, macaroni (cooked, no salt)

Starchy Vegetables

These foods contain more potassium than other foods in this group. If potassium is controlled in the diet, the number of servings of these foods will be limited.

3 to 5 mEq of Potassium

1/3 cup	Corn
1 small ear	Corn on the cob, 3 1/2-in long
10 (1 1/2 oz)	French fried potatoes, 2 to 3 1/2-in long
1/3 cup	Lima beans
1/2 small	Sweet potato, baked
1/4 cup	Sweet potato or yam, canned

5 to 10 mEq of Potassium

$^1/_2$ cup	Mashed potato
1 small	Potato, peeled, boiled

10 to 15 mEq of Potassium

$^2/_3$ cup	Parsnips
1 small	Potato, baked
1 cup	Pumpkin
$^3/_4$ cup	Squash: acorn, butternut, or winter

Other Bread Products

$2^1/_2$ Tbsp	Cornmeal, dry
3 Tbsp	Flour
$1^1/_2$ cups	Popcorn (popped, no salt)

Salted: 5 to 10 mEq of Sodium (Average, 8 mEq)

Bread: .5 mEq of Potassium

$^1/_2$	Bagel
1 slice	Bread: white (including French or Italian), whole-wheat, rye, raisin
4	Breadsticks, unsalted tops (4-in long)
$^1/_2$	Hamburger bun
1	Plain roll

Bread: 3 to 5 mEq of Potassium

$^1/_2$	English muffin
1 slice	Pumpernickel bread

Cereal: 1.5 mEq of Potassium

$^3/_4$ cup	Cereals, ready to eat
$^1/_2$ cup	Cereals (cooked, with $^1/_8$ tsp of salt)
$^1/_2$ cup	Barley (cooked, with $^1/_8$ tsp of salt)
3 Tbsp	Grapenuts
$^1/_2$ cup	Grits (cooked, with $^1/_8$ tsp of salt)

Crackers: 1.5 mEq of Potassium

10	Animal crackers
6	Arrowroot
3	Graham crackers, $2^1/_2$-in square
$^3/_4$	Matzo, 4-in by 6-in
5	Melba toast, 2-in by $3^3/_4$-in
3	Rye wafers, 2-in by $3^1/_2$-in
6	Round butter or whole-wheat crackers (low sodium)
6	Saltines, unsalted tops, $2^1/_2$-in square

Rice and Pasta

$^1/_3$ cup	Rice (cooked, with $^1/_8$ tsp of salt)
$^1/_2$ cup	Pasta: spaghetti, noodles, macaroni (cooked, with $^1/_8$ tsp of salt)

Starchy Vegetables

These foods contain more potassium than other foods in this group. If potassium is controlled in the diet, the number of servings of these foods will be limited.

3 to 5 mEq of Potassium

¹/₃ cup	Corn
1 small ear	Corn on the cob, 3¹/₂-in long
10 (1¹/₂ oz)	French fried potatoes, 2 to 3¹/₂-in long
¹/₃ cup	Lima beans
¹/₂ small	Sweet potato, baked
¹/₄ cup	Sweet potato or yam, canned

5 to 10 mEq of Potassium

¹/₂ cup	Mashed potato
1 small	Potato, peeled, boiled

10 to 15 mEq of Potassium

²/₃ cup	Parsnips
1 small	Potato, baked
1 cup	Pumpkin
³/₄ cup	Squash: acorn, butternut, or winter

Other Bread Products

¹/₂ cup	Chow mein noodles*
1 square	Cornbread, 2-in by 2-in by 1-in*
1 oz	Corn chips, unsalted†
1 small	Croissant†
¹/₂ cup	Croutons
¹/₄ cup (4 Tbsp)	Dried bread crumbs
2	Pancakes from mix, 4-in diameter*
1	Pita bread, 6-in diameter
1 small	Plain muffin, biscuit, 2-in diameter*
1 oz	Potato snack chips, unsalted†
³/₄ oz (25 sticks)	Pretzels, unsalted
2	Taco shells, 6-in diameter*
1	Tortilla, 6-in diameter
1	Waffle, 5-in diameter*

Desserts (Nutrient Content Varies with Recipe)

¹/₁₆ of 10-in cake	Angel food cake, plain
1	Cake doughnut, plain
2 small	Cookies, 1³/₄-in diameter
5	Gingersnaps
2	Ice cream cones (cone only)
2	Shortbread cookies
¹/₁₆ of 10-in cake	Sponge cake, plain
5	Vanilla wafers

---

*These foods contain one additional fat exchange.
†These foods contain two additional fat exchanges.

Vegetables

Each exchange equals approximately 1 g of protein. Unsalted vegetables are prepared without salt (less than 1 mEq of sodium). Salted vegetables are canned with added salt or prepared with $1/8$ tsp of salt per serving (approximately 12 mEq of sodium).

One serving of vegetable equals $1/2$ cup cooked or 1 cup raw unless otherwise specified. There are no "free" vegetables.

Moderate Potassium: 3 to 5 mEq of Potassium (Average, 4 mEq)

Avocado ($1/8$ med)	Dandelion greens	Peas, green ($1/4$ cup)
Alfalfa sprouts	Eggplant	Pea pods or snow peas
Bean sprouts	Endive	Radishes
Beets	Escarole	Rhubarb
Broccoli	Green pepper	Rutabaga
Cabbage	Green string beans	Summer squash
Carrots	Kale	Turnips
Chard	Lettuce	Water chestnuts
Chinese cabbage	Mustard greens	Watercress
Collards	Onion	Yellow string beans
Cucumbers	Parsley, raw (1 Tbsp)	Zucchini

Higher Potassium: 5 to 10 mEq of Potassium (Average, 7 mEq)

Artichokes	Cauliflower	Mushrooms	Tomatoes
Asparagus	Celery	Okra	Tomato juice (no salt)
Bamboo shoots	Chicory greens	Parsley	Turnip greens
Brussels sprouts	Kohlrabi	Spinach	Vegetable juice cocktail (no salt)

Fruit

Each exchange contains 0.5 g of protein, a trace of sodium, and averages of 2, 4, or 7 mEq of potassium.

Low Potassium: Less Than 3 mEq of Potassium (Average, 2 mEq)

1 small	Apple, fresh, 2-in diameter	$1 1/4$ cup	Cranberries
$1/2$ cup	Apple juice or cider	$1/3$ cup	Cranberry juice cocktail
$1/2$ cup	Applesauce	$1 1/4$ cup	Cranberry juice cocktail
$3/4$ cup	Blueberries		(low calorie)

Moderate Potassium: 3 to 5 mEq of Potassium (Average, 4 mEq)

$1/2$ cup	Cherries, canned	$1/2$ small	Mango	2 med	Persimmons,
12	Cherries, fresh	3 med	Passion fruit		native
2 large	Dates	$1/2$ cup	Peaches, canned	$1/3$ cup	Pineapple, canned
$1/2$ cup	Fruit cocktail	2 halves	Peaches, dried	$3/4$ cup	Pineapple, fresh
$1/2$ med	Grapefruit, fresh	1 med	Peach, fresh	$1/2$ cup	Pineapple juice
$1/2$ cup	Grapefruit juice	$1/2$ cup	Peach nectar	3 or $1/2$ cup	Plums, canned
$3/4$ cup	Grapefruit sections	$1/2$ cup	Pears, canned	2	Plums, fresh, 2-in
15 small	Grapes, fresh	1 half	Pear, dried	2 Tbsp	Raisin
$1/3$ cup	Grape juice	1 small	Pear, fresh	1 cup	Raspberries
5 med	Kumquats	$1/2$ cup	Pear nectar	1 cup	Rhubarb

High Potassium: 5 to 10 mEq of Potassium (Average, 7 mEq)

¹/₂ cup or 4 halves	Apricots, canned	¹/₂	Nectarine, 3-in
7 halves	Apricots, dried	1 small	Orange, fresh, 2¹/₂-in
4 med	Apricots, fresh	¹/₂ cup	Orange juice
¹/₂ cup	Apricot nectar	³/₄ cup	Orange sections
¹/₂	Banana, 9-in	1 cup	Papaya
³/₄ cup	Blackberries	1¹/₂ med	Pomegranate
¹/₄ small or 1 cup	Cantaloupe, 6-in	1 med	Prickly pear
1¹/₂	Figs, canned	3 med	Prunes
1 med	Figs, dried	¹/₃ cup	Prune juice
2 med	Figs, fresh	1¹/₄ cup	Strawberries
1 med	Guava	1 med	Tangelo
¹/₈ med or 1 cup	Honeydew	2 med	Tangerines, fresh
1 large	Kiwi fruit	¹/₂ cup	Tangerine juice
1 cup	Lemon juice*	1¹/₄ cup	Watermelon

*Up to 2 Tbsp of lemon juice may be used per day without being considered as part of the fruit group.

Low-Protein Products

Each exchange contains 0.2 g of protein, 0.5 mEq of sodium, a trace of potassium, and 100 kcal.

1 slice (1¹/₂ oz)	Low-protein bread
2 slices	Low-protein rusks
¹/₂ cup, cooked (¹/₄ cup dry)	Low-protein macaroni, ring macaroni, or noodles
¹/₂ cup, prepared	Low-protein gelatin (negligible protein, 1 mEq of sodium, 2 mEq of potassium, 85 kcal)
2 (2¹/₂-in diameter)	Low-protein cookies (0.2 g of protein, 2 mEq of sodium, 1 mEq of potassium, 1 fat serving, and 140 kcal)

Fats and Oils

Each exchange contains negligible amounts of protein and a trace of potassium. Sodium varies.

Unsalted: Trace of Sodium

1 tsp	Butter, unsalted
2 Tbsp	Gravy (meat drippings with fat thickened with cornstarch), unsalted
1 tsp	Margarine, unsalted
1 tsp	Mayonnaise, low sodium
1 tsp	Oil
1 tsp	Shortening

Salted: 2 mEq of Sodium

1 tsp	Butter
1 Tbsp	Cream cheese (limit to 1 serving/day)
1 tsp	Margarine
1 tsp	Mayonnaise
2 Tbsp	Nondairy creamer
2 Tbsp	Sour cream (limit to 1 serving/day)

Carbohydrate Supplements

Each exchange contains negligible amounts of protein, sodium, and potassium and 100 kcal.

Sugar and Syrups

2 Tbsp	Sugar
2 Tbsp	Honey
2 Tbsp	Jelly or jam
2 Tbsp	Syrup, pancake or light corn

Candy

3 large	Fondant or sugar mints
5 large	Marshmallows
8 small	Gumdrops
6 pieces	Hard candy, unfilled
10 large, 30 small	Jelly beans
11	Lifesavers™
2 med	Lollipop, unfilled

Fruit Desserts

1/4 cup	Cranberry sauce or relish
1/2 cup	Fruit ice (sherbert made without milk)
1 twin bar	Popsicle™ (2 1/2 oz bar)

Flavored Beverages

1 cup (8 oz)	Carbonated, fruit flavored Kool Aid™, artificially flavored lemonade

Flour Products

1/4 cup	Cornstarch or tapioca (may be used to thicken sauces and gravies)

Other Carbohydrate Supplements

1/4 cup	Polycose™ powder or liquid (contains 2 mEq of sodium, use as suggested)

Beverages

One cup (8 oz) of the following beverages contains only a trace of protein and sodium. The relative potassium content is noted.

Trace of Potassium

Cola	Orange soda
Gingerale	Postum™
Kool Aid™	Root beer
Lemonade	Seven Up
Limeade	Strawberry soda

2 mEq of Potassium

Coffee, instant and freeze-dried
Coffee, decaffeinated, instant, and freeze-dried
Decaffeinated coffee, brewed
Tea

4 mEq Potassium

Coffee, brewed

1.5 oz of liqueur contain a trace of sodium and a trace of potassium.

1.5 oz of rum, whiskey, or vodka contain no sodium and a trace of potassium.

12 oz of beer contain 1.5 mEq of sodium and 3 mEq of potassium.

4 oz of wine contain a trace of sodium and 3 mEq of potassium.

References

79. AmericanDiabetes Association and American Dietetic Association. Exchange lists for meal planning. Alexandria, VA, and Chicago, IL, 1986.

80. Pennington JAT, Church HN. Bowes and Church's food values of portions commonly used. 16th ed. Philadelphia: JB Lippincott, 1994.

81. Renal Dietetic Practice Group of the American Dietetic Association. National Renal Diet: professional guide. Chicago, IL, 1993.

POTASSIUM CONTROL

General Description

Potassium is widely distributed in foods but is highest in fruits and vegetables. General guidelines are given for increasing or decreasing potassium intake.

Indications and Rationale

Hypokalemia. Hypokalemia is associated most often with the use of diuretics but also may be induced by other drugs (such as corticosteroids), gastrointestinal disturbances (such as diarrhea, vomiting, and laxative abuse), some renal disturbances, some adrenal disorders, and burns.[82-88] In many instances, parenteral or oral administration of potassium supplements is warranted.

Treatment of hypokalemia that occurs with diuretic therapy for hypertension may consist of (1) restriction of dietary sodium to lessen urinary potassium wastage, (2) substitution of a potassium-sparing diuretic for a potassium-wasting one, (3) reduction of the dosage of potassium-wasting medications, if adequate blood pressure control can be maintained at a lower dosage, (4) use of potassium chloride supplements or potassium chloride salt substitutes, or (5) use of foods high in potassium.[84,85]

Many potassium chloride supplements are poorly accepted because of their unpleasant taste. Supplements of potassium citrate and potassium bicarbonate are better tolerated but less effective than potassium chloride.

Salt substitutes that contain potassium chloride may be a reasonable alternative since they generally cost less and are more palatable than prescription potassium chloride supplements.[89] Some patients develop a tolerance over time to the bitter, metallic taste of salt substitutes.[84] Although there is some variation among brands of potassium chloride salt substitutes, the usual potassium content is 10 to 13 mEq of potassium per gram.* Therefore, 5 g (1 tsp) of these salt substitutes would provide

---

*Potassium chloride provides 13.4 mEq of potassium per gram.

50 to 65 mEq of potassium. If a potassium chloride salt substitute is recommended to the patient, a specific dose should be indicated since excessive amounts can be harmful.[90] Many dietetic "low sodium" products use potassium chloride instead of sodium chloride, a substitution that substantially increases their potassium content.

Potassium intakes vary considerably depending upon the individual's food selection. For example, people who eat large amounts of fruits and vegetables have a higher potassium intake.[91]

The usual American diet provides 50 to 150 mEq of potassium daily.[91] It is difficult for most patients to consistently and reliably increase dietary intake of potassium to the desired therapeutic level. A range of 40 to 60 mEq of potassium from potassium chloride supplements is a frequently prescribed dose. When a similar increase in potassium is attempted with food, the total intake of calories or sodium (or both) is often appreciably increased also. Attempts to increase dietary potassium may be successful if the patient requires only minimal potassium supplementation to prevent hypokalemia, if the patient's usual diet is habitually low in potassium, or if therapy adjunctive to potassium supplements is required.

Hyperkalemia. A decrease in urinary output of potassium and an increase in serum potassium levels occur in advanced renal failure, hypoaldosteronism,[92] and adrenal insufficiency. The elderly are also more prone to hyperkalemia.[93,94] Excessive use of potassium-sparing diuretics may result in hyperkalemia.[95] Also, use of medications such as nonsteroidal anti-inflammatory drugs and angiotension-converting enzyme (ACE) inhibitors can result in hyperkalemia in patients with mild to moderate renal insufficiency. Treatment includes dietary restriction of potassium and reduction of the dosage or discontinuation of the use of these medications.

Both endogenous and exogenous sources can increase input of potassium to the serum.[96] Typically, the exogenous sources include a high dietary intake and excess intake of salt substitutes that contain potassium chloride. Treatment includes dietary restriction and discontinuation of salt substitutes or other dietetic foods containing potassium chloride. The low protein diet used for the predialysis patient is inherently restricted in potassium. In the usual diet, high protein foods contribute significant amounts of potassium. Restricting protein generally reduces dietary potassium intake as well.

The primary endogenous source of potassium is muscle and tissue catabolism.[96] One of the primary objectives in the dietary management of chronic renal failure is the prevention of muscle catabolism.

Physicians: How to Order Diet

Hypokalemia. The physician should specify the level of dietary potassium desired.
Hyperkalemia. The diet order should specify a low potassium diet: *60 mEq of potassium.*

FOOD SOURCES OF POTASSIUM[97]

The following foods are grouped by potassium content and may be used for planning potassium controlled diets. This list provides potassium content of foods according to their specific form (e.g., fresh, canned, dried, juice).

This list varies from the Food Exchange list for Protein, Sodium, and Potassium Control (see pp. 348–352). This list is according to potassium content only. Also the previous list groups foods together regardless of form and assigns the value to the form with the highest potassium content.

Low Potassium (Less Than 3 mEq of Potassium per Serving)

Meats, meat substitutes (such as eggs), breads, pasta, and cereals are generally low in potassium.

Fruits

Apple, fresh	1 small (2-in diam)	Figs, canned	2 med
Applesauce	1/2 cup	Grape juice	1/3 cup
Blueberries	3/4 cup	Peach nectar	1/2 cup
Cranberries	1 1/4 cup	Pears, canned	1/2 cup
Cranberry juice cocktail	1/3 cup	Pears, dried	1 half
Cranberry juice cocktail		Pear nectar	1/2 cup
(low calorie)	1 1/4 cup	Pineapple, canned	1/3 cup

Vegetables

All portions are 1/2 cup cooked or 1 cup raw unless otherwise indicated.

Alfalfa sprouts	Green pepper, cooked
Bamboo shoots, canned (1/2 cup)	Radishes, raw (10)
Beans sprouts,	Turnip, cooked
cooked or canned (1/2 cup)	Waterchestnuts, canned (1/2 cup)
Endive, raw (1/2 cup)	Watercress, raw

Nuts

Almonds	6 whole	Pecans	5 halves
Brazil nuts	2 med	Pumpkin seeds	2 tsp
Cashews, roasted	4 large	Sunflower seeds	1 Tbsp without shell
Filberts or hazelnuts	5	Walnuts	4 halves
Mixed nuts	8-12		

Dairy Foods

Cheese	1 oz
Cottage cheese	1/4 cup

Beverages

Coffee (instant or freeze-dried, decaffeinated and regular)	1 cup
Tea	1 cup
Lemonade	1 cup

Miscellaneous

Olives, black	5 med
Olives, green	9-10 med
Sweet, semisweet chocolate	1 oz
Tofu, fermented	4 oz
Wheat germ	1 Tbsp

Moderate Potassium (3 to 5 mEq of Potassium per Serving)

Most milk and dairy products and most fruits and vegetables contain moderate amounts of potassium.

Fruits

Apple juice or cider	¹/₂ cup	Mango	¹/₂ small
Apricots, canned	¹/₂ cup or 4 halves	Passion fruit	3 med
Apricot nectar	¹/₂ cup	Peaches, fresh	1 med (2³/₄-in diam)
Berries		Peaches, canned	¹/₂ cup
Blackberries, canned, frozen	³/₄ cup	Pears, fresh	1 small or ¹/₂ large
Raspberries	1 cup	Persimmon	2 med
Cherries, canned	¹/₂ cup	Pineapple, fresh	³/₄ cup
Cherries, fresh	12 large	Pineapple juice	¹/₂ cup
Dates	2¹/₂ med	Plums, fresh	2 small (2-in diam)
Fruit cocktail	¹/₂ cup	Plums, canned	¹/₂ cup or 3
Grapes, fresh or canned	15 small	Prunes, canned	3 med
Grapefruit, fresh	¹/₂ med	Prunes, dried	3 med
Grepefruit juice	¹/₂ cup	Raisins	2 Tbsp
Kumquats	5 med		

Vegetables

All portions are ¹/₂ cup cooked or 1 cup raw unless otherwise indicated.

Asparagus	Dandelion greens, cooked	Peas
Bean sprouts, raw	Eggplant	Peapods or snow peas
Beets	Escarole	Rhubarb
Broccoli, cooked	Green beans	Summer squash, cooked
Cabbage	Green pepper, raw	Sweet potato or yam,
Carrots, cooked	Kale	canned, cooked (¹/₄ cup)
Cauliflower, cooked	Lettuce	Turnip greens
Chinese cabbage, raw	Mustard greens	
Cucumbers	Onion, cooked	

Dairy Foods

Milk	¹/₂ cup
Yogurt, whole milk	¹/₂ cup

Miscellaneous

Brewed coffee	1 cup	Peanut butter	2 Tbsp
Canned soup	1 cup	Peanuts	1 oz or 25
Chocolate chips	¹/₄ cup	Postum	1 cup
Cocoa powder	2 Tbsp	Tofu, raw	4 oz (¹/₂ cup)

High Potassium (5 to 10 mEq of Potassium per Serving)

The following foods are high in potassium. Many low sodium dietetic foods, such as canned soups, are also high in potassium because the sodium chloride is replaced with potassium chloride.

Fruits

Apricots, dried	7 halves
Banana	$1/2$ (9-in long)
Berries	
Blackberries, raw	$3/4$ cup
Strawberries	$1^1/4$ cup
Figs, fresh or dried	2 med
Grapefruit, sections	$3/4$ cup
Guava	1 med
Kiwi	1 large
Lemon juice	1 cup
Melons	
Cantaloupe	$1/3$ (5-in diam) or 1 cup cubed
Honeydew	$1/8$ med or 1 cup cubed
Watermelon	$1^1/4$ cup cubed
Nectarine	$1/2$ (3-in diam)
Orange, fresh	1 ($2^1/2$-in diam)
Orange juice	$1/2$ cup
Papaya	$1/2$ med or 1 cup
Peaches, dried	2 halves
Pomegranate	$1/2$ med
Prickly pear	1 med
Prune juice	$1/3$ cup
Tangerine, fresh	2 ($2^1/2$-in diam)
Tangerine juice	$1/2$ cup
Tangelo	1 med

Vegetables

All portions are $1/2$ cup cooked or 1 cup raw unless otherwise indicated.

Artichoke (1 med)	Okra, cooked
Asparagus	Onion, raw
Bamboo Shoots, raw or boiled	Parsley
Broccoli, raw	Parsnips ($1/3$ cup)
Brussels sprouts	Potato, mashed
Carrots, raw (1 med)	Rutabaga, cooked
Cauliflower, raw	Spinach, raw
Celery, cooked	Summer squash, raw
Chinese cabbage, cooked	Sweet potato or yam, fresh, cooked ($1/4$ cup)
Collards	Tomatoes (med)
Corn, cooked ($1/2$ cup or 1 ear)	Tomato juice salted and unsalted ($1/2$ cup)
Dandelion greens, raw	Vegetable juice cocktail salted and unsalted ($1/2$ cup)
Kohlrabi	Yellow beans
Mushrooms	Zucchini

Dairy Foods	
Yogurt, custard style	$\frac{1}{2}$ cup
Yogurt, low fat	$\frac{1}{2}$ cup

Miscellaneous	
Chocolate, bitter	1 oz
Sunflower seeds	$\frac{1}{4}$ cup
Tofu, raw (firm)	4 oz ($\frac{1}{2}$ cup)
Low sodium canned soups	1 cup

Very High Potassium (10+ mEq of Potassium per Serving)

The following foods contain very high amounts of potassium.

Fruits	
Apricots, fresh	4 med

Vegetables

All portions are $\frac{1}{2}$ cup cooked or 1 cup raw unless otherwise indicated.

Bamboo shoots, raw	Pumpkin (1 cup)
Beet greens, cooked	Spinach, cooked
Chard, cooked	Squash: acorn, hubbard, butternut,
Chicory, raw	winter ($\frac{3}{4}$ cup)
Potato, baked or boiled (1 small, 2-in diam)	Waterchestnuts, raw

Miscellaneous

Salt substitute (potassium chloride) ($\frac{1}{4}$ tsp)
Low sodium baking powder (1 tsp)

References

82. Podrid PJ. Potassium and ventricular arrhythmias. Am J Cardiol 1990;65:33E–43E.
83. Calhoun KA. Serum potassium concentration abnormalities. Crit Care Nurse 1990;13(3): 34–38.
84. Longford HG. Potassium in hypertension: the case for its role in pathogenesis and treatment. Postgrad Med 1983;73:227–233.
85. Fischer RG. Managing diuretic-induced hypokalemia in ambulatory hypertensive patients. J Fam Pract 1982;14:1029–1036.
86. Edes TE. Hyperkalemia. Postgrad Med 1990;87:104–106.
87. Rude RK. Physiology of magnesium metabolism and the important role of magnesium in potassium deficiency. Am J Cardiol 1989;63:31G–34G.
88. Zull DN. Disorders of potassium metabolism. Emerg Med Clin North Am 1989;7(4):771–794.
89. Sopko JA, Freeman RM. Salt substitutes as a source of potassium. JAMA 1977;238:608–610.
90. Schim van der Loeff HJ, Strack van Schijndel RJM, Thijs LG. Cardiac arrest due to oral potassium intake. Intensive Care Med 1988;5:58–59.
91. Food and Nutrition Board Research Council. Recommended Dietary Allowances, 10th ed. Washington, DC: National Academy of Science, 1989:173.
92. Fulop M. Hyperkalemia in ketoacidosis. Am J Med Sci 1990;299:164–169.
93. Kleinfield M. Hyperkalemia in the elderly. Compr Ther 1990;49–53.
94. Michaelis MF. Hyperkalemia in the elderly. Am J Kidney Dis 1990;16:296–299.

95. Madias NE, Zelman SJ. What are the metabolic complications of diuretic treatment. Geriatrics 1982;37:93–99.
96. Elms JJ. Potassium imbalance: causes and prevention. Postgrad Med 1982;72:165–171.
97. Pennington JAT. Bowes and Church's food values of portions commonly used, 16th ed. Philadelphia: JB Lippincott, 1994.

15 / *Nutritional Management and Transplantation*

NUTRITION IN TRANSPLANTATION

Transplantation of healthy organs and tissues for diseased ones has become an increasingly effective and common therapy. Advances made in immunosuppression have dramatically reduced the rejection of transplants. Whether the transplanted organ or tissue is allogenic (from one person to another), autologous (from within the same person), or even xenogenic (from an animal to a person), transplant recipients have many common nutritional problems and concerns. Attention to and optimal nutritional intervention prior to transplant, immediately post-transplant and long term after transplant can reduce complications and improve patient morbidity. Nutritional assessment and management of patients at each of these stages will be discussed in this section.

Nutrition Assessment and Management

Nutritional assessment and management of the transplant patient may be viewed in three phases: (1) pretransplantation; (2) immediate post-transplantation (approximately 2 months); and (3) long-term post-transplantation.

Pretransplantation. Nutritional status of the patient can substantially affect surgical outcome, length of hospital stay, morbidity (which includes episodes of sepsis and respiratory failure), and mortality. Transplant candidates are at increased risk of becoming malnourished. Mechanisms for malnutrition appear in Table 15-1. The registered dietitian should perform nutritional assessment prior to transplantation. The goal of nutritional therapy during the pretransplantation phase is to optimize nutrient intake within any necessary dietary modifications. For those patients having liver transplantation, a low bacteria diet, sometimes in combination with prophylactic oral antibiotics, has been utilized at some centers to reduce the incidence of infections. Frequent monitoring, reassessment, and encouragement are essential in the care of these patients. Enteral or parenteral nutrition support may be necessary to ensure adequate nutrient intake.

363

TABLE 15-1   Mechanisms for Malnutrition in Transplant Patients

Inadequate oral intake—anorexia, nausea, vomiting, early satiety, esophagitis, thick saliva, dysgeusia, dyspnea, ascites

Iatrogenic—dietary restrictions resulting from the disease

Increased nutrient losses—dialysis, diarrhea, vomiting, malabsorption

Hypermetabolism and/or hypercatabolism

Inability to remove waste products

Medication side effects

Given the likely compromise in nutritional status prior to transplant and the increased nutritional requirements immediately post-transplant, it is recommended that the patient take a multiple vitamin and mineral supplement to ensure that nutrient requirements are satisfied.

Immediately Post-Transplantation.   Nutritional requirements following transplantation are influenced by the nutritional status prior to transplantation, degree of hypermetabolism and/or hypercatabolism, and allograft function. Energy requirements may be difficult to determine in the stressed or septic patient. In this case indirect calorimetry can be used to measure caloric expenditure. See Chapter 3, Nutritional Screening and Assessment.

Those who experience ventilator dependence, infections, impaired gastrointestinal function, poor oral intake, or frequent interruptions in intake due to medical procedures may need enteral or parenteral feedings. Concentrated solutions of enteral or parenteral feedings may be needed if fluid restrictions are required. Combining two or more nutritional support modalities (such as oral and enteral feedings) provides flexibility and a greater chance of meeting energy and protein needs in patients whose intake is suboptimal.

Immunosuppressive therapy prevents rejection of the transplanted organ or tissue. Because the immune system is also responsible for fighting infection, a delicate balance between preventing rejection and avoiding infection is necessary. A variety of drugs may be used to suppress the immune response, but a common maintenance regimen includes cyclosporine, azathioprine, and prednisone. The patient must continue to take such medications indefinitely. These immunosuppressive drugs have a number of well-recognized nutrition-related side effects (Table 15-2).[1] When immunosuppression is at its peak, a low bacteria type diet is often utilized; thereafter those activities that minimize the risk of food poisoning are continued. On-going monitoring for drug-nutrient interactions should be routinely performed. The diet can then be adjusted as needed to prevent potential nutritional problems and meet the patient's immediate and long-term needs.

Long-Term Post-Transplantation.   The long-term nutritional management for all patients who have received organ transplantation is quite similar, but there are a few issues unique to each type of allograft. Therefore, refer to the various tables within this section for specific nutritional guidelines for each type of transplant.

TABLE 15-2 Examples of Drugs Used in Transplantation and Their Nutrition-Related Side Effects

Drug (Mechanism)	Transplant Procedure(s)	Nutrition Related Side Effect(s)	
		Acute	Chronic
Prednisone			
(Anti-inflammatory, immunosuppressive, enhances other immuno-suppressives)	BMT, kidney, liver, pancreas, thoracic	Fluid/sodium retention Increased appetite Hyperglycemia	Weight gain Calcium/phosphorus wasting osteoporosis GI ulceration
Azathioprine (Imuran)			
(Anti-inflammatory, immunosuppressive, depresses delayed hypersensitivity reactions)	BMT, kidney, liver, pancreas, thoracic	Nausea/vomiting Diarrhea Macrocytic anemia Mucositis	Esophagitis Pancreatitis Increased risk of infection
OKT3			
(Inhibits T-cell effector function)	Kidney, liver	Fever/chills Nausea/vomiting Diarrhea Hypertension Fluid retention	Increased risk of infection with multiple exposures
Cyclosporine			
(Decreases IL-2 production, spares T-suppressor cells)	BMT, kidney, liver, pancreas, thoracic	Nephrotoxicity Hyperkalemia Hypomagnesemia Hyperuricemia	Hypertension Hyperglycemia Hyperlipidemia
Tacrolimus (FK 506/Prograf)			
(Decreases IL-2 production, spares T-suppressor cells—more potent than cyclosporin)	Kidney, liver	Nausea Vomiting with IV doses Abdominal pain Pancreatitis (?) Neurotoxicity (?) Nephrotoxicity Hyperkalemia	Hyperglycemia
Methotrexate (MTX)			
(Antimetabolite, inter-feres with DNA synthesis, repair and cellular replication)	BMT	Anorexia Nausea Stomatitis Diarrhea Fever/chills	—

BMT = Bone marrow transplant; GI = gastrointestinal.

Excessive weight gain during the first year after organ transplant is a common nutritional problem. This weight gain is attributed to an increased appetite (partially due to corticosteroid therapy). Other contributing factors include lack of exercise, enhanced nutrient absorption, and the freedom of a varied diet after what may have been a highly restricted pretransplant regimen. Prior to allograft placement, many patients suffer from anorexia due to their primary illness and possibly other complicating conditions. Patients who are below their ideal body weight at the time of transplant need to gain weight, but excessive gain should be avoided to help minimize hyperlipidemia, hypertension, and diabetes due to corticosteroid use.

Given the catabolic effects of stress and post-transplant medications, an adequate protein intake is recommended to avoid reduction of protein stores.

Reduction of fat intake to less than 30% of total kilocalories with 10% or less of total kilocalories as saturated fat and less than 300 mg of cholesterol per day is recommended to control the hyperlipidemia effects of corticosteroid therapy.

Most patients are encouraged to follow a no-added salt diet once they have stabilized after transplant. However, if hypertension or fluid retention persists or develops, a further reduction in sodium intake is warranted.

Other considerations include limitation of simple carbohydrates to help control weight and hyperlipidemia. A high fiber diet with emphasis upon adequate soluble fiber intake is recommended because it may be beneficial in the presence of hypercholesterolemia and diabetes. Electrolyte requirements, such as potassium, phosphorus, and calcium, vary with organ function and medication side effects. Therefore, routine monitoring of serum levels post-transplant is recommended.

Body image problems including concern about the development of obesity, moonface, and other characteristics of steroid-induced Cushing's syndrome can develop. Adolescent transplant patients may be at risk for developing anorectic or bulimic behaviors to control their weight. The dietitian provides appropriate nutrition education to patients and their families. In many cases this is an ongoing process because patients may have a variety of nutritional concerns. Behavior modification techniques may help patients with weight control.

A regular exercise program is essential for weight control post-transplant. Pretransplant and immediate post-transplant exercise as tolerated will help the patient maintain or regain muscle strength. The benefits of exercise include weight control, cardiovascular conditioning, and maintenance of bone density. These benefits should be reviewed with the patient and exercise strongly encouraged.

The following sections present guidelines for provision of a low bacteria diet to transplant patients as well as specific nutritional considerations for various types of transplants: bone marrow, liver, kidney, pancreas/pancreas-kidney, and thoracic organs.

Reference

1. Ohara MM. Immunosuppression in solid organ transplantation: a nutrition perspective. Top Clin Nutr 1992;7(3):6–11.

LOW BACTERIA DIETS

General Description

Various types of low bacteria diets are commonly used to assist in the prevention of infection in transplant patients. While the use and content of such diets (Table 15-3) is somewhat controversial and differs for the various types of transplants, these diets follow three general principles:

1. Avoiding foods that may contain gram-negative bacteria (and certain yeasts)
2. Practicing safe food handling and preparation techniques to avoid contamination of food
3. Avoiding foods that are inherently contaminated with microbes such as raw eggs, raw or undercooked meat, fish and seafood, and unpasteurized milk.

Nutritional Inadequacy

Low bacteria diets are similar to the general hospital diet and are not inherently lacking in nutrients as compared to the Recommended Dietary Allowance (RDA). A daily multiple vitamin supplement, which provides nutrients at a level equivalent

TABLE 15-3 Low Bacteria Diets—Foods to Avoid

Food Groups	Type of Transplant			
	Thoracic Organs	Bone Marrow*	Liver†	Pancreas-Renal‡
Meats and eggs	Any undercooked	Any undercooked	Any undercooked; all cheese and cottage cheese products	Any undercooked; all cheese and cottage cheese products
Fat	—	—	—	—
Milk	—	—	—	—
Starch	—	—	—	—
Vegetables	—	All raw vegetables (including salads and garnishes)	All raw vegetables (including salads and garnishes)	All raw vegetables (including salads and garnishes)
Fruit	—	All fresh fruits	Fresh fruit with peels that are consumed (e.g., grapes, cherries, berries)§	Fresh fruit with peels that are consumed (e.g., grapes, cherries, berries)§
Beverages	—	—	—	—
Condiments/ Seasonings	Pepper, dried herb packets	—	—	—

*To be followed whenever neutrophil count is $<0.5 \times 10^9$/L.

†To be followed while activated, a minimum of 21 days post-orthotopic liver transplant and whenever taking oral selective bowel decontamination solution.

‡To be followed only after pancreas-renal transplant and whenever taking oral selective bowel decontamination solution.

§Fresh fruit that can reasonably be peeled and rinsed is allowed (e.g., apples, oranges, banana, grapefruit, pears, melon, pineapple, peaches, nectarines, kiwi).

to the RDA, is recommended for persons who consume diets of 1,200 kcal or less or for those individuals with food aversions or intolerances that greatly limit the variety of food choices. During the transition from parenteral nutrition to oral intake, vitamins and minerals at levels that meet the RDA are provided parenterally.

Indications and Rationale

Infection is a major cause of morbidity and mortality in transplant recipients. Diet therapy is often used as an adjunct to bowel decontamination, antibiotic therapy, and/or controlled environments (ranging from simple isolation to sterile laminar flow rooms) to prevent infection.[2-5] The goal of low bacteria diets is to help minimize the incidence of infection by avoiding various types of foods associated with a high gram-negative bacterial content and situations where a significant risk of food-borne illness exists.[2,3,5,6] The use of these diets is accepted even though the diets are based more on theory than on randomized controlled trials. Due to the unpalatability and cost of sterile diets, many institutions use more liberal low bacterial type diets without apparent sacrifice in effectiveness.[3,4]

For patients receiving liver or pancreas-renal transplants, the low bacteria diet is used in conjunction with an oral selective bowel decontamination solution (OSBD) containing Polymyxin E, Gentamicin, and Nystatin. Liver transplant patients take the OSBD 4 times daily while activated pretransplant and for at least 3 weeks post-transplant to eradicate the gram-negative and fungal flora in the gastrointestinal tract.[2] Pancreas-renal transplant patients take OSBD and follow the low bacteria diet in the initial post-transplant period (approximately 3 weeks).[7]

For all other transplant patients the actual restriction of foods is generally limited to the initial post-transplant period when immunosuppression is at its peak. In the long-term post-transplant period, the objective becomes one of safe food handling in addition to dietary selections that minimize the risk of food poisoning.

Physicians: How to Order Diet

The diet order should indicate:
Bone marrow: *general— no fresh fruits or vegetables*
Liver or pancreas-renal: *low bacteria diet*
Thoracic: General— *no pepper or herb packet*
Additional dietary modifications that may be necessary (e.g., sodium restriction) should be indicated. The dietitian determines the appropriate caloric level and other characteristics of the diet based on nutritional assessment, patient tolerance, and discussion with the physician.

References

2. Wiesner RH, Hermans P, Rakela J, Washington J, Perkins J, DiCecco S, Krom RAF. Selective bowel decontamination to prevent gram-negative aerobic bacterial and candida colonization and prevent infection following orthotopic liver transplantation. Transplantation 1988;45:570–574.

3. Aker SN, Cheney CR. The use of sterile and low-microbial diets in ultra isolation environments. JPEN 1983;7:390–397.

4. Anon. Low-microbial vs. sterile diets for immunocompromised patients. Nutrition and the M.D. 1989;15:1.

5. Moe G. Enteral feeding and infection in the immunocompromised patient. Nutr Clin Prac 1991;66:55–64.

6. Remington JS, Schimpff SC. Occasional notes: please don't eat the salads. N Engl J Med 1981;304:433–435.

7. Perkins JD, Frohnert PP, Service FJ, Wilhelm MP, Keating MR, DiCecco SR, Johnson JL, Munn SR, Velosa JA. Pancreas transplantation at Mayo: III. Multidisciplinary management. Mayo Clinic Proc 1990;65:496–508.

KIDNEY TRANSPLANTATION

Kidney transplantation is the most common solid organ transplantation performed. It is accepted therapy for many patients with end-stage renal disease. Diseases that most frequently lead to kidney transplantation include those that cause irreversible chronic renal failure, such as glomerulonephritis, chronic pyelonephritis, polycystic kidney disease, diabetic nephropathy, and hypertensive nephrosclerosis. Medical contraindications agreed upon by most transplant centers include malignancy, severe coronary artery disease, or an active infection. Kidney transplantation is considered a high risk procedure for individuals with diabetes or obesity.

Accurate nutritional assessment is difficult in patients with renal disease and transplantation because common assessment parameters are affected by the disease itself. Actual body weight and anthropometric measurements are affected by edema and diuretic therapy. Techniques used to assess protein status (nitrogen balance, albumin, transferrin) are typically depressed in patients with renal failure and may be affected by hydration, iron stores, or infection. An in-depth nutrition history (including nutrient intake and restrictions, vitamin and mineral supplementation, relative weight change with attention to wasting, appetite, and food intolerances) is helpful. When performed routinely, appropriate dietary intervention may slow deterioration of renal function and help to minimize nutritional risks of transplantation.[8,9]

Pretransplant

Prior to kidney transplantation, it is advised that a patient with declining renal function follow a protein- and sodium-controlled diet. Limitation of potassium and/or further reduction in phosphorus intake may also be necessary as the patient progresses toward end-stage renal disease. See Chapter 14, Renal Diseases and Disorders—Chronic Renal Failure, Nephrotic Syndrome, Peritoneal Dialysis, and Hemodialysis.

Immediate and Long-Term Post-transplant

Guidelines for the nutritional care of patients immediately post-transplant and their long-term follow-up can be found in Table 15-4.

Kilocalories.   The caloric requirement in the immediate post-transplant period is high due to surgical stress and catabolism. Indirect calorimetry may be used when a patient may benefit from an accurate assessment, but it may not be warranted for the patient who does not present a nutritional risk. Caloric require-

TABLE 15-4   Nutritional Care Guidelines for Kidney Transplantation[9,10,12]

	Immediately Post-transplant*	Long-Term Post-transplant
Kilocalories†	Basal Harris-Benedict + 30%	Basal Harris Benedict + 10–20% (to avoid excessive weight gain)
Protein†	1.3–1.5 g/kg/day	1 g/kg/day
Sodium	90–135 mEq/day	No added salt 90 mEq if hypertension is present
Potassium	No restriction 70 mEq/day if hyperkalemia is present	Same
Calcium	1,200 mg/day	Same
Cholesterol	≤ 300 mg/day	Same
Fat	30% of kilocalories; emphasis on unsaturated fat	Same
Simple carbohydrate	Limit	Same
Fiber	Emphasize	Same
Alcohol	Avoid	Same

*Approximately first 2 mo after transplant.

†Harris-Benedict equation and protein requirements are based on actual (dry) weight.

ments may be estimated using the Harris-Benedict equation and a stress factor of 1.3. The patient's dry weight should be used or an adjusted weight if the patient is obese (see Chapter 3, Nutritional Screening and Assessment). From 6 to 8 weeks after transplant, nutrient needs decrease. Caloric requirements should be established to achieve maintenance or desirable body weight.

Protein.   Following transplantation, restriction of dietary protein is no longer required. The primary focus is to provide adequate kilocalories and protein to maintain proper nutritional status or correct any preoperative deficiencies. Large doses of steroids typically used in the immediate post-transplant period, along with the stress of surgery, markedly increase protein catabolism.[10] The optimal dietary protein requirement is less clear for stable renal transplant patients on maintenance dose steroids. Conflicting goals exist for optimizing protein status and maintaining long-term renal function. More studies are needed to best determine protein needs for the stable transplant patient.[10]

Carbohydrates and Fats.   Glucose intolerance is common in patients with uremia and may continue to be problematic after kidney transplantation. Surgical stress, sepsis, and corticosteroid therapy contribute to this intolerance. Restriction of simple carbohydrate may be helpful in improving glucose tolerance and reducing the cushingoid side effects of steroid administration.

During the immediate post-transplant period, fat modification or restriction may need to be tempered in order to achieve caloric requirements. Hypercholesterolemia and hypertriglyceridemia are the two most common lipid abnormalities found in transplant patients. Factors that may contribute include steroid therapy, renal dysfunction, basal hyperinsulinism with glucose intolerance, and diuretic therapy. Besides infection, atherosclerotic diseases (ischemic heart disease, cerebrovascular accidents) are a major cause of death for these patients. Because of this, kidney transplant patients are encouraged to follow the American Heart Association's dietary recommendations. In addition to dietary restriction, pharmacologic therapy and regular exercise may also be necessary.[11,12]

Electrolytes and Minerals.   In the immediate post-transplant phase and until renal function improves, strict monitoring of fluid balance, electrolytes, and blood pressure is critical. Sodium restriction to 2 g may be necessary if antihypertensive medication is required. This may be liberalized as edema resolves and blood pressure improves.

Recommendations regarding potassium and calcium should be individualized for each patient. Because near normal kidney function is expected, potassium restriction is seldom necessary. Potassium levels should be monitored, however, because hyperkalemia may occur due to cyclosporine use. Cyclosporine use may also deplete magnesium levels; supplementation may be required. Calcium supplements may benefit renal transplant patients because chronic renal disease may result in the depletion of bone mineral calcium.[10,13] Also, the use of corticosteroids post-transplant may aggravate osteopenia.[10,14] If calcium supplements are prescribed to help maintain bone mass, the physician may want to monitor urine and serum levels in order to detect hypercalcuria and hypercalcemia if they should occur. Hypophosphatemia can occur when antacids are used to prevent steroid-induced gastritis. Patients may need to be reminded to increase their intake of phosphorus-containing foods and to discontinue phosphate binders previously prescribed. (It should be noted that calcium and phosphorus balance is a complex issue. A patient may have hyperparathyroidism secondary to kidney failure prior to transplant and improve after transplant, or the hyperparathyroidism may persist and require further surgery. Diet in these cases does not determine outcome.)

References

8. Blue LS. Nutritional considerations in kidney transplantation. Top Clin Nutr 1992;7(3):17–23.
9. Pagenkemper JJ, Foulks CJ. Nutritional management of the adult renal transplant patient. J Renal Nutr 1991;1:119–124.
10. Pruchno CJ, Hunsicker LG. Nutritional requirements of renal transplant patients. In: Mitch WE, Klahr S, eds. Nutrition and the kidney. Boston: Little, Brown, 1993:346–364.
11. Nelson J, Beauregard H, Gelinas M, St Louis G, Daloze P, Smeisters C, Corman J. Rapid improvement of hyperlipidemia in kidney transplant patients with a multifactorial hypolipidemic diet. Transplant Proc 1988;20:1264–1270.
12. Moore RA, Callahan RF, Cody M, Adams PL, Litchford M, Buckner K, Galloway J. The effect of the American Heart Association Step One Diet on hyperlipidemia following renal transplantation. Transplantation 1990;49:60–62.

13. Liddle VR, Walker PJ, Johnson HK, Ginn HE. Diet in transplantation. Dialysis Transplant 1977;6:9–11.
14. Hoy WE, Sargent JA, Hall D, McKenna BA, Pabico RC, Freeman RB, Yarger JM, Byer BM. Protein catabolism during the postoperative course after renal transplantation. Am J Kidney Dis 1985;5:186–190.

PANCREAS TRANSPLANTATION AND PANCREAS-KIDNEY TRANSPLANTATION

Pancreas transplantation can offer patients with diabetes mellitus long-term glucose control, improved quality of life, and may prevent the progression of neuropathy, retinopathy, and nephropathy.[15,16] A combined pancreas-renal transplant is done for diabetic patients with renal failure. With a successful transplant the diabetic and renal failure dietary restrictions can be liberalized. The patient has freedom from the portioning of food and the timing of meals to an insulin program.[17-19] Guidelines for the nutritional care of patients prior to, immediately following, and long-term post-transplant appear in Table 15-5.

Pretransplant

Factors affecting pretransplant nutritional status include duration of diabetes and degree of control, duration of renal failure, compliance with diet, and/or presence of gastroparesis. A dietitian should assess the individual's current intake and emphasize the importance of maintaining or improving nutritional status prior to transplant. (See Chapter 8, Diabetes Mellitus, Chapter 14, Chronic Renal Failure, and Chapter 9, Delayed Gastric Emptying.)

Immediately Post-transplant

Immediately post-transplant, the patient will need to follow the low bacteria diet (pancreas-renal) for 21 days. This is used in conjunction with the OSBD solution to help eradicate the gram-negative and fungal flora in the gastrointestinal tract.

Kilocalories. No conclusive studies are available that clearly establish the nutritional requirements of patients needing pancreas or pancreas and renal transplants. One may assume that caloric requirements in the immediate post-transplant phase are high due to surgical stress and catabolism. Indirect calorimetry may be used to accurately assess energy needs and to avoid overfeeding and glucose intolerance. For the patient not at nutritional risk, caloric requirements may be estimated by using the Harris-Benedict equation and a stress factor of 1.2. In our experience, ideal weight is used when calculating nutrient needs.

Protein. Following transplantation, protein requirements are also increased due to catabolism. Needs are estimated to be 1.2 to 1.5 g/kg of ideal body weight. These estimates are for patients with adequate kidney or graft function.

Carbohydrates and Fats. After transplantation, glucose intolerance may result from steroid therapy, surgical stress, and sepsis. Simple carbohydrate is de-emphasized and fiber is encouraged. As time progresses, this measure also helps to control weight and hyperlipidemia.

TABLE 15-5 Nutritional Care Guidelines for Pancreas and Pancreas-Renal Transplantation

	Pretransplant	Immediately Post-transplant*	Long-Term Post-transplant
Kilocalories†	Basal + 20%; increase if needed to maintain weight	Basal + 30%	Basal + 20% to avoid excess weight gain
Protein†	Restrict if needed; otherwise 1 g/kg/day	1.2–1.5 g/kg/day	1 g/kg/day
Fat	30% of kilocalories; limit saturated fat (in renal failure, increase fat as needed)	30% of kilocalories; limit saturated fat	30% of kilocalories; limit saturated fat
Cholesterol	≤ 300 mg/day (in renal failure, increase cholesterol as needed)	≤ 300 mg/day	≤ 300 mg/day
Fiber/simple carbohydrate	Emphasize fiber as tolerated; deemphasize simple carbohydrate	Emphasize fiber as tolerated; deemphasize simple carbohydrate	Emphasize fiber as tolerated; deemphasize simple carbohydrate
Sodium	No added salt or ≤ 90 mEq for edema or hypertension	No added salt or ≤ 90 mEq for edema or hypertension	No added salt or ≤ 90 mEq for edema or hypertension
Potassium	60 mEq if indicated	60 mEq if indicated	60 mEq if indicated
Calcium	800–1,200 mg	800–1,200 mg	1,200–1,500 mg
Alcohol	Avoid	Avoid	Avoid
Low bacteria diet	Not used	21 days post-transplant	As indicated

*Approximately first 2 mo after transplantation.

†Harris-Benedict equation and protein requirements are based on ideal body weight.

Because of the tendency of transplant patients toward hyperlipidemia, fat should be limited to 30% or less of kilocalories, with a restriction in saturated fat.[20]

Fluid and Electrolytes. Post-transplant patients may be volume overloaded. Depending upon renal function, fluid and electrolytes may or may not be restricted. Monitoring of fluid, electrolytes, and blood pressure will determine the need for dialysis and thus the restriction or liberalization of potassium, sodium, or fluid.[20]

Long-Term Post-transplant

As with kidney transplantation, long-term nutritional management focuses on prevention of hyperlipidemia and excessive weight gain due to continued use of steroids (see Chapter 15, Kidney Transplantation). There may also need to be adjustments to deal with symptoms of diabetic gastroparesis (see Chapter 8, Diabetes Mellitus, and Chapter 9, Delayed Gastric Emptying).

Dietary recommendations for pancreas and pancreas-renal transplantation are summarized in Table 15-5.

References

15. Perkins JD, Frohnert PP, Service FJ, Wilhelm MP, DiCecco SR, Johnson JL, Munn SR, Velosa JA. Pancreas transplantation at Mayo: III. Multidisciplinary management. Mayo Clinic Proc 1990;65:496–508.
16. Corry RJ. Status report on pancreas transplantation. Transplant Proc 1991;23: 2091–2094.
17. Luzi L, Facchini F, Secchi A, Battezzati A, Alemagna S, Ferrari G, Staudacher C, DiCarlo V, Pozza G. Glucose metabolism in patients after combined kidney-pancreas transplantation. Transplant Proc 1990;22:661.
18. Tibell A, Linder R, Larsson M, Tydén G, Groth CG, Bolinder J, Östman J. Long-term glucose control after pancreatic transplantation. Transplant Proc 1990;22:645–646.
19. Frohnert PP, Velosa JA, Munn SR, Marsh CL, Perkins JD. Morbidity during the first year after pancreas transplantation. Transplant Proc 1990;22:577.
20. Vizioli TL, Ishkanian I. Nutrition in pancreas-renal transplantation. J Renal Nutr 1992; 2(4):161–164.

LIVER TRANSPLANTATION

Liver transplantation is considered an appropriate treatment modality and is no longer an experimental procedure for many types of liver disease.[21,22] Advances in immunosuppressive and medical therapies and in surgical techniques have greatly reduced morbidity and mortality and widened the applicability of the procedure.

The four main criteria that should be met by candidates for liver transplantation are (1) irreversible progressive liver disease, (2) unavailable, exhausted, or less beneficial alternate therapies, (3) absence of absolute contraindications, and (4) patient and family acceptance of the transplant.[23] Table 15-6 lists the most common liver diseases that often require transplantation.[23]

Most patients with chronic end-stage liver disease requiring liver transplantation show some signs of malnutrition.[24-27] Accurate nutritional assessment of these patients is difficult because the effects of chronic liver disease can not be separated from those of malnutrition.[26,27] Therefore, pretransplant nutritional assessment should be a combination of the usual laboratory analysis and anthropometric measurements along with subjective parameters such as appearance, thorough nutrition and weight history, and the degree of ascites and/or edema.[27] Guidelines for nutritional care of all three phases of liver transplantation are listed in Table 15-7.[27-31]

Pretransplant

Nutritional support of the pretransplant patient focuses on management of any eating problems within the dietary restrictions so that optimal intake can be achieved. The primary objectives are to provide adequate kilocalories and protein in order to decrease the rate of protein catabolism, and to correct any macro- and micronutrient deficiencies (see Chapter 10, Hepatobiliary Diseases).[26] A low bacteria diet is initiated while the patient is awaiting surgery and is taking an OSBD solution.

TABLE 15-6 Liver Disease Candidates for Transplantation[23]

Genetic

Wilson's disease
Crigler-Najjar syndrome, type 1
Protoporphyria
α^1-Antitrypsin
Metabolic liver diseases

Extrahepatic biliary atresia

Hepatobiliary cancer

Chronic parenchymal liver disease

Budd-Chiari syndrome
Chronic active hepatitis and cirrhosis
Primary biliary cirrhosis
Sclerosing cholangitis
Alcoholic liver disease

Fulminant (acute) liver failure

Viral-induced
Drug-induced
Wilson's disease

With permission from: Schenker S. Medical treatment vs. transplantation in liver disorders. Hepatology 1984;4:102s-106s.

Immediately Post-transplant

In the immediate post-liver transplantation period (4 to 8 weeks) the focus of nutritional support is to provide adequate kilocalories and protein to meet the needs of these hypercatabolic (but not necessarily hypermetabolic) patients and to begin the repletion process.[28-30] Calorie and protein requirements are calculated using the patient's ideal or estimated lean weight (rule of thumb). This is based on data collected comparing calculated needs at ideal and actual weights versus resting energy expenditure (indirect calorimetry) and urine urea nitrogen output.[29] Other institutions may base their calculations on the patient's estimated dry weight.[31] Actual weight should only be used if the patient does not have ascites, edema, or fluid overload. Nutritional support may be provided by a combination of parenteral, enteral, and oral means. Central parenteral nutrition is often begun 24 to 36 hours after transplantation and continued until an adequate oral intake is established. Enteral feedings are used when parenteral nutrition is no longer appropriate or desirable, yet when adequate oral intake cannot be achieved. Patients are quickly advanced to an oral diet that is low in bacteria and high in protein (with other restrictions as indicated). Early satiety and altered taste perception may limit oral intake initially. Between meal feedings and/or supplements may be needed to meet goals for nutrient intake, especially protein.

TABLE 15-7 Nutritional Care Guidelines for Liver Transplantation[27-31]

	Pretransplant	Immediately Post-transplant*	Long-Term Post-transplant
Kilocalories†	Basal + 20% or more	Basal + 15–20%	Basal + 10–20% to maintain goal weight
Protein†	1 g/kg/day (minimize need for restriction)	1.2–1.75 g/kg/day	1 g/kg/day
Fat	As needed	30% of kilocalories	30% of kilocalories; low in saturated fat
Carbohydrate	As needed	50–60% of kilocalories	Reduced simple sugars
Sodium	90 mEq or less	90–180 mEq	90–135 mEq
Fluid	1,000–1,500 ml	As needed	As needed
Calcium	800–1,200 mg	800–1,200 mg	1,200–1,500 mg
Vitamins/other minerals	To meet RDA Water-soluble form of vitamins A, D, and E	To meet RDA	To meet RDA
Low bacteria diet	While activated	For at least 21 days	As indicated

*Approximately first 2 mo after transplantation.

†Harris-Benedict equation and protein requirements are based on ideal body weight pre- and immediately post-transplant and actual (dry) weight for long-term post-transplant.

Long-Term Post-transplant

Nutritional care in the long-term post-liver transplant phase focuses on returning to a healthy, well-balanced diet. However, modifications are often needed to deal with the long-term problems that commonly occur post-transplantation.[26] Excessive weight gain, hypertension, and hyperlipidemia are common post-transplantation. Osteoporosis (osteopenia) is common prior to transplant in many patients who have had cholestatic liver disease or who have been on long-term steroids. This often worsens during the first 6 months after transplant but then improves with return of good liver function, tapering of steroids, and adequate nutrition (especially calcium) and exercise.[32] Steroid-induced diabetes or insulin resistance also occurs occasionally after transplantation.

References

21. National Institutes of Health. Consensus development conference statement: liver transplantation—June 20–23, 1983. Hepatology 1984;4:1075–1105.
22. More liver transplants recommended by NIDDK consensus development panel. NIH Record 1983;35(14):1,9.
23. Schenker S. Medical treatment vs. transplantation in liver disorders. Hepatology 1984;4: 1025–1065.

24. DiCecco SR, Wieners EJ, Wiener RH, Southorn PA, Plevak DJ, Krom RAF. Assessment of nutritional status of patients with end-stage liver disease undergoing liver transplantation. Mayo Clin Proc 1989;64:95–102.

25. Hehir DJ, Jenkins RL, Bistrian BR, Blackburn GL. Nutrition in patients undergoing orthotopic liver transplant. JPEN 1985;9:695–700.

26. Porayko MK, DiCecco SR, O'Keefe SJD. Impact of malnutrition and its therapy on liver transplantation. Semin Liver Dis 1991;11:305–314.

27. Hasse JM. Nutritional implications of liver transplantation. Henry Ford Hosp Med J 1990;38:235–240.

28. Shanbhogue RLK, Bistrian BR, Jenkins RL, Randall S, Blackburn GL. Increased protein catabolism without hypermetabolism after human orthotopic liver transplantation. Surgery 1987;101:146–149.

29. Plevak DJ, DiCecco SR, Wiesner RH, Porayko MK, Janzow DJ, Hammel K. Nutritional support for liver transplantation: identifying caloric and protein requirements. Accepted for publication, Mayo Clinic Proceedings (March 1994).

30. O'Keefe SJD, Williams R, Calne RH. "Catabolic" loss of body protein after human liver transplantation. BMJ 1980;1:1107–1108.

31. Hasse JM. Nutrition considerations in liver transplantation. Top Clin Nutr 1992;7(3): 24–33.

32. Porayko MK, Wiesner RH, Hay JE, Krom RAF, Dickson ER, Beaver S, Schwerman L. Bone disease in liver transplant recipients: incidence, timing and risk factors. Transplant Proc 1991;23(1):1462–1465.

THORACIC ORGAN TRANSPLANTATION

Thoracic organ transplantation (heart, heart and lung, or lung) has become effective treatment for end-stage cardiac and pulmonary diseases. Patients who undergo this procedure present nutritional challenges.[33] Although the importance of nutrition in the long-term success or failure of thoracic transplantation has not been fully defined, certain nutritional efforts seem prudent in order to minimize known complications.

Pretransplant

Prior to transplant, candidates may be malnourished.[34] Poor cardiopulmonary function results in impaired delivery of oxygen and nutrients to tissues and in elevated caloric needs for increased respiratory and cardiac work. Anorexia secondary to dyspnea; medication side effects; and prescribed or self-imposed dietary prescriptions may also be contributing factors. Malabsorption may also occur as the intestinal tract becomes edematous, leading to reduced absorption of essential nutrients, which in turn perpetuates cardiac and gut atrophy.[34,35] Cardiac cachexia (protein-caloric malnutrition associated with severe congestive heart disease) has been cited as a risk factor for poor outcome after heart transplantation.[36] It has been suggested that nutritional intervention before (and after) transplantation may help reduce operative complications and improve outcome.[37]

Nutritional management of malnourished pretransplant patients involves the provision of adequate kilocalories, protein, and other nutrients. The hypermetabolism of congestive heart failure may increase energy requirements by 20 to 30%

due to greater cardiac and pulmonary energy expenditure.[38] A diet that meets or slightly exceeds the RDA for protein satisfies the needs of most cardiac transplant patients; higher protein and higher kilocalories may be needed for patients requiring nutritional repletion. However, caution is warranted because excessive nutritional support may induce metabolic or respiratory distress.[39] Restriction of fluid and sodium may be necessary to control edema. These should be adjusted according to the severity of cardiopulmonary failure and diuretic sensitivity. Restriction of caffeine may also be advised. In most cases, intake of sufficient calories and nutrients becomes more critical than limiting dietary fat and cholesterol prior to surgery.[38] Vitamin and mineral supplementation may be needed due to inadequate intake or poor absorption.[36,40] Dietary recommendations for patients receiving thoracic organ transplantation appear in Table 15-8.

TABLE 15-8   Nutritional Care Guidelines for Thoracic Organ Transplantation

	Pretransplant	Immediately Post-transplant*	Long-Term Post-transplant
Kilocalories†	Basal + 20–30%; Appropriate to maintain or obtain desirable body weight	Basal to Basal + 20%	Basal + 20%; Appropriate to maintain desirable body weight
Protein†	0.8–1.2 g/kg/day	1.2–1.5 g/kg/day	0.8–1.5 g/kg/day as indicated by protein status and renal function
Fat	< 30% of kilocalorie; limit saturated fat (liberalized as needed)	< 30% of kilocalories; limit saturated fat	< 30% of kilocalories; limit saturated fat
Carbohydrate	As needed	As needed	50–60% of kilocalories; deemphasize simple carbohydrate
Cholesterol	200–300 mg/day	200–300 mg/day	200–300 mg/day
Sodium	60–90 mEq/day	90–135 mEq/day	90–180 mEq/day
Calcium	800–1,200 mg/day	800–1,200 mg/day	1,200–1,500 mg/day
Fluid	1–3 L/day	1–3 L/day	Not restricted except for impaired renal output
Caffeine	Restrict if patient has arrhythmias	Restrict if patient has arrhythmias	Restrict if patient has arrhythmias
Low bacteria diet	Not used	90 days post-transplant	Use only if indicated

*Approximately first 2 mo after transplantation.

†Harris-Benedict equation and protein requirements are based on actual (dry) weight.

Six small meals are usually best tolerated because larger feedings may place excessive demand on cardiorespiratory function by increasing metabolic rate (thermogenic effect) and thus increasing the amounts of oxygen needed and carbon dioxide produced.[41] Crowding of diaphragmatic action by a large meal also impairs respiratory function. Smaller meals and frequent snacks may also help to counteract early satiety.

Immediately Post-transplant

Post-transplant patients are in a catabolic state and have increased nutrient requirements to promote wound healing. In addition to considering preoperative nutritional status, assessment should include the transplanted organs' functions and the effects of immunosuppressive medications.

Energy needs may be difficult to determine in stressed and septic patients, and indirect calorimetry can be a valuable tool in setting calorie goals. For most patients, postoperative recovery increases caloric requirements by 20% above basal; however, basal kilocalories are provided immediately post-surgery.[40] Adequate dietary protein at levels of 1.2 to 1.5 g/kg of body weight may help offset protein catabolism and muscle wasting associated with high doses of prednisone in the immediate post-transplant phase. Other nutrition-related side effects of prednisone and a multiple-drug immunosuppressive regimen should be anticipated, and their prevention or other intervention should be part of the nutritional care plan.[41,42]

Patients often resume oral intake within 3 to 5 days of surgery. During this period, intake proceeds slowly. Cool, soft foods or liquids are often preferred.[35] Small, frequent meals and liquid nutritional supplements may help to achieve nutrient needs.[38] A low bacteria diet is generally prescribed after transplant, but the benefits of this practice are still under investigation (see Chapter 15, Low Bacteria Diets).

Nutritional support may be considered for individuals whose intake remains inadequate. Enteral nutrition is preferred over the parenteral route due to increased risk of infection in the immunosuppressed patient.[40] Concentration of parenteral or enteral feedings is often necessary to prevent fluid overload. Lung transplant recipients may also have decreased ability to cough and clear secretions due to denervation of allografted organs. These individuals are at increased risk for aspiration,[40] and antiaspiration measures should be followed as with all patients receiving enteral nutrition support.[43]

Long-Term Post-transplant

The major medical problem for cardiac transplant patients in the long-term post-transplant phase is graft atherosclerosis.[44] Although this is thought to be due to an immunological process, hypercholesterolemia,[45] hypertriglyceridemia,[46] hypertension,[47] smoking[47] and obesity[48] play a part. Hypercholesterolemia—specifically, elevated low-density lipoprotein—is commonly observed. Although the mechanisms involved in this hyperlipidemia remain to be more clearly defined, a lipid-lowering diet may be of some benefit, particularly if the diet modifications do not impose undue hardship.[49] As with other types of transplants, the long-term use of prednisone may potentiate bone loss, so attention to dietary factors that influence bone mass is indicated (see Chapter 8, Osteoporosis). Glucose intolerance and obesity due to prednisone therapy are also problematic, and preventive dietary measures are prudent. Likewise the long-term use of cyclosporine may result in hypertension, hyperkalemia, hypomagnesemia, and nephrotoxicity. The long-term nutritional care plan may be altered according to these nutrition-related drug effects.[41,42]

References

33. Poindexter SM. Nutrition support in cardiac transplantation. Top Clin Nutr 1992;7(3):12–16.

34. Heymsfield SB, Hoff RD, Gray TF, Casper K. Heart disease. In: Kinney JM, Jeejeebhoy KN, Hill GL, Owen OE, eds. Nutrition and metabolism in patient care. Philadelphia, PA: WB Saunders, 1989:477–509.

35. Schocken DD, Holloway JD, Powers PS. Weight loss and the heart. Arch Intern Med 1989;149:877–881.

36. Moore C, Chowdhury Z, Young JB. Heart transplantation programs: a national survey. J Heart Lung Transplant 1991;10(1):50–55.

37. Mullen J, Buzby G, Matthews D, Smale BF, Rosato EF. Reduction of operative morbidity and mortality by combined preoperative and postoperative nutritional support. Ann Surg 1980;192:604–613.

38. Rock CL, Leonard LB. Nutrition care of cardiac transplant patients. Top Clin Nutr 1990;5(2):1–9.

39. De Meo MT, Van De Graaff W, Gottlieb K, Sobotka P, Mobarhan S. Nutrition in acute pulmonary disease. Nutr Rev 1992;50(1):320–328.

40. Frazier OH, VanBuren CT, Poindexter SM, Waldenberger F. Nutritional management of the heart transplant recipient. Heart Transplant 1985;4(4):450–452.

41. Maurer JR. Therapeutic challenges following lung transplantation. Clin Chest Med 1990;11(2):279–290.

42. Gilbert-Barness EF, Barness LA. Pathologic consequences of immunosuppressive therapy used in treating transplant rejection. Perspect Pediatr Pathol 1989;13:146–193.

43. Kirk AJB, Colquhoun IW, Corris PA, Hilton CJ, Dark JH. Impaired gastrointestinal motility in pulmonary transplantation. Lancet 1990;336(8717):752.

44. Kriett JM, Kay MP. The registry of the international society for heart and lung transplantation: eighth official report—1991. J Heart Lung Transplant 1991;10:491-498.

45. Eich D, Thompson JA, Ko D. Hypercholesterolemia in long-term survivors of heart transplantation: an early marker of accelerated coronary artery disease. J Heart Lung Transplant 1991;10:45–49.

46. Billingham M. Cardiac transplant atherosclerosis. Transplant Proc 1987;19(4)(Suppl 5):19–25.

47. Radovancevic B, Poindexter S, Birovljev S. Risk factors for development of accelerated coronary artery disease in cardiac transplant recipients. Eur J Cardiothorac Surg 1990;4:309–313.

48. Winters GL, Kendall TJ, Radio SJ. Post-transplant obesity and hyperlipidemia: major predictors of severity of coronary arteriopathy in failed human heart allografts. J Heart Lung Transplant 1990;9:364–371.

49. Keogh A, Simons L, Spratt P, Esmore D, Chang V, Hickie J, Baron D. Hyperlipidemia after heart transplantation. J Heart Transplant 1988;7:171–175.

BONE MARROW TRANSPLANTATION

Bone marrow transplantation (BMT) is a therapy for certain hematologic disorders such as aplastic anemia, acute leukemia, some forms of lymphoma, and, more recently, solid tumors such as breast cancer. Critical to a successful transplant is a donor with closely matched histocompatible antigens. The closest match is that of a genetically identical twin (syngeneic). The more common match is a human leukocyte antigen (HLA) identical sibling (allogeneic). In certain cases, the patient's own marrow is aspirated and infused later (autologous).[50]

Pretransplant

Prior to transplantation, patients are generally in adequate nutritional status. Patients are assessed by a dietitian upon admission to the hospital. A diet history that includes food preferences and dislikes is helpful for reference in the post-transplant phase when oral feeding is resumed. Pretransplant counseling may include a discussion on food and nutrition services provided, avoidance of fresh fruits and vegetables due to bacterial content, potential side effects of "conditioning" (chemotherapy and radiation), and use of central parenteral nutrition (CPN).

Prior to transplantation, the patient is given several days of high dose chemotherapy and possibly total body irradiation to eradicate to the extent possible the leukemia or lymphoma and prevent possible graft rejection and/or relapse.[51]

Nutritional consequences of the conditioning phase may include nausea, vomiting, mucositis, esophagitis, xerostomia, thick viscous saliva, dysgeusia, anorexia, early satiety, diarrhea, and steatorrhea. The duration and intensity of these symptoms and the stress of the treatments are such that protein-calorie malnutrition in some degree is almost a certainty. Strategies for dealing with these problems are a major focus of nutritional care in the post-transplant phase. (See Chapter 12, Cancer, for methods of dealing with eating problems.) Another consequence of the conditioning is impaired immune function and reduced ability of the patient's body to deal with bacterial and fungal pathogens. Fresh fruits and vegetables contain gram-negative bacteria and are ordinarily no hazard to the healthy person, but may provoke a serious infection in the BMT patient. Therefore a low bacteria diet is indicated.[52,53] (See Chapter 15, Low Bacteria Diets.)

The patient undergoing BMT is often unable to maintain an adequate oral intake owing to the mucosal ulceration and severe anorexia induced by the transplantation conditioning programs, infection, or graft versus host disease (GVHD). GVHD is characterized by development of an immune response by the grafted tissue or organ against the host—a sort of reverse rejection. Frequent monitoring of nutrient intake and the encouragement of adequate kilocalorie and protein intake are essential in the care of the BMT patient. Specific nutritional care guidelines for BMT patients appear in Table 15-9.

Immediately Post-transplant

Severe oropharyngeal mucositis and anorexia result in a significantly decreased oral intake due to the conditioning regimen. This can last for up to 1 month. CPN is instituted to meet nutritional needs. Daily nutrient (kilocalories, protein, fat) intake from oral and parenteral routes is monitored closely. Literature has shown that estimated energy needs may be 20 to 30% above basal, and protein needs increase to 1.5 to 2.0 g/kg per day.[54-60] Our experience has confirmed that provi-

TABLE 15-9   Nutritional Care Guidelines for Bone Marrow Transplantation

	Pretransplant (Includes Conditioning Phase)	Immediately Post-transplant*	Long-Term Post-transplant
Kilocalories†	Basal + 10–20%	Basal + 20%	Basal + 10–15%
Protein†	1 g/kg/day	1.2–1.5 g/kg/day	1 g/kg/day
Fat	As needed	As needed	As needed
Carbohydrate/fiber	As needed	As needed	As needed
Sodium	As needed	As needed	As needed
Fluid	As needed	As needed	As needed
Calcium	800–1,200 mg/day	800–1,200 mg/day	800–1,200 mg/day
Vitamins/other minerals	To meet RDA	To meet RDA	To meet RDA
Low bacteria diet	During conditioning phase	Whenever neutropenic	Whenever neutropenic

*Approximately first 2 mo after transplantation.

†Harris-Benedict equation and protein requirements are based on actual (dry) weight.

sion of kilocalories at 20% above basal has been adequate to minimize weight loss. Standard CPN monitoring practices are followed (see Chapter 16, Parenteral Nutritional Support) as long as CPN therapy continues.

Oral intake is encouraged as early as possible. The patient and the family are informed of protein and kilocalorie intake goals. Cooperation and encouragement from family members to assist the patient in meeting nutrient intake goals is an important part of the recovery process. However, it is not recommended that food be brought in from outside the hospital while the patient is neutropenic. When the patient has engrafted but oral intake remains inadequate, food may be brought in if approved by the physician.

A major complication of BMT may be GVHD, which can present as an acute or chronic state. It is thought that the newly grafted bone marrow recognizes the host's cells as foreign. GVHD may cause multiple organ damage but especially involves the skin, the gastrointestinal tract, and the liver.[54,61,62]

Gastrointestinal GVHD is a major nutritional complication. Its signs and complications can include abdominal pain, nausea, vomiting, diarrhea, bloody stools, malabsorption, altered intestinal motility, and ileus.

The dietary protocol for management of gastrointestinal GVHD appears in Table 15-10.

The low bacteria diet (no fresh fruits and vegetables) restriction instituted upon admission is maintained until dismissal from the hospital. If the neutrophil count is adequate (greater than 0.5×10^9 per liter), consumption of carefully washed fresh fruits and vegetables may be resumed. Upon dismissal, the patient should be able to maintain weight on oral intake alone. The patient is counseled regarding nutritional needs and how to meet them at home or in another outpatient setting.

TABLE 15-10 Dietary Management of Gastrointestinal Graft Versus Host Disease[54,62]

Step 1

Bowel rest and no food by mouth until the stool volume is less than 500 ml/day for 2 days or more. Nutrition is provided by CPN.

Step 2

The introduction of low residue, low lactose (preferably isosmotic) beverages in small, frequent feedings. When symptoms improve, advance to Step 3. CPN support is provided to meet nutrient and kilocalorie goals.

Step 3

The introduction of solid foods that are low in residue, lactose, and fat (approximately 30 g of fat per day) and that have no gastric irritants (see Chapter 9, Peptic Ulcer Disease). These foods should be taken as tolerated. The slow introduction of foods, one at a time, in frequent, small meals, is necessary. CPN support continues as needed as a nutrient supplement.

Step 4

Gradually liberalize the previous dietary restrictions until a normal diet is tolerated asymptomatically.

CPN = Central parenteral nutrition.

Patients are required to maintain food intake records after dismissal from the hospital for a period of up to 4 weeks. The records are reviewed and evaluated by the dietitian as part of the outpatient follow-up. Patients are counseled as needed to assure an adequate oral intake and weight maintenance.

Long-Term Post-transplant

Weight loss is a common nutritional consequence for 3 to 12 months after BMT. Patients with no or limited GVHD tend to regain their weight by their 1 year evaluation. Patients with extensive GVHD are less likely to regain the lost weight. The use of immunosuppressive therapy for extensive GVHD may offset weight loss due to fluid retention and appetite enhancement.[63,64]

Common problems affecting oral intake include oral sensitivity, taste changes, xerostomia, and anorexia. Less frequently occurring problems include esophageal stricture, diarrhea, and steatorrhea. A diet as tolerated using nutritional supplements is recommended.

Weight should be monitored on a monthly basis. Those patients with an inappropriate weight loss and/or eating problems should be referred to the dietitian for counseling.

References

50. Thomas ED. Bone marrow transplantation in hematologic malignancies. Hosp Pract 1987;Feb 15:77–91.
51. Letendre L, Hoagland HC, Moore SB, Chen MG, Gastineau DA, Gertz MA, Habermann TM, Litzow MR, Noël P, Solberg LA, Tefferi A. Mayo Clinic experience with syngeneic bone marrow transplantation, 1982 through 1990. Mayo Clin Proc 1992;67:109–116.

52. Aker SN, Cheney CL. The use of sterile and low microbial diets in ultraisolation environments. JPEN 1983;7:390–397.

53. Anon. Low-microbial vs. sterile diets for immunocompromised patients. Nutrition and the MD 1989;87(7):1.

54. Aker SN. Bone marrow transplantation: nutrition support and monitoring. In: Bloch SA, ed. Nutrition management of the cancer patient. Rockville MD: Aspen Pubs 1990:199–225.

55. Peters E, Beck J, LeMaistre C. Changes in resting energy expenditure (REE) during allogeneic bone marrow transplantation. Am J Clin Nutr 1990;51:521. Abstract.

56. Szeluga DJ, Stuart RK, Brookmeyer R, Utermohlen V, Santos GW. Energy requirements of parenterally fed bone marrow transplant recipients. JPEN 1985;9(2):139–143.

57. Weisdorf SA, Lysne J, Wind D, Haake RJ, Sharp HL, Goldman A, Schissel K, McGrave PB, Ramsay NK, Kersey JH. Positive effect of prophylactic total parenteral nutrition on long-term outcome of bone marrow transplantation. Transplantation 1987;43(6): 833–838.

58. Lenssen P, Cheney CL, Aker SN, Cummingham BA, Darbinian J, Gauvreau JM, Barale KV. Intravenous branched chain amino acid trial in marrow transplant recipients. JPEN 1987;11(2):112–118.

59. Szeluga DJ, Stuart RK, Brookmeyer R, Utermohlen V, Santos GW. Nutrition support of bone marrow transplant recipients: a prospective, randomized clinical trial comparing total parenteral nutrition to an enteral feeding program. Cancer Res 1987;47:3309–3316.

60. Geibig CB, Owens JP, Mirtallo JM, Bowers D, Nahikian-Nelms M, Fatschka P. Parenteral nutrition for marrow transplant recipients: evaluation of an increased nitrogen dose. JPEN 1991;15(2):184–188.

61. Beck J. Allogenic bone marrow transplantation in chronic myelogenous leukemia and its nutrition implications: a case study. Top Clin Nutr 1992;7(3):34–40.

62. Gauvreau JM, Lenssen P, Cheney CL, Aker SN, Hutchinson ML, Barale KV. Nutritional management of patients with intestinal graft-versus-host disease. J Am Diet Assoc 1981; 79:673–677.

63. Lenssen P, Sherry ME, Cheney CL, Nims JW, Sullivan KM, Stein JM, Moe G, Aker SN. Prevalence of nutrition-related problems among long-term survivors of allogeneic marrow transplantation. J Am Diet Assoc 1990;90(6):835–842.

64. Boock CA, Reddick JE. Taste alterations in bone marrow transplant patients. J Am Diet Assoc 1991;91(9):1121–1122.

16 / *Nutritional Support of Adults*

ENTERAL NUTRITIONAL SUPPORT OF ADULTS

General Description

Enteral nutrition is defined as the provision of liquid formula diets by mouth or by tube into the gastrointestinal tract.[1] Patients unable or unwilling to take adequate nutrients by mouth require an alternative form of nutritional support. Some patients may need nutritional support via the intravenous route. Others are capable of digesting and absorbing nutrients delivered through feeding tubes introduced into the alimentary tract. Enteral tube feeding has been shown to be an effective method for treating and for preventing nutritional deficiencies.[2]

The approach to enteral tube feeding should be a cooperative team effort and include the physician, dietitian, nurse, and pharmacist. When enteral tube feedings are to continue beyond the hospitalization period, a multidisciplinary discharge and follow-up plan is needed for the patient.

Indications and Rationale

Any disease process that adversely affects oral intake may ultimately lead to significant nutritional deprivation and depletion. Patients who cannot eat, will not eat, or should not eat, yet who have adequate function of the gastrointestinal tract, are candidates for enteral tube feeding (Table 16-1).

Enteral feeding has a number of distinct advantages over parenteral feeding. The route of feeding is more physiologic. Other advantages include maintenance of gastrointestinal immune and barrier function, avoidance of central catheter related complications, and lower cost.[3-5]

Enteral tube feeding is contraindicated in patients with peritonitis, distal intestinal obstruction, intractable vomiting or severe diarrhea. Parenteral nutrition should be considered when a properly managed trial of tube feeding fails to meet

385

TABLE 16-1 Indications for Tube Feeding

Nutritional Disorder	Cause
Oral intake inadequate or contraindicated	Mechanical: stroke, central nervous system disorders, coma, oropharyngeal and esophageal disorders, partial or complete esophageal or gastric obstruction Poor appetite: chemotherapy, radiation therapy, drug effect, nausea Transitional feeding: advance from parenteral to oral intake Psychological: anorexia nervosa, depression, Alzheimer's disease
Increased nutritional requirements	Burns, trauma, sepsis, surgical or medical stress
Digestive and absorptive disorders	Inflammatory bowel disease, short bowel syndrome, pancreatitis, irradiated bowel, proximal and distal intestinal fistulae, immunocompromised syndromes
Metabolic and excretory disorders	Glycogen storage disease Hepatic encephalopathy Renal disease

nutritional goals, aggravates the primary condition, or creates secondary problems such as pulmonary aspiration or unmanageable diarrhea.

Determination of Nutrient Needs

Assessment of the nutritional status of every patient is fundamental and includes four key components: nutritional history screen, anthropometric procedures, clinical examination, and biochemical data. Nutritional assessment is a process that documents the presence of malnutrition, aids the clinician in selecting the best method for providing nutrients, and allows for objective monitoring of nutritional support efforts. It is also needed to estimate nutritional requirements in order to select the correct type and amount of formula, and to estimate the need for vitamin, mineral, and fluid modifications. (See Chapter 3, Nutritional Assessment.)

Kilocalories. The estimation of the patient's caloric requirement helps determine the quantity of formula needed daily. Most tube feeding formulations provide 1.0 kcal/ml, although there are formulations providing up to 2.0 kcal/ml. Patients' sensitivity to volume and their overall fluid requirements may necessitate the selection of a more concentrated or more dilute formula.

Protein. The amount of protein provided by a formula depends on the amount of formula administered daily and on the concentration of protein in the formula. The patient's protein requirements can be met by adjusting the quantity of formula, by selecting a formula with a different protein density, or by adding a protein module to the formula. Most commercial formulas contain a nonprotein kilocalorie-to-nitrogen ratio of 150:1 (with a range between 100:1 and 200:1), which is thought to be optimal for nonstressed patients.

Vitamins, Minerals, and Trace Elements. It is important to note the quantity of an enteral formula necessary to meet the Recommended Dietary Allowances (RDA) for vitamins and minerals. Most commercial formulations provide 100% or more of the RDA for vitamins and essential minerals in 1,300 to 1,900 ml. Supplemental vitamins and minerals should be given when the quantity of formula does not provide the full requirement. The individual's nutritional status should also be monitored and the amounts of vitamins and minerals adjusted accordingly. Known essential trace elements are present in many commercial formulas, and current clinical practice is to supplement with additional trace elements only if a deficiency is detected.

Water. Fluid balance in patients receiving enteral tube feeding should be monitored. In general, the daily water requirement for a healthy adult is 1 ml/kcal taken[6] or approximately 30 to 32 ml/kg.[7] However, the fluid requirement of the hospitalized patient varies and must be determined in each individual situation.[6,7] Most commercial tube feeding formulations contain 700 to 850 ml of water per liter. Water given in addition to that provided by the formula is usually given as a flush at intervals throughout the day. A minimum of 30 ml of water every 6 hours is recommended as a flush for tube patency alone.

Nutritional Formulations

A wide variety of commercially prepared formulas with variable sources and concentrations of protein, carbohydrate, and fat are currently available. The formulas differ in caloric density; nutrient source; kilocalorie-to-nitrogen ratio; electrolyte, vitamin, mineral, and fiber content; and osmolality. Commercial products offer many distinct advantages over hospital or home-blended mixtures, including a known nutrient composition, controlled osmolality and consistency, ease in preparation and storage, bacteriological safety, and in most instances lower cost.[8,9]

Appendix 10 displays the nutrient content of many of the formulas that are available. Data are derived from manufacturers' analyses and are presented on the basis of nutrients per 1,000 ml. The volumes needed to assure 100% of the RDA for vitamins should be noted and supplements provided if needed. These formulas are often categorized as polymeric, predigested (elemental or semielemental), special disease-specific formulas, and modular nutrient sources.

Polymeric Formulas. (Appendix 10.) Polymeric formulas are composed of intact proteins, disaccharides and polysaccharides, and variable amounts of fat, residue, and lactose. The osmolality of polymeric formulas is usually lower than the osmolality of "elemental" formulas. In general, these formulas require a functioning gastrointestinal tract for digestion and absorption of nutrients.

Polymeric formulas can be subdivided into blended food products, lactose-containing products, hypercaloric lactose-free products, and normocaloric lactose-free products. Normocaloric lactose-free formulas can be subdivided into those that are isosmotic, those that are hyperosmotic, those that are higher in nitrogen content, and those that contain fiber.

Predigested Formulas. (Appendix 10.) Predigested formulas are composed of low molecular weight nutrients, have minimal residue, are thought to lead to less stimulation of pancreatic and gastrointestinal secretions, and are less allergenic than other formulas.[10] These products usually have a greater osmolality than polymeric formulas because of the small molecular weight of the nutrients. These formulas have a relatively poor palatability and are therefore best suited to tube administration. However, flavoring options are available, which increase palatability and patient acceptance.

Protein sources include short-chain peptides and/or free amino acids. Studies have shown that the small peptides are better absorbed when presented to the intestinal mucosa than are free amino acids. However, further studies are needed to confirm the ideal peptide-containing nitrogen source in predigested diets.[11] Carbohydrate sources in predigested formulas include oligosaccharides and sucrose.

Fat sources are usually medium-chain triglycerides (MCTs) and/or polyunsaturated oils such as safflower, corn, soy, or sunflower. The elemental formulas have a low long-chain fat content and thus are beneficial for patients with significant fat malabsorption or severe exocrine pancreatic insufficiency. MCTs can be effectively absorbed intact without bile salt and pancreatic lipase activity. They pass directly into the portal system rather than through the lymphatic circulation. However, MCTs are not a source of essential fatty acids. (See Chapter 9, Fat Malabsorption, for further information on MCTs.)

Modular Products.   (Appendix 10.) Individual macronutrient modules such as glucose polymers, protein, and lipids are available as additives to food and enteral formulas to change overall fuel composition.

Individually customized enteral solutions may also be formulated from modular products to yield nutritionally complete formulas that meet the needs of patients with fluid restrictions, electrolyte imbalances, or specific nutrient requirements. Vitamins, minerals, and trace elements in amounts appropriate for each patient must be added. Therefore modular formulas require labor-intensive custom formulation.[12,13]

Special Disease-Specific Formulas.   (Appendix 10.) These products are designed for patients who have specific medical conditions that may require nutrient modification. In patients with hepatic encephalopathy, the use of formulas high in branched-chain amino acids (BCAAs: leucine, isoleucine, and valine) and low in aromatic amino acids (AAAs: phenylalanine, tyrosine, and tryptophan) and methionine may increase the ratio of serum BCAAs to AAAs. This BCAA:AAA ratio is thought to help reverse abnormally high serum levels of AAA and thereby control the severity of encephalopathy, but study results are thus far inconclusive.[14-16] (See also Chapter 10, Hepatobiliary Disease.)

The use of specific amino acids for the hypermetabolic and stressed patient is a relatively new area, which requires further study.[10,17] Information on metabolic processes during stress has led to the development of formulas specifically designed with increased BCAA content.[18] These high BCAA (44% to 50% of total amino acids) formulas are not restricted in AAA, unlike the formulas marketed for hepatic encephalopathy. Theoretically, the BCAA, especially leucine, may support protein synthesis and improve nitrogen balance in the hypermetabolic and stressed patient.

There are formulas currently available that contain arginine, ribonucleic acids, and fish oils (omega-3 fatty acids). This combination of nutrients appears to enhance T-lymphocyte function and overall immune response and promote positive nitrogen balance in immunocompromised, stressed patients. Studies have been completed that suggest these formulas may benefit cancer, postsurgical,[19,20] and burn patients.[21] However, widespread use of these products should await further research in other patient populations.

Formulas are also available that are designed for patients with specific conditions such as pulmonary disease, glucose intolerance, or renal failure. Patients with chronic renal failure may benefit from the use of formulas containing nitrogen in the form of essential amino acids and histidine. However, conventional protein sources should be given if patients are receiving hemodialysis. The use of formulas with only essential amino acids is not recommended for patients with acute renal failure due to depletion of the nonessential amino acids responsible for ammonia detoxification.[22] Many of the special disease-specific formulas are also controlled for minerals, vitamins, and electrolytes to minimize complications.

Intestinal Fuels. Numerous studies have investigated dietary components that are trophic to intestinal cells and may thereby enhance gut barrier function. These include glutamine and short-chain fatty acids (SCFAs).

Glutamine, a nonessential amino acid, is the most abundant amino acid in circulation. In spite of this, intracellular stores may be depleted by more than 50% following severe illness. In animals, the metabolism of glutamine by enterocytes is an important regulatory mechanism of nitrogen metabolism in normal and catabolic states. Therefore, glutamine may be considered to be an essential amino acid during critical illness and stress. It comprises 4% to 6% of dietary protein and is present in varying quantities in enteral formulas.[23-26]

SCFAs (acetate, butyrate, and propionate) are important fuels for colonocytes. Enteral infusion of SCFAs has been shown to speed intestinal healing and support mucosal integrity in animal and human studies.[27] Fiber-containing enteral formulas are thought to support bowel integrity by supplying polysaccharides, which are fermented by colonic bacteria to yield SCFAs.[28] Numerous fiber-containing formulas are currently available, most of which contain soy polysaccharides. Oat, fruit, and vegetable fibers are also used in several formulas. In addition to enhancing colonic mucosal integrity, fiber-containing formulas may help normalize intestinal motility. They are therefore helpful for use in patients requiring long-term tube feeding for control of constipation.[29] Fiber-containing formulas may also help prevent diarrhea by promoting colonic water and sodium absorption and by adding bulk to the stool. Optimal applications in critically ill patients remain to be established.[30]

Formula Selection. Selection of the appropriate formula is based on the individual patient's medical and nutritional status. Digestive and absorptive capabilities indicate whether a predigested or polymeric formula is needed. Individual nutrient requirements further specify the type and the amount of formula necessary to provide adequate nutritional support and whether supplemental sources of nutrients are required. An ongoing assessment of nutritional status while the patient is receiving tube feeding will determine the effectiveness of the nutritional program.

Tube Feeding Access Routes

The route for tube feeding depends on the anticipated duration of feeding, the condition of the gastrointestinal tract (e.g., esophageal obstruction, prior gastric or small bowel resections), and the potential for aspiration. Access to the gut can be accomplished at the bedside (nasoenteric tube), through specialized procedures (percutaneous endoscopic gastrostomy, percutaneous endoscopic jejunostomy), or in the operating room (surgical gastrostomy or jejunostomy).

Nasal Intubation.   Nasal intubation for placement of a feeding tube is the simplest and most commonly used approach to tube feeding. This technique is preferred for patients in whom eventual resumption of oral feeding is anticipated. Patient comfort and acceptance is greater when a small-diameter, soft silicone rubber feeding tube is used.[31] Access to the duodenum and the jejunum is possible with long weighted tubes.

Tube Enterostomies.   In general, tube enterostomies are preferred when long-term tube feeding is anticipated, when obstruction makes nasal intubation impossible, or during planned abdominal surgery.[32] Conventional gastrostomies require a surgical procedure with the use of general anesthesia. For high risk patients, morbidity and mortality rates may be high. Percutaneous endoscopic placement of a gastrostomy has advantages and can be performed with minimal sedation. Potential complications are usually minor and infrequent.[33,34]

Postpyloric access is preferred for patients in whom gastric feeding is contraindicated. Jejunal or duodenal access permits early postoperative feeding because the small bowel is less affected than the stomach and colon by postoperative ileus. Intestinal feedings are also thought to minimize the risk of vomiting and aspiration from the infusion, but this has yet to be proven conclusively. Percutaneous endoscopic jejunostomy tubes have been placed either directly or through an existing gastrostomy.[35,36] Needle catheter jejunostomy placed at the time of laparotomy provides access for postoperative nutritional support in patients who are malnourished preoperatively, who may undergo major upper abdominal operations, or who will receive postoperative chemotherapy or radiation therapy. The development of skin-level nonrefluxing gastrostomy tubes has provided a desirable option for alert, ambulatory patients who are on long-term enteral nutritional support.[37,38] Tubes with dual gastric and jejunal ports are available for those patients who require both intestinal feedings and gastric decompression.

Administration of Tube Feeding

Proper administration of enteral formulas ensures safe delivery of desired nutrients, enhanced patient tolerance, and optimum nutritional support. Choice of the specific method for administration of tube feeding (e.g., intermittent or continuous infusion), control of the initial rate and concentration of the formula, and a systematic progression to reach nutrient requirements are all important factors for tube feeding administration.

Methods of Feeding.   Tube feeding may be administered by continuous, intermittent, or bolus infusion. The choice of technique depends mainly on gastrointestinal function, feeding site, and, ultimately, patient response.

Continuous infusion.   Continuous infusion is the controlled delivery of a prescribed volume of formula at a constant rate over a continuous period of time (e.g., 12 to 24 hours) using an infusion pump. This method is considered to be advantageous since gastric pooling is minimized and fewer gastrointestinal side effects are experienced.[39] Continuous infusion into the jejunum is more analogous to normal gastric emptying. Additionally, daily energy requirements may be less during continuous formula infusion than during intermittent infusion because of a decrease in diet-induced thermogenesis.[40]

Continuous infusion is most often indicated in patients who have taken nothing by mouth for a significant period of time, who are debilitated, who have impaired gastrointestinal function, or who have uncontrolled insulin-requiring diabetes mellitus. The continuous method is particularly favored for intestinal feeding, although some patients tolerate intermittent infusion. A constant infusion rate can be ensured by using an infusion pump. Continuous drip by gravity is possible, but accuracy is less easily achieved.

Intermittent infusion.   In intermittent feeding, the total quantity of formula needed for a 24 hour period is divided into equal portions, and the required fractions are administered in 3 to 6 feedings. Each feeding is usually administered by gravity over a 30 to 90 minute period. Individual tolerance may vary, with some patients tolerating a more rapid rate. Rate of intermittent infusion (rather than volume) has been cited as a major reason for symptoms of intolerance.[41] A volume of 480 ml per feeding can be achieved in a number of patients. Prolongation of the feeding time can often accommodate the increased volume per feeding.

An advantage of the intermittent feeding method is that it requires only simple equipment. It works particularly well in the home care setting because it allows patients greater freedom to accommodate lifestyles. Intermittent infusion may be more physiologic than continuous infusion since it represents a more normal feeding pattern. However, in the absence of infusion pumps, feedings must be monitored closely. The procedure may become quite time-consuming when multiple feedings are scheduled each day.

Bolus feeding.   Bolus feeding is the intermittent, rapid administration of large volumes of formula (240 to 480 ml) over a very short period of time, usually by syringe. This method of feeding is least cumbersome to the patient but is associated with an increased possibility of aspiration, regurgitation, and gastrointestinal side effects. A rate of 30 ml/minute or a volume of 500–750 ml per feeding appears to mark physical tolerance limits.[41] This method of infusion is generally not appropriate for postpyloric feeding.

Initiation of Tube Feeding.   Regardless of the choice of feeding technique, a systematic approach to initiating tube feeding is mandatory to ensure patient tolerance. Generally, the initial infusion rate should be slow. Standardized order forms may facilitate the initiation and monitoring of tube-fed patients (see Appendix 11).

Rate.   Infusion rates should not exceed the patient's ability to manage the volume provided. An initial administration rate of 20 ml/hour of an isotonic formula is recommended. Lower rates may be necessary for critically ill patients, those with impaired absorption, and those who are receiving hypertonic formulas. Patients should be monitored for symptoms of intolerance. For gastric feedings, gastric residual should be measured routinely during continuous feedings or before each intermittent feeding.

Concentration.   It is not necessary to dilute isosmotic formulas for initiation of enteral feedings. Hypertonic formulas may be administered in the stomach at full strength at an initially low rate. In fact, some studies show that net nutrient intake and nitrogen balance can be improved by using undiluted hypertonic diets, without exacerbation of intestinal symptoms.[42,43] However, hypertonic formulas delivered into the jejunum may require dilution. If the volume is large enough, formulas of high osmolality can lead to intestinal distention and increased motility by stimulating secretion into the intestinal lumen. The diarrhea that is often associated with initiation of enteral feedings is, however, multifactorial in most cases.[44-46] (See Chapter 9, Diarrhea.) The initial diarrhea can generally be alleviated by diluting the formula or by decreasing the flow rate.

Progression of Feeding.   The site of feeding (gastric versus intestinal), previous length of time without enteral feeding, and formula osmolality are important in determining the rate of advancement of enteral feedings. Most patients can tolerate a standard advancement of 10 ml every 12 hours. Rate and concentration should not be altered simultaneously. If the feeding is not tolerated, reduce the rate or the concentration to the level of tolerance, then gradually increase again.

Patients started on low volumes of dilute formulas receive only a fraction of their nutritional requirements. Therefore, progression to a goal level of feeding should be performed as diligently as is possible for the patient. Most patients with a normal intestinal tract tolerate advancement to maintenance needs within 48 hours. Patients with shortened or compromised small bowel, severe debilitation, or lack of oral feedings for a week or more may benefit from a less aggressive advancement. Prolonged disuse of the gastrointestinal tract results in both functional and anatomical atrophy. These changes can be reversed by slow and gradual challenges in the form of small, then progressively larger, feedings.

Complications and Their Prevention

Mechanical Complications.   Mechanical problems are often associated with the tube type and its position. Examples of mechanical complications include nasal catheter dislocation or obstruction, lower esophageal sphincter incompetence, reflux of gastric contents leading to aspiration pneumonia, and gastrostomy or jejunostomy tube leakage resulting in skin erosion.[45]

Tubes that are small in diameter (e.g., 8 or 9 Fr) and pliable are associated with reduced irritation and improved patient tolerance. However, small lumen tubes are more likely to become occluded, from residual of the feeding or from pulverized medication. In an attempt to prevent obstruction of the tubes, irrigation with 30 ml of warm water should occur every 6 hours. Irrigation should also be done with medications, whenever the feeding is interrupted, and before and after each intermittent feeding.[46] If the tube becomes obstructed and the warm water flush is unsuccessful in clearing it, the use of a commercial enzyme solution or cola may clear the obstruction.[47]

One must also be aware of the medications given via a feeding tube. Whenever possible, liquid forms of medications should be administered. Pharmacological activity of the medications administered with tube feedings may be either enhanced or diminished. For example, if phenytoin is administered while the patient is receiving continuous tube feeding, the effect of the drug may be diminished. Therefore, the patient's feeding schedule may need to be adjusted to allow for optimum effect of the medication.[48-50]

Inadvertent tube placement in the respiratory system is a potential complication when placing small nasoenteric tubes. Thus, placement of these tubes should be verified by chest X-ray prior to administration of feedings. Periodic verification of gastric tube location by aspiration of gastric contents is recommended.[45] Tubes can be displaced by altered gastric motility, vomiting, coughing, or inadvertently by confused patients. When the dislodged tube has been repositioned, its location should be reconfirmed by X-ray.

Mechanical complications observed most frequently with enterostomy feedings include leakage of gastrointestinal contents around the stoma site with subsequent skin erosion, wound infection, and tube dislodgement. Proper tube maintenance and routine site care should help control such complications.[51]

Gastrointestinal Complications. Gastrointestinal side effects of tube feeding may include one or more of the following: delayed gastric emptying, constipation, nausea, vomiting, cramping, abdominal pain, malabsorption, and diarrhea (see Table 16-2).[52] Such problems are sometimes related to the rate and/or concentration of the formula being administered. A systematic progression in the feeding rate or concentration and use of a feeding pump may decrease the risk of gastrointestinal side effects.[45] It is important to remember that the tube feedings may not always be the cause of a gastrointestinal complication, so other possible causes should be evaluated.

Vomiting and pulmonary aspiration are more likely to occur when gastric emptying is delayed. This risk can be lessened by elevating the upper part of the patient's body to a 30 degree angle and by checking for gastric residuals every 4 to

TABLE 16-2   Common Tube Feeding Problems and Causes

Vomiting	Diarrhea	Constipation
Improper tube placement	Rapid advance of tube feeding rate	Lack of bulk in the diet
Tube too large		Inadequate fluid
Rate of feeding too fast	Intolerance to formula ingredients (e.g., lactose)	Lack of activity
Residual volume from previous feeding too great	Intestinal atrophy	Neuromuscular injuries
Osmolality of feeding too high	Medications (e.g., antibiotics, hyperosmolar sorbitol-containing elixir medications)	Medications affecting GI motility (narcotics, anticholinergics)
Medications given with feeding		
Head of bed not elevated	Severe protein and calorie malnutrition	
Gastric dysmotility	Malabsorption	
	Bacterial overgrowth	

GI = Gastrointestinal.

6 hours or before each intermittent feeding. The residual should not exceed the amount infused during the preceding 2 hours (for pump feedings), or 100 ml (for intermittent feedings).[46,53] If the residual is excessive, the feeding should be held and the residual rechecked in 1 hour. The residuals should be replaced to avoid depletion of electrolytes.[54] If large volume residuals persist, the physician should be contacted and the patient's condition should be evaluated. Reduction in the rate of administration of the formula may alleviate the problem.[55] Pharmacological intervention with metaclopramide also may be employed.[56] Positioning the tip of the tube beyond the pylorus may also lessen the risk of aspiration.

Diarrhea is often listed as a complication of enteral nutrition. There are many potential causes for diarrhea occurring in patients receiving enteral feeding. Some are related to the nutrients in the formulas (such as lactose), temperature of the formula, bacterial contamination, osmolality of the formula, method of delivery, and inadequate fiber content of the formula. Other causes are not related to the tube feeding, most notably drug therapy, such as antibiotics, or hypertonic medications given postpylorically. Elixir medications that contain sorbitol have also been implicated as frequent causes of diarrhea. Other causes not related to tube feeding are intestinal villous atrophy resulting from malnutrition or prolonged disuse of the intestinal tract, hypoalbuminemia, fecal impaction, and other gastrointestinal disorders.[57-60]

Persistent diarrhea may lessen with a reduction in the rate of administration or the concentration of solution. Adherence to feeding at a low infusion rate may promote intestinal mucosal adaptation, with a return to more normal villous absorptive surface area, intestinal enzyme production, and motility. If formulas are changed while adaptation is taking place, the second formula used is likely to be credited with being less prone to produce diarrhea. Antidiarrheal agents can be used with the objective of maintaining optimal delivery of nutrients. Medications that slow gastrointestinal motility include deodorized tincture of opium, paregoric, diphenoxylate hydrochloride (Lomotil™), and loperamide hydrochloride (Imodium™).[61] However, if antibiotic-induced diarrhea is suspected, stool toxin assays and stool cultures should be evaluated for pseudomembranous colitis caused by *Clostridium difficile*. It is dangerous to give antidiarrheal agents in this case because they slow transit time and increase exposure to toxins.[46] Food-borne infectious diarrhea can be prevented by paying close attention to technique in the preparation and handling of formulas. Any formula manipulation at the time of preparation or administration should be carried out with clean technique.

Most commercial formulas are in ready-to-feed form and are packaged in sterile containers. Feeding sets or containers should be changed daily. In general, enteral formulas should not be opened and maintained at room temperature for longer than 12 hours.[54] However, this recommendation may be more limited for specific products. Any remaining formula that is opened and unused should be refrigerated and then discarded after 24 hours. Tube feeding containers should be labeled with the expiration time and date.

Metabolic Complications.   Metabolic complications observed during enteral nutrition are similar to those that may occur during parenteral nutrition but are usually less severe because of the adaptive capacity of the gut. Metabolic complications that may occur include hyperglycemia, hypertonic dehydration, hyperna-tremia, hyperkalemia, hypokalemia, and hypophosphatemia.

Another complication may occur in patients who are chronically malnourished or who have been without nutrition for a great length of time. This complication, termed the "refeeding syndrome," is marked by shifts in fluid balance and by shifts of phosphorus, potassium, glucose, and magnesium to the intracellular space to allow energy synthesis.[62] Peripheral edema and congestive heart failure are possible manifestations.

Metabolic complications can be avoided or managed easily when patients are routinely monitored. Routine monitoring of patients receiving enteral nutrition should include but is not limited to (1) close attention to intake and output and daily measurement of weight to assure adequate hydration and (2) frequent monitoring of electrolyte levels, glucose levels, and other appropriate laboratory checks.

Tube Feeding at Home

The demand for tube feeding at home, with the consequent need to coordinate its application, has been growing steadily owing to many factors. Acknowledgment of nutrition as a strong component of medical care and recognition that continued nutritional support is frequently needed at the time of hospital dismissal have led to an increasing number of patients using enteral nutrition in the outpatient or home setting. The rapid development of sophisticated enteral formulas and delivery systems have made home tube feeding feasible and practical. Changing health care reimbursement patterns have also increased the emphasis on home care. Industry has responded with the appearance of a multitude of private home nutritional support companies, each offering to manage home care services on behalf of the medical center with varying degrees of intensity and scope.

Patient Education

Education of the patient who is receiving home enteral tube feeding is a joint healthcare team effort. The dietitian and the nurse provide individualized training of the patient and family members. Instructional responsibilities should be identified, and a timetable for implementation should be established. The techniques for instruction include oral instruction, written guidelines, staff demonstration, return demonstration by the patient and family, and their assumption of full responsibility for tube feeding prior to dismissal from the hospital.[63]

A source for receiving supplies such as formula, administration equipment, and site care items is arranged for the patient prior to dismissal. Avenues for financial assistance with the costs of the home nutrition program are also identified.[64] Responsibility for the patient receiving home enteral tube feeding continues following dismissal from the hospital. Frequent telephone contact and return appointments are used to follow the progress of nutritional rehabilitation, to assist with solving problems, and to adjust the enteral program according to changes in needs. Follow-up of patients referred into the Mayo Clinic program reveals that, although many problems with tube feeding are experienced, the majority can be resolved at home. Also, most patients report that they can maintain or improve their level of function.[65]

Physicians: How to Order Diet

See Appendix 11: Physicians Adult Enteral Nutrition Order Sheet and Appendix 11: Considerations for Ordering Adult Enteral Nutrition Solutions. The order sheet should indicate:

1. The standard formula, or brand name from the hospital formulary.
2. The method of feeding (e.g., continuous, or number of and times for intermittent feedings).
3. The initial flow rate, duration, progression to goal and water flushes. According to the preceding guidelines, the dietitian will determine the amount of formula required to provide an appropriate caloric and protein level.

If tube feeding is to continue beyond hospitalization, the dietitian and nutrition support service should also be notified.

References

1. ASPEN Board of Directors. Guidelines for the use of parenteral and enteral nutrition in adult and pediatric patients. JPEN 1993;17(4 supplement):1sa–52sa.
2. Heymsfield SB, Bethel RA, Ansley JD, Nixon DW, Rudman D. Enteral hyperalimentation: an alternative to central venous hyperalimentation. Ann Intern Med 1979;90:63–71.
3. Bower RH, Talamini MA, Sax HC, Hamilton F, Fischer JE. Postoperative enteral vs parenteral nutrition: a randomized controlled trial. Arch Surg 1986;121:1040–1045.
4. McArdle AH, Palmason C, Morency I, Brown RA. A rationale for enteral feeding as the preferable route of hyperalimentation. Surgery 1981;90:616–623.
5. Bethel RA, Jansen RD, Heymsfield SB, Ansley JD, Hersh T, Rudman D. Nasogastric hyperalimentation through a polyethylene catheter: an alternative to central venous hyperalimentation. Am J Clin Nutr 1979;32:1112–1120.
6. Food and Nutrition Board, National Research Council. Recommended dietary allowances, 10th ed. Washington, DC: National Academy of Science, 1989:249–250.
7. Randall HT. Water, electrolytes and acid-base balance. In: Shils ME, Young VR, eds. Modern nutrition in health and disease, 7th ed. Philadelphia: Lea & Febiger, 1988:108–141.
8. Keighley MR, Mogg B, Bentley S, Allan C. "Home brew" compared with commercial preparation for enteral feeding. BMJ 1982;284:163.
9. Gormican A, Liddy E. Nasogastric tube feedings: practical considerations in prescription and evaluation. Postgrad Med 1975;53:71–76.
10. Heimburger DC, Weinsier RL. Guidelines for evaluating and categorizing enteral feeding formulas according to therapeutic equivalence. JPEN 1985;9:61–67.
11. Silk DB, Fairclough PD, Clark ML, Hegarty JE, Marrs TC, Addison JM, Burston D, Clegg KM, Matthews DM. Use of a peptide rather than free amino acid nitrogen source in chemically defined "elemental" diets. JPEN 1980;4:548–553.
12. Matarese LE. Standardized enteral nutritional support. Nutritional Support Services 1983;3:27–30.
13. Ideno KT. Enteral nutrition. In: Gottschlich MM, Matarese LE, Shronts EP, eds. Nutrition support dietetics core curriculum. Silver Spring, MD: ASPEN, 1993:71–104.
14. Skipper A. Specialized formulas for enteral nutrition support. J Am Diet Assoc 1986;86: 654–658.
15. McGhee A, Henderson JM, Millikan WJ, Bleier JC, Vogel R, Kassouny M, Rudman D. Comparison of the effects of hepatic-aid and a casein modular diet on encephalopathy, plasma amino acids, and nitrogen balance in cirrhotic patients. Ann Surg 1983;197: 288–293.

38. Shike M, Wallach C, Gerdes H, Hermann-Zaidins M. Skin-level gastrostomies and jejunostomies for long-term enteral feeding. JPEN 1989;13:648–650.

39. Woolfson AMJ, Ricketts CR, Hardy SM, Saour JN, Pollard BJ, Allison SP. Prolonged naso-gastric tube feeding in critically ill and surgical patients. Postgrad Med J 1976;52:678–682.

40. Heymsfield SB, Casper K, Grossman GD. Bioenergetic and metabolic response to con-tinuous v. intermittent nasoenteric feeding. Metabolism 1987;36:570–575.

41. Heitkemper ME, Martin DL, Hansen BC, Hanson R, Vanderberg V. Rate and volume of intermittent enteral feeding. JPEN 1981;5:125–129.

42. Keohane PP, Attrill H, Love M, Frost P, Silk DBA. Relation between osmolality of diet and gastrointestinal side effects in enteral nutrition. BMJ 1984;288:678–680.

43. Zarling EJ, Parmar JR, Mobarhan S, Clapper M. Effect of enteral formula infusion rate, osmolality and chemical composition upon clinical tolerance and carbohydrate absorp-tion in normal subjects. JPEN 1986;10:588–590.

44. Brinson RR, Kolts BE. Hypoalbuminemia as an indicator of diarrheal incidence in criti-cally ill patients. Crit Care Med 1987;15:506–509.

45. Cataldi-Betcher EL, Seltzer MH, Slocum BA, Jones KW. Complications occurring dur-ing enteral nutrition support: a prospective study. JPEN 1983;7:546–552.

46. Bockus S. Troubleshooting your tube feedings. Am J Nurs 1991;9:24–30.

47. Marcuard SP, Stegall KL, Trogdon S. Clearing obstructed feeding tubes. JPEN 1989;13:81–83.

48. Parr MD, Record KE, Griffith GL, Zeok JV, Todd EP. Effect of enteral nutrition on war-farin therapy. Clin Pharm 1982;1:274–276.

49. Wright B, Robinson L. Enteral feeding tubes as drug delivery systems. Nutritional Support Services 1986;6:33–48.

50. Saklad JJ, Graves RH, Sharp WP. Interaction of oral phenytoin with enteral feedings. JPEN 1986;10:322–323.

51. Torosian MH, Rombeau JL. Feeding by tube enterostomy. Surg Gynecol Obstet 1980; 150:918–927.

52. Silk DBA, Payne-James JJ. Complications of enteral nutrition. In: Rombeau JL, Caldwell MD, eds. Enteral and tube feeding. Philadelphia: WB Saunders, 1990:510–531.

53. Heitkemper MM, Williams S. Prevent problems caused by enteral feeding. J Gerontol Nurs 1985;11:25–30.

54. Guenter P, Jones S, Jacobs DO, Rombeau JL. Administration and delivery of enteral nutrition. In: Rombeau JL, Caldwell MD, eds. Enteral and tube feeding. Philadelphia: WB Saunders, 1990:192–203.

55. Rombeau JL, Barot LR. Enteral nutritional therapy. Surg Clin North Am 1981;61:605–620.

56. Lindor KD, Malagelada JR. Symposium on upper gastrointestinal motility disorders: gas-tric motility disorders: an overview. South Med J 1984;77:943–946.

57. Heimburger DC. Diarrhea with enteral feeding: will the real cause please stand up. Am J Med 1990;88:89–93.

58. Broom J, Jones K. Causes and prevention of diarrhoea in patients receiving enteral nutritional support. J Hum Nutr 1981;35:123–127.

59. Anderson BJ. Tube feeding: is diarrhea inevitable? Am J Nurs 1986;86:704–706.

60. Kohn CL, Keithley JK. Techniques for evaluating and managing diarrhea in the tube-fed patient. Nutr Clin Pract 1987;2:250–257.

61. Breach CL, Saldanha LG. Tube feeding complications: Part I. Gastrointestinal. Nutritional Support Services 1988;8:15–19.

62. Havala T, Shronts E. Managing the complications associated with refeeding. Nutr Clin Pract 1990;5:23–29.

63. Nelson JK, Weckwerth JA. Home enteral nutrition. In: Skipper A, ed. Dietitian's hand-book of enteral and parenteral nutrition. Rockville, MD: ASPEN, 1989:311–325.

16. Eriksson LS, Persson A, Wahren J. Branched-chain amino acids in t̄ chronic hepatic encephalopathy. Gut 1982;23:801–806.

17. Cerra FB, Mazuski J, Teasley K, Nuwer N, Lysne J, Shronts E, Kon̄ Nitrogen retention in critically ill patients is proportioned to the branché Crit Care Med 1983;11:775–778.

18. Mobarhan S, Thurabore LS. Enteral tube feeding: a clinical perspectiv̄ advances. Nutr Rev 1991;49:129–140.

19. Lieberman MD, Shou J, Torres AS, Weintraub F, Goldfine J, Sigal R, Daly JM̄ nutrient substrates on immune function. Nutrition 1990;6:88S–91S.

20. Cerra FB, Lehman S, Konstantinides N, Konstantinides F, Shronts EP, Holman̄ of enteral nutrition on in vitro tests of immune function in ICU patients: a pr̄ report. Nutrition 1990;6:84S–87S.

21. Gottschlich MM, Jenkins M, Warden GD, Baumer T, Havens P, Snook JT, Alex̄ JW. Differential effects of three enteral dietary regimens on selected outcome var̄ in burn patients. JPEN 1990;14:225–236.

22. Hirschberg RR, Kopple JD. Enteral nutrition and renal disease. In: Rombeau̇ Caldwell MD, eds. Clinical nutrition: enteral and tube feeding. Philadelphia: Saunders, 1990:400–415.

23. Andrassy RJ. Preserving the gut mucosal barrier and enhancing immune respons̄ Contemp Surg 1988;32:1–7.

24. Bulus N, Cersosimo E, Ghishan F, Abumrad NN. Physiologic importance of glutaminē Metabolism 1989;38:1–5.

25. Smith RJ, Wilmore DW. Glutamine nutrition and requirements. JPEN 1990;14:94S–99S.

26. Souba WW, Herskowitz K, Austgen TR, Chen MK, Salloum RM. Glutamine nutrition: theoretical considerations and therapeutic impact. JPEN 1990;14:237S–243S.

27. Rombeau JL, Kripke SA. Metabolic and intestinal effects of short-chain fatty acids. JPEN 1990;14:181S–185S.

28. Scheppach W, Burghardt W, Bartram P, Kasper H. Addition of dietary fiber to liquid formula diets: the pros and cons. JPEN 1990;14:204–209.

29. Slavin J. Commercially available enteral formulas with fiber and bowel function measures. Nutr Clin Prac 1990;5:247–250.

30. Koruda MJ. Controlling diarrhea in the tube fed patient. Support Line (Newsletter of Dietitians in Nutrition Support) 1991;13:10–14.

31. Herrmann ME, Liehr RM, Tanhoefner H, Emde C, Riecken EO. Subjective distress during continuous enteral alimentation: superiority of silicone rubber to polyurethane. JPEN 1989;13:281–285.

32. Sitzmann JV. Nutritional support of the dysphagic patient: methods, risks and complications of therapy. JPEN 1990;14:60–63.

33. Shike M, Berner YN, Gerdes H, Gerold FP, Bloch A, Sessions R, Strong E. Percutaneous endoscopic gastrostomy and jejunostomy for long-term feeding in patients with cancer of the head and neck. Otolaryngol Head Neck Surg 1989;101:549–554.

34. Larson DE, Burton DD, Schroeder KW, DiMagno EP. Percutaneous endoscopic gastros̄ tomy: indications, success, complications and mortality in 314 consecutive patients̄ Gastroenterology 1987;93:48–52.

35. Kaplan DS, Murthy UK, Linscheer WG. Percutaneous endoscopic jejunostomy: lonḡ term follow-up of 23 patients. Gastrointest Endosc 1989;35:403–406.

36. Rosenblum J, Taylor FC, Lu CT, Martich V. A new technique for direct percutaneoū jejunostomy tube placement. Am J Gastroenterol 1990;85:1165–1167.

37. Foutch PG, Talbert GA, Gaines JA, Sanowski RA. The gastrostomy button: a prospect̄ assessment of safety, success, and spectrum of use. Gastrointest Endosc 1989;35:41–44

64. Regenstein M. Reimbursement for nutrition support. Nutr Clin Pract 1989;4:194–202.
65. Nelson JK, Palumbo PJ, O'Brien PC. Home enteral nutrition: observations of a newly established program. Nutr Clin Pract 1986;1:193–199.

PARENTERAL NUTRITIONAL SUPPORT OF ADULTS

General Description

Parenteral nutrition (PN) is a form of intravenous therapy that provides the opportunity to replenish or to maintain nutritional status.[66] Nutrients include amino acids (nitrogen), dextrose (carbohydrate), lipids, electrolytes, minerals, vitamins, and trace elements that are in an appropriate volume of fluid. Central parenteral nutrition (CPN) is delivered through a large diameter vein, usually the subclavian or the superior vena cava. Peripheral parenteral nutrition (PPN) is delivered through a smaller vein, usually in the forearm. There are also catheters that are inserted in a peripheral location but that deliver the PN centrally into a large diameter vein. These are called PICC, or peripherally inserted central catheters.

Indications and Rationale

In general, the dictum "If the gut works, use it" should be heeded whenever possible. PN should be utilized whenever nutritional support is needed and the enteral route is not available, is inadequate, or is contraindicated. It must be recognized that it is difficult to establish absolute criteria for the utilization of PN in hospitalized patients.[67] Variations in the nature and the extent of individual nutritional problems demand the exercise of clinical judgment.

CPN is indicated when the gastrointestinal tract cannot be used, when the volume and concentration of the solution preclude peripheral administration, when the anticipated duration of therapy is greater than 7 days to 2 weeks, and when substantial depletion of body fat and protein has occurred or is anticipated. The central venous route is often utilized to provide complete patient nutrition. PPN is preferred when the solution concentration is less than 1,000 mOsm/L and duration of therapy is expected to be less than 10 days to 2 weeks.

Parenteral Nutrition Component Products

Hospital pharmacies compound PN solutions just prior to their administration because of the relative chemical instability of the formulations. Component products of PN formulations typically include water, amino acids, dextrose, electrolytes, vitamins, and trace elements. Fat emulsions are infused concurrently with the PN solution by means of a "piggyback" administration system or are added directly to the PN solution as a total nutrient admixture or 3-in-1 solution. Tables 16-3 to 16-5 display the content of standard PN formulas that are available for routine use in the Mayo Medical Center.

Amino Acids.   In the United States, the source of nitrogen typically used in PN is a synthetic crystalline amino acid solution, which is available with or without

TABLE 16-3   Adult Parenteral Nutrition Formulary for the Mayo Medical Center

Standard Formulas	CPN* per Liter (Final Concentration)	PPN† per Liter (Final Concentration)
Dextrose concentration	10%, 15%, 20%, or 25%	5%
Amino acid concentration	4.25%	4.25%
Nitrogen	7.15 g	7.15 g
Sodium	36.5 mEq	36.5 mEq
Potassium	30.0 mEq	30.0 mEq
Calcium	4.7 mEq	4.7 mEq
Magnesium	5.0 mEq	5.0 mEq
Chloride	35.0 mEq	35.0 mEq
Phosphorus	15.0 mmol	15.0 mmol
Acetate	70.5 mEq	70.5 mEq

*Central parenteral nutrition with standard electrolytes.

†Peripheral parenteral nutrition with standard electrolytes.

TABLE 16-4   Standard Adult Multivitamin Injection

Multivitamin	Amount per Standard Dose per Day
A (retinol)	3,300 IU
D (ergocalciferol)	200 IU
E (DL-alpha tocopherol acetate)	10 IU
C (ascorbic acid)	100 mg
B_1 (thiamine)	3.0 mg
B_2 (riboflavin)	3.6 mg
B_6 (pyridoxine)	4.0 mg
B_{12} (cyanocobalamin)	5 µg
Folic acid	400 µg
Niacinamide	40 mg
B_5 dexpanthenol	15 mg
Biotin	60 µg

TABLE 16-5   Fat Emulsions

	250 ml	500 ml
10% (1.1 kcal/ml)	275 kcal	550 kcal
20% (2.0 kcal/ml)	500 kcal	1000 kcal

added electrolytes and minerals. The products available for adults may be categorized by use, such as for general use, for renal disease, for hepatic disease, and for use in the traumatized patient. A comparison of amino acid products and their contents can be found in Appendix 12.

General amino acid preparations are patterned to the amino acid profile of egg albumin. Although these products differ somewhat in composition, in general they may be considered to be therapeutically equivalent.

The efficacy of essential amino acid products for use in renal failure patients and the use of solutions that contain increased concentrations of branched chain amino acids (BCAAs) and decreased aromatic amino acids (AAAs) for hepatic encephalopathy and for stress or trauma are controversial.

Dextrose. Solutions of dextrose in concentrations of 10% through 70% are mixed with the appropriate amount of amino acids to obtain the desired solution. The dextrose used in formulating intravenous solutions is dextrose monohydrate. Because of the hydrated form, it provides 3.4 kcal/g of dextrose.

Electrolytes. Electrolytes and minerals are provided as part of the general amino acid product, as a combined electrolyte concentrate, or they may be added separately as individual salts. Appendix 12 lists the electrolyte products typically used in the compounding of PN solutions.

The requirements for electrolytes vary according to individual patient needs. For most patients, the electrolytes provided with the amino acid products or as combined electrolyte concentrates are adequate in maintenance amounts. (Note that neither calcium nor phosphorus is provided as part of an amino acid product in the combined electrolyte concentrates.) To correct derangements of plasma electrolyte concentrations and to compensate for losses, changes are made in the amounts of individual electrolytes that are provided in the parenteral solution. If deficits are extensive, corrections may be made more effectively by using separate replacement solutions.

Vitamins. Multivitamin products for intravenous use have been formulated according to the recommendations of the American Medical Association Nutrition Advisory Group (AMA-NAG).[68] One adult and one pediatric multivitamin formulation are available commercially from several manufacturers (see Appendix 12). These formulations are used as a daily maintenance dosage for patients who receive PN when intravenous vitamin supplementation is required. Patients with multiple vitamin deficiencies or with markedly increased requirements may be given multiples of the daily dosage as indicated by the clinical status. Supplementation of the daily multivitamin dosage with a single vitamin may be necessary for a specific vitamin deficiency.

Trace Elements. Trace elements are those nutrients that make up less than 4.0 g (or 0.01%) of the total body content. Trace elements are available commercially as combination products or as single entity injections. The multiple trace element injection that is currently used in the Mayo Medical Center is listed in Table 16-6; 1 ml of the injection supplies trace elements in the amounts suggested for daily administration by the AMA-NAG for stable adult patients.[69-70] Individual trace elements may be supplemented in appropriate daily doses as specific patient deficiencies dictate.

TABLE 16-6   Standard Adult Trace Element Injection

Trace Element	Amount per Standard Dose per Day
Zinc	4 mg
Copper	0.8 mg
Manganese	400 µg
Chromium	8 µg
Selenium	48 µg

Fat Emulsions.   Intravenous fat emulsions are routinely used in PN therapy as a calorically dense energy substrate (9 kcal/g) and to prevent essential fatty acid deficiency. Fat emulsions are available in 10% and 20% concentrations of soybean oil or a combination of soybean and safflower oils with an emulsifying agent (egg yolk phospholipid) and glycerol for isotonicity. The calorie content of each fat emulsion is determined by the amount of lipid present as well as the kilocalories added by glycerol. Fat provides 9 kcal/g; therefore, in a 10% lipid emulsion there are 0.9 kcal/ml and in a 20% lipid emulsion there are 1.8 kcal/ml. The glycerol adds 0.2 kcal/ml, which means the total caloric content for the 10% emulsion is 1.1 kcal/ml and for the 20% emulsion is 2.0 kcal/ml.

A comparison of fat emulsion products is found in Appendix 12.

Because fat emulsions are isotonic, they may be administered through a peripheral vein. Alternatively, they may be added directly to the PN solution (total nutrient admixture) or piggybacked into the PN line. If an in-line filter tubing system is used, the fat emulsion must be piggybacked below the filter.

The minimum dose of lipid to prevent linoleic acid deficiency has been estimated to be 2 to 4% of the daily caloric requirement. The daily adult dosage of intravenous fat should not exceed 2.5 g/kg, and a continuous, rather than an intermittent, infusion is better tolerated. The use of fat emulsions is contraindicated in patients with disturbances of normal fat metabolism such as familial hypertriglyceridemia, and they should be used cautiously in patients with an egg allergy.

"Missing Nutrients."   Total parenteral nutrition (TPN) is the provision of nutrients totally by the intravenous route. All essential nutrients are not provided. We do not add iron, iodine, vitamin K, or molybdenum to standard PN formulas. Patients who receive PN formulas should be assessed for the need for these nutrients.

Drug Vehicle.   PN solutions are frequently used as a vehicle for medication administration. Medications can be piggybacked into the PN line via a "Y" site or added directly to the PN solution. The advantages of direct medication addition include the ability to restrict fluid, limit vascular access, contain cost, and reduce the time required to administer medications.

Compatibility of a medication with a PN solution must be proven prior to addition and is dependent on physical and chemical stability with respect to time, temperature, and pH. Physical compatibility refers to the absence of precipitate for-

Text continued on p. 408.

TABLE 16-7 Adult Parenteral Nutrition Laboratory Monitoring Guidelines

The laboratory tests and frequencies listed below are suggested for the routine monitoring of adult patients receiving parenteral nutrition. Additional laboratory monitoring tests at more frequent intervals may be necessary during periods of patient stress or metabolic instability.

	Baseline*	Day of Therapy								
		2	3	4	7	14	21	28	35	42
Chem Group										
Albumin	X				X	X	X	X	X	X
Alkaline phosphatase	X				X	X	X	X	X	X
Aspartate aminotransferase	X				X	X	X	X	X	X
Bilirubin	X				X	X	X	X	X	X
Calcium	X				X	X	X	X	X	X
Creatinine	X				X	X	X	X	X	X
Glucose	X	X	X	X	X	X	X	X	X	X
Potassium	X				X	X	X	X	X	X
Sodium	X				X	X	X	X	X	X
Phosphorus	X				X	X	X	X	X	X
Total protein	X				X	X	X	X	X	X
Uric acid	X				X	X	X	X	X	X
Electrolyte Panel										
Creatinine	X				X	X	X	X	X	X
Chloride	X				X	X	X	X	X	X
HCO$_3$	X				X	X	X	X	X	X
Potassium	X	X	X	X	X	X	X	X	X	X
Sodium	X	X	X	X	X	X	X	X	X	X
Urea	X				X	X	X	X	X	X
Essential Element Screen										
Copper	X				X	X		X		X
Iron	X				X	X		X		X
Magnesium	X				X	X		X		X
Zinc	X				X	X		X		X
Individual										
Prothrombin time	X				X	X		X		X
Heme group†	X									
Triglycerides†‡	X									
Selenium	X							X		

*Baseline tests preceding initiation of parenteral nutrition.

†Baseline. Additional test frequency determined by primary service.

‡Repeat level prior to start of second bottle of fat emulsion.

TABLE 16-8 Complications of Parenteral Therapy[71]

Complication	Etiology	Signs and Symptoms	Treatment	Prevention
MAJOR TECHNICAL COMPLICATIONS				
Catheter Insertion				
1. Pneumothorax	Subclavian venipuncture Unusual anatomy	Dyspnea Chest pain Cyanosis	Observation if small	Use internal jugular for high risk patients
	Improper training		Chest tube if large or progressive	Trained and approved doctor
	Multiple punctures			Stop after three to four attempts and get help
	Failure to remove respirator			Ambu bag during procedure except during thrust of needle
	Slow leak			Repeat chest X-ray
2. Malposition	Anatomical	Pain or tingling in the ear or the neck area on the side of insertion or none	Reposition with guidewire or fluoroscopy or new puncture	Proper position if possible
	Needle passed through vein	No free reflux of blood	Catheter removal	
3. Subclavian artery puncture	Incorrect insertion	Return of bright red blood under high pressure	Remove needle Elevate head of bed	Strict adherence to technique
		Hematoma	Pressure to puncture site Close patient observation	
4. Carotid artery puncture	Internal jugular catheterization	Hematoma untreated may lead to tracheal obstruction	Local application of direct pressure	
5. Catheter embolism	Shearing off section of catheter	Cardiac irritability	Radiologic or surgical removal	Never pull back catheter through needle
6. Air embolism	During catheter threading	Dyspnea Chest pain Tachycardia Tachypnea Cyanosis Paresis Cardiac arrest	Needle aspiration of heart Left side down in steep Trendelenburg position	Trendelenburg position during insertion Keep hub covered at all times Valsalva maneuver each time catheter open to air

Catheter Maintenance

Complication	Cause	Signs/Symptoms	Treatment	Prevention
1. Air embolism	Tubing disconnection Patent tract after removal of catheter	Dyspnea Chest pain Tachycardia Tachypnea Cyanosis Disorientation Paresis Cardiac arrest	As above Reconnect tubing Contact physician	Tape tubing connections Use Luer-loks Ointment and/or occlusive dressing for 12–24 hr
2. Catheter obstruction	Mechanical (pump) failure Kink in catheter	Solutions stop running Occlusion alarm	Adjust pump Reset alarm Aspiration of catheter	Hourly monitoring of solution Close observation during dressing change
3. Thrombosis	Mechanical irritation Patient's hypercoagulable state	Distended collateral veins and chest wall Acute unilateral edema of arm, neck, and face Pleuritic chest pain Inability to thread catheter	Catheter removal Intravenous heparin Venogram	Not always possible Heparin in TPN solution Do not cycle TPN if low AT-III*

MAJOR SEPTIC COMPLICATIONS

Catheter-Related Sepsis

Complication	Cause	Signs/Symptoms	Treatment	Prevention
Catheter-Related Sepsis	Inadequate asepsis during catheter insertion, inadequate dressing care and solution maintenance or solution preparation Immunosuppression	Glucose intolerance Spiking temperature Elevated white count Hypotension Disorientation Inflammation or drainage from catheter exit site	Removal of catheter Culture of solution Chest X-ray Cultures of urine, sputum, draining wounds Blood culture (central and peripheral) Catheter removal with tip culture (new puncture or guidewire) Antimicrobial therapy when indicated	Rigid adherence to specific policies and procedures Inspection of catheter site for each dressing change procedure

Septic Thrombosis

Complication	Cause	Signs/Symptoms	Treatment	Prevention
Septic Thrombosis	Untreated catheter sepsis Bacteremic seeding from unknown or other source	Same as catheter-related plus unilateral pain and swelling in arm, shoulder, and neck area	Venogram Remove catheter and culture tip Intravenous heparin Antimicrobial therapy	Immediate response to suspected sepsis Periodic changes of catheter (i.e., new puncture or over a guidewire) when other septic source known

Continued.

*TPN = Total parenteral nutrition; AT-III = antithrombin III; CNS = central nervous system.

TABLE 16-8 Complications of Parenteral Therapy[71]—cont'd

Complication	Etiology	Signs and Symptoms	Treatment	Prevention
MAJOR METABOLIC COMPLICATIONS				
Hyperglycemia	Diabetes mellitus	Elevated blood glucose Glycosuria	Regular insulin subcutaneously or intravenously	Coordinate initiation and insulin requirement
	Too rapid initiation		Slow rate	Start slow with step increments (i.e., day 1—1 L, day 2—2 L, day 3—2 or 3 L)
	Infection or sepsis		Addition of regular insulin Slow rate until blood glucose stable	
	Drug related (i.e., steroids)		(May increase fat source for calories)	Advance more slowly
	Stress from major surgery		Slow rate or stop infusion	Halve infusion rate during surgery Stop hypertonic solution and infuse dextrose solution or lactated Ringer's solution several hours to 24 hr pre- and postoperatively
Hyperglycemic Hyperosmolar Nonketotic Dehydration	Uncontrolled hyperglycemia	Elevated blood glucose level (500–1,000 mg/100 ml or higher) Glycosuria Osmotic diuresis Metabolic imbalances Lethargy Coma Death	Stop hypertonic solution Hydration with free water Judicious doses of IV insulin and potassium Close laboratory and patient monitoring	Immediate and proper control of blood glucose level to <200
Hypoglycemia	Sudden decrease or stop of infusion due to mechanical problem	Blood glucose in range of 40 mg/100 ml Lethargy	Bolus dextrose infusion Monitor serum glucose	Accurate administration with hourly patient monitoring
Hyperkalemia	Inability to utilize administered potassium Decrease in renal function Low cardiac output Systemic sepsis	Cardiac arrhythmias Bounding or diminished pulses	Stop infusion Change to low potassium solution	Close metabolic monitoring

Condition	Cause	Clinical Signs and Symptoms	Treatment	Monitoring
	Increased requirement with anabolism; Excessive GI losses	Cardiac arrhythmias, Muscle weakness, Impaired respiratory function	Increase potassium in solution; Measure and replace losses	Close metabolic monitoring
Hypophosphatemia	Lack of phosphate supplementation; Excessive use of phosphate binders (i.e., antacids); Increased demand during anabolism	Lethargy, Altered speech, Peripheral paresthesias, Increased respirations, Coma	Add phosphate to solution; May require peripheral repletion; Adjust amount per patient	Close metabolic monitoring; Standardized solutions
Hypocalcemia	Lack of or insufficient supplementation	Paresthesia twitching positive Chvostek's sign	Add or adjust calcium in solution	Close metabolic monitoring
Hypomagnesemia	Lack of or insufficient amounts of magnesium in solution	Tingling sensation around mouth, Paresthesia, Dizziness, Disorientation	Add or adjust magnesium in solution	Standardized solutions; Close metabolic monitoring
Essential Fatty Acid Deficiency	Lack of fat supplement	Dry, scaly skin, Hair loss	IV administration of 10% or 20% fat emulsion	Routinely include fat emulsion infusion each week (i.e., twice a week)
Vitamin K Deficiency	Deficient oral intake, severe diarrhea, obstructive jaundice, prolonged antibiotic therapy	Hematuria, ecchymoses, bleeding, purpura, increased prothrombin time	Weekly administration PO or IM of vitamin K	Monitoring prothrombin level
Iron Deficiency	Excessive blood loss	Pallor, fatigue, listlessness, exertional dyspnea, headache, paresthesia	IM or IV iron dextran or whole blood	Serial determination of hemoglobin and mean cell volume, serum iron
Zinc Deficiency	Chronic illness; Diseases that predispose to excessive gastrointestinal loss	Diarrhea, CNS* disturbances, skin lesions, poor wound healing, alopecia, anorexia, growth retardation	Refeed and treat illness; Addition of zinc to solution	Serial determination of serum zinc

Reprinted with permission: Griggs BA, Ingalls M, Ayers N, Champagne C. A basic nursing guide to providing TPN for the adult patient. Washington, DC: American Society for Parenteral and Enteral Nutrition, 1984: 12-15.

mation or fat emulsion changes. Chemical stability is the preservation of bioavailability/activity of the medication and each nutrient in the PN solution.

Patient Monitoring

Patients who receive PN require thoughtful monitoring. The assessed nutrient needs are compared with the PN solution and adjustments are made as needed. Initial height and weight, daily weight, daily intake and output, twice daily temperature, daily whole blood glucose (at the bedside), and quantity of food intake during the transition from PN to enteral or oral diet are the criteria that are monitored. These data should be documented in the medical record.

Serum laboratory tests are also monitored on a routine basis. Table 16-7 lists the tests and the frequencies that are suggested for baseline and routine monitoring. Additional tests at more frequent intervals may be necessary during periods of patient stress or metabolic instability.

Complications

The complications of CPN therapy can be divided into three categories: technical, septic, and metabolic. With proper patient monitoring and with scrupulous technique, most of these complications can be prevented or minimized. Table 16-8 describes the most common complications in each category with the possible cause, signs and symptoms, recommended treatment, and guidelines for prevention.[71]

Physicians: How to Order Parenteral Nutrition

Before PN is initiated, several questions should be considered. What are the indications for PN? Can enteral feedings be used? What is the anticipated duration of therapy? Should central or peripheral administration be employed? Has the position of the central catheter been verified radiologically? Baseline laboratory measurements should also be requested and the nutritional needs of the patient estimated.

The Physician's Adult Parenteral Nutrition Order Sheet (Appendix 13), in use at the Mayo Medical Center, lists the contents and describes the standard PN formulas that are available for patients with normal metabolic needs. A CPN formula is intended for administration through a central vein (e.g., subclavian). A PPN formula may be administered through a peripheral (e.g., forearm) vein. In general, the use of PPN should be limited to shorter therapy (less than 7 days to 2 weeks) and less than 1,000 mOsm/L of formula. Patient tolerance of PPN decreases markedly as the duration of the therapy or the concentration of the solution increases.

On initiating PN, the indications for PN should be indicated in the medical history and laboratory monitoring should be initiated (Table 16-7). The order sheet (see Appendix 13) lists various options for the final dextrose concentration. Most patients can be adequately nourished with dextrose concentrations of 15 or 20% in a standard electrolyte formula. Fat should be provided on a daily basis and is best limited to 30% of total kilocalories and infused continuously over 24 hours. The standard multivitamin and trace element injections should be provided on a daily basis.

Additional electrolytes may be added to the standard formulas in the space provided. Formulas with less than standard electrolyte concentrations or alterations in dextrose or amino acids must be ordered in the nonstandard formula section. Medications may be added to PN formulas only when compatible and chemically stable, and when their continuous intravenous dosing is appropriate and consistent with the continuous infusion of PN. Nutrient requirement guidelines for adult patients with normal metabolic needs are indicated on the order sheet (see Appendix 13). PN should be ordered daily.

References

66. Fleming CR, Nelson JK. Nutritional options. In: Kinney JM, Jeejeebhoy KN, Hill GL, Owen OE, eds. Nutrition and metabolism in patient care. Philadelphia: WB Saunders, 1988:752–772.
67. A.S.P.E.N. Board of Directors. Guidelines for the use of parenteral and enteral nutrition in adult and pediatric patients. JPEN 1993;17(4 supplement):1sa–52sa.
68. American Medical Association Department of Foods and Nutrition. Multivitamin preparations for parenteral use: a statement by the nutrition advisory group. JPEN 1979;3: 258–262.
69. Fleming CR. Trace element metabolism in adult patients requiring total parenteral nutrition. Am J Clin Nutr 1989;49:573–579.
70. American Medical Association Department of Foods and Nutrition. Guidelines for essential trace element preparations for parenteral use: a statement by an expert panel. JAMA 1979;241:2051–2054.
71. Griggs BA, Ingalls M, Ayers N, Champagne C. A basic nursing guide to providing TPN for the adult patient. Silver Spring, MD: American Society for Parenteral and Enteral Nutrition, 1984:12–15.

17 / *Diets in Preparation for Diagnostic Tests*

BREATH HYDROGEN CONCENTRATION

The breath hydrogen analysis test is used in the study of carbohydrate maldigestion and malabsorption and, most commonly, in the assessment of lactose intolerance. In addition, this test can indicate the presence of small bowel bacterial overgrowth or of intestinal stasis syndromes, as in pseudo-obstruction.[1,2]

Ordinarily, lactose is broken down by small intestine enzymes into galactose and glucose, and these are absorbed. When maldigestion exists, ingested lactose is not absorbed, and bacteria in the colon metabolize the lactose to form hydrogen. The hydrogen is then absorbed into the bloodstream and, finally, expired in the breath. The appearance of hydrogen in any significant amount in expired air is abnormal and is a useful indication of lactose (or other carbohydrate) malabsorption.

Hydrogen breath analysis is performed after an overnight fast. Individuals are instructed not to eat or to drink anything except water after midnight. For the test, oral lactose (or other carbohydrate) is given, and serial samples of breath are collected and measured for hydrogen.

Studies have shown that the fasting breath hydrogen concentration can be affected by the meal preceding the fast.[3] As little as 100 g of breadstuffs or pastas made from wheat flour can significantly elevate breath hydrogen concentration for up to 10 hours postprandially.[4] Legumes contain substantial amounts of carbohydrates that cannot be digested and absorbed in the small intestine but that are fermented by bacteria in the colon. As little as 2 to 5 g of these carbohydrates can elevate breath hydrogen.

Patients scheduled for hydrogen breath testing should be instructed to avoid dietary sources of breath hydrogen that may interfere with test results. The meal preceding the fast should not contain the foods listed at the top of the next page.

411

Wheat-Containing Foods

Breads	Spaghetti
Rolls	Noodles
Breadsticks	Breaded items, such as breaded fish
Crackers	Desserts, such as cake and cookies
Macaroni	

Legumes

Beans such as butter, navy, pinto, kidney, baked, string, soya, and mung beans
Peas such as garden, chick, and split peas
Peanuts
Lentils

Physicians: How to Order Diet

The diet order should indicate diet for *breath hydrogen test.*

References

1. Calloway DH, Murphy EL, Bauer D. Determination of lactose intolerance by breath analysis. Am J Dig Dis 1969;14:811–815.
2. Levitt MD, Donaldson RM. Use of respiratory hydrogen (H_2) excretion to detect carbohydrate malabsorption. J Lab Clin Med 1970;75:937–945.
3. Perman JA, Modler S, Barr RG, Rosenthal P. Fasting breath hydrogen concentration: normal values and clinical application. Gastroenterology 1984;87:1358–1363.
4. Anderson IH, Levine AS, Levitt MD. Incomplete absorption of the carbohydrate in all-purpose flour. N Engl J Med 1981;304:891–892.

CARBOHYDRATE METABOLISM

Patients scheduled for glucose tolerance testing (oral and intravenous) or for tolbutamide response testing should receive a diet with ample carbohydrate for at least 3 days before the test is performed. The diet should contain adequate protein, adequate kilocalories (for weight maintenance), and at least 150 g of carbohydrate. Although 300 g carbohydrate diets have traditionally been used in preparation for tests of carbohydrate metabolism, valid testing results have been reported with intakes of 150 to 200 g.[5]

The purpose of the diet is to condition the insulin-releasing mechanism and the glucose-disposing enzyme systems to respond fully to a glucose or tolbutamide challenge. This diet also helps assure adequate stores of hepatic glycogen to provide a source of glucose for restoration of plasma glucose levels after the initial hypoglycemic response to tolbutamide. The response to challenge by a glucose load or by tolbutamide may be abnormal in normal persons who have fasted, who have missed meals during the several days before testing, or who have followed a diet very low in carbohydrate.[6] Results of glucose tolerance tests in hospitalized patients are commonly invalid because of the stress of current or recent illness, inactivity, drugs, or the supine position assumed during the test.

Hospitalized patients are served a general diet (which contains 200 to 300 g of carbohydrate) or a modified diet with at least 150 g of carbohydrate. The physician should be notified if the patient's intake is inadequate.

Outpatients should be advised to eat their usual diet and some additional sweets and desserts. It is particularly important that a dietitian discuss with the patient an appropriate diet to follow in preparation for the test if the patient has been following a weight reduction diet, a diet very low in carbohydrate, or other unusual dietary practices.

Physicians: How to Order Diet

The diet order should indicate diet in preparation for *glucose tolerance test.*

References

5. Wilkerson HLC, Hyman H, Kaufman M, McCuistion AC, Francis JOS. Diagnostic evaluation of oral glucose tolerance tests in nondiabetic subjects after various levels of carbohydrate intake. N Engl J Med 1960;262:1047–1053.
6. Marble A, Ferguson BD. Diagnosis and classification of diabetes mellitus and the nondiabetic melituria. In: Marble A, Kroll LP, Bradley RF, Christlieb AR, Soeldner JS, eds. Joslin's diabetes mellitus, 12th ed. Philadelphia: Lea & Febiger, 1985:339.

FAT ABSORPTION

The test diet is used to determine the presence of steatorrhea, an indication of gastrointestinal maldigestion or malabsorption. Fat intake is controlled, and stools are collected during the test period, which is usually 48 to 72 hours in duration.

In the hospital setting, food intake is monitored, and fat intake can be accurately estimated. In the outpatient setting, patients are advised to control fat intake as closely as possible. However, there is likely to be greater variance in the diet owing to inaccuracies in fulfilling instructions coupled with difficulties in tolerating a daily intake of 100 g of fat. Actual fat consumption can be estimated through diet recall.

The diet is generally planned to provide 100 g of fat per day. An average intake of 100 plus or minus 10 g of fat is usually considered acceptable. Ordinarily, stool fat for normal adult subjects who are consuming the 100 g fat test diet is 4 to 5 g per day.[7] A value greater than 7 g per day is considered to indicate steatorrhea.* Because of the large variation in total fecal solids, fat excretion expressed as a percentage of the dry weight of the stool is not a satisfactory measure of steatorrhea. Average stool fat increases with increased dietary fat. Some patients find it extremely difficult to eat a diet containing 100 g of fat. In some instances, it may be more reasonable to set a goal of 60 to 80 g of fat.

Normal standards for the lower fat intake are then computed by the formula at the top of the next page.

---

*In children, steatorrhea is defined as fecal fat excretion of 5 g or more per day with a diet containing 40 to 65 g of fat. See p. 558 for additional guidelines for test diets for steatorrhea in children.

$$(0.021 \times \text{Grams of Dietary Fat per 24 Hours}) + 2.93 = \text{Grams of Fecal Fat per 24 Hours*}$$

This formula may permit the interpretation of fecal fat analysis, even when fat intake differs considerably from that in the standard test diet. The dietitian can determine the expected average amount of stool fat for this level of intake in addition to reporting the amount of fat actually consumed.

Stool nitrogen remains remarkably constant over a wide range of protein intake, although a high fiber diet tends to increase stool nitrogen somewhat. Mean stool nitrogen on the standard 100 g fat test diet was 1.7 g per 24 hours (a range of 0.8 to 2.5 g) in the studies by Wollaeger et al.[7,8] Other studies suggest a somewhat lower range, with means of 1.2 to 1.3 g of nitrogen per 24 hours.[8,9] Stool nitrogen, like stool fat, is increased in malabsorption and in maldigestion and can be used to confirm stool fat data.

Stool fat and nitrogen data should be viewed not only as numbers to confirm or to disprove a diagnosis but also as a means of assessing the nutritional consequences of an intestinal disorder. Stool fat in excess of 7 g per day can be multiplied by the factor of 9 kcal per gram to obtain kilocalories wasted by steatorrhea. Stool nitrogen in excess of 2 g per day multiplied by the factor of 6.25 g of protein per gram of nitrogen gives the equivalent amount of protein wasted. This figure multiplied by the factor of 4 kcal per gram yields protein kilocalories wasted by malabsorption or by maldigestion.

Physicians: How to Order Diet

The diet order should indicate *test diet for steatorrhea* or *100 g fat test diet* and the date the diet is to begin. The dietitian will calculate the normal value for fat excretion based on the estimated fat consumption if actual fat intake is outside the range of 100 plus or minus 10 g per day.

Suggestion for Meal Planning

When portion sizes can be measured reliably, any food may be served as long as fat content can be determined. In an outpatient setting, the diet may be more accurately fulfilled if fat-free and low fat foods are used and if measured amounts of fat are added. Table 17-1 gives three examples of daily meal plans that allow for 100 g of fat.

*According to this formula, an average amount of stool fat of 5.03 g would be expected after a dietary fat intake of 100 g, and a stool fat of 3.98 g would be expected after a dietary fat intake of 50 g. Example: $(0.021 \times 50 \text{ g of dietary fat}) + 2.93 = 3.98 \text{ g of stool fat.}$

TABLE 17-1 Three Possible Meal Plans to Achieve a Daily Intake of 100 g of Fat

Whole Milk	Skim Milk	Vegetable	Fruit	Bread	Meat†	Fat	Low Fat Dessert	Low Fat Sweets
2	—	Ad lib	Ad lib	Ad lib	6	10	Ad lib	Ad lib
—	2	Ad lib	Ad lib	Ad lib	6	14	Ad lib	Ad lib
—	—	Ad lib	Ad lib	Ad lib	8	12	Ad lib	Ad lib

†Calculations are based on values for medium fat meats.

The Food Exchange Lists (see Chapter 8, Diabetes Mellitus–Food Exchange Lists) can be used as a tool for meal planning.

References

7. Wollaeger EE, Comfort MW, Osterberg AE. Total solids, fat and nitrogen in the feces: III. A study of normal persons taking a test diet containing a moderate amount of fat; comparison with results obtained with normal persons taking a test diet containing a large amount of fat. Gastroenterology 1947;9:272–283.

8. Wollaeger EE, Comfort MW, Weir JF, Osterberg AE. The total solids, fat and nitrogen in the feces: I. A study of normal persons and of patients with duodenal ulcer on a test diet containing large amounts of fat. Gastroenterology 1946;6:83–92.

9. Reifenstein EC Jr, Albright F, Wells SL. The accumulation, interpretation and presentation of data pertaining to metabolic balances, notably those of calcium, phosphorous and nitrogen. J Clin Endocrinol Metab 1945;5:367–395 .

5-HIAA

The presence of 5-hydroxyindoleacetic acid (5-HIAA) in the urine is an indication of an abnormal production of serotonin. An excess of 5-HIAA may indicate that the patient has a carcinoid tumor. For 24 hours before urine collection, patients scheduled for 5-HIAA testing should avoid ingesting exogenous sources of serotonin, which increase urinary 5-HIAA, and medications that interfere with the test.

Foods to Avoid[10-12]

Alcohol	Pecans
Avocado	Pineapple
Bananas	Plantain
Butternuts	Plums
Eggplant	Tomatoes
Hickory nuts	Walnuts, black and English
Kiwi fruit	

Medications to Avoid

Acetaminophen (Tylenol™)
Cough syrup containing glyceryl guaiacolate
Phenacetin

Physicians: How to Order Diet

This diet may be ordered as *diet in preparation for 5-HIAA testing*.

References

10. Wegener LT. 5-Hydroxyindoleacetic acid (5-HIAA) urine. In: Wegener LT, ed. Mayo medical laboratories handbook. Rochester, MN: Mayo Clinic, 1983:116.

11. Feldman JM, Lee EM. Serotonin content of foods: effect on urinary excretion of 5-hydroxyindoleacetic acid. Am J Clin Nutr 1985;42:639–643.

12. Feldman JM, Lee EM, Castleberry CA. Catecholamine and serotonin content of foods: effect on urinary excretion of homovanillic and 5-hydroxyindoleacetic acid. J Am Diet Assoc 1987;87(8):1031–1035.

Normal Nutrition and Therapeutic Diets for Infants, Children, and Adolescents

18 / *Pediatric Nutritional Assessment*

PEDIATRIC NUTRITIONAL ASSESSMENT

A nutritional assessment program can increase the quality of care given to pediatric patients by identifying patients at risk for developing nutritional deficiencies and by promoting early nutritional intervention. Nutritional assessment provides an objective basis for dietary recommendations and for evaluation of nutritional support. This information provides data to evaluate the nutritional status of the individual at a given point in time. Serial assessments are essential for facilitating optimal intervention and for monitoring growth and nutritional status over longer periods of time.

Nutritional assessment includes clinical assessment, anthropometric evaluation, dietary evaluation, and biochemical data. Selection of parameters, techniques, and standards relevant to a specific population is important in order to minimize cost and to maximize benefit effectiveness. Table 18-1 presents guidelines for three levels of nutritional assessment.

Clinical Assessment

In general, clinical assessment of nutritional status in children is similar to that for adults (see Chapter 3, Nutritional Screening and Assessment). Clinical signs of nutritional deficiencies are nonspecific and should lead to further laboratory assessment.

Anthropometric Evaluation

Accurately determined anthropometric measurements are one of the best indicators of nutritional status in children. Height (or length if the child is less than 2 years old) and weight are generally considered to be the most important measures of normal growth and nutritional status in children because the standards available are based on large groups of healthy growing children and have been used successfully for a number of years. Head circumference is measured when children are less than 2 years of age. Skinfold and midarm circumference measure-

419

TABLE 18-1   Guidelines for Selection of Nutritional Assessment Techniques

	Indications	Anthropometrics	Clinical	Laboratory Data	Dietary
Screening	All children	Height (or length) Weight Weight for height (or length) Head circumference in children less than 2 yr	Health history and general physical appearance	Hemoglobin and/or hematocrit (at least once in first 15 mo) Mean corpuscular volume (MCV)	Dietary history of usual intake, feeding skills, and behaviors Use of supplements
*Intermediate (add)**	Child at risk identified from screening or with disease known to affect nutritional status	Body composition including triceps skinfold (TSF) and arm muscle circumference measurements, if indicated	Physical exam for evidence of nutritional deficiency or excess	Serum albumin	3–7 day food record
*In-depth (add)**	Identification of specific nutrient deficiency or excess Child with severe nutritional deficiencies Evaluation of response to nutritional therapy	Growth velocity, if indicated (see Chapter 20, Failure to Thrive)		Specific vitamin and mineral levels; prealbumin	

*Add indicates that the techniques recommended at a given level should be in addition to those recommended at the previous level.

ments require reliable equipment, considerable skill, and practice for accuracy. In addition, interpretation of the results can be complex, and the norms currently available are not universally accepted.[1-3]

Measurements of Height and Length.   Growth graphs from the National Center for Health Statistics (NCHS) (see Pediatric Appendix 28) are used to assess a child's growth progress over time. The graphs are based on a cross-sectional sample of healthy children from the United States from 1963 to 1975.[4] Proper technique in obtaining the measurements and exact age are essential for valid use of the graphs.

Measurement technique from birth to 36 months.   Record the weight of the nude child. Recumbent length, without shoes, should be measured using a length board with a fixed headboard and a movable right angle footboard. This requires two people—one to position the child and the other to obtain the measurement. Values on the birth to 36 month graph are based on recumbent length. Therefore, standing height should not be recorded on this graph.

Measurement technique from 2 to 18 years.   Weight should be taken in light clothing without shoes. Height should be measured without shoes with the child standing against a fixed scale on a rigid surface wide enough to provide back and heel support. A right angle movable headboard should be lowered until it touches the head. Values on the 2 to 18 year graph are based on standing height. Therefore, recumbent length should not be recorded on this graph.

Interpretation.   Measurements that consistently fall between the 5th and 95th percentiles generally indicate normal growth. Crossing percentiles within the 25th to 75th percentiles is not unusual and most likely represents normal growth. However, crossing percentiles in a progressively upward or downward direction, or measurements near the upper or lower end of the normal percentiles, may indicate nutritional or health problems.

Measurements below the 5th and above the 95th percentiles may indicate a need for further evaluation and follow-up. Weight for length or height indicates how much the child weighs in relation to other children of the same sex and length (or height). When weight for length or height is greater than the 95th percentile, it is suggestive of obesity.[5] Follow-up measurements should be done every 1 to 3 months for infants and young children and every 3 to 6 months for older children.

Decreased weight for height or length may suggest a state of acute or chronic malnutrition, whereas decreased height for age may suggest chronic undernutrition. Weight for height has replaced weight for age as the criterion by which acute protein-calorie malnutrition (PCM) is determined because the latter failed to account for the effect of height differences. Weight for height or length is independent of age and is useful mainly before the onset of puberty. Standard growth charts after the age of 10 years in girls and 11.5 years in boys should be used cautiously since the pubescent growth spurt occurs at different ages and may result in deviations from the norm in heights and weights. Ideal weight for height and age is not necessarily at the same percentile on the growth chart as the height percentile.

Measurements of Head Circumference.   Head circumference is closely related to growth in body length up to 2 years of age. After this age, slower head circumference growth makes it an ineffective measurement of nutritional status. It is primarily a screening measurement for micro- and macrocephaly owing to nonnutritional abnormalities. However, a small head circumference in infants or in older children with failure to grow may indicate severe and long-term caloric deficit during the first 2 years of life.[6]

Growth Graphs and Evaluation for Special Groups.

Developmental disabilities.   For children with genetic abnormalities that result in growth retardation and developmental delay, weight for height or length may be more useful in assessing growth adequacy and nutritional needs than height or weight for age. The Baldwin-Wood Tables (see Pediatric Appendix 29) can be used to assess weight for height among these children.[7] Baumgartner et al have published incremental growth tables that may be useful in assessing short-term changes in the growth rate of a child in relation to disease or therapy.[8]

"Height-age" can be useful in estimating advisable weight when children are at less than the 5th percentile for height. Height-age is the age at which the child's height would be at the 50th percentile. Advisable weight would be the 50th percentile weight for that age with a range of 25th to 75th percentile.

Cronk has developed growth graphs for children with Down's syndrome. These graphs correct for the slower growth rate of children with Down's syndrome (see Pediatric Appendix 30, and Chapter 20, Developmental Disability for further discussion).[9] Butler and Meaney have reported standards for children with Prader-Willi syndrome, which provide a means for assessing these children, who typically have short stature and excessive weight for height.[10] Lyon et al have developed a growth curve for girls with untreated Turner syndrome.[11]

Premature infant.   Growth progress of the premature infant (less than 38 weeks of gestation) can be followed either by the child's "adjusted age" or on a growth graph for premature infants developed by Babson.[12] Adjusted age is the infant's birth age minus the number of weeks of prematurity. This age should be used for approximately the first 18 months of life or until catch-up growth is completed. The use of Babson's growth chart allows growth progress to be monitored prior to 40 weeks from conception and can be used for 12 months postterm (see Pediatric Appendix 31, and Chapter 20, Low Birth Weight Infant for further discussion).

Growth Graphs and Evaluation for Ethnic Groups.   Size differences between ethnic groups appears to be due to genetic or environmental factors or the interaction between them.[13]

Mexican-American children.   Similar stature is expected for Mexican-Americans and non-Hispanic white preadolescent children. Deviations from these should be seen as a marker of nutritional status rather than an ethnic marker. For Mexican-American adolescents, the interpretation of small stature is not clear, because genetic potential for growth or cohort effects may account for differences.[14]

Southeast Asian children.   Growth patterns of Asian children appear to be different from those of other population groups.[13] Growth graphs based on Thai children can be useful in monitoring growth in children with Southeast Asian ancestry.[15,16] Growth patterns of first generation Southeast Asian infants appear to differ from NCHS standards for United States children.[17]

International standards.   When NCHS standards are used for populations outside the United States, many children will be found to be very small, so it may be necessary to construct curves below the 3rd percentile, using standard deviations below the mean.[13]

Estimation of Body Fat and Protein Status.   Children with decreased weight for height (less than 5th percentile) have increased morbidity and longer hospitalizations.[18] Further nutritional assessment may be beneficial in identifying how decreased body weight has altered total body composition and how body composition is changed by nutritional therapy. Measurements of body fat and body protein may indicate the area(s) and the severity of compromise.

Body fat.   Since approximately 50% of body fat is subcutaneous fat, a simple and fairly reliable measurement of body fat, and thus of caloric reserves, is triceps skinfold. Measurement techniques, which have been published by Frisancho, should be followed.[19] The average of three triceps skinfold measurements should be compared to the triceps skinfold percentile tables published by Frisancho (see Pediatric Appendix 32).

Edema may falsely increase the skinfold measurement. Measurements of infants can be quite difficult and require frequent practice and much patience.

Values below the 5th percentile are considered abnormally low, and nutritional intervention should be considered. Measurements greater than the 90th percentile for age indicate a need for close medical supervision and for dietary counseling. Those greater than the 95th percentile may need to be treated.[19]

Body protein.   Upper arm circumference and triceps skinfold are necessary for estimating arm muscle circumference and arm muscle area. The nomogram (see Pediatric Appendix 33) can be used for making these calculations.[19] These values can then be compared with arm muscle circumference and arm muscle area percentile tables (see Pediatric Appendix 34, and Pediatric Appendix 35) to estimate body muscle mass relative to other children of the same age and sex.[20] Height-age standards, instead of those for chronological age, should be used for children with decreased height for age since these measurements are to a certain extent height-dependent.

Values below the 5th percentile are considered abnormal. Further evaluation or intervention is recommended.[18]

Dietary Assessment

Dietary assessment may include a retrospective or prospective estimation of the child's intake. Information regarding the child's development, socioeconomic status, eating attitudes and behavior, and those of his or her family is useful. Assessment of parent-child interaction and the psychosocial environment of the family are also valuable components in the overall evaluation.

Qualitative information on dietary intake, food frequency, and usual meal and snack patterns is generally adequate for screening purposes. The diet should be evaluated for adequacy of food sources of key nutrients.

For infants on formula and solids, an accurate estimation of typical dietary intake is usually obtainable from the parents. Kilocalories, protein, and other key nutrients can be calculated. The diet history should include formulas and/or breast milk used, age at introduction of solids, variety of solids used, how the formula is prepared, vitamin and mineral supplements given, and problems such as vomiting, diarrhea, constipation, and colic.

Quantitative information about the older child's typical intake is extremely difficult to get from the child or from parents. Parents of preschoolers are more likely to underestimate rather than overestimate the amount of food their child ate. When a parent does not care for the child full time, it is necessary to obtain information from all caregivers.[21] Children of school age and older may or may not be able to give accurate nutritional histories and should be evaluated individually as to maturity and level of dietary awareness. Third to sixth grade children may be able to record food intake most accurately by food frequency.[22] Frequently, it is helpful to interview the parents and child separately. A prospective food intake record should be initiated under the supervision of a dietitian if quantitative information is warranted by other indices of the nutritional assessment.

Evaluation of Nutritional Adequacy.   Key nutrients for growing children include kilocalories, protein, iron, calcium, and vitamins A, D, and C. The diet should also be evaluated for the content of foods with low nutrient density, for the interference of these foods with intake of other more nutritious foods, and for adverse effects of these foods on dental health. The dietary history should also include information about past diets, including vegetarian diets, diets for chronic disease, and diets for weight reduction. Food aversions, sensitivities, vitamin and mineral or food supplements, and medications also need to be evaluated because these factors can enhance or pose a risk to nutritional and health status.

Assessment of Feeding Skills and Attitudes.   Feeding skills and attitudes are an integral part of normal physical and psychosocial development. An initial assessment of the child's ability to feed himself and of the appropriateness of the texture of food eaten for the age of the child should be made. A more detailed discussion of the assessment of feeding skills is included in Chapter 19, Healthy Infants, Children, and Adolescents, and Chapter 20, Developmental Disability.

Knowledge of child and adolescent behavior, especially as it relates to food and eating habits, is essential. Periods of increased or decreased appetite, food jags, binges, disinterest, willingness to try new foods, or lack of it are common at various stages throughout childhood and adolescence. Dietary assessment should include the age-appropriateness of the child's attitudes and behaviors.

Biochemical Data

Biochemical data may either confirm nutrient excesses or deficiencies suspected from other nutritional assessment parameters or identify clinically unapparent nutritional abnormalities. There is no one simple set of tests that can give an estimate of overall or individual nutrient stores, nor are the tests uniformly precise and accurate. Laboratory studies should be selected on the basis of the patient, level of assessment, evaluation of other nutritional assessment parameters, and risk factors determined from the family history with consideration of the amount of blood volume needed for testing in relation to the infant or child's size. Pediatric Appendix 36, presents selected references for pediatric laboratory values.

Iron Deficiency Anemia.   Screening for iron deficiency is a reasonable part of all routine nutritional assessment since it is one of the most common nutritional problems of children in our society. Hemoglobin and hematocrit can be used to screen for iron deficiency anemia, and mean corpuscular volume (MCV) should be added whenever possible. All three measures require the use of age-specific norms. Of the three, hematocrit, which measures the percent of packed red cells in whole blood, is the least sensitive indicator for identifying children with iron deficiency anemia, and MCV is the most sensitive.[5] In addition, it must be recognized that anemia is a late manifestation of iron deficiency but may also be attributable to other nutritional or non-nutritional factors. When hemoglobin, hematocrit, and/or MCV are below normal for age, a treatment trial with an iron supplement may be initiated, with follow-up laboratory studies to assess the response. Differential diagnosis of iron deficiency anemia, however, would require measurement of ferritin or serum iron, total iron binding capacity, percent saturation, and transferrin. In iron deficiency anemia, ferritin, which is a measure of body reserves, is low, serum iron and transferrin may be low to low normal, total iron binding capacity is above normal, and percent saturation is low.

Protein Status.   Serum albumin is an appropriate screening test to measure visceral protein status in the hospitalized patient. In the stressed patient, however, hypoalbuminemia may indicate metabolic response to injury rather than nutritional status. Because serum-albumin has a half-life of approximately 20 days, it is considered a good indicator of long-term body protein nurture. Liver secretory proteins with shorter half-lives, such as prealbumin (about 2 days) and creatinine height index,[23] can be useful in assessing treatment progress when nutritional intervention is initiated.

Other Studies.   Other biochemical studies can be used to further identify the extent and severity of malnutrition. Assessment of the vitamin and mineral status of a malnourished child is essential in the rehabilitation process. When biochemical data are outside the normal range, the studies may need to be repeated for confirmation before additional studies are ordered or treatment is initiated. The types of studies and/or treatment are dependent on the biochemical abnormalities.

References

1. Owen GM. Measurement, recording and assessment of skinfold thickness in childhood and adolescence: report of a small meeting. Am J Clin Nutr 1982;35:629–638.
2. Bishop CM, Bowen PE, Ritchey SJ. Comparison of two newly developed sets of upper arm anthropometric norms for American adults (letter). Am J Clin Nutr 1982;36: 554–557.
3. Frisancho AR. Reply to letter by Bishop et al. Am J Clin Nutr 1982;36:557–560.
4. Hamill PVV, Drizd TA, Johnson CL, Reed RB, Roche AF, Moor WM. Physical growth: National Center for Health Statistics percentiles. Am J Clin Nutr 1979;32:607–629.
5. Hubbard VS, Hubbard LR. Clinical assessment of nutritional status. In: Walker WA, Watkins JB, eds. Nutrition in pediatrics. Boston: Little, Brown, 1985:121.
6. Fomon SJ. Nutritional status. In: Fomon SJ, ed. Infant nutrition, 2nd ed. Philadelphia: WB Saunders, 1974:459.
7. Jelliffe DB. The assessment of the nutritional status of the community. Monograph No. 53. Geneva: World Health Organization, 1966.
8. Baumgartner RN, Roche AF, Himer JH. Incremental growth tables: supplementary to previously published charts. Am J Clin Nutr 1986;43:711–722.

9. Cronck C, Crocker AC, Pueschel SM, Shea AM, Zackai E, Pickens G, Reed RB. Growth charts for children with Down's syndrome: 1 month to 18 years of age. Pediatrics 1988;81:102–110.

10. Butler MB, Meaney FJ. Standards for selected anthropometric measurements in Prader-Willi syndrome. Pediatrics 1991;88:853–860.

11. Lyon AJ, Preece MA, Grant DB. Growth curve for girls with Turner syndrome, Arch Dis Child 1985;60:932–935.

12. Babson SG, Benda GI. Growth graphs for the clinical assessment of infants of varying gestational age. J Pediatr 1976;89:814–820.

13. Falkner F. Growth monitoring: fetus to the first two postnatal years. In: Brunser O, Carrazza JR, Gracey M, Nichols BL, Senterre JC, eds. Clinical nutrition of the young child. New York: Raven Press, 1991:23–38.

14. Martorell R, Mandoza FS, Castillo RO. Genetic and environmental determinants of growth in Mexican Americans. Pediatrics 1989;84:864–871.

15. Chavalittamrong B, Vathakanon R. Height and weight of Bangkok children. Standards of height and weight of Bangkok children. J Med Assoc Thailand 1977;61(Suppl 2): 1–28.

16. Khanjanasthiti P. The anthropometric nutritional classification in Thai infants and preschool children. J Med Assoc Thailand 1977;60(Suppl 1):1–19.

17. Baldwin LM, Sutherland S. Growth patterns of first generation Southeast Asian infants. Am J Dis Child 1988;142:526–531.

18. Merritt RJ, Blackburn GL. Nutritional assessment and metabolic response to illness of the hospitalized child. In: Suskind RM, ed. Textbook of pediatric nutrition. New York: Raven Press, 1981:285.

19. Frisancho A. New norms of upper limb fat and muscle areas for assessment of nutritional status. Am J Clin Nutr 1981;34:2540–2545.

20. Gurney JM, Jelliffe DB. Arm anthropometry in nutritional assessment: nomogram for rapid calculation of muscle circumference and cross-sectional muscle and fat areas. Am J Clin Nutr 1973;26:912–915.

21. Baranowski T, Sprague D, Henshe Baranowski J, Harrison JA. Accuracy of maternal dietary recall for preschool children. J Am Diet Assoc 1991;91:669–674.

22. Baranowski T, Dworkin R, Henshe JC, Clearman DR, Dunn JK, Nader PR, Heads PC. The accuracy of children's self reports of diet: Family Health Project. J Am Diet Assoc 1986;86:1381–1385.

23. Viteri FE, Jorge A. The creatinine height index: its use in the estimation of the degree of protein depletion and repletion in protein/calorie malnourished children. Pediatrics 1970;46:696–706.

19 / *Normal Nutrition*

HEALTHY INFANTS, CHILDREN, AND ADOLESCENTS

General Description

The nutrient needs of normal infants are based on estimations of intake of breast-fed infants with satisfactory growth (see Chapter 2, Recommended Dietary Allowances). There are few data on the nutritional requirements of preschoolers, school age children, and adolescents. The recommended allowances for these groups are based on extrapolations from infant and adult data with estimations for growth. Beyond the recommended allowances, the nutritional needs of the child for prevention of disease and promotion of health must be considered.[1]

Nutritional Requirements of Infants

Energy. The average intake of healthy, growing infants (see Chapter 2, Recommended Dietary Allowances) is one of the best measures of caloric need. The higher caloric demand of infants, as compared with adults, is related to increased heat loss due to a relatively greater body surface area relative to weight and to the larger percentage of metabolically active tissue. During the first year, approximately 85 to 90% of the estimated energy intake is used for body maintenance and growth, while an average of 10 to 15% is used for physical activity.[2]

Protein, Carbohydrates, and Fat. The Recommended Dietary Allowances (RDA) for protein at birth is 2.2 g/kg/day.[3] This decreases to 1.6 g/kg/day during the latter half of the first year as growth decelerates.[3] The requirements for carbohydrates and fats have not been specifically determined. The usual caloric distribution of the diet of infants drinking human milk or infant formulas is approximately 40 to 50% from fat and 40 to 45% from carbohydrate. However, of the total caloric intake, a maximum of 60% from carbohydrates and a minimum of 30% from fat is recommended in order to ensure adequate caloric intake and satiety.[4] The recommended intake of fat in the form of long-chain triglycerides to provide essential fatty acids is 3% of total kilocalories.[5]

Fluid.   In neonates, the daily turnover of water is approximately 15% of body weight. Since the immature kidneys of young infants are less able to concentrate urine, more fluid is required, particularly in warm climates. A fluid intake of 120 to 150 ml/kg/day is recommended.[5] This recommendation is ordinarily met by human milk or by commercial formulas.

Minerals.   Estimations of the minerals needed for infants, except for iron and fluoride, are based on averages from breast milk. Breast milk may provide inadequate iron and fluoride in some situations.[6] Iron fortified commercially prepared formula contains adequate amounts of all minerals except fluoride.

Approximately 50% of iron is absorbed from human milk compared with 7% from iron fortified formula and 4% from infant cereals.[6]

Supplemental iron is recommended after 6 months of age for breast-fed term infants and after 4 months of age for infants fed noniron-containing formulas.[6] An iron fortified cereal introduced at this time provides the additional iron needed. An intake of 1 mg/kg/day maintains hemoglobin levels in term infants.[3] The recommended allowance for 6 months to 3 years is set at 10 mg/day and is considered adequate for most healthy children.[3]

Estimated safe and adequate intakes of fluoride have been set at 0.1 to 0.5 milligram from birth to 6 months of age and 0.2 to 1.0 mg from 6 to 12 month.[3] A fluoride supplement of 0.25 mg/day is recommended for all breast-fed infants who are not living in an area where the water is adequately fluoridated.[6] Infants fed commercial ready-to-feed formulas should also receive a fluoride supplement. The amount of fluoride in human milk varies only slightly with the amount in the mother's diet. However, unsupplemented breast-fed infants of mothers drinking fluoridated water have been shown to have a rate of dental caries comparable to that of formula-fed infants with adequate fluoride intake.[7] When powdered or concentrated formulas are used, the requirement for fluoride depends on the fluoride content of local water. If the water and fluoride concentration is less than 0.3 parts per million, 0.25 mg/day of fluoride should be supplemented. Formulas mixed with fluorinated water do not need further supplementation. Excessive fluoride ingestion, 0.1 to 0.3 mg/kg of body weight, causes dental fluorosis, a brownish mottling of the teeth.[8]

Vitamins.   Human milk provides adequate levels of all vitamins when the mother's diet is nutritionally balanced. However, there have been reports of rickets in breast-fed black infants, in infants who consumed or whose nursing mothers consumed vegan diets, and in infants who had minimal sunlight exposure.[9,10] In addition, unsupplemented breast-fed infants have been shown to have decreased bone mineral concentrations by 12 weeks of age compared to babies receiving 400 IU of vitamin D per day.[10,11] The long-term outcome of the degree of bone mineralization attained during infancy is unknown and warrants further study.[13] Therefore, a daily supplement of 400 IU is recommended for breast-fed infants who are not exposed regularly to sunlight.[7,12] When adequate vitamin D was provided, bone mineralization was comparable for infants given human milk, cows' milk formula, or soy formula.[13] Commercial infant formulas are supplemented with all the necessary vitamins.

TABLE 19-1   Vitamin and Mineral Supplementation for Infants

Type of Feeding	Iron	Vitamin D	Fluoride	Other
Breast	Additional iron from a supplement or an iron fortified infant cereal is needed after 6 mo of age	Supplementation may be recommended if the infant has little exposure to sunlight	Supplementation may be recommended based on the fluoride content of the water supply	None
Formula	Supplementation is needed by 4 mo of age if the formula does not contain iron	No supplementation needed	Supplementation is recommended for infants receiving ready-to-feed formulas. It may be recommended for powdered formulas, based on the fluoride content of the water supply	None
Cows' milk plus solid food (after 1 yr of age)	Additional iron from a supplement or from an iron fortified infant cereal is needed	No supplementation needed	Supplementation may be recommended	None

Table 19-1 provides information on types of feeding and the recommended vitamin and mineral supplementation.

Human Milk.   Breast-feeding provides numerous benefits to the infant and the mother. These include the nutritional and immunological benefits of human milk for the infant and the psychological, physiological, social, and hygienic benefits of the breast-feeding process for both mother and infant.[14] Human milk is ideally suited for the infant.[14] Its composition averages 7% protein, 55% fat (4% as essential fatty acids), and 38% carbohydrate. The composition varies with the stage of the feeding (i.e., there is a higher proportion of fat at the end of the feeding), with the time of day, and with the length of nursing. Human milk supplies approximately 20 kcal/oz, or 67 kcal per 100 ml.

The advantages of human milk are numerous.[6] Human milk has a solute concentration compatible with the infant's immature kidneys. The fat in human milk is better absorbed because of its higher concentration of bile salt–stimulated lipase. Human milk contains antibodies and other immune factors that may reduce the incidence or severity of certain infections and conditions in the infant. The incidence of gastroenteritis, otitis media, and asthma has been shown to be less frequent among breast-fed infants, even in industrialized countries, than among formula-fed infants.[6] However, the incidence of upper respiratory infections and eczema appears to be equally common in breast-fed and formula-fed infants.[15,16]

Most drugs are excreted into breast milk at concentrations that are not harmful to the infant. Breast-feeding is contraindicated only when the medications or chemicals that are taken by the mother and transmitted to the infant via breast milk are harmful to the infant. A detailed listing of medications that are transferred via breast milk is available.[17] These medications include anticoagulants, some antibiotics, anticancer drugs, tranquilizers, antidepressants, and sedatives. Nicotine from heavy cigarette smoking, alcohol, marijuana, and other illicit drugs are also harmful to the nursing infant. Also listed are medications that are compatible with breast-feeding.[17] Nursing mothers should contact their physicians before taking any medications. Concern has been raised about the transmission of environmental contaminants, especially pesticide residues, in breast milk. Thus far no harmful effects have been shown, although investigations are being continued and extended to include contamination of cows' milk and other infant foods.[17]

Occasionally, certain circumstances may inhibit breast-feeding. Breast-feeding may not be possible if the mother is chronically ill. If the infant needs a modified infant formula (see Infant Formulas and Feedings, Appendix 25) or if the infant is unable to nurse, a special formula or feeding device may be necessary.

Formulas. Commercially prepared formulas are patterned after human milk and are adjusted to meet the recommended allowances. The protein is slightly higher than in human milk and has been treated to produce a fine, easily digested curd. Vegetable oils are used instead of butterfat as the fat source. Subsequently, the cholesterol content is extremely low, less than 3 mg per 100 ml. (Cows' milk has about 20 mg of cholesterol per 100 ml, and human milk has about 30 mg per 100 ml.) Studies of infants who received either breast or bottle feedings have not shown differences in plasma cholesterol concentration or in the incidence of arteriosclerosis.[5] The major disadvantage of commercial formulas is the absence of immunological properties in human milk.

Staged formulas (i.e., "start-up" formulas for 1- to 6-month-olds and "follow-up" formulas for 6- to 12-month-olds) have received increased attention recently but offer no benefit.[18] A standard infant formula, plus iron fortified cereal and the introduction of other solid foods, is satisfactory for the 6- to 12-month-old infant.[18]

The use of soy based formulas for infants has increased, and studies comparing infants fed soy protein formulas versus cows' milk protein formulas found no significant differences in growth.[17] However, the use of soy formulas in the prevention of allergic disease in infancy is controversial, and various studies show conflicting results.[17] Soy protein formulas might be recommended for vegetarian families, for the management of children with galactosemia, and for infants with a family history of infantile eczema.[12]

Cows' Milk. Cows' milk is not recommended for infants under 6 months of age, because it contains higher proportions of nutrients that are not well tolerated by the infant. The protein content of cows' milk is three times greater than in human milk. The higher protein and mineral content of cows' milk causes a higher renal solute load, which increases obligatory water loss. Supplementary water may lessen the effects of the increased solute load, but adequate water consumption is difficult for the infant to achieve. Newborn infants are at risk for development of hypernatremia and irreversible central nervous system damage because of their limited capacity for renal solute excretion. In addition, the protein in cows' milk is not well utilized, and the fat is not absorbed as efficiently as the fat in human milk.[6] Furthermore, only about 1% of the total kilocalories is in the form of essential fatty acids.[5,19] Another disadvantage of cows' milk is a curd that is larger, tougher, and more slowly digested. This can result in gastrointestinal blood loss, and the protein may cause a higher incidence of allergic reactions. In addition, heating cows' milk concentrates the protein and electrolytes because of water evaporation and therefore further potentiates dehydration and hypernatremia.

There is a higher incidence of iron deficiency in infants fed cows' milk in the second 6 months of life. Even though solid foods are providing some iron at this time, the incidence of iron deficiency is twice as high in infants fed cows' milk as in infants fed iron fortified formulas.[20] After the infant is 6 months old, if cows' milk is used it should be whole milk, because infants fed skim milk or 2% milk receive insufficient energy to support maintenance requirements.[20] Growth is achieved but at a reduced rate. Energy is obtained by the mobilization of body fat as clinically evidenced by a substantial reduction in triceps and subscapular skinfold thicknesses. A further consideration may be whether an infant who is required to mobilize stores of body fat in order to supply energy requirements is able simultaneously to synthesize the lipids essential for myelination of the nervous system.[21] Therefore, whole cows' milk of any fat content is not recommended for infants during the first 6 months of life and strongly discouraged until 1 year of age.[22] Table 19-2 provides a comparison of the RDA for normal infants with the composition of human milk, cows' milk, and commercial formula.

Introduction of Solid Foods.   The newborn infant has a number of primitive adaptive reflexes, such as suckling, swallowing, and rooting, that probably developed as survival mechanisms and that help to promote the acquisition of liquid foods. Most primitive reflexes disappear by 3 to 4 months of life. Table 19-3 correlates the infant's digestive and neuromuscular development with nutritional requirements and implications for feeding during the first year of life.

The age to introduce solids cannot be definitely determined, since each infant matures at a different rate. However, by 4 to 6 months most infants are physiologically and developmentally ready for semisolid foods. Feeding solids before this time may lead to poor eating habits and overfeeding since infants are unable to communicate when they are full. In addition, when solid foods are introduced earlier, the infant may be fed a diet that varies from the recommended caloric distribution of 7 to 16% of kilocalories from protein, 35 to 55% from fat, and the rest from carbohydrates.[4]

A reasonable schedule for the introduction of solid foods is presented in Table 19-4.

Starting with iron fortified cereal, 1 to 2 tsp of a single ingredient baby food are introduced at 4 to 5 day intervals so that food sensitivities can be readily determined. Semisolids and solids should both be given at a feeding. As foods other than milk or formula are introduced, the composition of the total diet should be considered (Table 19-5). For example, the infant may receive fewer kilocalories and other nutrients required for growth and development when certain strained foods, like fruit or vegetables, are substituted for human milk or formula.[4] The infant's acceptance of specific foods should be considered when planning a nutritionally balanced diet.

Text continued on p. 436.

TABLE 19-2 Comparison of Recommended Dietary Allowances for Normal Infants with Composition of Human Milk, Cows' Milk, and Milk Based (Commercial) Formula

Nutrient	Recommended Dietary Allowances[a]		Human Milk[b] (per 1,000 ml)	Whole Cows' Milk[b] (per 1,000 ml)	Commercial Milk Based Formula[c] (per 1,000 ml)
	0–6 Mo	6–12 Mo			
Weight, kg	6	9			
lb	13	20			
Height, cm	60	71			
in	24	28			
Water, ml			871	876	875
Energy, kcal	kg × 108	kg × 98	747	701	670
Protein, g	kg × 2.2	kg × 1.6	10.6	33	15–16
Fat, g			45	38	36–37
Carbohydrate, g			72	47	70–72
Vitamin A, RE	375	375	610	270	340–500
Vitamin D, IU	400	400	20	400[d]	400–425
Vitamin E, mg TE	3	4	2.4	0.6	5.7–8.5
Ascorbic acid, mg	30	35	52	11	55
Thiamin, mg	0.3	0.4	0.142	0.43	0.4–0.7
Riboflavin, mg	0.4	0.5	0.373	1.56	0.6–1.0
Niacin, mg NE	5	6	1.83	0.74	79
Vitamin B6, mg	0.3	0.6	0.18	0.51	0.3–0.4
Vitamin B12, µg	0.3	0.5	trace	6.6	1.5–2.0
Folacin, µg	25	35	33	51.6	50–100
Calcium, mg	400	600	307	1,370	550–600
Phosphorus, mg	300	500	141	910	440–460
Sodium, mg	115–350[e]	250–750[e]	180	768	250–390
Potassium, mg	350–925[e]	425–1,275[e]	532	1,430	620–1,000
Magnesium, mg	40	60	35	130	40–50
Iodine, µg	40	50	61	116	40–70
Iron, mg	6	10	0.5	0.45	1.4–12.5[f]
Zinc, mg	5	5	1.2	3.9	2.0–4.0

Key:

RE = Retinol equivalents - 1 RE = 1 µg retinol or 6 µg β-carotene

IU = International units - 1 IU = 0.25 µg cholecalciferol

TE = Tocopherol equivalents - 1 TE = 1 mg α tocopherol equivalent

NE = Niacin equivalents - 1 NE = 1 mg niacin

[a]From Food and Nutrition Board. Recommended Daily Allowances, 10th ed. National Research Council—National Academy of Sciences, Washington, DC, 1989.

[b]American Academy of Pediatrics Committee on Nutrition. Pediatric nutrition handbook, 3rd ed. Elk Grove Village, IL: AAP, 1993, 354–359. Mean data for mature milk (15 days to 15 months postpartum).

[c]Manufacturer's information.

[d]Assumes fortification of cows' milk with 400 IU of vitamin D.

[e]Allowances for sodium and potassium are ranges considered to be safe and adequate.

[f]Values for formula not fortified and fortified with iron.

TABLE 19-3 Developmental Patterns, Nutritional Needs, and Implications for Feeding*

	Birth	1 Mo	2 Mo	3 Mo	4 Mo	5 Mo	6 Mo	7 Mo	8 Mo	9 Mo	10 Mo	11 Mo	12 Mo
Nutritional Requirements													
	Rapid growth requires greater quantity of protein, energy, and other essential nutrients.												
					Iron stores depleted.								
							Begin fluoride if necessary.						
	Human milk meets nutritional requirements for term infants. Commercially prepared formulas are the approved alternative.												
								Amount of milk needed is diminished. Meats are an important source of protein and iron. Actual meat intake is usually low, iron fortified cereal or formula also remains an important source of iron.					
Digestion													
	Enzymes present to digest milk. Little saliva. Butterfat poorly utilized.												
			Starches poorly digested, utilized.										
										Stomach acid volume increases.			
Developmental Abilities													
	Rhythmic suck. Infant will stick out tongue when spoon introduced (tongue protrusion reflex).												
				Drooling.									
					Starts to chew. Can use tongue to put food in back of mouth. Opens mouth to spoon. Feeds self cracker.								
									Will turn face away when full. Easily chews soft table foods.				

*Every child is an individual. This chart is meant as a guideline.

Continued.

TABLE 19-3   Developmental Patterns, Nutritional Needs, and Implications for Feeding—cont'd

Birth	1 Mo	2 Mo	3 Mo	4 Mo	5 Mo	6 Mo	7 Mo	8 Mo	9 Mo	10 Mo	11 Mo	12 Mo
Developmental Abilities—cont'd												
Infant will turn head to the same side, open mouth, and may begin to suck when cheek is stroked (rooting reflex).		Sleeps 5–8 hr at night.		Sleeps 8–12 hr at night.			Drinks from cup.					
			Hands to mouth constantly.							Child will use thumb and fore-finger to pick up objects (pincer grasp).		
								Child will use thumb and fingers to pick up objects (thumb-finger grasp).				
		Lifts head.	Reaches for objects.	Sits with support.	Reaches for objects out of reach.	Transfers objects hand-to-hand. Sits alone.						
Implications for Feedings												
Breast milk or commercially prepared formula only. No solids necessary.				May begin iron fortified cereals.				Finger foods. Gradually add and increase foods from all food groups.		Regular meal times. Adjust quantity of intake.		
				Can sit in high chair.		Begin fruits, vegetables. Begin to use cup.			Offer juices, milk from cup.		Allow weaning from the bottle; wean from breast if desired.	

TABLE 19-4 Food Introduction by Age

Age	Food to Introduce
4–6 mo	Infant cereal
5–7 mo	Vegetables, fruits (and their juices if drinking from a cup)
6–8 mo	Protein foods*—cheese, yogurt, cooked beans, meat, fish, chicken, turkey, egg*

*Emphasize lean meat with more frequent use of fish and poultry and less frequent use of egg yolks.

TABLE 19-5 Dietary Guidelines for the First Year of Life*

Basic Food Groups	Major Nutrients Supplied	Number of Servings Recommended per Day
MILK		
Whole milk, cheese, cottage cheese, yogurt, ice cream, creamed soups	Protein, calcium, riboflavin, B_{12}	By 4–6 mo: 30–32 oz of breast milk or formula By 9 mo: 24 oz of breast milk or formula 9–12 mo: 16–24 oz of breast milk or formula After 12 mo: whole milk 1 oz cheese = $^3/_4$ cup milk $^1/_2$ cup cottage cheese = $^1/_4$ cup milk $^1/_2$ cup ice cream = $^1/_4$ cup milk $^1/_4$ cup pudding = $^1/_4$ cup milk
MEAT		
Beef, lamb, veal, fish, poultry, eggs, dry beans, peanut butter	Protein, niacin, iron, thiamin	4–6 mo: none 6–8 mo: 1–2 servings 9–12 mo: 2 servings 1 serving = 1 oz lean meat, poultry, fish; 1 egg; $^1/_4$ cup cooked dried beans, peas, or lentils; 2 Tbsp peanut butter
GRAIN		
Whole-grain enriched or fortified breads, cereal, crackers, rice, spaghetti, noodles, rolled oats, or tortillas	Carbohydrates, thiamin, iron, niacin	4–6 months: 1–2 servings of cereal 6–12 mo: 2–3 servings 12 mo: 4 servings 1 serving = $^1/_2$ slice bread; $^1/_4$ cup cooked cereal
FRUITS AND VEGETABLES		
Should include vitamin C every day, vitamin A every other day Sources of vitamin C: Citrus fruit, strawberries, fortified juices, tomato, broccoli Sources of vitamin A: Carrots, spinach, sweet potato, apricots, winter squash	Carbohydrates, vitamins A and C	4–6 mo: 1 serving fruit 6–8 mo: 2 servings fruit, 1–2 servings vegetable 9–12 mo: 4 servings; 1 or more from each vitamin group 1 serving = $^1/_4$ cup juice, $^1/_2$ piece of fruit, $^1/_4$ cup cooked vegetables

*These are general guidelines for the average child.

By the end of the first year of age, the infant consumes about 300 to 450 g (10 to 15 oz) of solid food each day, and thus the amount of human milk or formula decreases to about 750 ml each day.[2] Total milk intake should not exceed 1 L/day.[5] Most children can be weaned from the breast or bottle to a cup by this time, although they may need assistance with drinking from the cup for several months beyond the first year.

Nutritional Needs of Preschool and School Age Children

Energy.   Energy needs vary widely, depending on the child's stage of growth and level of activity. During the first 3 years, the caloric requirement is 102 kcal/kg of body weight.[39] Caloric requirements until puberty are similar for boys and girls, ranging from 90 kcal/kg of body weight for children 4 to 6 years old to 70 kcal/kg for 7 to 10 year-olds (see Chapter 2, Recommended Dietary Allowances).

Protein.   The current RDA for protein is based on the maintenance requirement for adults (0.8 g/kg) plus an additional amount for growth and for adjustment of protein utilization efficiency. The protein allowance decreases from 1.2 g/kg at ages 1 to 3, to 1.1 g/kg for 4- to 6-year-olds, to 1.0 g/kg for 7- to 10-year-olds. Normally, the preschool and school age child consumes approximately 10 to 15% of total kilocalories from protein sources. Generally this results in a protein intake of almost twice the recommended amount.[23] The protein allowance for school age children is 1.0 g/kg of body weight, or 5.7% of the caloric recommendation.[3]

Other Nutrients.   There are no allowances established for carbohydrates or fats. However, it has been recommended that 1 to 2% of total kilocalories be from linoleic acid to assure an adequate essential fatty acid intake.[3]

The recommendations for minerals and vitamins have been determined by interpolation, with arbitrary allowances for growth (see Chapter 2, Recommended Dietary Allowances). Several dietary surveys have shown low intakes of iron, vitamin A, and ascorbic acid in certain population groups, but clinical symptoms of deficiency are rare or are not a major nutritional problem.[24,25] Because deficiencies of vitamins and minerals (except for iron) are not common in normal, well-fed children, supplementation is usually not necessary after infancy.[26]

Meeting Nutritional Requirements.   The 1-year-old begins to show an increasing curiosity about his or her expanding world while exhibiting a decreasing interest in food at mealtimes. The child is beginning to discern flavors and textures and so may suddenly decide to dislike foods that were liked before. Children of this age also like to feel and explore foods with their fingers and to feed themselves.

By 2 to 3 years of age, the child struggles to do many things independently. Food jags are common, and dislikes may change from day to day and week to week. Parents report a high degree of dissatisfaction with the appetite and interest in food shown by this age group.

The 4- to 5-year-old child is usually more interested in play activities than eating and so may dawdle at mealtime. The child is a great imitator and may quickly follow the example set by a parent or an older brother or sister. These changes are considered normal for these age groups and should be expected. Consequently, time and patience are required by parents during meals.

TABLE 19-6 Guide to Recommended Food Intake for Children and Teens

Food Group	Servings/Day	Average Size of Serving For Child's Age				
		1–2 Yr	3–4 Yr	5–6 Yr	7–10 Yr	11–Teen
MILK	4					
Milk (whole, skim, dry, evaporated, buttermilk)		1/2 cup*	1/2–3/4 cup	3/4 cup	3/4–1 cup	1 cup
Yogurt		1/2 cup	1/2–3/4 cup	3/4 cup	3/4–1 cup	1 cup
Cheese		3/4 oz	3/4 oz	1 oz	1 oz	1 1/2 oz
MEAT	3 or more					
Egg		1/2–1	1	1	1	1
Lean meat, fish, poultry		1/2 oz (2 Tbsp)	1/2 oz (2 Tbsp)	3/4 oz (3 Tbsp)	1 1/2–2 oz	2–3 oz
Peanut butter		—	1 Tbsp	2 Tbsp	2–3 Tbsp	2–3 Tbsp
Legumes (dried peas and beans)		—	1/2 cup	1/2–3/4 cup	1/2–3/4 cup	1/2–3/4 cup
Cottage cheese		2–4 Tbsp	4–6 Tbsp	6 Tbsp	1/2 cup	1/2 cup
FRUITS AND VEGETABLES	4 or more					
Vegetables		3 Tbsp	3 Tbsp	1/4 cup	1/3 cup	1/2 cup
Fruits		3 Tbsp	3 Tbsp	1/4 cup	1/3 cup	1/2 cup
Juice		1/4 cup	1/3 cup	1/3 cup	1/2 cup	1/2 cup
BREADS AND CEREALS	4 or more					
Whole-grain bread		1/2 slice	1 slice	1 1/2 slices	1–2 slices	1–2 slices
Ready-to-eat cereals		1/2 oz	3/4 oz	1 oz	1 oz	1 oz
Cooked cereals		1/4 cup	1/3 cup	1/2 cup	1/2 cup	1/2 cup
Spaghetti, macaroni, noodles, rice		1/4 cup	1/3 cup	1/2 cup	1/2 cup	1/2 cup
Crackers		2	3–4	3–4	4–6	4–6
FATS AND OILS	To meet energy needs					
Margarine, butter, oil, mayonnaise, salad dressing		1/2 tsp	1 tsp	1 tsp	1 Tbsp	2 Tbsp
DESSERTS AND SWEETS	To meet energy needs					
Pudding or ice cream		1/3 cup	1/3 cup	1/2 cup	3/4 cup	1 cup
Cake		1/2 piece	1/2 piece	3/4 piece	1 piece	1 piece
Cookies		1	1–2	2	2–3	2–3
Pie		1/3 piece	1/3 piece	1/2 piece	1 piece	1 piece
Jelly, jam, honey, sugar, syrup		2 tsp	2 tsp	2 tsp	1 Tbsp	1 Tbsp

*Do not use skim milk before 2 yr of age.

The school age child needs guidance in the selection of foods that are good sources of minerals and vitamins and that provide adequate protein and kilocalories so that nutrient needs are met. Normal weight children are able to balance their energy intake with their energy requirement via appetite regulation.

A child's nutrient requirements in relation to body size are greater than adults. Therefore, care givers need to be creative when planning meals and snacks in order to provide an interesting yet nutritionally balanced diet. Serving guidelines to help ensure a nutritionally adequate diet for children are listed in Table 19-6.

Establishing Good Eating Habits.   Eating habits and attitudes about food learned during childhood are likely to become lifelong practices. As the child gains more independence and as the peer group exerts increasing influence, healthy eating habits and a positive attitude toward food can provide the basis for proper food selection. Optimal eating habits can be developed by considering the following suggestions:

1. Parental and sibling attitudes have an impact on the child's request for and attitude toward food. Parents need to establish regular mealtimes, encourage breakfast, and provide nutritious snacks in a pleasant atmosphere. It has been reported that in this age group, snacks provide approximately one-fourth of the total energy intake.[27] New foods should be introduced gradually, at the beginning of the meal when the child is hungry, and in a form easily handled. Vegetables and meat are the foods most frequently reported as disliked by children, but these foods provide important nutrients.[27]

2. Growth rate, mastery of fine and gross motor skills, and personality development affect what and how much the child eats. Utensils needed and portion sizes must be consistent with the child's developmental level. Undernutrition and skipping meals reduce the quality of physical and mental effort available to participate in learning experiences.[19]

3. Emotional stresses or involvement with other activities that conflict with mealtimes may influence food and nutrient intake. These situations should be minimized or eliminated whenever possible.

4. Negative eating behaviors should be ignored; positive behaviors should be encouraged and praised; and favorite foods should not be used as a reward.

5. If the child does not eat at mealtime, wait for the next regularly scheduled snack or meal.

6. It is important to recognize the tendency for developing obesity during childhood (see Chapter 23, Weight Control).

The American Heart Association has made general dietary recommendations for healthy American children above 2 years of age and for adolescents. They include dietary fat and cholesterol control and decreased salt intake (see Chapter 22, Hyperlipidemia).

Nutritional Requirements of the Adolescent

No period of growth is less predictable than adolescence. Because of the wide variability in rates of growth and their timing, there are no norms for adolescent growth as it relates to chronological age.[28] For practical purposes, however, the RDA are convenient and are satisfactory when applied to the general population.[3] Individual needs can be verified through dietary interview and follow-up.

The greatest demand for energy and nutrients occurs during the peak in the growth spurt, which varies according to gender and with each individual. Limitations of either kilocalories or protein during this stage have been shown to inhibit growth.[3] Each adolescent must be evaluated according to his or her unique maturation stage and biological age. Tanner's stages of maturity (see Chapter 23, Weight Control) can be helpful for estimating the caloric needs of the child.

Caloric and protein requirements are summarized in Table 19-7.

TABLE 19-7   Recommended Dietary Allowances for Kilocalories and Protein for Adolescents[3]

Age	Kcal/kg/day	Protein g/kg/day
Males		
11-14	55	1.00
15-18	45	0.90
19-24	40	0.80
Females		
11-14	47	1.00
15-18	40	0.80
19-24	38	0.80

Vitamin requirements of adolescents are best correlated not with age but with rate and stage of growth, the highest demand being at peak velocity of growth. Recommended allowances for minerals are usually estimated to meet the needs of the adolescent who is growing at the fastest rate. Levels less than that may be quite adequate for some adolescents.[29]

Meeting Nutritional Requirements.   Nutrients most often consumed in low or marginal amounts in the adolescent diet are iron, calcium, riboflavin, and vitamin A.[25] Adolescents' need for iron increases as the result of expanding blood volume and increased muscle mass. In addition to increased needs, females must replace iron lost through menstruation. Many weight-conscious adolescent females consume low kilocalorie diets, which makes it even more difficult to achieve iron requirements. Insufficient intakes of calcium and riboflavin have been associated with decreased dairy food and increased soft drink consumption. This trend affects calcium absorption by altering the calcium-to-phosphorus ratio of 1:1 at a time when increased calcium is needed for bone mineralization. Although low intakes or low plasma levels of vitamin A are often cited, evidence of a clinical deficiency is rare.[30,31]

Nutrient needs can best be met when the diet contains a wide variety of foods. The recommended allowances of all nutrients (with the possible exception of iron) can be met by following the Food Guide Pyramid, as indicated in Chapter 2.

Eating Habits.   Newly acquired independence and decision making result in adolescents spending more time outside the home, thus making independent food choices. Trying to understand the adolescent's ideas about food and food choices makes it more likely that the positive aspects of their practices can be emphasized and recommendations be accepted.

Adolescence is a period of alteration in life style and self-concept, as well as a time of physical growth and increased nutritional needs. The typical adolescent is involved in a busy school schedule, extracurricular activities, and perhaps part-time employment. Time schedules may lead to the omission of some meals, especially breakfast, or to increased frequency of eating (2 to 6 times per day). A greater number of meals are eaten away from home, especially fast foods and vending machine snacks.[32] Altered body image may cause intermittent stress and may therefore make adolescents more vulnerable to abnormal eating habits, such as overeating, weight reduction, and anorexia nervosa or bulimia nervosa. Greater independence from the family and the desire to be accepted by peers often lead to altered eating practices, such as vegetarianism, changing the diet in hopes of improving athletic performance, fad dieting, and indulging in alcohol. All of these factors put adolescents at risk for suboptimal nutrition.

Nutritional Implications of Substance Abuse by the Adolescent

Alcohol is the drug of choice among teens and is generally not viewed as illegal by most. In one survey, 46% of students reported drinking alcohol while only 5% were using cocaine and fewer than 2% reported using LSD, PCP, or heroin.[33] About 22% of boys and 30% of girls reported smoking tobacco at least monthly, with a slightly greater percentage of boys smoking marijuana than tobacco.[33]

Substance abuse in adolescents appears to be related more to poor dietary habits and symptomatic deterioration in general health than to specific effects on growth or nutritional status.

Elevated serum iron concentration in boys and girls and elevated transferrin saturation and hemoglobin concentration in boys are associated with frequency of alcohol use.[34] The nutrients most likely to be deficient because of adolescent alcohol abuse are pyridoxine, folic acid, vitamin A, and thiamine.

Adolescent alcohol and marijuana users as compared to nonusers showed significant differences in the presence of symptoms of nutritional deficiency such as muscle weakness, bleeding gums, and tiredness. Other significant differences were not seen among these groups except in plasma zinc concentration, which was low in marijuana abusers.[35] All adolescents reported consuming adequate nutrients, although alcohol and marijuana abusers reported eating more snack foods and less fruits, vegetables, and milk.

Although alcohol and marijuana users reported considerable intake of energy in the form of alcohol, they also reported eating sufficient food to provide adequate levels of all nutrients measured.

Generally, adolescents appear to protect themselves from nutritional deficiency by adequate consumption of key nutrients so that their overall physical health is compromised in a general way but not in a way specifically related to the effects of alcohol and marijuana, as has been described in adults. Behaviors that correlate significantly with the level of substance use in adolescents are risk-taking, poor school performance, use of diet pills, laxatives, diuretics or self-induced vomiting for weight control, and lack of seat belt use.[36] Knowledge of these correlations is useful in the clinical setting.

Nutritional intervention is an essential component of an alcohol-drug dependency treatment program. Nutritional assessment identifies eating habits and provides information needed for counseling and educating the adolescent about healthy food choices.

References

1. Winick M. The role of early nutrition in subsequent development and optimal future health. Bull N Y Acad Med 1989;65(10):1020–1025.
2. Kien CL. Energy metabolism and requirements in disease. In: Walker WA. Nutrition in pediatrics: basic science in clinical application. Boston: Little, Brown, 1985:87.
3. Food and Nutrition Board. Recommended daily allowances, 10th ed. National Research Council—National Academy of Sciences. Washington, DC: 1989.
4. Fomon SJ. Infant nutrition. Philadelphia: WB Saunders, 1974:152,182.
5. Krieger I. Pediatric disorders of feeding, nutrition and metabolism. New York: John Wiley and Sons, 1982:1,31.
6. Institute of Medicine. U.S. Subcommittee on Lactation. Nutrition during lactation. Washington, DC: National Academy of Sciences, National Academy Press, 1991.
7. Committee on Nutrition. Fluoride supplementation. Pediatrics 1986;78:758–760.
8. Fomon SJ, Filer LJ, Anderson TA, Ziegler EE. Recommendations for feeding normal infants. Pediatrics 1979;63:52–59.
9. Bachrach SB, Fisher J, Parks JS. An outbreak of vitamin D deficiency rickets in a susceptible population. Pediatrics 1979;63:871–877.
10. Edidin DV, Levitsky LL, Schey W, Dumbovic N, Campos A. Resurgence of nutritional rickets associated with breast feeding and special dietary practices. Pediatrics 1980;65: 232–235.
11. Greer FR, Scarey JE, Levin RS, Steechen JJ, Asch PS, Tsang RC. Bone mineral content and 25-hydroxyvitamin D concentration in breast-fed infants with and without supplemental vitamin D. J Pediatr 1981;98:696–701.
12. American Academy of Pediatrics Committee on Nutrition. Pediatric nutrition handbook, 3rd ed. Elk Grove Village, IL: AAP, 1993:37.
13. Hillman LS. Mineral and vitamin D adequacy in infants fed human milk or formula between 6 and 12 months of age. J Pediatr 1990;117:134–142.
14. American Dietetic Association. Position paper: promotion and support of breast feeding. JADA 1993; 93:467–469.
15. Pipes PT. Nutrition in infancy and children, 3rd ed. St. Louis: Mosby, 1985:57,175,229.
16. Kovar MG, Serdula MK, Marks JS, Fraser DW. Review of the epidemiologic evidence for an association between infant feeding and infant health. Pediatrics 1984;74(suppl): 615–638.
17. American Academy of Pediatrics Committee on Drugs. Transfer of drugs and other chemicals into human milk. Pediatrics 1989;84(5):924–936.
18. Ziegler E. Milks and formulas for older infants. J Pediatr 1990;117:76–79.
19. Pipes PL. Nutrition in infancy and childhood, 4th ed. St. Louis: Mosby , 1989.
20. Ernst JA, Brady MS, Rickard KA. Food and nutrient intake of 6 to 12 month old infants fed formula or cows' milk: a summary of four national surveys. J Pediatr 1990;117:86–100.
21. Fomon SJ, Filer LJ, Ziegler E, Bergmann K, Bergmann RL. Skim milk in infant feeding. Acta Paediatr Scand 1977;66:17–30.
22. American Academy of Pediatrics Committee on Nutrition. The use of whole cows' milk in infancy. Pediatrics 1992;89:1105–1109.
23. Robinson CH. Nutrition during infancy. In: Robinson CH, Lawler MR, Chenoweth WL, Garwick AE. Normal and therapeutic nutrition, 17th ed. New York: MacMillan, 1986:280.
24. Ad Hoc Committee to Review the Ten-State Nutrition Survey. Nutrition, growth, development and maturation: findings from the ten-state nutrition survey of 1968–1970. Pediatrics 1973;51:1095–1099.
25. Abraham S, Carroll MD, Dresser CM, Johnson CL. Dietary intake findings, United States 1971–1974. DHEW Publication. No. (HRA) 77–1647. Washington, DC: U.S. Government Printing Office, 1977.

26. Fahey PJ, Boltri JM, Monk JS. Key issues in nutrition during childhood and adolescence. Postgrad Med 1987;82(4):301–305.

27. Stanek K, Abbott D, Cramer S. Diet quality and the eating environment of preschool children. JADA 1990;90(11):1582–1584.

28. Heald FP. New reference points for defining adolescent requirements. In: McKigney JI, Munro HN, eds. Nutrient requirements in adolescence. Cambridge, MA: MIT Press, 1978:295.

29. Milner JA. Trace minerals in the nutrition of children. J Pediatr 1990;117(2 Pt 2):147–155.

30. Heald FP. The adolescent. In: Jelliffe DD, Jelliffe EFP, eds. Nutrition and growth. New York: Plenum Press, 1979:239.

31. Greenwood CT, Richardson DP. Nutrition during adolescence. World Rev Nutr Diet 1979;33:1–41.

32. American School Health Association. The national adolescent student health survey: a report on the health of America's youth. Bethesda MD: U.S. Department of Health and Human Services, Public Health Service, Office of Disease Prevention and Health Promotion, Centers for Disease Control, National Institute on Drug Abuse, 1989.

33. Robinson TN, Killen JD, Taylor CB, Telch MJ, Bryson SW, Saylor KE, Maron DJ, Maccoby N, Farquhar JW. Perspectives on adolescent substance use: a defined population study. JAMA 1987;258(15):2072–2076.

34. Friedman IM, Kraemer HC, Mendoza FS, Hammer LD. Elevated serum iron concentration in adolescent alcohol users. Am J Dis Child 1988;142:156–159.

35. Farrow JA, Rees JM, Worthington-Roberts BS. Health developmental and nutritional status of adolescent alcohol and marijuana abusers. Pediatrics 1987;79(2):218–223.

36. Joffe A, Radius S, Gall M. Health counseling for adolescents: what they want, what they get, and who gives it. Pediatrics 1988;82(3 Pt 2):481–485.

YOUNG ATHLETES

Nutrition is very important for both competitive and recreational adolescent athletes. Estimation of the adolescent athlete's nutritional needs must consider not only the increased kilocalorie and nutrient requirements for exercise but also the requirements to support normal growth. The nutritional assessment of the adolescent athlete involves evaluation of fluid, energy, protein, and vitamin and mineral needs.

Fluid and Electrolyte Replacement

Adequate fluid and electrolyte intake is one of the most important nutritional considerations for the young athlete. There are a number of physiological differences between the adolescent and the adult. The adolescent is less able to control body temperature, particularly when environmental temperatures exceed body temperature, and has a larger body surface area in relation to weight, lower sweating capacity, lower cardiac output, higher heat production and a slower rate of acclimation to warm temperatures.[37]

Hydration during sporting events and strenuous training should be monitored. Since thirst is not a reliable indication of hydration, cool liquids should be administered before, during, and after prolonged exercise. A weight loss of 1 lb indicates a need for intake of 16 oz of water. Table 19-8 presents fluid replacement guidelines for the adolescent athlete. Individual fluid requirements vary depending upon environmental conditions and the intensity of physical activity. Excessive

TABLE 19-8 Fluid Replacement Guidelines for Adolescents

Timing	Amount	Type of Beverage
BEFORE ACTIVITY		
1–2 hr	18–24 oz	Cool water
DURING ACTIVITY		
Every 15–20 min	9–12 oz	Cool water
AFTER ACTIVITY		
Begin immediately	Replace each pound of body weight lost by sipping 16 oz of fluid, or enough to quench thirst plus 6–8 oz	Cool water

water intake during prolonged exercise may result in hyponatremia. (For fluid requirements for postpubescent athletes, refer to Chapter 4, Nutritional Needs for Physical Performance.)

Controversy exists regarding the ideal fluid replacement for consumption by athletes. Electrolyte- or carbohydrate-containing beverages offer no advantage over water in maintaining plasma volume, plasma electrolyte concentration, or in improving intestinal absorption under most circumstances.[38] Consumption of carbohydrate-containing beverages during prolonged exercise (over 60 to 90 minutes) may enhance performance, but for the majority of young athletes water remains the ideal fluid replacement.[38] (For fluid needs of young athletes involved in prolonged exercise, see Chapter 4, Nutritional Needs for Physical Performance.)

Energy

Determination of caloric requirements for young athletes involves consideration of a number of variables, including age, sex, type of activity, and degree and duration of exertion. To date, there are no generally accepted guidelines for calculating energy costs of activities for this age group. The average daily requirement during adolescence is 40 to 50 kcal/kg/day.[39] Depending on the level of activity, the growing athlete may require an additional 500 to 1,000 kcal/day. Athletes in endurance sports such as marathoning, cycling, or cross-country skiing may have caloric requirements in excess of 5,000 kcal/day.[40]

In general, physical activity increases caloric expenditure and automatically increases the appetite, with the result that more food is ingested. In most instances, sufficient kilocalories are consumed to maintain appropriate body weight and support growth. However, approximately one-third of female athletes struggle with eating disorders, obsessions about food, or distorted eating patterns.[41] Although it is unlikely that a teenager engaged in heavy physical training will gain too much weight, caloric intake greater than the daily expenditure is not recommended, because it results in unnecessary fat deposition. The increased caloric requirements are best met by increasing food servings from each of the major food groups (see Chapter 2, Food Guide Pyramid) without significantly altering the proportions of the micro- or macronutrients of the diet.[42] The distribution of total kilocalories should be approximately 55 to 60% carbohydrate, 30 to 40% fat, and 15 to 20% protein.[37,43]

Protein

For many years it has been generally believed that physical activity does not significantly increase the need for dietary protein. The RDA for protein for teens are 45 to 59 g/day for males and 44 to 46 g/day for females.[39] Because the diet consumed by this population usually exceeds the RDA, supplementation of the diet with extra protein is usually not necessary.[37]

Results of research on the importance of protein relative to the energy needs for building muscle have been inconsistent.[43,44] Studies suggest that the protein requirement for the adolescent active in weight training is greater than the RDA.[43] Because most adolescents consume more than the RDA for protein, these increased requirements can be readily obtained through ingestion of ordinary food without the use of special protein supplements.[42]

Vitamins and Minerals

Vitamin supplements are generally not recommended for the young athlete for several reasons. First, excess water-soluble vitamins cannot be stored in the body effectively and thus are rapidly excreted in the urine when tissue saturation occurs. Second, fat-soluble vitamins are retained and stored in the body, and daily high potency supplements of vitamins A and D are known to be toxic and sometimes fatal. Third, a nutritionally balanced diet that contains approximately 1,800 kcal/day usually provides satisfactory levels of all vitamins.

The most significant effect of exercise on mineral nutrition is loss of the electrolytes, sodium, and potassium through sweat.

Sodium requirements for the young athlete have not been determined. Deficits can be replaced on a regular basis by salting foods to a satisfying taste. Salt tablets are rarely needed and, if ingested, may cause gastrointestinal disturbances from fluid movement into the gut.

The amount of potassium lost through sweat is negligible when the environmental temperature is mild and the exercise level is moderate. However, potassium losses may occur under conditions of moderate to extreme heat with profuse sweating. Usually, normal food intake is sufficient to replace losses.

Iron is a mineral of major importance for maintenance of optimal athletic condition. Iron is an essential component of hemoglobin, which is necessary for oxygen transport; therefore, the adequacy of iron status significantly affects endurance and physical performance. Inadequate intake is the major cause of iron deficiency in athletes. In some athletes, hematuria, gastrointestinal blood loss, iron loss in sweat, or intravascular hemolysis caused by mechanical trauma may contribute to iron deficiency anemia.[45] It should be recognized that highly trained athletes may have relatively low levels of hemoglobin without iron deficiency.

The iron deficient teen should be identified and provided with iron supplements and dietary counseling regarding food sources of iron. There are no documented daily recommended iron requirements for the growing teen. However, the RDA of 10 mg for preadolescents (7 to 10 years of age) and 12 mg for male adolescents and 15 mg for female adolescents (11 to 14 years of age) appear to be reasonable goals. One recommendation suggests that the athlete with iron deficiency should be treated with 50 to 100 mg of elemental iron 3 times daily until testing indicates iron sufficiency. Therapy should continue for an additional 6 months to ensure that body iron stores are replenished.[46]

Studies have indicated that athletes who are in sports that require low body weight or body fat often consume fewer vitamin-rich foods than are recommended.[42] Calcium, zinc, and B vitamins are frequently inadequate in the typical adolescent diet.[42] Individual counseling should consider the adolescent's requirements and need for supplementation after thoroughly assessing the diet history.[47] A multiple vitamin and/or mineral supplement that provides 100% of the RDA for age may be appropriate to ensure adequate intake.[42]

Pregame and Postgame Meal

The consumption of a special pregame meal is controversial. Since individuals differ with regard to food preferences, psychological needs, and digestive responses to stress, a variety of foods and eating schedules may be thought of as "supportive." A pregame meal should be eaten about 2 to 3 hours prior to the start of an athletic event and should include complex carbohydrate.[47] The consumption of foods with a high sugar content approximately 20 to 40 minutes before the start of the event can result in an increased osmotic effect and may cause retention of fluids in the gastrointestinal tract. The athlete may experience nausea, stomach cramps, and, during endurance events, dehydration.[42]

After competition, fluids and carbohydrate-rich foods should be offered. Parents and coaches should be advised that special treats or meals should not be given to reward the athlete who does well or withheld to punish one who does not do well. Doing so may potentiate an unnecessary value on food and eating.[37]

Achieving Competing Weight

Weight loss for athletes who participate in such sports as wrestling and gymnastics may be wrongfully encouraged to achieve competitive weight. Studies have shown that cutting weight can have adverse effects on body composition, nutrient intake, renal function, electrolyte balance, thermal regulation, testosterone level, and strength.[48]

A young athlete who wants to reduce body fat to a level desired for competition needs a well-planned program of exercise and a prescribed diet that is sufficient to support the needs of training while protecting muscle tissue from being used as a source of energy. The amount of fat to be lost is estimated by assessing the existing level of body fat and projecting the optimal level of fat desired for the specific sport. The optimal level for the elite young male athlete is estimated at between 8 to 10% and for the elite female athlete, between 14 to 16%. Laboratory techniques such as underwater weighing may produce the smallest errors in body fat estimates. In most cases the only available anthropometric measurements are skinfold measurements and body weight. These can be used to make reasonably accurate estimates providing the minimal weight standard is not changed after the season has begun.[49] For the average teen athlete, a desired rate of fat reduction to achieve an appropriate level of fat is a maximum of 2 lb/week.[43] This fat reduction can be accomplished by creating a negative energy balance of approximately 1,000 kcal/day.[48] Energy expenditure is increased in training activities, so the desired negative energy balance can occur while the average male athlete has a food intake of no less than 2,000 kcal/day and the average female athlete's food intake is no less than 1,800 kcal/day.[48] This restricted caloric intake is maintained for the few weeks that are required to reduce weight or fat to the desired level. Once the desired level has been achieved, caloric intake is increased to maintain a desired competing weight and to satisfy the energy needs of athletic training and normal growth. Weight and level of fat should be monitored and should remain stable during the competing season.

Athletes attempting to gain weight should increase weight as muscle mass, not fat. Muscle mass is increased only through muscle strength training supported by an appropriate increase in food intake. The addition of 750 to 900 kcal to a diet that is known to maintain the athlete's stable weight will support the energy demands for a gain of approximately 1 to 1½ lb of muscle weight. It is recommended that the high kilocalorie diet required to support muscle growth from increased work be low in saturated fats and cholesterol.[48] No food or vitamin increases muscle mass. Some steroid drugs and hormones do increase muscle mass, but their use should be strongly discouraged for a number of well-publicized reasons.[37]

In summary, as physical training increases, the young athlete needs more energy. Therefore, food intake must be adjusted and consideration given to the appropriate balance of fats (30 to 40%), carbohydrates (55 to 60%), and proteins (15 to 20%). Supplements of vitamins and minerals are not needed, since the athlete usually meets these needs by increasing kilocalories and by eating a variety of foods. Hydration during sports events and strenuous training should be monitored. A weight loss of 1 lb indicates a need for intake of 16 oz of water. Weight loss and weight gain for the young athlete should be supervised by a qualified health professional.

References

37. Steen SN. Nutritional assessment and management of the school-aged child athlete. In: Benning JR, Steen SN, eds. Sports nutrition for the 90s: the health professional's handbook. Rockville, MD: Aspen Publishers, 1991.

38. Squire DL. Heat illness: fluid and electrolyte issues for pediatric and adolescent athletes. Pediatr Clin North Am 1990:37(5):1085–1097.

39. Recommended Dietary Allowances, 10th ed. Committee on Dietary Allowances, Food and Nutrition Board, National Research Council, Washington, DC:1989.

40. Harvey JS. Nutritional management of the adolescent athlete. Clin Sports Med 1984; 3(3):671–679.

41. Clark N. How to approach eating disorders among athletes. Top Clin Nutr 1990;5(3):41–47.

42. Worthington-Roberts R. Nutritional considerations for children in sports. In: Pipes P, ed. Nutrition in infancy and childhood. St. Louis; Mosby, 1989:223–267.

43. Loosli GR, Benson J. Nutritional intake in adolescent athletes. Pediatr Clin North Am 1990;37(5):1143–1152.

44. National Dairy Council. Food power: a coach's guide to improving performance. National Dairy Council, Rosemont, IL, 1991.

45. Risser W. Iron deficiency in adolescents and young adults. Phys Sports Med 1990; 18(2):87–101.

46. Nickerson HJ, Holubets MC. Causes of iron deficiency in adolescent athletes. J Pediatr 1989;114(pt 1):657–663.

47. McKeag DB. Adolescents and exercise. J Adolesc Health Care 1986;7:1215–1295.

48. Smith NJ. Weight control in the athlete. Clin Sports Med 1984;3(3):693–704.

49. Thorland WG, Johnson GO, Cesar CJ, Housh, TJ. Estimation of minimal wrestling weight using measures of body build and body composition. Int J Sports Med 1987;8: 365–370.

VEGETARIAN DIET

General Description

The reasons for adopting a vegetarian diet are many and include religion, ethics, and economics. Increased interest in a healthy life-style that lowers serum lipid levels and prevents obesity may also result in adoption of a vegetarian diet.[50]

Vegetarianism is a term that embraces a variety of dietary practices. The diet is classified according to the extent by which animal foods are excluded (see Chapter 4, Vegetarian Diet, Table 4-12).

Infants, children, and adolescents who follow the more restrictive vegetarian dietary practices are at high risk for the development of nutritional deficiencies because of their rapid growth rates and the need for kilocalories and nutrients to support growth.[50]

Nutritional Adequacy

The American Dietetic Association recognizes that well-planned vegetarian diets are consistent with good nutrition status.[51] The extent to which food selection and feeding patterns meet the dietary recommendations for infants, children, and adolescents is dependent on the type of vegetarian diet chosen and on the degree of careful meal planning by the caregivers.

The primary indicator of nutritional adequacy is normal growth and development. Evidence shows that diets of children containing animal protein will likely grow normally (i.e., lacto- or lacto-ovovegetarians).[52,53] Although it is possible for a more restrictive vegan diet to support normal growth, children who adhere to this dietary practice are at increased nutritional risk. They tend to be shorter in stature and lighter in weight than the normal pediatric population.[54,55] Some catch-up growth may occur during the preschool years if a less restrictive diet is provided.[50]

Energy. Adequate caloric intake for vegetarian infants and children is seldom a problem when some animal protein is used. However, if the diet is high in fiber and complex carbohydrate, the result may be a diet so low in caloric density that the infant or child may have difficulty consuming adequate kilocalories. The limited capacity of the stomach cannot tolerate a sufficient volume of these low energy foods to meet caloric needs.

Protein. The quantity and quality of protein consumed in a vegetarian diet is important, since protein requirements are higher per kilogram of body weight throughout periods of growth. When caloric needs are met with a good variety of foods, the quantity of protein should be adequate.

The quality of protein, or the amino acid composition of a food, is rarely a concern when some animal foods are consumed at each meal. In a vegetarian regimen, it is necessary to combine vegetable proteins that complement each other at each meal since all vegetable proteins contain relatively limited quantities of one or more essential amino acids. See Chapter 4, Vegetarian Diet, Table 4-13 for a scheme for combining complementary proteins.

Vegan children often fail to grow as well as children following less restrictive vegetarian regimens despite protein intakes that exceed the RDA.[56] The bioavailability of amino acids may be decreased by a high fiber intake, by processing and storage of foods or inadequate intake. Lysine, methionine, and threonine intakes may be particularly inadequate as the bioavailability of these amino acids may be less than the digestibility of the protein in the product. Vegan children may require considerably more protein than the RDA standard for normal growth.[56]

Vitamins and minerals. The most successful way to meet vitamin and mineral needs is through dietary diversity. The possibility of deficiency states is a concern primarily when all foods of animal origin are excluded. The most common deficiencies include the vitamins B_{12}, D, and riboflavin and the minerals calcium, iron, and zinc.[50] Mineral deficiency can occur for two reasons: inadequate intake and low bioavailability. Table 19-9 presents vegetarian sources of these critical nutrients.

Low vitamin B_{12} intakes during pregnancy and lactation by vegan mothers may produce a B_{12} deficiency in the infant. Both fetal stores and breast milk supply limited amounts of B_{12} and must be supplemented by additional B_{12}. A B_{12} supplement, or the consumption of B_{12}-fortified foods, is considered essential for all veg-

TABLE 19-9   Vegetarian Sources of Critical Nutrients[60]

Nutrient	Source
Calcium	Dairy products, dark leafy greens, fortified soy milk, legumes, peanuts, almonds, and seeds.
Iron	Legumes, dark leafy greens torula yeast, dried fruits, whole and enriched grains, blackstrap molasses, consuming food that contains vitamin C (citrus fruits, peppers, tomatoes) with any iron-rich food.
Zinc	Eggs, cheese, milk, legumes, nuts, wheat germ, and whole grains.
Riboflavin	Dairy products, eggs, whole and enriched grains (if eaten daily), brewer's yeast, dark leafy greens, legumes.
Vitamin B_{12}	Dairy products, eggs, nutritional yeast, foods fortified with B_{12}, fermented soy products, supplements.
	Fortified milk, fortified soy milk, exposure of skin to sunshine.

With permission from: Lifshitz F, Finch NM, Lifshitz JZ, eds. Children's Nutrition. 1991. Boston: Jones and Bartlett Publishers;246.

ans (Table 19-9). Sea plants, such as seaweeds and algae, may contain some B_{12}, but this source is too variable to be considered a reliable source of B_{12}.[57]

Potentially vitamin B_6 deficiency may develop because its bioavailability may be severely compromised by the presence of pyridoxine glycoside, found only in plants.[50]

Newborn infants of vegan mothers are predisposed to vitamin D deficiency. A vitamin D supplement or the consumption of fortified foods is imperative (see Table 19-9) for pregnant women, infants, and children who consume no foods of animal origin. Reliance on sunshine alone, particularly in northern climates or in cultures where most of the body is covered by clothing may not provide all of the vitamin D needed to protect children against rickets.[51]

There have been no reported cases of riboflavin deficiencies in vegans. However, when milk products are not used, other food sources of riboflavin must be consumed (see Table 19-9).

A diet low in calcium and high in fiber also can contribute to long-term depletion in calcium stores.[58] Since calcium is necessary for normal growth, an inadequate calcium intake compounded with insufficient vitamin D jeopardizes growth potential. Therefore, the vegan diet must include plant foods with high calcium content (see Table 19-9). Calcium bioavailability appears to be inhibited by oxalic acid, dietary fiber, and phytates, but this effect may not be significant.[50]

Iron from foods is absorbed as either heme (animal sources) or nonheme (plant sources) iron. Heme iron is absorbed much better than nonheme iron. Nonheme iron absorption is significantly improved when some heme iron or a source of ascorbic acid is consumed at the same meal.[51] Phytic acid, oxalic acid, large amounts of plant fiber, phosvitin in egg yolks, and tannic acid in tea decrease absorption.[51] It is important to emphasize the consumption of at least one food high in iron and one high in ascorbic acid for each meal (see Table 19-9). Infants who are exclusively breast fed after 4 to 6 months require an iron supplement.[51]

The bioavailability of zinc from vegan food sources is questionable.[50] Few researchers have assessed zinc intake or status of vegetarian children. Phytate and fiber present in some cereals may reduce zinc availability and the bioavailability of zinc from legumes is not known.[58] Refer to Table 19-9 for food sources.

As the prime sources of dietary carnitine are found in dairy products and meats, vegan children consume a low carnitine diet. They have lower plasma carnitine concentrations than those consuming a mixed diet, but little is known about the risks this poses.[59]

Goals of Dietary Management

The nutritional goal in vegetarian diets for infants, children, and adolescents is to achieve an intake that meets all known nutrient needs and that supports normal growth and development.

The use of food groups may be beneficial when devising meal patterns to assure proper meal planning. Table 19-10 presents a basic food guide for infants and children on lacto-ovo diets.[60]

In addition, the following dietary practices and meal plan (Table 9-11) should be encouraged for vegan infants and children:

TABLE 19-10   Basic Food Guide for Infants and Children on Lacto-Ovo Diets[60]

	Serving Size					
	Infant		Toddler	Preschooler	Pre-adolescent	Adolescent
Food Items	0–$^1/_2$ yr	$^1/_2$–1 yr	1–3 yr	4–6 yr	7–10 yr	11–18 yr
MILK AND MILK PRODUCTS (4 servings per day)						
Infant formula	$^3/_4$–1 C	$^3/_4$–1 C	—	—	—	—
or						
Milk	—	—	$^1/_2$–$^3/_4$ C	$^3/_4$ C	1 C	1 C
or						
Cheese	—	—	$^3/_4$–1 oz	1 oz	1$^1/_2$ oz	1$^1/_2$ oz
or						
Yogurt	—	$^3/_4$–1 C	$^1/_2$–$^3/_4$ C	$^3/_4$ C	1 C	1 C
EGGS (1 serving per day)						
Egg	—	$^1/_2$	1	1	1	1$^1/_2$
PLANT PROTEIN (2 or more servings per day)						
Legumes	—	1–6 T	0–$^1/_4$ C	$^1/_2$ C	$^1/_2$ C	$^1/_2$–$^3/_4$ C
or						
Meat analogues	—	—	$^1/_4$–$^1/_2$ oz	$^3/_4$–1 oz	$^3/_4$–1 oz	1–1$^1/_4$ oz
or						
Textured vegetable protein (TVP)	—	—	0–$^1/_8$ oz	$^1/_2$ oz	$^1/_2$ oz	$^1/_2$–$^3/_4$ oz
NUTS AND SEEDS (2 or more servings per day)						
Nuts and seeds	—	—	—	$^1/_4$–$^1/_2$ oz	$^1/_2$ oz	$^1/_2$–$^3/_4$ oz
or						
Nut butters	—	—	$^1/_4$ T	$^3/_4$ T	1–1$^1/_4$ T	1–1$^1/_2$ T
CEREALS, BREADS AND WHOLE GRAINS (4 or more servings per day)						
Whole grain bread	—	—	$^1/_4$–$^1/_2$ slice	$^3/_4$–1 slice	1–1$^1/_2$ slices	1$^1/_2$–2 slices
or						
Cooked cereal	0–1 T	$^3/_4$ C	$^1/_4$ C	$^1/_4$–$^1/_2$ C	$^1/_2$–$^3/_4$ C	$^3/_4$–1 C
or						
Dry cereal	—	$^3/_4$–$^3/_4$ C	$^1/_2$ C	$^3/_4$ C	$^3/_4$–1 C	1–1$^1/_2$ C
FRUIT AND VEGETABLES (4 or more servings per day)						
Juice	0–1 oz	$^3/_8$–$^3/_4$ C	$^1/_4$–$^1/_2$ C	$^1/_2$ C	$^1/_2$–1 C	$^1/_2$–1 C
or						
Raw	—	—	$^1/_2$ C	$^1/_2$–1 C	1–1$^1/_2$ C	1–1$^1/_2$ C
or						
Cooked	1–1$^1/_2$ T	1–2 T	$^1/_4$–$^1/_2$ C	$^1/_2$ C	$^1/_2$–$^3/_4$ C	$^1/_2$–$^3/_4$ C

FATS, OILS AND SWEETS

The amount of these foods that should be included in the diet depends on the individual's caloric needs.

With permission from: Lifshitz F, Finch NM, Lifshitz JZ, eds. Children's nutrition. Boston: Jones and Bartlett Publishers, 1991:244.

TABLE 19-11   Basic Food Guide for Infants and Children on Vegan Diets[60]

Food Items	Infant 0–$\frac{1}{2}$yr	Infant $\frac{1}{2}$–1 yr	Toddler 1–3 yr	Preschooler 4–6 yr	Pre-adolescent 7–10 yr	Adolescent 11–18 yr
FORTIFIED SOY MILK (4 servings per day)						
Isomil	$\frac{1}{2}$–$\frac{3}{4}$ C	$\frac{3}{4}$–1 C	$\frac{3}{4}$	$\frac{3}{4}$ C	1 C	1 C
or						
Prosobee	—	—	—	—	—	—
or						
Soyalac	—	—	—	—	—	—
or						
Nursoy	—	—	—	—	—	—
PLANT PROTEIN (2 or more servings per day)						
Legumes	—	1–6 T	$\frac{1}{4}$–$\frac{1}{2}$ C	$\frac{1}{2}$–$\frac{3}{4}$ C	$\frac{3}{4}$–1 C	$\frac{1}{2}$–$\frac{3}{4}$ C
or						
Meat analogues	—	—	$\frac{1}{2}$–$\frac{3}{4}$ oz	$\frac{3}{4}$–1 oz	1 oz	$\frac{3}{4}$–1 oz
or						
Textured vegetable protein (TVP)	—	—	$\frac{1}{8}$–$\frac{1}{4}$ oz	$\frac{1}{2}$ oz	$\frac{3}{4}$ oz	$\frac{1}{2}$–$\frac{3}{4}$ oz
NUTS AND SEEDS (2 or more servings per day)						
Nuts and seeds	—	—	—	$\frac{1}{4}$–$\frac{1}{2}$ oz	$\frac{1}{2}$ oz	$\frac{1}{2}$–$\frac{3}{4}$ oz
or						
Nut butters	—	—	$\frac{1}{4}$ T	$\frac{3}{4}$ T	1–1$\frac{1}{4}$ T	1–1$\frac{1}{2}$ T
CEREALS, BREADS AND WHOLE GRAINS (4 or more servings per day)						
Whole grain bread	—	$\frac{1}{4}$–$\frac{1}{2}$	$\frac{1}{2}$–1 slice	$\frac{3}{4}$–1 slice	1–1$\frac{1}{2}$ slices	1$\frac{1}{2}$–2 slices
or						
Cooked cereal	0–1 T	—$\frac{1}{4}$ C	$\frac{1}{4}$–$\frac{1}{2}$ C	$\frac{1}{2}$ C	$\frac{1}{2}$–1 C	$\frac{3}{4}$–1 C
or						
Dry cereal	—	—	$\frac{1}{2}$–$\frac{3}{4}$ C	$\frac{3}{4}$ C	$\frac{3}{4}$–1 C	$\frac{3}{4}$–1 C
FRUIT AND VEGETABLES (4 or more servings per day)						
Juice	0–1 oz	$\frac{1}{4}$ C	$\frac{1}{4}$–$\frac{1}{2}$ C	$\frac{1}{2}$ C	$\frac{1}{2}$–1 C	$\frac{1}{2}$–1 C
or						
Raw	—	—	$\frac{1}{2}$ C	$\frac{1}{2}$–1 C	1–1$\frac{1}{2}$ C	1–1$\frac{1}{2}$ C
or						
Cooked	1–1$\frac{1}{2}$ T	2 T	$\frac{1}{4}$–$\frac{1}{2}$ C	$\frac{1}{2}$ C	$\frac{1}{2}$–$\frac{3}{4}$ C	$\frac{1}{2}$–$\frac{3}{4}$ C
BREWER'S YEAST (1 serving per day)						
	—	—	1 T	1 T	1 T	1 T
MOLASSES (1 serving per day)						
	—	—	1 T	1–2 T	1–2 T	1–2 T

FATS, OILS AND SWEETS

The amount of these foods that should be included in the diet depends on the individual's caloric requirements.

With permission from: Lifshitz F, Finch NM, Lifshitz JZ, eds. Children's nutrition. Boston: Jones and Bartlett Publishers, 1991:244.

1. Breast feed infants for at least 6 months and preferably longer (one must pay careful attention to the mother's diet).
2. Toddlers should use fortified soy formulas or milk whenever possible.
3. Supplemental vitamins and minerals may be necessary in the older child or adolescent when soy milk is not used.
4. Vitamin B_{12} must be supplemented.
5. Certain foods may be considered unsafe for infants and toddlers: honey; home canned fruits and vegetables, owing to the potential for food-borne illness; vegetable juices, such as carrot or spinach, which have high nitrate content; whole nuts (nut butters may be used); and granolas, because of the potential for choking.
6. Reduce fiber intake to increase calcium absorption by partly replacing whole grain cereals with lower fiber grains.[61]

Physicians: How to order diet

The diet order should indicate *vegetarian diet*. The dietitian determines food preferences and establishes a nutritionally adequate diet.

REFERENCES

50. Jacobs C, Dwyer JT. Vegetarian children: appropriate and inappropriate diets. Am J Clin Nutr 1988;48:811–818.
51. Position of the American Dietetic Association: vegetarian diets. J Am Diet Assoc 1993; 93:1317–1319.
52. Tayter M, Stanek KL. Anthropometric and dietary assessment of omnivore and lacto-ovo-vegetarian children. J Am Diet Assoc 1989;89:1161–1163.
53. Sabat J, Lindsted KD, Harris RD, Johnston PK. Anthropometric parameters of school-children with different life-styles. AJDC 1990;144:1159–1163.
54. Sanders TAB. Growth and development of British vegan children. Am J Clin Nutr 1988; 48:822–825.
55. van Staveren WA, Dagnelie PC. Food consumption, growth and development of Dutch children fed on alternative diets. Am J Clin Nutr 1988;48:819–821.
56. Acosta PB. Availability of essential amino acids and nitrogen in vegan diets. Am J Clin Nutr 1988;48:868–874.
57. Dagnelie PC, van Staveren WA, Vergote FJVRA, Dingjan PG, van den Berg H, Hautvast JGAJ. Increased risk of vitamin B12 and iron deficiency in infants on macrobiotic diets. Am J Clin Nutr 1989;50:818–824.
58. Dagnelie PC, Vergote FJVRA, van Staveren WA, van den Berg H, Dingjan PG, Hautvast JGAS. High prevalence of rickets in infants on macrobiotic diets. Am J Clin Nutr 1990; 51:202–208.
59. Lombard KA, Olson AL, Nelson SE, Rebouche CJ. Carnitive status of lactoovovegetarians and strict vegetarian adults and children. Am J Clin Nutr 1989;50:301–306.
60. Anon. Alternative eating styles. In: Lifshitz F, Finch NM, Lifshitz JZ, eds. Children's nutrition. Boston: Jones and Bartlett Publishers, 1991:232–246.
61. Fanelli MT, Kuczmarski RJ. Food selection for vegetarians. Dietetic Currents 1983; 10:1–4.

20 / *Other Nutritional Considerations*

DEVELOPMENTAL DISABILITY

Children with developmental disabilities require the same nutrients as normal, healthy children; however, the amounts needed may vary. These children are at risk for altered growth, poor weight gain or obesity, anemia, food intolerances, adverse nutrient and drug interactions, constipation, and poor dental health. In addition, they have many feeding problems, both physical and psychosocial in origin, that may affect nutritional intake and status.[1] The goals of nutritional care are to assure adequate nutritional intake to promote maximum growth potential and feeding skills. Developmental disability includes a wide variety of conditions, each of which has a different impact on nutritional needs, feeding skills, and problems. The dietitian should have knowledge of normal development and behaviors and of how each condition or its treatment affects nutritional status.

Nutritional Assessment

Lack of standards, particularly for growth, make nutritional assessment of the developmentally delayed child difficult.[2] It is important, therefore, that nutritional status be evaluated at about 6 month intervals, after infancy, so that full growth potential and nutritional health are optimized. Nutritional assessment should include feeding assessment, in addition to the more traditional parameters discussed in Chapter 18, Pediatric Nutritional Assessment.

Anthropometrics. Growth is difficult to evaluate. There are few standards for developmentally delayed children, and obtaining accurate measurements is often difficult due to the spasticity or lack of cooperation of the child. Measurement of recumbent length, sitting height, arm span, or tibia length, rather than standing height, may be used for estimation of total length. Crown-rump length can be used for infants. Appropriate adjustment should be made before the measurement is plotted on a height graph. In some conditions,

---

TABLE 20-1   Syndromes Associated with Growth Retardation

Cerebral palsy
de Lange's syndrome
Down's syndrome
Hurler's syndrome
Prader-Willi's syndrome
Silver's syndrome
Trisomy 13 and 18
Turner's syndrome
William's syndrome

---

growth retardation and abnormal body composition are attributable to genetic or biological defect.[1] Syndromes in which growth retardation is frequently seen are presented in Table 20-1.

Height-age (see Chapter 18, Pediatric Nutritional Assessment) can be used to estimate a child's ideal weight range and caloric need. However, it is important to assure that malnutrition is not contributing to the growth deficit. Weight for height ratio is also helpful in the evaluation of weight control for those children below normal height for age.[3] The Baldwin-Wood Tables (Pediatric Appendix 29) are useful for evaluating weight for height in the older child. The Turner growth chart can be useful for evaluating girls with Turner's syndrome aged 2 to 19 years.[4] Cronk's growth graphs can be used for children with Down's syndrome aged 1 month to 18 years (Pediatric Appendix 30). The graphs reflect the relatively slower growth of these children, which begins at about 6 months of age, and can aid in early detection of failure-to-thrive or tendency to be overweight among Down's syndrome children.[5]

Dietary Assessment.   Dietary assessment should include an evaluation of caloric and nutrient intake for growth stage, consistency and texture of the diet for the child's feeding skill level, and medications being used. For children on anticonvulsant medication, attention should be given to adequacy of folic acid, calcium, phosphorus, ascorbic acid, vitamins B_6, B_{12}, and D, zinc, and magnesium.[6] Diets of children with reduced caloric requirements should be assessed carefully for nutrient adequacy because these diets need to be more nutrient dense than normal. Children with severe mental retardation who cannot feed themselves are at risk for inadequate caloric and nutrient intake. Care should be taken to estimate the amount and type of food actually consumed, as opposed to the amount offered, since a significant portion of the food may be refused or spilled.[6] Children who receive the majority of their kilocalories from milk or milk-based supplements may be at risk for iron deficiency anemia. Dietary adequacy may also be affected by bizarre eating habits such as pica, poor appetite and early satiety, food allergies, and rumination. Rumination is the chronic regurgitation of ingested food, which may or may not be reswallowed, and frequently results in chronic undernutrition.[7]

TABLE 20-2 Factors Influencing Development of Feeding Skills

Sitting balance
Head and neck control
Jaw, lip, and tongue control
Sucking, swallowing, chewing, and drinking abilities
Persistence of primitive reflexes
Arm, eye, and hand control
Grasp

Food is often used for behavior modification. The impact of the amount, frequency, and type of food on nutritional and dental status should be evaluated.[7] Care providers should be encouraged to use things other than food for behavior modification.

Feeding Assessment. Feeding assessment involves the evaluation of feeding skills and behaviors that may influence nutritional status.[2] Occupational, physical, and speech therapists can aid in assessing feeding skills, problems, and capabilities.[2]

The development of feeding skills in developmentally delayed children usually proceeds in the same sequence as that of normal children. However, the chronological age at which the developmental stages occur is unpredictable.[1] Self-feeding impairment, oral-motor dysfunction, and psychosocial factors can interfere with the development of feeding skills.[8] Some developmentally delayed children are hypersensitive in the oral area and may require a desensitization program before more textured food or spoon feeding can be introduced. Factors influencing the development of feeding skills are presented in Table 20-2.

The degree of motor dysfunction that involves the mouth area and the degree of the developmental disability that interferes with self-feeding have been found to correlate with inadequate dietary intake and growth. Pneumonia, due to repeated aspiration of food, is a problem for some of those children that may necessitate a feeding gastrostomy (see Chapter 29, Enteral Nutritional Support). Table 20-3 describes appropriate textures and foods for various feeding skills.[3]

Developmentally delayed children can present with many of the same food-related behaviors as normal children, though perhaps at a different age. They can be expected to have periods of reduced food intake, food jags, and attempts to control their parents or care providers by the acceptance or the rejection of food.[1] In addition, some feeding problems can develop as a result of feedings being associated with unpleasant circumstances in children who must be fed frequently or whose feeding is time-consuming due to chewing and swallowing dysfunction.[3] Feeding assessment should evaluate what are normal and abnormal behaviors and how these behaviors interfere with the development of feeding capabilities and adequate nutrient intake.

TABLE 20-3 Guidelines for Selection of Food for Feeding Skill Level

Feeding Skill Level	Type of Food Indicated	Examples
Sucking	Use fluids	Milk/formula
Elevation of tongue: moves food to back of mouth	Continue using fluids	Milk/formula
Swallowing (with head forward and no gagging; elevation of back and tongue)	Introduce blended diet	Baby food, thick purees, mashed potatoes, applesauce, custard, ice cream, yogurt, mashed banana
Up-and-down chewing with jaw control and minimal drooling	Start finely ground foods	Oatmeal: cottage cheese, finely ground meat, scrambled egg, well-mashed cooked vegetables, egg salad, peanut butter if no tongue thrust
Lateral tongue movement	Begin coarsely ground foods	Ground meats in gravy, tuna fish, chopped fruits and vegetables, fine coleslaw, cheese, rice, liverwurst, banana slices, flavored yogurt
Rotary chewing	Use chopped foods	Crackers, finely chopped meats, fruits and vegetables, salad greens, coleslaw, macaroni, dry cereal
Reaches for and grasps objects; brings hands to mouth	Begin finger feeding with large pieces	Crackers, teething biscuit, oven-dried toast, cheese sticks
Voluntary release	Finger feeding with small pieces	Dry cereal, small pieces of meat, cottage cheese
Puts lips on cup rim	Begin cup feeding	
Reaches for spoon; ulnar deviation of wrist	Self-feeding	Foods that adhere to spoon, cooked cereal, mashed potato, applesauce, cottage cheese
Increased rotary movement of jaw	Increase texture and variety	Chopped meats, raw vegetables and fruits

Adapted from Zeman FJ. Nutrition care in neurological, muscular, and skeletal disorders. In: Zeman FJ, ed. Clinical nutrition and dietetics. New York: Macmillan, 1991:711; reprinted with permission.

Dietary Recommendations

Energy.   Children with developmental disabilities have varied kilocalorie needs. Children with Down's syndrome, spastic cerebral palsy, Prader-Willi's syndrome, myelomeningocele, and other disorders that limit activity usually have decreased energy needs, and obesity is a common problem. Children with hyperactivity, hypertonia, and athetoid cerebral palsy frequently have greatly increased requirements for kilocalories. Generally, caloric recommendations based on height or height-age are more appropriate than those based on age or weight alone.[1] In addition, the stage of sexual maturation of the older child should be considered because some of these children undergo early pubescence and others delayed puberty. Tanner's stages of maturity and their effect on caloric requirements are discussed in Chapter 23, Weight Control. The guidelines in Table 20-4 are useful for making an initial estimate of caloric need. Any estimate of caloric need must be individualized, however, and must have periodic follow-up to assess growth progress and possible need for dietary change.

Protein.   Protein requirements are thought to be the same as for normal children of the same height-age.

Fluids.   The developmentally delayed child may not be able to respond to thirst or to express a need to drink. Some children may not be able to close their lips adequately to hold and swallow liquids easily. These children are at risk for dehydration and constipation. Special attention needs to be paid to the amount of fluids intended versus the amount actually consumed, which commonly falls below expectation. Thickened fluids, such as milkshakes, sherbet, gelatin, and soups, may be helpful to assure adequate fluid intake. (See also Chapter 5, Dysphagia.)

TABLE 20-4   Guidelines for Estimating Caloric Requirements in Children with Developmental Disabilities

Condition	Caloric Recommendation
Ambulatory, ages 5 to 12 years	13.9 kcal/cm of height
Nonambulatory, ages 5 to 12 years	11.1 kcal/cm of height[3]
Cerebral palsy with severely restricted activity	10 kcal/cm of height[6]
Cerebral palsy with mild to moderate levels of activity	15 kcal/cm of height[6]
Athetoid cerebral palsy, adolescence	Up to 6,000 kcal[1]
Down's syndrome, boys ages 1 to 14 years	16.1 kcal/cm of height
Down's syndrome, girls ages 1 to 14 years	14.3 kcal/cm of height[6]
Myelomeningocele	Approximately 50% of RDA for age after infancy. May need as little as 7 kcal/cm of height to maintain normal weight[1,6]
Prader-Willi's syndrome	10 to 11 kcal/cm of height for weight maintenance; 8–9 kcal/cm of height for weight loss[1]

Fiber.   Many developmentally delayed children cannot chew raw or fibrous foods. Lack of fiber in the diet, coupled with low fluid intake and immobility, frequently results in constipation. In addition, diets that consist primarily of dairy-based supplements, rather than a well-balanced diet, may result in constipation. Unprocessed bran (which can be soaked or cooked in a liquid or baked into muffins), whole-grain cereals, and prunes or prune juice may help prevent constipation.[6] (See Chapter 24, Constipation and Encopresis, for further discussion of dietary recommendations.)

Nutrient-Drug Interactions.   Drug therapy is frequently used in the treatment of children with developmental or behavioral problems or seizures and may affect nutritional requirements. Anticonvulsants may increase the requirements for folic acid, vitamin B_{12}, and D and may affect bone and dental health. However, supplementation should not be given routinely, but rather individualized based on biochemical and/or radiological data with frequent review and adjustments. Central nervous system stimulants can result in appetite suppression and decreased growth. Growth rate of children on these drugs should be monitored frequently. Steroids can cause increased appetite and obesity.[6] The pharmacist can assist in determining possible drug-nutrient interactions, timing of medications to reduce anorectic effects, and so forth.[2]

Nutrition Education.   Nutrition education of parents, care providers, and the child, if possible, should be anticipatory and preventive in focus. The diet should be palatable and as close to normal as possible in terms of texture, taste, and variety. Eating is frequently one of the few pleasures in the life of a severely disabled child. In addition, it is easier to teach proper feeding behaviors than to try to change bad habits. Education should include feeding methods, food preparation, nutritional needs, and special diets when appropriate. It requires a team effort that includes the dietitian, physician, nurse, and occupational, speech, and physical therapists. Due to the prevalence of psychosocial feeding problems among handicapped children, parents and care providers need to be educated about normal feeding behaviors and appropriate strategies to prevent or resolve feeding problems.[9] Inability to recognize developmental readiness to acquire new skills can result in failure to provide the child with appropriate stimuli.[1,3] For example, failure to progress from pureed foods to a more textured diet at the appropriate time may result in the child refusing lumpy foods at a later date. In addition, limited expectations for the developmentally delayed child can affect how the care provider interacts with the child during feeding and can therefore hinder development of full capabilities. Whenever possible, the child should be taught adequate food selection by good role modeling, particularly if the child is to be largely responsible for his or her own food selection.

Obesity prevention should be discussed with care providers or parents of children. Ideally, this education should begin, for parents of a child with myelomeningocele, during the first hospitalization to close the spinal cord defect. When the infant's weight for height exceeds 10 to 20% over ideal body weight, parents should be advised to limit high kilocalorie, low nutrient foods in order to slow the rate of weight gain.[6] Children with Down's syndrome are also at risk for obesity, and parents or care providers should be educated regarding obesity prevention at the first signs of inappropriate weight gain.

References

1. Pipes PL, Pritkin R. Nutrition and feeding of children with developmental delays and related problems. In: Pipes PL, ed. Nutrition in infancy and childhood. St Louis: Mosby, 1989:361–386.
2. Wodarski LA. An interdisciplinary nutrition assessment and intervention protocol for children with disabilities. J Am Diet Assoc 1990;90:1563–1568.
3. Zeman FJ. Nutrition care in neurological, muscular and skeletal disorders. In: Zeman FJ, ed. Clinical nutrition and dietetics. New York: Macmillan, 1991;703–722.
4. Lyon AJ, Grant DB. Growth curve for girls with Turner syndrome. Arch Dis Child 1985; 60:932–935.
5. Cronk CE, Crocker AC, Pueschel SM, Shea AM, Zackai E, Pickens G, Reed RB. Growth charts for children with Down syndrome: 1 month to 18 years of age. Pediatrics 1988; 81:102–109.
6. Anon. Developmental disabilities. In: Lawrence KE, Nell DiLima S, eds. Dietitian's patient education manual. Gaithersberg, MD: Aspen, 1991;20-1 to 20-60.
7. Rast J, Ellinge-Allen JA, Johnston JM. Dietary management of rumination: four case studies. Am J Clin Nutr 1985;42:95–101.
8. Thommessen M, Riis G, Kase BF, Larsen S, Heiberg A. Energy and nutrient intakes of disabled children: do feeding problems make a difference? J Am Diet Assoc 1991;19: 1522–1525.
9. Krick J, VanDuyn MS. The relationship between oral-motor involvement and growth: a pilot study in a pediatric population with cerebral palsy. J Am Diet Assoc 1984; 84:555–559.

FAILURE TO THRIVE

Failure-to-thrive (FTT) is a term used to describe physical growth failure in infants and young children that may be accompanied by retarded motor and social development. It may be caused by an identifiable disease process and then is commonly called "organic"; it may be psychosocial in origin, referred to as "non-organic"; or multiple causes may be present.

Numerous guidelines have been proposed to define FTT. Fomon defines it as a rate of gain in length and/or weight falls more than two standard deviations below the mean for at least 56 days in infants under 5 months of age or for at least 3 months in older infants.[10] Other criteria used to define FTT utilize the National Center for Health Statistics (NCHS) growth curves (see Pediatric Appendix 28) and include the following:

1. Weight less than 80% of the 50th percentile for age[11]
2. Weight less than the 3rd percentile of the NCHS growth curve[11]
3. A drop of 2 or more percentile ranks in weight for height[11]
4. Weight for height less than 80% based on the calculation of:[12]

$$\text{Percent Weight for Height} = \frac{\text{Actual Weight}}{\text{Median Weight for Height-Age}} \times 100$$

5. Height-age[13] for chronologic age less than 80%:

$$\frac{\text{Height-Age}}{\text{Chronologic Age}} = < 0.8$$

Growth deficits are usually manifested in weight first, then height, and finally head circumference.

Common organic causes that either increase nutritional requirements or result in diminished intake or excessive losses of kilocalories include congenital heart disease,[14] gastrointestinal disorders,[15] cystic fibrosis, central nervous system disturbances, and, rarely, endocrine disorders.[16] Children with renal disease[17] or with constitutional short stature also may present as FTT. A detailed patient, family, and growth history, physical examination, and nutritional history can frequently rule out obvious organic causes.

Children with nonorganic FTT may exhibit physical symptoms associated with feeding, such as vomiting, foul-smelling stools, diarrhea, poor appetite, falling asleep during feeding, and rumination. Nonorganic FTT can be accidental, neglectful, or deliberate. Accidental FTT may occur through errors in formula preparation, diet selection, or feeding technique. Deliberate underfeeding is rare. Neglectful FTT often occurs because the mother is emotionally overwhelmed or psychologically disturbed.[18]

In cases without obvious organic cause, a feeding trial that provides adequate kilocalories is usually initiated on either an outpatient or inpatient basis. Organic causes may be investigated after failure of the feeding trial or simultaneously, provided the diagnostic procedures do not interfere with the feeding trial.

Dietary Recommendations

Nutrition Assessment. A detailed nutritional history taken from the child's parents or caretakers should include a recent or prospective dietary food intake record and a history of food intake that includes whether the child was breast- or bottle-fed, types of formulas given, when solids were introduced, and age at weaning. The nutrition history should also include eating patterns and habits, food allergies, excessive losses of nutrients via vomiting or diarrhea, food likes and dislikes, family eating patterns, method of formula preparation, understanding of child size portions, and how the family views the feeding behaviors and problems. The food intake record should be evaluated for adequacy of kilocalories, protein, and other key nutrients for which suspected deficiencies might exist. In cases of suspected inadequate or inappropriate offering of feedings, the diet history may not be reliable, and hospitalization for observation is usually warranted. The practitioner should unobtrusively observe the parents while they are feeding the child.

Anthropometric procedures performed with care are essential and include, at a minimum, height or length, weight, and head circumference (in infants). Measurements should be plotted over time on the NCHS growth curve.

Feeding Trial. A feeding trial of adequate kilocalories is initiated to determine the cause of the FTT when there are no obvious organic causes. On an outpatient basis, the parents are instructed in the amount, type, and frequency of feedings to be given and on how to keep a food diary. Close follow-up to evaluate growth progress and dietary intake is conducted by the physician and the dietitian. In the hospital, daily kilocalories and protein intake, weight, feeding frequency and duration, special techniques required to feed, and losses from vomiting or diarrhea are recorded. The diet offered should be appropriate for the child's developmental age and should be as close to the home diet, in terms of types of food, as possible. The patient is initially fed amounts as desired on a regular schedule. If the intake is not adequate, further steps are taken to increase intake, such as increasing the caloric density of the feedings and more frequent feedings.

There are many differences of opinion in the literature as to what constitutes an adequate caloric intake for the child recovering from FTT. Recommendations range from caloric levels adequate to promote normal rates of growth in most healthy infants of similar age[10] to caloric levels 50% higher than normal for age.[19] An initial caloric goal based on the Recommended Dietary Allowances (RDA) for the patient's height-age (age at which the child's height is at the 50th percentile of the NCHS growth curve) and weight is usually adequate to produce weight gain in the child who does not have increased energy requirements or excessive losses. Weight gain can be expected to begin in 2 to 17 days in infants less than 6 months. The lag time is greater for older infants and children.[12,20]

Evaluation of feeding trials results in the following three classifications:

1. *Adequate intake with weight gain.* Many factors affect weight gain in relation to energy intake, even in the normal healthy infant. However, some guidelines are available to evaluate whether the weight gain is appropriate for the energy intake. In the first 6 months of life, the average weight gain per unit of energy intake is estimated to be 3.6 g per 100 kcal. It is about 1.4 g per 100 kcal in the second 6 months.[12]

   This classification suggests psychosocial and/or environmental problems. The parents are then instructed in how to provide adequate nutrition for their child.

2. *Adequate intake with no weight gain.* In this scenario one must increase caloric intake to that estimated for catch-up growth and/or investigate for nonorganic causes of the FTT.

3. *Inadequate intake with no weight gain.* When this is found, one must investigate whether the poor intake is attributable to poor feeding techniques, to the use of inappropriate foods, or to specific mechanical or neuromotor dysfunction.

Catch-up Growth.   The diet should be increased to provide for catch-up growth once weight gain is established. Catch-up growth requires kilocalories and protein far in excess of those normal for age. Peterson et al[11] have formulated the following method of estimating caloric and protein requirements for catch-up growth.

1. Plot height and weight on NCHS growth curves (see Pediatric Appendix 28).
2. Determine weight-age (age at which present weight is at the 50th percentile).
3. Determine ideal weight (50th percentile for present age).
4. Calculate:

$$\text{Predicted kcal per kg for catch-up growth} = \frac{(\text{RDA kcal per kg for Weight-Age}) \times (\text{Ideal Weight in kg})}{\text{Actual Weight in kg}}$$

5. Repeat the process to determine protein catch-up requirements using RDA for grams of protein per kilogram in place of RDA for kilocalories per kilogram.

Ellerstein and Ostrov[20] have developed the concept of "growth quotient" (GQ) to evaluate the patient's rate of growth. The GQ can be used to determine if catch-up growth is occurring.

$$GQ = \frac{\text{Mean Daily Weight Gain (for a Specified Time)}}{\text{Normal Daily Weight Gain for Age}}$$

NCHS growth curves or incremental growth normal tables[21] can be used to determine normal weight increments for age. A GQ of 1.00 represents the average growth rate. This expression of growth rate is especially helpful in the evaluation of catch-up growth in older children recovering from FTT whose actual weight gains appear small.[20]

Patient Education and Follow-up.   In the outpatient setting, parent education should begin as soon as the diagnosis is made. Appropriate community resources should be contacted, and close follow-up should be arranged. For the hospitalized child, parent education should be initiated by the healthcare team while the patient is in the hospital. The dietitian educates the parents about what the child's nutritional needs are and how to provide them. The parents should be advised that their child's appearance will change dramatically with catch-up growth. The child may even appear fat at first, but the child's weight for height should normalize with time. Frequently, the caloric density of the child's food needs to be increased because most children have a limited capacity for volume of food; specific instructions should be given to the parents. A nutritional care referral should be sent to a nutritionist at the public health agency or an outpatient dietitian.

References

10. Fomon SJ. Infant nutrition, 2nd ed. Philadelphia: WB Saunders, 1974:81.
11. Peterson KE, Washington J, Rathbun J. Team management of failure-to-thrive. J Am Diet Assoc 1984;84:810–815.
12. Kien CL. Failure-to-thrive. In: Walker WA, Watkins JB, eds. Nutrition in pediatrics: basic science and clinical application. Boston: Little, Brown, 1985:757.
13. Fiser RH, Meredith PD, Elders MJ. The child who fails to grow. Am Fam Physician 1975;11:108–119.
14. Ehlers KH. Growth failure in association with congenital heart disease. Pediatr Ann 1978;7:35–57.
15. Lavy U, Bauer CH. Pathophysiology of failure-to-thrive in gastrointestinal disorders. Pediatr Ann 1978;7:20–33.
16. Abrams CA. Endocrinologic aspects of failure-to-thrive. Pediatr Ann 1978;7:58–72.
17. Friedman J, Lewy JE. Failure-to-thrive associated with renal disease. Pediatr Ann 1978;7:73–82.
18. Schmitt BD, Mauro RD. Nonorganic failure to thrive: an outpatient approach. Child Abuse Negl 1989;13:235–248.
19. Whitten CF, Pettit MG, Fischhoff J. Evidence that growth failure from maternal deprivation is secondary to undereating. JAMA 1969;209:1675–1682.
20. Ellerstein NS, Ostrov BE. Growth patterns in children hospitalized because of caloric-deprivation failure to thrive. Am J Dis Child 1985;139:164–166.
21. Baumgartner RN, Roche AF, Himes JH. Incremental growth tables: supplementary to previously published chart. Am J Clin Nutr 1986;43:711–722.

LOW BIRTH WEIGHT INFANT

General Description

Generally, the smaller and/or more malnourished the infant at birth, the greater the nutritional requirements in the early months of life, but all infants of low birth weight (less than 2,500 g) are not alike. Infants who are normally grown, but premature, differ from infants who are malnourished in utero and gestationally more mature. The nutritional requirements of similar weight infants in the two groups are usually considered to be similar, except perhaps for kilocalories, but their ability to feed and their feeding tolerance may vary considerably. More mature infants who are small may be able to suck and to swallow feedings on their own, whereas premature infants who are less than 34 weeks of gestation usually cannot. Small-for-date infants are at greater risk for hypoglycemia in the early days after birth since they have minimal glycogen stores, and they usually require more kilocalories for growth than their age-matched counterparts.[22] Very-low-birth-weight (VLBW) infants (less than 1,200 g) and sick larger infants may need special nutritional support that combines parenteral and enteral nutrition, regardless of their gestational age.

Nutritional Considerations

There has been a significant increase in the survival of preterm infants. With major advances in respiratory and other life support measures, some feel that ensuring adequate nutrition has replaced respiratory difficulties as the major limiting factor for survival of these infants.[23]

Much remains unknown about the nutritional requirements of premature infants. A useful, though arbitrary, goal of nutritional care is the maintenance of in utero growth rates and body composition. Babson[24] has published growth curves based on the growth of healthy premature infants from birth to 12 months from term (see Chapter 18, Pediatric Nutritional Assessment, and Appendix 31). These growth curves can be used to evaluate the premature infant's progress in terms of both rate of incremental change in height, weight, and head circumference and rate of growth. The nutritional goal for small-for-date infants is to provide for catch-up growth in order for the infants to reach their growth potential as quickly as possible.[25]

Nutritional requirements are believed to be higher for the low-birth-weight infant than for the healthy term infant for many reasons, including fewer nutrient reserves, less efficient absorption and utilization of nutrients, greater losses of nutrients, less body fat insulation, and more rapid rate of growth.[22] Thus, preterm infants are characterized by rapid growth, poor reserves, and immaturity of numerous biological functions, and they are vulnerable to any excess or deficiency in nutritional intake.[23] Actual requirements for most nutrients remain unknown, but useful estimates have been proposed from the research data.

Goals of Dietary Management

Estimation of requirements and advisable intakes for energy protein and major minerals and electrolytes have been calculated by a factorial method. This method

TABLE 20-5 Advisable Enteral Intakes[26-28]

Nutrient	Intake for 800–1,200 g Infant (per kg/day)	Intake for 1,200–1,800 g Infant (per kg/day)
Kilocalories	120–130	120–130
Protein (g)	4	3.5
Sodium (mEq)	3.5	3
Potassium (mEq)	2.5	2.3
Chloride (mEq)	3.1	2.5
Calcium (mg)	210	185
Phosphorus (mg)	140	123
Magnesium (mg)	10	8.5

was based on the composition of fetal weight gain in the third trimester with adjustments for dermal and urinary losses, intestinal absorption, and growth.[26] These estimations are summarized in Table 20-5.

Kilocalories. Estimations of caloric requirements are approximately 50 kcal/kg/day for basal expenditures plus 70 to 75 kcal/kg/day for activity, specific dynamic action, fecal loss, cold stress, and growth.[26] We have generally found that healthy low-birth-weight infants gain an average of 20 to 30 g per day on intakes of 120 to 130 kcal/kg/day. Bronchopulmonary dysplasia (i.e., increased work of breathing), congenital heart defects, frequent seizure activity, and intrauterine growth retardation may increase caloric requirements.

Protein. The advantages of high protein quality are well recognized, but more work is necessary to determine the quantity of protein needed. Protein quality and quantity should be considered when feedings for the premature infant are planned. In addition to the eight amino acids known to be essential to adults, histidine, tyrosine, cystine, and taurine may be essential to premature infants because of the infants' immature enzyme systems.[26] Whey-predominant protein appears to result in fewer serum amino acid disturbances,[27] less risk of late metabolic acidosis,[25,28] and greater efficiency of nitrogen retention.[29] Whey protein eliminates the risk of lactobezoar formation when compared to casein-predominant milk protein.[30]

Fat. The premature infant is at risk for the development of essential fatty acid deficiency as early as 5 to 8 days after birth due to low endogenous reserves at birth.[31] As soon as possible after birth, at least 3% of the caloric intake should be provided by linoleic acid. However, large amounts of polyunsaturated fats cause an increase in vitamin E requirement, which must be met by supplementation. Long-chain saturated fats are not well absorbed by the premature infant's gut. Medium-chain triglycerides are better absorbed, presumably because they are not dependent on duodenal intraluminal bile salts, which are inadequate in the premature infant. Human milk fat, though mainly saturated, is well absorbed due to its unique triglyceride configuration and to the presence of bile salt–activated lipase in the milk.[28] Fat usually makes up approximately 50% of the energy intake for the premature infant.[28]

TABLE 20-6 Advisable Daily Intakes for Selected Vitamins and Trace Elements for Low-Birth-Weight Infants[26,28,33,34]

Nutrient	Ziegler*	AAP†	Tsang‡
Vitamin D (IU)	600	500	400
Vitamin E (IU)	30	5–25 plus 0.7/100 kcal, and 1.0 IU of vitamin E/g linoleic acid	25 for 2–4 wk, then 5
Vitamin C (mg)	60	35	30
Folic acid (µg)	60	30	15/kg
Copper (µg)	60/100 kcal	90/100 kcal	100–200/kg
Zinc (mg)	0.5/100 kcal	0.5/100 kcal	0.8–1.2/kg
Iron (mg)	2–3/kg (begin at 2 wk)	2–3/kg (begin at 1–2 mo)	2/kg (begin when birth weight doubled)

*Data from Ziegler EE, Biga RL, Fomon SJ. Nutritional requirements of the premature infant. In: Suskind RM, ed. Textbook of pediatric nutrition. New York, Raven Press, 1981: 29–39.

†Data from American Academy of Pediatrics Committee on Nutrition. Nutritional needs of low-birth-weight infants. Pediatrics 1985; 75:976–986.

‡Data from Tsang RC, ed. Vitamin and mineral requirements in preterm infants. New York: Marcel Dekker, 1985.

Carbohydrate. Lactose may not be efficiently absorbed in the early days of postnatal life, because lactase activity does not mature until near term. Glycosidases, which facilitate the absorption of glucose polymers, are active in even the very premature infant's gut. Thus, glucose polymers are absorbed well and offer the additional advantage of adding less osmotic load to the feeding than lactose or monosaccharides.[32]

Minerals. Two-thirds of fetal bone mineralization takes place in the last trimester of pregnancy. Bone mineral content is low in both premature and small-for-date infants, even at term.[32] The fetal accretion rates and the advisable intakes (see Table 20-5) to achieve those rates for calcium and phosphorus are approximately four and five times higher, respectively, than is provided by human milk. Adequate vitamin D is also necessary for good bone mineralization and growth after birth. Deficiencies of vitamin D, calcium, and phosphorus have been associated with osteopenia, rickets, and decreased bone mineral content in these infants.[27] In order to ensure adequate bone growth and mineralization in these infants, close attention should be given to providing the levels of calcium and phosphorus that are estimated to achieve fetal accretion rates and to providing adequate vitamin D.[26]

Vitamins and Trace Elements. Nutritional requirements for vitamins and trace elements remain largely undefined for premature infants. Advisable intakes based on current data have been published.[26,28,33,34] The levels recommended are generally the same as for term infants except that greater amounts are recommended for vitamins C, D, and E, folic acid, zinc, copper, and iron. Recommendations for those nutrients are compared in Table 20-6.

The requirement for vitamin E increases with the amount of polyunsaturated fatty acid and iron in the diet. The premature infant is born relatively deficient in vitamin E and is at risk for subsequent hemolytic anemia. While the need for vitamin E supplementation is generally agreed upon, the amount recommended varies from 5 to 30 IU or more per day.[26,27,33-36] At least 1.0 IU of vitamin E per gram of linoleic acid should be maintained to prevent hemolytic anemia in the premature infant.[28] In addition, the use of pharmacological doses of vitamin E to reduce the severity of retrolental fibroplasia and bronchopulmonary dysplasia is the subject of much controversy and research.[37,38] While the data are yet inconclusive, it seems desirable to provide sufficient vitamin E from birth to raise the infant's serum level to normal as quickly as possible and to maintain that level.

Negative balances of zinc and copper among premature infants in the early weeks of life[28] and reports of late deficiencies of these two trace elements have raised concern over what the requirements for these nutrients are in these infants.[38] Current recommendations range from approximately 0.6 to 1.2 mg/kg/day for zinc and 70 to 200 µg/kg/day for copper.[26,28,33]

The low-birth-weight infant is at risk for the development of iron deficiency anemia due to relatively low iron stores at birth, rapid growth rate, and diagnostic phlebotomies. However, iron is not utilized for hemoglobin synthesis in the early weeks of life, and the administration of iron may predispose the infant to vitamin E deficient hemolytic anemia.[26,30] Provision of 2 to 3 mg/kg/day of ferrous iron, beginning at approximately 1 month of age and continuing until 1 year of age, appears safe and aids in establishing adequate iron reserves in the premature infant.[26]

Provision of adequate nutrition for the low-birth-weight infant requires careful selection of the type of feeding to be given and monitoring for adequacy of nutrient intake. Supplements of 400 IU of vitamin D and 25 IU of vitamin E are usually given until the infant reaches 2 kg. Other nutrients may need to be supplemented as well, depending on the nutrient content of the feeding given. The nutritional requirements of premature infants is just beginning to be understood. Thus, feeding programs and protocols need to be frequently updated and revised.

Fluid

Water is quantitatively the most important nutrient, and the volume of water required in daily feedings is the basis for the nutritional management of the premature infant. The water requirement is determined by water losses from the body. This includes water lost insensibly, in obligatory renal losses, and in feces. Considering these losses, water needs vary widely for these infants. The minimum water requirement of a growing preterm infant in optimum conditions is about 130 ml/kg/day.[39]

Types of Feedings

Human Milk. Whenever possible, mothers of low-birth-weight infants should be encouraged to breast-feed. The advantages of human milk include its anti-infection factors, improved absorption of fat, more desirable protein composition, low renal solute load, presence of epidermal growth factor, improved digestibility relative to cow's milk formula, possible protection against necrotizing enterocolitis, and psychological benefit to mother and infant.[40,41]

There is, however, controversy about whether human milk alone is adequate for premature infants, particularly those less than 1,500 g at birth. Protein levels in human milk have generally been considered too low to support adequate growth. Studies have shown that the milk of mothers of preterm infants is slightly higher in protein than that of mothers of term infants,[27] but the level of protein falls rapidly during the first weeks of lactation. The initially higher level of protein may only be a function of the smaller volume of milk produced by these mothers.[39] Studies comparing the milk of mothers of term and preterm infants on sodium, chloride, magnesium, and caloric content have produced variable results.[27] Calcium and phosphorus levels are the same in milk of mothers of preterm and term infants and are not considered adequate for the preterm infant. Bone fractures, rickets, and decreased bone mineral content have been seen in premature infants fed breast milk exclusively.[28,38] Supplementation with calcium, phosphorus, and vitamin D is warranted, particularly for the breast-fed VLBW infant.

Whether or not human milk can result in adequate growth in the premature infant is also a topic of controversy. Most researchers agree that pooled milk of mothers of term infants is not adequate for the preterm infant and should not be used. Studies have shown that adequate growth can be achieved by using the milk from the infant's own mother.[27,42] However, many preterm infants cannot tolerate sufficient volumes of human milk for growth and require caloric supplementation of the milk. Considering all the possible inadequacies of human milk, even from the preterm infant's own mother, we choose to supplement the milk with one of two commercially available human milk supplements until the infant reaches 2 kg (see Appendix 25, Infant Formulas and Feedings).

Formulas. Special formulas designed to meet the expected nutritional needs of low-birth-weight infants have been developed. These formulas provide greater concentrations of certain nutrients in more readily absorbable forms than standard formulas for term infants. In these formulas, the protein is predominantly whey, fat content is part long-chain fatty acids and part medium-chain triglycerides, and carbohydrate is part lactose and part glucose polymers. Calcium and phosphorus content is designed to achieve intrauterine bone accretion rates in the infant. The exact composition of the formulas varies, and they should be supplemented with nutrients as needed (see Appendix 25, Infant Formulas and Feedings, or manufacturer's information). Higher caloric concentrations are available to enable the infant to consume adequate calories in limited fluid volumes. We have found that most infants who weigh less than 2,000 g need formula concentrations of at least 24 kcal/oz for adequate growth without excess fluid intake.

The use of soy-protein formulas in feeding premature infants has been associated with lower nitrogen retention, lower phosphorus levels, osteoporosis, and rickets. These formulas are not advisable except for specific therapeutic indications, and then should not be used for more than 3 to 4 weeks.[43]

Feeding Technique: Oral—Enteral—Parenteral. The immaturity of the gastrointestinal tract and the limited ability of other organ systems to metabolize and excrete nutrients and waste products are challenges to the provision of adequate nutrition for the low-birth-weight infant. Establishment of adequate nutrition is hindered by the infant's small stomach capacity, slow gastrointestinal motility, and the immature enzyme systems of the gastrointestinal tract, as well as by the risk of necrotizing enterocolitis. Preterm infants can respond to oral nutrition as early as 25 weeks of gestational age.[44] The use of enteral feedings in preterm infants may be warranted to avoid total parenteral nutrition–related complications such as cholestasis and to promote an earlier transition to oral feedings.[45] The immaturity of intestinal motor activity may result in the preterm infant's being unable to handle frequent feedings until motor activity becomes better coordinated.[45]

As discussed, small-for-date infants are different from premature infants with regard to feeding. The more mature infant who is small for gestational age usually feeds more vigorously and more actively than the gestationally immature infant and requires less special support, particularly at weights above 1,800 g. Small and/or immature infants usually do not suck and swallow well enough to meet their nutritional needs and require continuous or intermittent orogastric or oroduodenal tube feedings. If the low-birth-weight infant is well and free of respiratory distress, the first feedings are begun within 4 to 6 hours of birth. Enteral feedings should be introduced slowly, according to tolerance (see also Chapter 29, Pediatric Enteral Nutrition). Feedings should begin with sterile water or, if available, maternal colostrum, then advance to half-strength formula or human milk, and, finally, to full strength. The volume of the feedings is increased gradually over 7 to 10 days to achieve approximately 120 to 130 kcal/kg/day. After 1 week of well-tolerated enteral feedings, the infant who weighs less than 2,000 g is advanced to premature infant formulas that are concentrated to 24 kcal/oz, or one of the commercially available human milk supplements is added to the breast milk from the premature infant's mother. Bottle or breast-feeding is introduced gradually as tolerated by the infant.

A 2 kg infant is usually able to ingest and tolerate sufficient quantities of human milk or regular infant formula for growth. A multivitamin supplement that provides the equivalent of the RDA for term infants is advisable, at least until the infant is consuming 300 kcal/day.[46]

Parenteral nutrition that supplies all or part of the nutritional needs may be necessary to nourish the low-birth-weight infant. The solutions and nutrient levels chosen should be designed to meet, as nearly as possible, the special needs of the premature infant. See Chapter 29, Pediatric Parenteral Nutrition, for further guidelines.

References

22. Rickard K, Gresham E. Nutritional considerations for the newborn requiring intensive care. J Am Diet Assoc 1985;66:592–599.

23. DeCurtis M, DeCurtis D, Ciccimarra F. Nutritional requirements of preterm infants. World Rev Nutr Diet 1989;58:33–60.

24. Babson SG, Benda GI. Growth graphs for the clinical assessment of infants of varying gestational age. J Pediatr 1976;89:814–820.

25. Fenton TR, McMillan DD, Sauve RS. Nutrition and growth analysis of very low birth weight infants. Pediatrics 1990;86:378–383.

26. Ziegler EE, Biga RL, Fomon SJ. Nutritional requirements of the premature infant. In: Suskind RM, ed. Textbook of pediatric nutrition. New York: Raven Press, 1981:29–39.

27. Reynolds JW. Nutrition of the low-birth-weight infant. In: Walker WA, Watkins JB, eds. Nutrition pediatrics. Boston: Little, Brown, 1985:649.

28. American Academy of Pediatrics Committee on Nutrition. Nutritional needs of low-birth-weight infants. Pediatrics 1985;75:976–986.

29. Darling P, Lepage G, Tremblay P, Collet S, Kien LC, Roy CC. Protein quality and quantity in preterm infants receiving the same energy intake. Am J Dis Child 1985;139:186–190.

30. Brady MS, Rickard KA, Ernest JA, Schreiner RL, Lemons JA. Formulas and human milk for premature infants: a review and update. J Am Diet Assoc 1982;81:547–555.

31. Anon. Development of essential fatty acid deficiency in the premature infant given fat-free TPN. Nutr Rev 1985;43:14–15.

32. Kien CL, Liechty EA, Mullett MD. Effects of lactose intake on nutritional status in premature infants. J Pediatr 1990;116:446–449.

33. Ehrenkranz RA. Mineral needs in the very-low-birth-weight infant. Semin Perenatol 1989;13:142–159.

34. Tsang RC, ed. Vitamin and mineral requirements in preterm infants. New York: Marcel Dekker, 1985.

35. Ehrenkranz RA. Vitamin E and the neonate. Am J Dis Child 1980;134:1157–1165.

36. Bell EF, Filer LJ. The role of vitamin E in the nutrition of premature infants. Am J Clin Nutr 1981;34:414–422.

37. Committee on Fetus and Newborn. Vitamin E and prevention of retinopathy of prematurity. Pediatrics 1985;76:315–316.

38. Hittner HM, Godio LB, Rudolph AJ, Adams JM, Garcia-Prats JA, Friedman Z, Kautz JA, Monaco WA. Retrolental fibroplasia efficacy of vitamin E in a double blind chemical study of preterm infants. N Engl J Med 1981;305:1365–1371.

39. Ziegler EE. Infants of low birth weight: special needs and problems. Am J Clin Nutr 1985;41:440–446.

40. Brooke OG. Nutritional requirements of low and very low birthweight infants. Annu Rev Nutr 1987;7:91–116.

41. Steichen JJ, Krug-Wispé SK, Tsang RC. Breastfeeding the low birth weight preterm infant. Clin Perinatol 1987;14(1):131–171.

42. Anderson DM, Williams FH, Merkatz RB, Schulman PK, Kerr DS, Pittard WB. Length of gestation and nutritional composition of human milk. Am J Clin Nutr 1983;37:810–814.

43. Narayanan I. Human milk for low birth weight infants: nutrition and newer practical technologies. Acta Paediatr Scand 1989;31:455–461.

44. Berseth CL. Neonatal small intestinal motility: motor responses to feeding in term and preterm infants. J Pediatr 1990;177:777–782.

45. American Academy of Pediatrics Committee on Nutrition. Soy-protein formulas: recommendations for use in infant feeding. Pediatrics 1983;72:359–363.

46. American Academy of Pediatrics Committee on Nutrition. Vitamin and mineral supplement needs in normal children in the United States. Pediatrics 1980;66:1015–1021.

SICK INFANTS, CHILDREN, AND ADOLESCENTS

General Description

The impact of illness on the nutritional requirements of children is extremely variable and can change during the course of an illness. In pediatric patients, the special nutritional requirements of the disease are superimposed on relatively high

TABLE 20-7 Maximum Number of Days to Start Full Nutritional Support [47,50]*

Size of Child	Days
Term infant	3–4
10 kg	5
30 kg	7
50 kg	7

*Assuming carbohydrate has been administered from the start of the illness or trauma.

Data from: Wesley JR, Coran AG. Intravenous nutrition for the pediatric patient. Semin Pediatr Surg 1992; 1(3):212–230; and Seashore JH. Nutritional support of children in the intensive care unit. Yale J Biol Med 1984; 57:111–134.

requirements for growth and limited endogenous reserves.[47] The nutritional goals for short-term acute illnesses include the prevention of significant losses of nutrients and the facilitation of recovery of body mass from losses caused by illness or trauma. Catch-up growth occurs in the days following the acute illness, provided adequate nutrition is available. The goal of nutritional care with chronic disease is to provide adequate kilocalories and nutrients for growth in addition to the kilocalories and nutrients needed to replace losses or to meet increased requirements due to the disease.

In addition to the parameters discussed in Chapter 18, Pediatric Nutritional Assessment, consideration should be given to the nature and severity of the illness or trauma and to the ability of the child to take in adequate nutrition by oral, enteral, parenteral, or any combination of these methods. In addition, there must be ongoing, frequent re-evaluation of the nutritional status of the patient and of the care plan. The following discussion is limited to general nutritional considerations that are not discussed elsewhere under specific disease states.

Malnutrition can develop rapidly in a seriously ill infant or child and can affect the rate of recovery from illness or injury.[47] The initial goal of nutrition for the acutely ill pediatric patient is to minimize protein losses and to meet the metabolic requirements of the brain for glucose by the provision of protein-sparing carbohydrate, either enterally or parenterally. How soon such therapy is instituted depends on the size of the child and on whether protein-sparing carbohydrate has been given from the onset of the illness or trauma (Table 20-7). Full nutritional support should be started promptly for children who have lost weight prior to the illness or whose metabolic requirements are increased by the disease.[47]

Nutritional Considerations

Energy Needs. The energy recommendations of the National Research Council for children are designed for normal, healthy, growing children and include a substantial allowance for activity. Activity is decreased with illness, but increased energy needs are imposed by the illness. Trauma (operative or accidental), thermal injury, sepsis with or without fever, and congenital heart disease all result in various degrees of hypermetabolism.[48] Increased requirements may be

TABLE 20-8 Maintenance or Hospital Energy Requirements for Children[47,48]

Weight	Energy Requirements
3–10 kg	100 kcal/kg
11–20 kg	1,000 kcal + 100 kcal/2 kg > 10 kg
> 20 kg	1,500 kcal + 100 kcal/5 kg > 20 kg

offset by decreased needs in some cases, so that the RDA for energy for age may be appropriate. Various formulas for estimating energy needs during illness have been proposed.[49] However, it is important to remember that there is a paucity of data regarding the metabolic response of the child to illness or trauma, and that much of the information is extrapolated from adult research data.

Table 20-8 presents guidelines for determining energy needs of the ill child based on weight. These formulas can also be used to determine fluid needs by substituting milliliters per kilogram for kilocalories per kilogram.

Established formulas for calculating energy requirements include the Harris-Benedict equation to determine basal energy expenditure (BEE) and Seashore's equation for determining basal metabolic rate (BMR).[50] Many centers use the Harris-Benedict equation for children over 10 years of age.[51] A newer equation has been developed for infants:[51]

$$\text{kcal/24 hr} = 22.1 + (31.05 \times \text{Weight in kg}) + (1.16 \times \text{Height in cm})$$

Seashore's formula for BMR is:

$$\text{BMR (kcal/day)} = [55 - (2 \times \text{Age in yr})] \times \text{Weight in kg}$$

This formula can be used for children who are between the 10th and 90th percentiles for weight. For under- or overweight children, weight-age should be used (see Chapter 18, Pediatric Nutritional Assessment) rather than chronological age. Table 20-9 presents Seashore's guidelines for the estimation of total daily energy needs using the formula for BMR plus adjustments for activity and stress. This method is appropriate for children up to age 15. After age 15, the Harris-Benedict equation can be used.[50]

Assessment of basal energy requirements by indirect calorimetry provides a more precise estimate of energy expenditure and is warranted in situations of more long-term critical illness.[47,51,52]

Protein Needs.   Protein requirements are increased by severe trauma or illness. The initial response of the body to illness or to stress is the mobilization of protein for the synthesis of proteins associated with the immune response. In addition, there is an increased use of amino acids in the liver for gluconeogenesis, which can result in a negative nitrogen balance.[47] Protein requirements are related to (1) the previous nutritional state of the infant or child, (2) the length and severity of the catabolic state, and (3) the amount of extrarenal losses that may be occurring.

TABLE 20-9   Estimation of Energy Requirements

		Add
BMR:	$[55 - (2 \times \text{Age in Years})] \times \text{Weight in kg}$	_____
Maintenance: (includes specific dynamic action and amount of energy needed for equilibrium in the resting but awake state with minimal muscular movements)	Basal + 20%	_____
Activity: (0% for comatose state, 25% for hospitalized child who ambulates 2 to 3 times a day, 50% for active non-hospitalized child)	Basal + 0–25%	_____
Sepsis:	Basal + 13% for Each 1°C above Normal	_____
Simple Trauma:	Basal + 20%	_____
Multiple Injuries:	Basal + 40%	_____
Burns:	Basal + 50–100%	_____
Growth and Anabolism: (100% for growth in infancy and adolescence; 50% for the years in between)	Basal + 50–100%	_____
TOTAL		_____

With permission from: Seashore JH. Nutritional support of children in the intensive care unit. Yale J Biol Med 1984; 57:111–134.

Vitamins and Mineral Needs.   Provision of levels of vitamins and minerals to meet the RDA for age is generally considered adequate except when there are large losses related to specific disease states, such as burns, renal disease, and malabsorption states. Additional supplementation of the nutrients involved is discussed in those sections.

Nutritional Support

Nutritional care planning for the sick child includes determination of the child's nutritional requirements, selection of the most appropriate avenue for the delivery of the kilocalories and nutrients necessary to prevent nutritional depletion, and selection of the most appropriate feeding or formula.[47]

Oral Feeding.   The gastrointestinal tract should be used whenever possible, preferably by oral ingestion. High protein and/or high kilocalorie supplements added to the diet may be useful, since children are rather limited in their ability and willingness to increase their volume of dietary intake. Small, frequent feedings of familiar foods rather than 3 large meals may result in greater intake. Close follow-up of intake is necessary to evaluate the success of the nutritional care plan and to make adjustments to ensure adequate nutritional intake.

Enteral Feeding.   Tube feeding, either alone or in conjunction with other avenues, may be necessary to achieve adequate intake when oral intake is inadequate. Commercially prepared formulas are preferred because of better sanitation and reliability of nutritional content. The product chosen should be evaluated for nutritional adequacy (see Appendix 25 for nutritional content of infant formulas and feedings), and appropriate supplements should be provided. See Chapter 29, Pediatric Enteral Nutrition.

Parenteral Nutrition.   Parenteral nutrition is appropriate only when the gastrointestinal tract cannot be used. In younger children, a parenteral nutrition solution designed for children, rather than adults, should be used (see Chapter 29, Pediatric Parenteral Nutrition).

References

47. Wesley JR, Coran AG. Intravenous nutrition for the pediatric patient. Semin Pediatr Surg 1992;1(3):212–230.
48. Kien CL. Energy metabolism and requirements in disease. In: Walker WA, Watkins JP, eds. Nutrition in pediatrics: basic science and clinical application. Boston: Little, Brown, 1985:87.
49. Hendricks KM. Estimation of energy needs. In: Walker WA, Hendricks KM, eds. Manual of pediatric nutrition. Philadelphia: WB Saunders, 1990:59–71.
50. Seashore JH. Nutritional support of children in the intensive care unit. Yale J Biol Med 1984;57:111–134.
51. Kerner JA. Parenteral nutrition. In: Walker WA, Durie PR, Hamilton JR, Walker-Smith JA, Watkins JB, eds. Pediatric gastrointestinal disease: pathophysiology, diagnosis, management. Vol 2, Part 7. Philadelphia: BC Decker, 1991:1645–1675.
52. Wesley JR. Nutrient metabolism in relation to the systemic stress response. In: Fuhrman B, Zimmerman JJ, eds. Pediatric critical care. St Louis: Mosby–Year Book, 1992:755–774.

PART IV

Nutritional Management of Diseases and Disorders for Infants, Children, and Adolescents

21 / *Allergy in Children*

ALLERGY

General Description

Symptoms of food allergy vary among individual children. Treatment involves elimination of the offending food(s) from the diet. Nutrient deficiencies may result from this reduced variety of foods in the child's diet. Therefore, the nutrient intake of the child with food allergies may need to be carefully monitored.

Nutritional Inadequacy

Vitamin or mineral supplements may be indicated, depending on the specific foods or groups of foods that must be eliminated from the diet. An assessment of the diet for nutritional adequacy should be done for each individual child.

Indications and Rationale

Despite the strides made in many areas of healthcare, much confusion still exists in the area of food allergy. This confusion may be explained first by the fact that the term "food allergy" is used incorrectly to describe any type of adverse reaction to foods. Secondly, the problem of food allergy is complex. Finally, although the diagnostic procedures and laboratory tests presently available are effective in diagnosing true food allergy, they are inadequate in identifying adverse but nonallergic reactions to food.

Adverse reactions to foods and food additives may be broadly classified into two types: immunological reactions (food allergy) and nonimmunological reactions (food intolerance). Nonimmunological reactions may be attributable to a pharmacological or a toxic action of the food or the result of an enzyme deficiency. Examples of food or food additive intolerances are lactose intolerance and reactions to tartrazine or to sulfite compounds. The exact incidence of all adverse reactions to foods is unknown. However, food intolerances outnumber immunological or food allergy reactions.

TABLE 21-1 Classification of Foods into Food Families

ANIMAL SOURCES

Mollusks
Abalone
Mussel
Oyster
Scallop
Clam
Squid

Amphibians
Frog

Mammals
Beef
Pork
Goat
Mutton
Venison
Horsemeat
Rabbit
Squirrel

Crustaceans
Crab
Crayfish
Lobster
Shrimp

Reptiles
Turtle

Birds
Chicken
Duck
Goose
Turkey
Guinea hen
Squab
Pheasant
Partridge
Grouse

Fish
Sturgeon
Hake
Anchovy
Sardine
Herring
Haddock
Bass
Trout
Salmon
Whitefish
Scrod
Shad
Eel
Carp
Codfish
Halibut
Catfish
Sole
Pike

Fish (cont'd)
Flounder
Drum
Mullet
Weakfish
Mackerel
Tuna
Pompano
Bluefish
Snapper
Sunfish
Swordfish

PLANT SOURCES

Grain Family
Wheat
  Graham flour
  Gluten flour
  Bran
  Wheat germ
Rye
Barley
  Malt
Corn
Oats
Rice
Wild rice
Sorghum
Cane

Mustard Family
Mustard
Cabbage
Cauliflower
Broccoli
Brussels sprouts
Turnip
Rutabaga
Kale
Collard
Celery cabbage
Kohlrabi
Radish
Horseradish
Watercress

Ginger Family
Ginger
Turmeric
Cardamon

Pine Family
Juniper

Orchid Family
Vanilla

Madder Family
Coffee

Tea Family
Tea

Pedalium Family
Sesame seed

Mallow Family
Okra
Cottonseed

Spurge Family
Tapioca

Arrowroot Family
Arrowroot

Arum Family
Taro

Buckwheat Family
Buckwheat
Rhubarb

Potato Family
Potato
Tomato
Eggplant

Gooseberry Family
Gooseberry
Currant

Honeysuckle Family
Elderberry

Citrus Family
Orange
Grapefruit
Lemon
Lime
Tangerine
Kumquat

Pineapple Family
Pineapple

Papaw Family
Papaya

Birch Family
Filbert
Hazelnut

Mulberry Family
Mulberry
Fig
Hop
Breadfruit

Maple Family
Maple syrup

Palm Family
Coconut
Date
Sago

Pomegranate Family
Pomegranate

Ebony Family
Persimmon

Rose Family
Raspberry
Blackberry
Loganberry
Boysenberry
Dewberry
Strawberry

TABLE 21-1 Classification of Foods into Food Families—cont'd

PLANT SOURCES—cont'd

Banana Family	**Poppy Family**	**Parsley Family**	**Morning Glory Family**
Banana	Poppy seed	Parsley	Sweet potato
Plantain		Parsnip	Yam
	Plum Family	Carrot	
Grape Family	Plum	Celery	**Sunflower Family**
Grape	Prune	Celeriac	Jerusalem artichoke
Raisin	Cherry	Caraway	Sunflower seed
	Peach	Anise	
Myrtle Family	Apricot	Dill	**Pepper Family**
Allspice	Nectarine	Coriander	Black pepper
Cloves	Almond	Fennel	
Paprika			**Nutmeg Family**
Guava	**Laurel Family**	**Heath Family**	Nutmeg
	Avocado	Cranberry	
Mint Family	Cinnamon	Blueberry	**Walnut Family**
Mint	Bay leaf		English walnut
Peppermint		**Legythis Family**	Black walnut
Spearmint	**Olive Family**	Brazil nut	Butternut
Thyme	Green olive		Hickory nut
Sage	Ripe olive	**Composite Family**	Pecan
Marjoram	Red pepper	Leaf lettuce	
Savory	Green pepper	Head lettuce	**Cashew Family**
	Bell pepper	Endive	Cashew
Gourd Family	Chili	Escarole	Pistachio
Pumpkin	Tabasco	Artichoke	Mango
Squash	Pimiento	Dandelion	
Cucumber		Oyster plant	**Beech Family**
Cantaloupe	**Lily Family**	Chicory	Beechnut
Muskmelon	Asparagus		Chestnut
Honeydew melon	Onion	**Legume Family**	
Persian melon	Garlic	Navy bean	**Fungi Family**
Casaba	Leek	Kidney bean	Mushroom
Watermelon	Chive	Lima bean	Yeast
	Aloe	String bean	
Apple Family		Soybean	**Sterculia Family**
Apple	**Goosefoot Family**	Lentil	Cocoa
Pear	Beet	Black-eyed pea	Chocolate
Quince	Spinach	Pea	
	Swiss chard	Peanut	
		Licorice	
		Acacia	
		Senna	

With permission from: Metcalfe DD. The diagnosis of food allergy: theory and practice. In: Spector SL, ed. Provocative challenge procedures: background and methodology. Mt. Kisco, NY: Futura Publishing Co., 1989.

Food allergy may appear at any age, but true allergic reactions to foods are most common in infants and young children and decrease in frequency with age.[1] Allergic reactions are most commonly caused by relatively few foods, which include milk, fish, eggs, nuts, soy, wheat, and peanuts.[2-4] The causative food is called an allergen. The allergic reaction is almost always immediate and may affect the skin (hives, itching, eczema), the respiratory system (swelling of the throat, sneezing, coughing, wheezing, nasal stuffiness), the gastrointestinal tract (vomiting, diarrhea, cramping), and the cardiovascular system (anaphylactic shock). Symptoms of food allergy are not uniform and may vary from child to child. There is a dose-response effect with food allergy: ingestion of small quantities of allergenic food may produce minimal or no symptoms, while ingestion of larger quantities may produce widespread symptoms. An anaphylactic shocklike reaction strongly suggests that exposure to that allergen will result in another shocklike reaction. A child who is allergic to one food may be allergic to foods in related food families. Peanuts, for example, belong to the pea family; persons who cannot eat peanuts may not be able to eat beans or peas. They usually are able to tolerate nuts because true nuts are in a different food family. The food family list[5] is shown in Table 21-1.

True food allergy is not difficult to diagnose. The diagnosis is usually made by history. Verification by allergic skin testing or by measurement of food-specific IgE (allergy-causing) antibodies in serum by radioallergosorbent testing, or RAST, is usually helpful in identifying a true allergic reaction.

Goal of Dietary Management

The goal of management is to design a diet that does not include the offending food(s) but ensures meeting the child's nutritional needs.

Dietary Recommendations

There is no standard procedure for identifying suspected food allergies in children. Offending foods can often be identified by the patient and by taking a diet history. A diet can be devised that does not include suspected foods.[6]

Children with suspected multiple food allergies or intolerances who appear to tolerate an extremely limited number of foods need intensive evaluation to determine which foods truly cannot be tolerated. It is very uncommon to be allergic to more than two foods from different food groups. After evaluation by an allergist, it may be necessary to hospitalize the child and provide an elemental diet to see if symptoms abate. If the symptoms resolve, suspected foods are added to the diet in a double-blind fashion to attempt to reproduce the clinical exacerbation of allergy. Results of challenge feeding may be correlated with results of testing for specific IgE by skin test or invitro methods, such as RAST.

Periodically, challenges with foods known to cause an allergic reaction should be done since a significant number of children are able to tolerate the food as they grow older. Challenge with foods believed to cause anaphylactic reactions should not be done.[4,7]

Physicians: How to Order Diet

The diet order should indicate *foods necessary to avoid due to food allergy(ies) and/or intolerances*. The dietitian designs and monitors the diet assuring nutritional adequacy. Specific guidelines to aid in management of various food allergies or intolerances are available.[6,8] Chapter 6, Adult Food Allergy and Intolerance, also provides guidelines for managing allergies and intolerances to foods.

References

1. Foucard T. Developmental aspects of food sensitivity in childhood. Nutr Rev 1984;42: 98–104.
2. May CD. Food allergy: perspective, principles, practical management. Nutr Today 1980;Nov–Dec:28–31.
3. Cant AJ. Food allergy in childhood. Hum Nutr 1985;39A:277–293.
4. Forbes GB, Woodruff CW. Hypersensitivity to food. In: Forbes GB, Woodruff CW, eds. Pediatric nutrition handbook. Elk Grove, IL: American Academy of Pediatrics, 1985: 257–266.
5. Metcalfe DD, Sampson HA, Simon RD. Food allergy: adverse reactions to foods and food additives. Oxford: Blackwell Scientific Publications, 1991.
6. Anon. Food allergy. In: DiLima SN, ed. Dietitian's patient education manual. Vol 1. Gaithersburg, MD: Aspen Pub, 1992:5:1–5:25.
7. Sachs MI, Yunginger JW. Food-induced anaphylaxis. Immunol Allergy Clin North Am 1991;11(4):743–755.
8. Olejer V. Managing food allergies in infants and toddlers. In: Perkin JE, ed. Food allergies and adverse reactions. Gaithersburg, MD: Aspen Pub 1990:117–128.

22 / *Cardiovascular Diseases in Childhood*

HYPERTENSION

General Description

Treatment should be individualized for children with hypertension. The least amount of intervention required to achieve blood pressure goals while maintaining a high degree of compliance is optimal treatment for elevated blood pressure in childhood. Nonpharmacological intervention is the initial treatment and focuses on dietary sodium modification, weight control, and exercise training. Even when, in the rare patient, antihypertensive drug therapy is used to control blood pressure, these intervention strategies should be maintained.

Indications and Rationale

Data linking cardiovascular risk with systolic and diastolic blood pressures in children are not available.[1] There is, however, growing concern about the possible relationship between minor elevations of blood pressure in youth and the subsequent development of adult essential hypertension with the associated risks of heart attack and stroke. There is strong indirect evidence supporting the benefit of blood pressure lowering in hypertensive children and adolescents. Blood pressure levels in the child and adolescent are dependent upon many factors both genetic and environmental. For example, blood pressure normally increases with age during the preadult years. Larger children (heavier and/or taller) have higher blood pressures than smaller children of the same age. Obese children have higher blood pressures than lean children. Therefore, the level of a child or adolescent's blood pressure must be considered with respect to both body size and age.

In order to identify and treat hypertension, the measurement of a child's blood pressure is necessary at each visit to the physician. Measurements above the 90 percentile of the distribution for age and sex should be a reason for further follow-up to determine whether there is a consistent trend toward hypertension.

483

TABLE 22-1   Definitions

Term	Definition
Normal BP	Systolic and diastolic BPs < 90th percentile for age and sex
High normal BP*	Average systolic and/or average diastolic BP between 90th and 95th percentiles for age and sex
High BP (hypertension)	Average systolic and/or average diastolic BPs ≥ 95th percentile for age and sex with measurements obtained on at least three occasions

BP = blood pressure.

*If the BP reading is high normal for age, but can be accounted for by excess height for age or excess lean body mass for age, such children are considered to have normal BP.

With permission from: Task Force on Blood Pressure in Children. Report of the Second Task Force on Blood Pressure Control in Children. Pediatrics 1987;79:1–25.

TABLE 22-2   Classification of Hypertension by Age Group*

Age Group	High-Normal (mm Hg; ≤ 90th Percentile)	Significant Hypertension (mm Hg; ≤ 95th Percentile)	Severe Hypertension (mm Hg; > 99th Percentile)
Newborn			
7 days (supine)	Systolic BP ≥ 90	Systolic BP ≥ 96	Systolic BP ≥ 106
8–30 days (supine)	Systolic BP ≥ 98	Systolic BP ≥ 104	Systolic BP ≥ 110
Infant (< 2 yr)	Systolic BP ≥ 105	Systolic BP ≥ 112	Systolic BP ≥ 118
	Diastolic BP ≥ 70	Diastolic BP ≥ 74	Diastolic BP ≥ 82
Children			
3–5 yr	Systolic BP ≥ 108	Systolic BP ≥ 116	Systolic BP ≥ 124
	Diastolic BP ≥ 70	Diastolic BP ≥ 76	Diastolic BP ≥ 84
6–9 yr	Systolic BP ≥ 114	Systolic BP ≥ 122	Systolic BP ≥ 130
	Diastolic BP ≥ 72	Diastolic BP ≥ 78	Diastolic BP ≥ 86
10–12 yr	Systolic BP ≥ 120	Systolic BP ≥ 126	Systolic BP ≥ 134
	Diastolic BP ≥ 75	Diastolic BP ≥ 82	Diastolic BP ≥ 90
Adolescents			
13–15 yr	Systolic BP ≥ 126	Systolic BP ≥ 136	Systolic BP ≥ 144
	Diastolic BP ≥ 78	Diastolic BP ≥ 86	Diastolic BP ≥ 92
16–18 yr	Systolic BP ≥ 132	Systolic BP ≥ 142	Systolic BP ≥ 150
	Diastolic BP ≥ 82	Diastolic BP ≥ 92	Diastolic BP ≥ 98

*Data should be interpreted with a knowledge of the child's height and weight.

With permission from: Task Force on Blood Pressure in Children. Report of the Second Task Force on Blood Pressure Control in Children. Pediatrics 1987;79:1–25.

Preventive measures include avoiding excessive sodium consumption, maintaining optimal weight, exercising regularly, and avoiding the use of tobacco.[2,3]

Definitions and classifications of hypertension are presented in Tables 22-1 and 22-2 respectively. These are modifications of those developed by the Second Task Force on Hypertension in Children[1] and are based not on risk data but on clinical judgment and consensus. An algorithm for the systematic identification of children with elevated blood pressure measurements in need of diagnostic evaluation and treatment is shown in Figure 22-1. This outline from the Second Task Force Report does not address all of the variables that affect blood pressure in the preadult years but makes the assessment more precise than when age alone is used. Just as it is important for children "probably at risk" to receive a therapeutic intervention, it is also important that children at "marginal risk" not receive potentially harmful treatment. Tables showing the percentile of blood pressure measurements as a function of age and sex are in the Report of the Second Task Force on Hypertension and Children.[1]

A national survey revealed substantial differences among physicians in managing cardiovascular disease risk factors in children aged 2 to 18 years.[2] Generally, counseling for cardiovascular risk factors such as family history, diet, overweight, lack of exercise, and use of tobacco should be the emphasis in treating children and adolescents with hypertension. Nonpharmacological intervention strategies including weight reduction, physical conditioning, and dietary modification should be the initial treatment.

Goals of Dietary Management

The primary goal is to achieve gradual reduction in children's sodium intake while maintaining nutritional adequacy for growth and development.[3] Weight control is essential for blood pressure control and should be included in the recommended dietary modifications if appropriate (see Chapter 23, Pediatric Weight Control). Emphasis is placed on modification of current dietary practices: substitution of more appropriate foods that are lower in sodium content and controlled in calories rather than recommending significant changes or complete elimination of favorite foods. The dietary modifications are to be made gradually over several months and at a pace identified as reasonable for each individual child or adolescent. The goal is long term, with emphasis on gradually developing a lifestyle that can be maintained into adulthood. The new eating habits must be implemented in a way that allows the child or adolescent to maintain a good self-image and must be flexible enough to accomodate a lifestyle that may include school lunch, fast foods, and other favorite foods.

Dietary Recommendations

Dietary factors probably make an important environmental contribution to blood pressure elevation in essential hypertension. Little information is available on the effects of changes in dietary habits as a means of preventing or treating high blood pressure.[4,5] It is likely that a trend toward elevated blood pressure in childhood predicts a greater chance for developing significant hypertension in adult life, while consistently normal blood pressure measurements in childhood may mean that hypertension in adult life is less likely.[1]

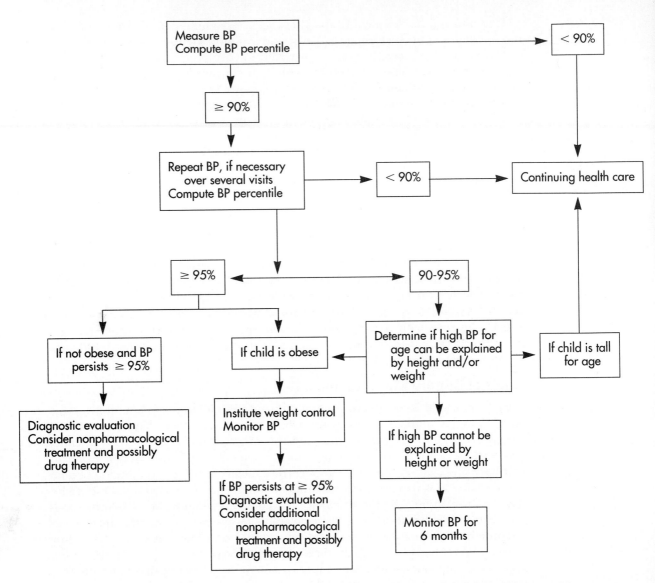

FIGURE 22-1 Algorithm for identifying children with high blood pressure (BP). Note: Whenever BP measurement is stipulated, the average of at least two measurements should be used. (With permission from: Task Force on Blood Pressure in Children. Report of the Second Task Force on Blood Pressure Control in Children. Pediatrics 1987;79:1–25.)

The sodium intake of children is far in excess of that required for health.[3] Therefore, the potential benefit of dietary sodium reduction appears to outweigh any potential risk from this form of intervention. The degree of sodium control required to effectively lower blood pressure has not been established, and a practical method for identification of sodium-sensitive subjects is not currently available. The Second Task Force and the American Heart Association Nutrition Committee recommendations limit dietary sodium to 85 to 100 mEq (2 to 2.3 g of dietary sodium or 5 to 6 g of sodium chloride) per day.[1] This would represent a significant reduction from the current average American sodium intake. In our practice, limiting dietary sodium to 90 to 150 mEq/day is common and still represents a significant decrease while perhaps enhancing compliance by not restricting the diet unnecessarily. Obtaining a profile of the child's usual sodium intake by considering types, amounts, and frequency of use of high sodium foods, methods of food preparation, and use of table salt is useful in individualizing the dietary recommendation. Improvement is the goal, so a stepwise progression in sodium control is recommended. There are no conclusive data concerning the roles of potassium, calcium, or magnesium supplementation in blood pressure control in children. (See also Chapter 7, Hypertension, for further information on sodium control.)

Physicians: How to Order Diet

The diet order should indicate a *diet for sodium control* for the hypertensive child or adolescent. Cholesterol and total fat control and/or weight control (dietitian will determine calorie levels) should also be stated in the diet order.

References

1. Task Force on Blood Pressure Control in Children. Report of the Second Task Force on Blood Pressure Control in Children. Pediatrics 1987;79:1–25.
2. Grobbee D. Interference with dietary habits in young hypertensive-prone subjects. J Hypertens 1989;7:525–528.
3. Mendoza SA. Hypertension in infants and children. Nephron 1990;54:289–295.
4. Kimm SYS, Payne GH, Lakatos E, Darby C, Sparrow A. Management of cardiovascular disease risk factors in children. Am J Dis Child 1990;144:967–972.
5. Witschi SC, Capper AL, Hosmer DW, Ellison RC. Sources of sodium, potassium, and energy in the diets of adolescents. J Am Diet Assoc 1987;87(12):1651–1655.

HYPERLIPIDEMIA

General Description

The initial management of children with hyperlipidemia should be a diet reduced in fat and cholesterol as recommended by the National Cholesterol Education Program's Expert Panel on Blood Cholesterol Levels in Children and Adolescents.[6] These "high-risk" children should be followed closely. The same diet is recommended for the general population of healthy children over the age of 2 years.

Nutritional Inadequacy

This diet is planned to meet the Recommended Daily Allowances (RDA) for calories and all nutrients. The diet may be inappropriate in children who are malnourished or who have special nutritional needs.[7] Care should be taken not to recommend severe restrictions in fat and cholesterol, because such diets may supply inadequate kilocalories and interfere with normal growth and development.[8] Children following low fat and cholesterol-restricted diets should be followed with periodic measurement of height and weight to assure that normal growth and development are taking place. If growth is less than desirable, an effort should be made to increase calorie and protein intake.

Indications and Rationale

The atherosclerotic process is accelerated by high blood cholesterol levels[6] and begins in childhood. It progresses in adolescence and young adulthood, even though serious clinical manifestations usually do not appear until middle age or later.[9] The evidence that establishes a causal relationship between blood cholesterol levels and coronary heart disease comes from genetic, experimental pathological, epidemiological, and intervention studies. However, it is clear that an elevated blood cholesterol level is not the only cause of coronary artery disease. Factors associated with risk for development of the disease are documented in adults. Whether or not these risk factors operate in children to exert influences over the atherosclerotic process is not firmly established.

There are some risk factors for cardiovascular disease that are nonalterable, such as sex and genetic differences. Risk factors potentially modifiable in childhood include cigarette smoking, sedentary lifestyle, obesity (see Chapter 23), hypertension (see Chapter 22), and elevated plasma total and low density lipoprotein cholesterol. Healthy food habits in early childhood are important. Unfavorable lifestyle and eating habits may be more easily correctable in youth than later in life, when both may be more intractable and self-perpetuating.

Goals of Dietary Management

The primary goal is to achieve moderate changes in children's cholesterol and fat intake while maintaining nutritional adequacy for growth and development. Excessive weight gain is to be avoided. Emphasis is placed on substitution and modification of current dietary practices rather than on inducing a drastic change or complete elimination of favorite foods. The dietary modifications are to be made gradually over several months and at a pace identified as reasonable for each individual child and adolescent. The goal should be long term, with emphasis on gradually setting a lifestyle that can persist into adulthood. The new eating habits must be implemented in a way that allows the child or adolescent to maintain a good self-image and must be flexible enough to accomodate a reasonable lifestyle.

Dietary Recommendations

Children at Risk for Coronary Artery Disease.   Children at high risk can often be identified from a family history of hyperlipidemia, premature coronary heart disease, hypertension, or stroke.[6,9] These children should have two total cholesterol, triglyceride, and high density lipoprotein cholesterol (HDLC) determinations. Low density lipoprotein cholesterol (LDLC) can be calculated using the Friedewald formula:[10]

$$LDLC = \text{Total Cholesterol} - \left(HDLC + \frac{\text{Triglycerides}}{5}\right)$$

If the calculated LDLC is between the 75th and 90th percentiles (approximately 110 to 129 mg/dl for ages 2 to 19 years), the child is counseled regarding diet and other cardiovascular risk factors and then followed at 3 to 6 month intervals. Those with LDLC levels above the 95th percentile (greater than 135 mg/dl) may have familial hypercholesterolemia; they should receive counseling for diet and cardiovascular risk factors and be reevaluated at 3 to 6 month intervals. Table 22-3 lists the National Cholesterol Education Program's dietary guidelines, which are used in treating children and adolescents at risk for cardiovascular disease.[6] Nonresponders to the Step One diet are counseled about a more controlled diet (Step Two). In this diet, 30% of calories are from fat, but with saturated fat levels reduced to less than 7% of total calories and cholesterol to less than 200 mg/day. Nonresponders to the second diet should be considered for treatment with a lipid-lowering agent. Again, counseling regarding cardiovascular risk factors is carried out. These children are usually followed at 3 to 6 month intervals.

If the child has hypertriglyceridemia and is overweight, a low fat and cholesterol-restricted diet is designed with calories for weight control[9] (see Chapter 23, Weight Control). Some children may require carbohydrate restriction in addition. Increased physical activity is essential.[10] If the child is of normal weight, then familial hypertriglyceridemia, alcohol use, other secondary causes, or laboratory error should be considered.[9]

TABLE 22-3 Characteristics of Step One and Step Two Diets for Lowering Blood Cholesterol

Nutrient	Recommended Intake	
	Step One Diet	Step Two Diet
Total fat	Average of no more than 30% of total calories	Same
Saturated fatty acids	Less than 10% of total calories	Less than 7% of total calories
Polyunsaturated fatty acids	Up to 10% of total calories	Same
Monounsaturated fatty acids	Remaining total fat calories	Same
Cholesterol	Less than 300 mg/day	Less than 200 mg/day
Carbohydrates	About 55% of total calories	Same
Protein	About 15–20% of total calories	Same
Calories	To promote normal growth and development and to reach or maintain desirable body weight	Same

With permission from: National Cholesterol Education Program: Report of the expert panel on blood cholesterol levels in children and adolescents. NIH Publication No. 91-2732. Washington DC: U.S. Department of Health and Human Services, September 1991.

TABLE 22-4   American Heart Association Dietary Guidelines for Healthy Children over 2 Years of Age

1. The diet should be nutritionally adequate, consisting of a variety of foods.

2. Caloric intake should be based on growth rate, activity level, and content of deposits of subcutaneous fat, so as to maintain desirable body weight.

3. Total fat intake should be approximately 30% of kilocalories, with 10% or less from saturated fat, about 10% from monounsaturated fat, and less than 10% from polyunsaturated fat. The emphasis should be on reducing total fat and saturated fat rather than on increasing polyunsaturated fat.

4. Daily cholesterol intake should be approximately 100 mg per 1,000 kcal, not to exceed 300 mg. This allows for differences in caloric intake in various age groups.

5. Protein intake should be about 15% of kilocalories derived from varied sources.

6. Carbohydrate kilocalories should be derived primarily from complex carbohydrate sources to provide necessary vitamins and minerals. Thus, the total percent of kilocalories from carbohydrates would be about 55%.

7. Excessive salt intake may be associated with hypertension in susceptible persons. On the whole, the American diet contains excessive amounts of salt. Therefore, a limitation on most highly salted processed foods and sodium-containing condiments and the elimination of added salt at the table are recommended.

With permission from: Weidman WH, Kwiterovitch P, Jesse MJ, Nugent E. Diet in the healthy child. Circulation 1983;67:1411A–1414A.

Healthy Children over 2 Years of Age.   The American Heart Association has advised a gradual shift from the current typical diet to one that is restricted in total fat, saturated fat, cholesterol, and sodium. The guidelines in Table 22-4 are recommended for healthy children over 2 years of age.[7] These recommendations are consistent with those of the National Cholesterol Education Program,[6] the U.S. Department of Agriculture and Department of Health and Human Services,[11] the Surgeon General,[12] the National Cancer Institute,[13] and the National Research Council.[14]

Physicians: How to Order Diet

The diet order should indicate, for the high risk child, *fat and cholesterol-restricted diet.* For the otherwise healthy child, the diet order should also indicate *fat and cholesterol-restricted diet.* If appropriate, weight control or reduction should also be stated (the dietitian will determine the caloric level). Other modifications should also be indicated (e.g., sodium restriction).

References

6. National Cholesterol Education Program. Report of the Expert Panel on Blood Cholesterol Levels in Children and Adolescents. NIH Publication No. 91-2732. Washington DC: U.S. Department of Health and Human Services, Sep 1991.

7. Weidman W, Kwiterovich P, Jesse MJ, Nugent E. Diet in the healthy child. Circulation 1983;67:1411A–1414A.

8. Fifshitz F, Moses N. Growth failure: a complication of dietary treatment of hyperlipidemia. Am J Dis Child 1989;143(5):537–542.

9. American Heart Association. Position statement: diagnosis and treatment of primary hyperlipidemia in childhood. Arteriosclerosis 1986;6(6):685A–692A.

10. Friedewald WT, Levy RI, Frederickson DS. Estimation of the concentration of low density lipoprotein cholesterol in plasma without use of the preparation ultracentrifuge. Clin Chem 1972;18(6):499–502.

11. Becque M, Katch VL, Rocchini AP, Marks CR, Moorehead C. Coronary risk incidence of obese adolescents: reduction by exercise plus diet intervention. Pediatrics 1988;82 (5):605–612.

12. USDA and USDHHS. Nutrition and your health: dietary guidelines for Americans, 3rd ed. Rev. November 1990. Home and Garden Bulletin No. 232. Washington, DC: USDA/USDHHS, Nov 1990.

13. Department of Health and Human Services. The Surgeon General's report on nutrition and health: summary and recommendations. DHHS Publication No. (PHS) 88-50211. Washington, DC: USPHS, 1988.

14. National Cancer Institute. Diet nutrition and cancer prevention: the good news. NIH Publication No. 87-2878. Bethesda, MD: USDHHS, Dec 1986.

15. Subcommittee on the Tenth Edition of the RDAs. Recommended Dietary Allowances, 10th ed. Washington, DC: National Academy Press, 1989.

PEDIATRIC CARDIAC SURGERY

General Description

The dietary progression for postoperative pediatric cardiac surgery patients is restricted in sodium and otherwise is similar to the progression for other types of surgery.

Nutritional Inadequacy

The diet for pediatric cardiac surgery patients is not inherently lacking in nutrients as compared to the RDA.

Indications and Rationale

Sodium intake is controlled as a precaution against congestive heart failure. (See Chapter 7, Hypertension; for the approximate sodium content of foods, see Tables 7-4 and 7-5.) The child follows the diet postoperatively until his or her dismissal from the hospital or for several weeks after dismissal. Depending on the child's progress, the sodium content of the diet is then increased, and this diet is followed for several weeks or longer. After this time, many patients may resume their usual dietary practices. The degree and duration of the sodium restriction vary with the type of surgery and with the response of the patient.[16]

Goals of Dietary Management

The goals of dietary management for children who have had cardiac surgery are aimed at providing the nutrients needed to support the healing process while controlling sodium to help prevent congestive failure.[17]

TABLE 22-5   Estimation of Energy Needs for Children Having Cardiac
Surgery[18]

Presurgical Body Weight (kg)	Suggested Kcal Intake
< 10	100 × kg of body weight
10–20	1,000 + 50 for each kg of body weight over 10 kg
> 20	1,500 + 20 for each kg of body weight over 20 kg

With permission from: Holliday HA, Segar WE. The maintenance need for water in parenteral fluid therapy. Pediatrics 1957;19:823–832.

Dietary Recommendations

Postoperatively there are two levels of sodium control. The first is a strict sodium restriction, the second is a mild sodium restriction:

Strict sodium restriction:	1 mEq/100 kcal
	(23 mg/100 kcal)
Mild sodium restriction:	4 mEq/100 kcal
	(92 mg/100 kcal)

Table 22-5 may be used to estimate the child's caloric needs.[18] (Also see Chapter 20, Sick Infants, Children, and Adolescents.)

Many pediatric cardiac patients are admitted for surgery with significant retardation of height and weight secondary to undernutrition caused by manifestations of their heart disease.[19] Catch-up growth may occur once the immediate effects of surgery are past and if the cardiac defect has been successfully corrected.

In the several weeks after cardiac surgery, patients may experience complications of gastrointestinal distress and decreased appetite (see Chapter 7, Cardiac Surgery for Adults), which may make it difficult to achieve recommended kilocalorie and protein intake.[20] During hospitalization the dietary intake should be carefully monitored and the nutrition plan of care changed as necessary. Daily weights and the type of surgical procedure will aid in deciding the degree of sodium restriction needed.

Small, frequent feedings and cool items are usually better tolerated and can result in greater caloric intake. Energy-dense foods and higher protein items that fit within the sodium restriction may be used to increase nutrient intake in order to prevent body protein catabolism.

Physicians: How to Order Diet

The diet order should specify either *strict or mild sodium restriction,* along with the patient's preoperative weight. This diet order will be used for each stage of the postoperative series (clear liquid, full liquid, and soft diet). Requests for instruction in the home-going diet should also indicate the duration of each sodium restriction.

References

16. Driscoll DJ. Evaluation of the cyanotic newborn. In: Gillette PC, ed. The pediatric clinics of North America. Philadelphia: WB Saunders, 1990:1–23.
17. Kern LS, O'Brien P. The Fontan procedure. Heart Lung 1985;14:457–467.
18. Holliday HA, Segar WE. The maintenance need for water in parenteral fluid therapy. Pediatrics 1957;19:823–832.
19. Gervasio MR, Buchanan CN. Malnutrition in the pediatric cardiology patient. Crit Care Q 1985;8(3):49–56.
20. O'Brien P, Elizson M. The child following the Fontan procedure: nursing strategies. Am Assoc Crit Care Nurs 1990;14:457–467.

23 / Endocrine Metabolism Diseases and Disorders in Children

DIABETES MELLITUS

General Description

The diet for children with diabetes is planned to be adequate in essential nutrients to ensure normal growth and development. The kilocalorie content of the diet must meet changing energy needs for growth and activity level yet should prevent obesity. Total fat, saturated fat, and cholesterol are modified in the diet in an effort to minimize vascular complications.

The diet for diabetes is planned with 5 or 6 feedings a day in an effort to distribute caloric intake in a way that minimizes fluctuations in blood glucose concentrations, and to provide nutrients at the time of maximal insulin action in order to ensure efficient energy utilization. The meal plan must be individualized to reflect the child's likes and dislikes and to be consistent with the personal, cultural, and/or ethnic food choices of the child and the family.

Nutritional Inadequacy

The diet for diabetes is planned to meet the Recommended Dietary Allowances (RDA) for kilocalories and all nutrients. The diet must be assessed and adjusted periodically to maintain a normal rate of growth.

Indications and Rationale*

The nutrient needs of the child with diabetes are the same as those of the child who does not have diabetes (see Chapter 19, Healthy Infants, Children, and Adolescents). However, greater attention must be given to the timing of meals and snacks, the consistency of intake from day to day, and the composition and caloric content of food intake. Regular and intermediate insulins are adminis-

---

*See Chapter 8, Diabetes Mellitus, for a more complete description and discussion of diabetes.

tered at specific times each day, and meal and snack times are planned to correlate with the peak action times of these insulins. Therefore, it is important that meals are eaten at regular times each day, with day-to-day variation not to exceed 30 minutes. A consistent distribution of kilocalories, carbohydrate, and protein among meals and snacks is recommended to stabilize changes in blood glucose and to allow more predictable results following changes in insulin dose. The carbohydrate in the diet is distributed so that 25 to 30% is provided at each meal and 8 to 10% at each snack. The diet for the infant and the young child is planned with mid-morning, mid-afternoon, and bedtime snacks. Diets for older children are planned with mid-afternoon and bedtime snacks; if needed, a mid-morning snack can also be included. Protein foods from the meat and/or milk exchange lists are included with each meal and snack. However, if breakfast and lunch or lunch and dinner are closely spaced, it may be appropriate to plan just a fruit or a starch exchange for the snack between these meals. The use of simple carbohydrates is not recommended for the child with diabetes, in order to minimize plasma glucose fluctuations. Moderate use of noncaloric artificial sweeteners is allowed. Extensive reviews of the available safety data for noncaloric artificial sweeteners were published in the Diabetes Task Force Report for the Committee on Nutrition of the American Academy of Pediatrics. These suggested that aspartame was the preferred sweetener in the meal plan of young children and adolescents with diabetes.[1,2]

The young child who has diabetes needs the help of a family member to plan and prepare the diet. As the child gets older, the child needs to be encouraged to make decisions at meal times, with parents available for support. This assists the child in becoming more independent with meal selections, both at home and away from home. One should avoid transferring responsibilities for self-care too early and placing unrealistic expectations on the child.[3]

The diet for diabetes is based on food exchange lists (see Chapter 8, Diabetes Mellitus, Food Exchange Lists, and Infant Formulas and Feedings in Pediatric Appendix 25).

Goals of Dietary Management

The goals of dietary management for children with diabetes are to provide nutrients and kilocalories to achieve normal growth and development, to maintain or attain an appropriate body weight for height and age, and to prevent hyperglycemia and hypoglycemia. The diet prescription should be individualized in the meal plan design, the educational component, and the follow-up program.

Nutritional management is an integral part of overall diabetes therapy, which also includes insulin administration, regular participation in physical activity, and emotional support and guidance (see Chapter 8, Diabetes Mellitus, Community Support Programs).

Determining Energy and Protein Needs.   Kilocalorie needs of the child are determined primarily from the present dietary intake, which is obtained by a thorough diet history. Supportive data for energy needs include the RDA for age and sex of the child (see Chapter 2, Recommended Dietary Allowances), and the Nomogram for Estimating Caloric Requirements (see Appendix 6), and the estimated level of activity. Prevention of excessive weight gain is important as a general health and psychological issue. Prevalence of obesity in childhood diabetes has been shown to be no greater than in nondiabetic children, and it is important to remember that diabetes is not as well controlled in those who are obese.[4] The protein level of the diet should meet the RDA for the child's age and weight and should represent about 15 to 20% of the total kilocalories of the diet.

Determining Dietary Fat and Sodium Needs. The American Heart Association has made general dietary recommendations for healthy American children above 2 years old and for adolescents. These recommendations are relevant to the child with diabetes since such persons are at greater risk for atherosclerosis than are nondiabetics. The recommendations include (1) the control of fat intake to no more than 30% of total kilocalories (10% saturated, 10% polyunsaturated, 10 percent monounsaturated), (2) the limitation of cholesterol to 100 mg/1,000 cal (not to exceed 300 mg/day), and (3) the elimination of salt at the table and the limitation of intake of high salt-containing foods.[5] When designing the diabetic meal plan, these recommendations should be considered as a means of slowing the disease process and of establishing eating habits that, in adulthood, may help to deter atherosclerosis. For children with elevated serum lipids whose diabetes is under good control, a diet should be used with the total fat controlled to less than 30% of total calories (equal amounts of the three types of fatty acids) and the cholesterol controlled to less than 200 mg/day.[6] While efforts to achieve this diet design should be made, it may be difficult to get a child or adolescent to adhere to the more rigorous schedule.

Fiber. Few studies have been reported of children with diabetes who have achieved improved blood sugar control from use of fiber-supplemented diets; the studies that have been reported have contradictory results.[7,8] However, as a general health measure, increased use of whole-grain breads and cereals, fresh fruits, and uncooked vegetables is appropriate for the child. (See Chapter 8, Diabetes Mellitus, Fiber.)

Changing Preferences and Needs. The diet history aids in planning the distribution of nutrients among meals and snacks. One should consider likes and dislikes, school and activity schedules, use of fast food and restaurant meals, use of convenience foods, and family eating patterns. The diet is planned to modify existing food practices as realistically as possible and to ensure optimal nutrition for activity and normal growth and development. The diet should be re-evaluated periodically to accommodate the child's changing nutritional needs and preferences.

School Lunch. The child with diabetes may choose to eat a school lunch or a lunch brought from home. If a school lunch is chosen, the child can learn to select foods from the school cafeteria menu. The school lunch menu is often published in local newspapers, or it can be obtained from the school. The child and the parents can plan the child's lunch by reviewing the menu and deciding which items should be eaten and which should be avoided. Many school districts have begun offering fat-, cholesterol-, and sodium-controlled menu items. The school food service can usually be contacted to get serving sizes of casseroles, pizza, and other menu items. A school lunch may have to be supplemented with foods from home to meet the needs of the diet.

TABLE 23-1   USDA School Lunch Pattern

Components	Minimum Daily Quantities
Meat or meat alternate	2 oz
Vegetable and/or fruit	3/4 cup
Bread or bread alternate	8 servings/wk
Milk	1/2 pint

To include school lunch in the meal plan, the following lunch meal plan usually works well:

2 meat exchanges
2–3 fat exchanges
3 starch exchanges
1 milk exchange
1–2 vegetable and/or fruit exchanges

The United States Department of Agriculture (USDA) has established a meal pattern for five age or grade groups that reduces the minimum portion size for children age 8 and under and offers more food to children age 12 and over.[9] The school lunch pattern established for ages 9 to 12 years is shown in Table 23-1. This pattern is used if portions are not adjusted for age or grade groups.

Skim milk is increasingly available in school lunch programs. If skim milk is not available, the meal plan should allow for the type of milk the school serves. If the school offers only one type of milk, USDA regulations state that it must serve low fat milk (either skim or 2%).

Eating for Extra Activity.   The diet probably needs to be adjusted when the child with diabetes engages in activities more strenuous than those in the normal daily routine.[10] The insulin dose may also need to be adjusted for increased activity. Because of individual tolerances and needs, the child may have to try different amounts of food for a given amount of exercise; too much may result in excessive elevation in blood glucose, too little may result in hypoglycemia.

The guidelines used at Mayo Clinic for planning additional snacks for activity are given in Table 23-2.[11]

The added carbohydrate is taken as a snack before starting the activity and is taken in addition to the normal meal plan. Use of these guidelines and observation of blood glucose patterns before and after activity periods should allow the child to identify more closely how much extra food is needed for specific types and durations of exercise.

Physical education and recess periods ideally should be scheduled early in the morning or after lunch. If this is not possible, changes in the composition and/or the timing of meals and snacks may be necessary.

The child with diabetes should be instructed to carry a readily available source of carbohydrate (sugar cubes, pure sugar candy) to be used in the event of an insulin reaction.

Diet During Illness.   The stress of illness, whether attributable to infection or to any other cause, can raise the blood sugar and thus cause diabetes to go out of

TABLE 23-2   Dietary Guidelines during Activities

Glucose Level (mg/dl)	Type of Activity		
	Light (walking, slow biking)	Moderate (tennis, swimming, jogging, biking)	Heavy (football, hockey, racquetball, basketball, strenuous biking or swimming)
< 80	1 fruit or starch per hr	1 meat, 1 starch, and 1 milk or 1 fruit initially, then 1 fruit or 1 starch per hr	2 meat, 2 starch, 1 milk, and 1 fruit initially; monitor glucose carefully, eat as needed
80–179	None	1 fruit or 1 starch per hr	1 meat, 1 starch and 1 milk or 1 fruit per hr
180–300	None	None	1 fruit or 1 starch per hr
> 300	Do not exercise	Do not exercise	Do not exercise

With permission from: Jensen MD, Miles JM. The roles of diet and exercise in the management of patients with insulin-dependent diabetes mellitus. Mayo Clin Proc 1986;61:813–819.

control.[12] Even when a child is unable to eat, the stress of illness can bring on hormonal changes that may raise the blood sugar and thereby change insulin requirements. Many diabetics feel that because they are unable to eat, they do not need to take insulin. Diabetics should take at least the usual amount of insulin when ill, especially if the blood glucose is normal or elevated. If the blood glucose is decreased, the amount of insulin may be decreased. Changes in appetite and in the ability to tolerate the usual meal plan may require that the child's diet be modified during times of illness. Insulin and carbohydrate are needed during these times to prevent ketoacidosis.

Eating and drinking are extremely important for the diabetic when he or she is ill. If eating is difficult, it may be helpful to modify food choices to those that are soft and easy to digest, such as canned fruits, eggs, toast, crackers, and hot cereal, especially if these foods are taken frequently in small amounts. If the child is unable to tolerate soft foods, a liquid diet can be used. Guidelines for these specific modifications should be included with the individualized meal plan. The soft foods or liquids should be taken in amounts to satisfy the carbohydrate content of each meal and snack in the meal plan. Table 23-3 presents the carbohydrate content of foods that may be used during illness. Eating 6 to 8 smaller meals rather than 3 to 4 normal meals is recommended.

When nausea, vomiting, or diarrhea are present, milk and milk products may not be tolerated as well as nondairy foods and should be avoided. Caution must be exercised with the child when nausea and vomiting are present because the child may be unable to tolerate and retain any carbohydrates, thus resulting in hypoglycemia. Although water, broth, tea, or other sugar-free fluids cannot be used to replace meals and snacks, they are needed to replace fluids that are lost by diarrhea, vomiting, and fever. These fluids should be encouraged throughout the day.

TABLE 23-3 Carbohydrate Content of Foods That May Be Used during Illness

MILK* (12 g of carbohydrate per exchange)
The following foods may be substituted for 1 milk exchange:

> $^1/_2$ cup *regular* carbonated beverage
> $^1/_2$ double stick popsicle
> 3 pieces hard candy
> 2 tsp corn syrup or honey
> 3 tsp granulated sugar
> 1 cup Gatorade
> 1 cup milk*
> milk shake* ($^1/_3$ cup milk and $^1/_4$ cup vanilla ice cream)*

STARCH AND FRUIT (15 g carbohydrate per exchange)
The following foods may be substituted for either 1 starch or 1 fruit exchange:

> 1 slice toast
> $^1/_2$ cup cooked cereal
> $^3/_4$ cup cream soup*
> 1 cup broth–based soup
> 6 saltines
> $^1/_2$ cup vanilla ice cream*
> $^1/_3$ cup sherbet
> $^1/_4$ cup pudding*
> $^1/_2$ cup *sweetened* gelatin
> $^1/_2$ cup orange juice
> $^1/_3$ cup grape juice

*Milk or milk products may not be tolerated when nausea, vomiting, or diarrhea are present.

It is imperative to monitor the blood sugar, regardless of the nature of the illness. The child should be in contact with a physician if the blood sugar is less than 80 mg percent in the presence of nausea or vomiting or greater than 240 mg percent on three subsequent blood sugar tests.

Physicians: How to Order Diet

The diet order should indicate a *diet for a child with diabetes mellitus.*

References

1. Brink SJ. Pediatric, adolescent, and young-adult nutrition issues in IDDM. Diabetes Care 1988;11(2):192–200.
2. American Diabetes Association. Nutritional recommendations and principles for individuals with diabetes mellitus: 1986. Nutrition Today 1987;Jan-Feb:29–35.
3. Daneman D. When should your child take charge? Diabetes Forecast 1991;44(5):61–66.
4. Abusrewil SS, Savage DCL. Obesity and diabetes control. Arch Dis Child 1989;64(9):1313–1315.

5. Weidman W, Kwiterovich P, Jesse MJ, Nugent E. Diet in the healthy child. Circulation 1983;67:1411A–1414A.

6. National Cholesterol Education Program. Report of the Expert Panel on Blood Cholesterol Levels in Children and Adolescents. Bethesda, MD. NIH Publication: 91-2732. September 1991.

7. Connell JE, Dobersen DT. Nutritional management of children and adolescents with insulin-dependent diabetes mellitus: a review by the diabetes care and education dietetic practice group. J Am Diet Assoc 1991;91(12):1556–1564.

8. Bruening KS, Luder E. Nutrition considerations in pediatric insulin-dependent diabetes mellitus. Top Clin Nutr 1991;7(1):33–43.

9. U.S. Department of Agriculture. School lunch patterns for various age/grade groups. Washington, DC, U.S. Government Printing Office. December 1983.

10. Franz MJ. Exercise and the management of diabetes mellitus. J Am Diet Assoc 1987;87(7):872–880.

11. Jensen MD, Miles JM. The roles of diet and exercise in the management of patients with insulin-dependent diabetes mellitus. Mayo Clin Proc 1986;61:813–819.

12. American Diabetes Association. Physician's guide to insulin-dependent diabetes: diagnosis and treatment. Alexandria, VA: ADA 1988:49.

INBORN ERRORS OF METABOLISM

General Description

Metabolic disorders are inherited traits that cause disease when the normal metabolism of a compound is impaired because of the absence or reduced activity of a specific enzyme or cofactor.[13] Some errors of metabolism result in no serious physical or mental limitations; others lead to rapid changes in the central nervous system and to severe mental retardation; still others may be lethal shortly after birth.[14]

Text continued on p. 506.

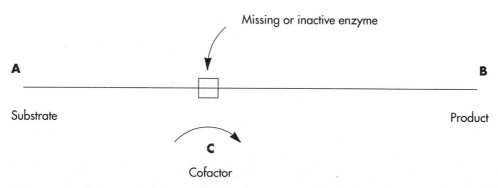

FIGURE 23-1 Defects seen in inborn errors of metabolism. (With permission from: Trahms CM. Nutritional care for children with metabolic disorders. In: Krause MV, Mahan LK, eds. Food, nutrition and diet therapy: a textbook of nutritional care. Philadelphia: WB Saunders, 1984:802.)

TABLE 23-4 Hereditary Metabolic Disorders Treated by Substrate Restriction

Disorder	Defective Pathway	Treatment	Selected Reference
AMINO ACIDS			
Maple syrup urine disease (branched-chain ketoaciduria)	α-Keto-iscocaproic acid (α-Keto-β-methylvaleric acid α-Ketoisovaleric acid) $\xrightarrow[- CO_2]{\alpha\text{-Ketodecarboxylase} + CoASH}$ BLOCK Isovaleryl CoA α-Methylbutyryl CoA Isobutyryl CoA	See p. 519 (nutritional therapy for classic maple syrup urine disease)	Essential amino acid requirements[16] (see Table 23-5)
Hypervalinemia	Valine $\underset{\text{Transaminase}}{\overset{- NH_2}{\rightleftarrows}}$ Valine BLOCK α-Ketoisovaleric acid	Diet low in branched-chain amino acids	Essential amino acid requirements[16] (see Table 23-5)
Isovaleric acidemia	Isovaleryl CoA $\underset{\text{Dehydrogenase}}{\overset{\text{Isovaleryl CoA}}{\rightleftarrows}}$ BLOCK β-Methylcrotonyl CoA	Low protein diet	
Leucinosis		Diet low in leucine, isoleucine, valine: milder variant responds well to massive doses of B_1, up to 20 mg/day	Essential amino acid requirements[16] (see Table 23-5)
Methylmalonic aciduria (acidemia)	Isoleucine, methionine, valine, threonine ↓ Methylmalonyl CoA → Methylmalonate $\underset{\text{Succinyl CoA}}{\overset{\text{Cobalamin}}{\rightleftarrows}}$ BLOCK Dependent	Dietary restriction of protein If vitamin B_{12} responsive, 1 mg/day IM Restrict protein containing isoleucine, threonine, valine, and methionine to amounts required for growth	

Homocystinuria	Defect in cystathionine synthase Homocysteine + serine $\longrightarrow$ Cystathionine	Restrict dietary methionine Lentils, gelatin, soya-protein sources low in methionine Low methionine diet supplemented with cystine or cysteine Folate or choline administration may lower homocystine Pyridoxine 150 to 200 mg/day may lower homocystine	Dietary management of inherited disease: phenylketonuria, galactosemia, tyrosinemia, homocystinuria, maple syrup urine disease[17]
Tyrosinosis	Defective p-hydroxyphenyl pyruvic acid oxidase activity in liver	Restrict dietary phenylalanine and tyrosine	Dietary management of inherited disease: phenylketonuria, galactosemia, tyrosinemia, homocystinuria, maple syrup urine disease[17]
Urea cycle Congenital lysine intolerance with periodic ammonia intoxication		Restrict protein to less than 1 g/kg body weight/day	
Carbamylphosphate synthetase defect	CO_2 + NH_3 $\xrightarrow{\text{defect}}$ Carbamylphosphate	Low protein diet, ketoacid mixture	
Citrullinemia	Citrulline $\longrightarrow$ Argininosuccinic acid Argininosuccinic acid Synthetase DEFECT	Low protein diet, ketoacid mixture	
Ornithine transcarbamylase deficiency	Ornithine $\xrightarrow{\text{defect}}$ Citrulline	Low protein diet, ketoacid mixture	
Argininosuccinic aciduria	Argininosuccinic acid $\longrightarrow$ Arginine Argininosuccinase DEFECT	Low protein diet, ketoacid mixture	

Continued.

TABLE 23-4 Hereditary Metabolic Disorders Treated by Substrate Restriction—cont'd

Disorder	Defective Pathway	Treatment	Selected Reference
CARBOHYDRATES			
Hereditary galactokinase deficiency	Galactose $\xrightarrow[\text{ATP}]{\text{Galactokinase DEFECT}}$ Galactose-1-P	Galactose-free diet	Common carbohydrate in food per 100 g edible portion (see Pediatric Appendix 27)
Galactosemia	Galactose-1-P + UDPG $\xrightarrow[\text{Galactose-1-P Uridyl transferase DEFECT}]{}$ UDP-galactose + glucose-1-P	Galactose-free diet	Dietary management of inherited metabolic disease: phenylketonuria, galactosemia, tyrosinemia, homocystinuria, maple syrup urine disease[17]
Hereditary fructose intolerance	Fructose-1-P $\xrightarrow[\text{Aldolase ALMOST ABSENT}]{}$ Glyceraldehyde + DHAP	Fructose-free diet	Common carbohydrate in foods per 100 g edible portion (see Pediatric Appendix 27)
Carbohydrate malabsorption Glucose-galactose malabsorption		Only fructose is tolerated Formula: protein hydrolysate, corn oil, and fructose Jerusalem artichoke is a useful carbohydrate source (contains insulin-fructose polymer)	
Sucrose-isomaltose malabsorption		Eliminate sucrose, dextrins, and starch from the diet	
Lactose malabsorption		Remove milk, certain milk products from diet Calcium is supplied by other sources	

Sucrase-isomaltase deficiency		Dietary fructose (up to 60% of total calories) as a form of therapy to increase sucrase activity Then, sucrose-restricted diet with approximately 20% of the total calories as fructose, permits occasional sucrose ingestion

GLYCOGEN DISEASES

Type O-glycogen synthetase deficiency	Liver has a very low glycogen content and virtual absence of glycogen synthetase	High protein diet Frequent carbohydrate feedings Extra meal at night
Type I: glucose-6-P defect (Van Creveld-Von Gierke's disease)	Glucose-6-P $\longrightarrow$ Glucose + P Glucose-6-phosphatase DEFICIENCY Glycogen mobilization-inhibited	See Glycogen Storage Disease, p. 508
Type III: debrancher enzyme defect (limit dextrinosis or Forbes disease)	Deficiency in enzymes needed for degradation of glycogen: amylo-1,6glucosidase and/or oligo-1,4 → 1,4 gluconyl-transferase	See Glycogen Storage Disease, p. 508
Type V: myophosphorylase deficiency (McArdle-Schmidt-Pearson disease)	Inability to mobilize glycogen from skeletal muscle	See Glycogen Storage Disease, p. 508
Type VI: hepatic phosphorylase deficiency glycogenosis (Hers disease)	Inability to mobilize glycogen from the liver to maintain homeostasis in glycose metabolism	See Glycogen Storage Disease, p. 508

With permission from: Nyhan WL. Nutritional treatment of children with inborn errors of metabolism. In: Suskind RM, ed. Textbook of pediatric nutrition. New York: Raven Press, 1981:563.

In many cases, nutritional treatment is available to modify the effect of the disorder by providing or by limiting the missing or inactive enzyme. Nutritional treatment can be used to restrict the amount of a substrate (A) available, to supplement the amount of product (B), to supplement the cofactor (C), or to combine two or all three of these approaches (Fig. 23-1).

Table 23-4 lists examples of inborn errors of metabolism that are treated with substrate restriction.[15]

Goals of Dietary Management

The goals of nutritional therapy are to maintain biochemical equilibrium for the specific pathway, to provide adequate nutrients to support normal growth and development, and to provide support for social and emotional development.[13]

Dietary Recommendations

Dietary management is a special challenge for the dietitian, the patient, and the patient's family. Accurate calculation of the meal plan is especially critical because in some instances excessive intake of the restricted nutrient can lead to neurologi-

TABLE 23-5   Essential Amino Acid Requirements*

	Infants 2–4 mo (mg/kg/day)	Boys 10–12 yr		Young Adults	
		(mg/day)	(mg/kg/day)	(mg/day)	(mg/kg/day)
Histidine	16–34				
Isoleucine	80–100	1,000	30	250–700	10–11
Leucine	76–150	1,000–1,500	45	620–1,100	11–13
Lysine	88–103	1,200–1,600	60	300–900	9–10
Methionine:					
No cystine		400–800	27	800–1,100	11–16
Cystine present	35–45			75–350	2–5
Phenylalanine:					
No tyrosine		400–800	27	800–1,100	11–16
Tyrosine present	47–90			220–500	3–7
Threonine	45–87	800–1,000	35	310–500	6–7
Tryptophan	15–22	60–120	3.7	160–225	3.1–3.2
Valine	85–105	600–900	33	650–800	11–14

*Exact information about amino acid requirements is deficient in that only three age groups have been investigated: infants under 3 months of age, boys 10 to 12 years old, and young adults of college age. Since the diets in these studies were mixtures of amino acids, they are very similar to the diets used in the treatment of metabolic errors.

The figures for adults are a composite of several studies; the values expressed in terms of body weight have used 60 kg for female and 70 kg for male subjects. It should be noted that expressed in terms of body weight, there is a reduction in quantities required with age. The greatest reduction occurs during the first year of life.

This table is from an advisory report prepared for the Food and Drug Administration; such reports do not necessarily represent AAP policy and may not reflect current knowledge and experience recognizing the evolving nature of pediatric science.

With permission from: The American Academy of Pediatrics Committee on Nutrition. Final report of the Task Force on the Dietary Management of Metabolic Disorders. Elk Grove Village, IL. Unpublished report. Dec 1985:19–21.

cal damage. On the other hand, insufficient amounts of kilocalories, protein (Table 23-5), vitamins, or minerals can impair growth and development.[14] Each clinic visit should usually include height and weight measurements, a thorough diet history, and, if possible, a food record. Particular attention should be paid to feeding problems or to unusual food habits that might suggest noncompliance with the diet.[16]

Treatment and monitoring should be conducted at a center that has specific knowledge and experience of metabolic disorders. A multidisciplinary approach is beneficial, including a pediatrition, pediatric social worker, psychologist, nutritionist, and nurse.[16]

A list of medical centers with expertise in the evaluation and treatment of inborn errors of metabolism is available from:

National Center for Education in Maternal and Child Health (NCEMCH)
2000 1st Street North
Suite 701
Arlington, VA 22201-2617
(703) 524-7802.

Suggested references for these disorders that may be of benefit for both parents and health professionals follow below.[16]

INFORMATION SOURCES FOR PARENTS AND HEALTH PROFESSIONALS

- Acosta PB, Boberg O, Silberstein F, Wenz E. Parent's guide to the child with PKU. Florida State University, Center for Family Services, 103 Sandels Building, Tallahassee, FL 32306. 1979.
- Acosta PB. A parent's guide to the child with maple syrup urine disease. Florida State University, Center for Family Services, 103 Sandels Building, Tallahassee, FL 32306. 1980.
- Acosta PB, Elsas LJ. Dietary management of inherited metabolic disease: phenylketonuria, galactosemia, tyrosinemia, homocystinuria, maple syrup urine disease. ACELMU Publishers, 1939 Westminister Way, Atlanta, GA, 30307. 1976.
- Schuett VE, Garda RH, Yandow JL. Treatment programs for PKU and other selected metabolic diseases in the United States. Publication No. (HRSA) 83-S206. Washington DC, U.S. Department of Health and Human Services.1983.
- Bell L. HSC equivalency system for dietary treatment of maple syrup urine disease. Clinical Investigation Unit, Nutrition Division, The Hospital for Sick Children, 555 University Avenue, Toronto, Ontario, Canada M5X 1G8. 1979.
- Bell L. Low protein equivalency system. Clinical Investigation Unit, Nutrition Division, The Hospital for Sick Children, 555 University Avenue, Toronto, Ontario, Canada M5X 1G8. 1981.
- Roberts RS, Meyer BA. Living with galactosemia: handbook for families. Metabolic Unit, James Whitcomb Riley Hospital for Children, Department of Pediatrics, Indiana University School of Medicine, 702 Barnhill Drive, Indianapolis, IN 46223. 1983.

- Amino acids. In: Pennington JAT, Church HN. Bowes and Church's food values of portions commonly used, 15th ed. Philadelphia: JB Lippencott, 1989:219.
- Dietary management of metabolic disorders. Evansville, IN 47721, Mead Johnson & Co., 1991.
- Schuett VE. Low protein food list: for phenylketonuria and metabolic diseases requiring a low-protein diet. 114 N Murray Street, Madison, WI 53713, University of Wisconsin Press, 1986.
- Schuett VE. Low protein cookery for phenylketonuria. 114 N Murray Street, Madison, WI 53713, Waisman Center, University of Wisconsin Press, 1988.
- Living with PKU: product handbook. Columbus, OH. Ross Laboratories, 1993.

References

13. Trahms CM. Nutritional care for children with metabolic disorders. In: Krause MV, Mahan LK, eds. Food, nutrition and diet therapy: textbook of nutritional care. Philadelphia: WB Saunders, 1984;802.
14. Robinson CH, Lawler MR, Chenowether WL, Garwick AE. Normal and therapeutic nutrition, 17th ed. New York: Macmillan, 1986:588.
15. Bradburn JM, Shapiro E. Nutritional treatment of children with inborn errors of metabolism. In: Suskind RM, Lewinter-Suskind L, eds. Textbook of pediatric nutrition, 2nd ed. New York: Raven Press, 1992:563–576.
16. American Academy of Pediatrics Committee on Nutrition. Final report, Task Force on the Dietary Management of Metabolic Disorders. Elk Grove Village, IL. Dec 1985:19–21 (unpublished report).
17. Acosta PB, Elsas LJ. Dietary management of inherited metabolic disease: phenylketonuria, galactosemia, tyrosinemia, homocystinuria, maple syrup urine disease. Atlanta: ACELMU Publishers, 1976.

GLYCOGEN STORAGE DISEASES

The glycogen storage diseases (GSD) are a group of disorders characterized by metabolic errors that lead to abnormal concentrations or structures of glycogen, primarily in liver or muscle tissue. GSD for which nutritional therapies have been identified are described in Table 23-6.

GLYCOGEN STORAGE DISEASE TYPE I

General Description

Type I glycogen storage disease (GSD-I) is a disorder that involves the enzyme glucose-6-phosphatase and results in difficulties in glucose synthesis from glyconeogenic precursors.[18] Frequent high starch feedings are prescribed during the day in conjunction with continuous tube feedings during the night or oral cornstarch therapy. The diet may also be limited in galactose and fructose.

TABLE 23-6 Nutritional Therapy for Glycogen Storage Diseases

Type	Defective Pathway	Abnormalities	Nutritional Therapy
I	Glucose-6-phosphatase deficiency	Hypoglycemia Hyperlipidemia Hepatomegaly Growth retardation Osteoporosis Metabolic acidosis	Frequent high starch feedings limited in lactose and fructose Nocturnal tube feeding or oral cornstarch feeding
IIB	Deficient activity of α-1,4-glucosidase (acid maltase deficiency)	Muscle weakness Hypotonia	May benefit from increased protein
III	Deficiency of amylo-1, 6-glucosidase (hepatic debrancher enzyme)	Hepatomegaly Growth failure Hyperlipidemia Fasting hypoglycemia	May benefit from increased protein Limited free sugar Frequent feedings 20–25% protein 40–50% carbohydrate 25–35% fat Nocturnal tube feedings or cornstarch may be useful
IV	Reduction in hepatic phosphorylase activity	Hepatomegaly Growth failure mild to moderate Hyperlipidemia Fasting hypoglycemia	Nocturnal cornstarch or high carbohydrate continuous enteral tube feedings may be of benefit
VI	Deficient activity of α-1,4-glycan 6-glycosyl transferase (branching enzyme)	Hepatic deterioration Failure to thrive Cirrhosis Portal hypertension Ascites, esophageal varices	Nocturnal tube feedings or oral cornstarch feedings may be beneficial

Nutritional Inadequacy

The meal plan and the nocturnal feedings provide adequate kilocalories for the child's age, size, and activity and adequate protein to meet the RDA for age. The diet needs to be evaluated for nutritional adequacy as compared with the RDA. Supplementation with a pediatric multivitamin-mineral supplement, including calcium, is required due to the limited intake of milk and fruit.

Indications and Rationale

The most common of the 12 recognized types of GSD is GSD-I, which represents about a quarter of the patients diagnosed with GSD.[19] Two types of GSD-I have been identified (Ia and Ib), and both are thought to be autosomal recessive disorders. Type Ia results from deficient activity of hepatic and renal glucose-6-phosphatase, the last enzymatic step in glucose production from hepatic glycogen and from the conversion of gluconeogenic precursors (such as amino acids and lactate) to glucose via gluconeogenesis.[20] Type Ib results from a defect in the transport of glucose-6-phosphate through the microsomal membrane, which is a necessary step for the substrate to gain access to glucose-6-phosphatase.

Physical examination reveals a protuberant abdomen with lumbar lordosis due to a very large increase in liver size. The untreated or poorly treated individual will have short stature. There is a tendency to adiposity, particularly of the cheeks, breasts, buttocks, and the backs of the arms and thighs. Fasting blood glucose concentration may be extremely low, but it is usually in the range of 36 to 54 mg/dl.[19]

The main causes of death are hypoglycemic convulsions and/or severe acidosis. In GSD-Ib, infections may be the most likely cause of death. Profound hypoglycemia may occur without clinical symptoms, however. This is currently explained by the high concentration of blood lactate, which is a substitute for glucose as an energy source for the brain.[19]

Serum lipids are greatly increased with hypertriglyceridemia and moderate increases in cholesterol and phospholipids. Hyperuricemia is a frequent finding, leading to gout if untreated. In older patients, proteinuria, indicative of progressive renal dysfunction, has been reported. Osteoporosis is a common finding.[19] Hepatic adenomas may develop during the second decade of life. Although they tend to regress after adequate dietary treatment, adenomas can undergo malignant degeneration.[19]

In addition to the above, type Ib patients exhibit a predisposition to infection related to neutropenia. White blood cell counts are normal, but the neutrophil count may be as low as one-tenth of the lowest normal value. Prolonged bleeding time in the absence of thrombocytopenia or coagulation factor deficiency has been documented in a large number of patients.[19]

Goals of Dietary Management

The goal of treatment is to minimize organic acidemia[22] and to maintain blood glucose levels above 70 mg/dl, thereby avoiding hypoglycemia from inadequate glucose (starch) intake.[18]

Dietary Recommendations

Recommended are high starch feedings spaced at $2^{1}/_{2}$ to $3^{1}/_{2}$ hour intervals[18] during the day depending upon the individual child's tolerance and combined with cornstarch therapy or nocturnal tube feedings of liquid formulas that contain glucose polymers. Treatment has been successful at improving survival and correcting abnormal growth and development.[19] Hepatomegaly is reduced due to decreases in triglyceride content and reduced but not normal lactate, uric acid, and triglyceride levels.[19] After initiation of treatment, a growth spurt of up to 1 cm/month may be seen the first year.[19] The improvement in blood chemistries and the growth spurt after the initiation of treatment may be attributable to the correction of hypoglycemia and of the chronic metabolic acidosis.

Patient response to treatment with frequent daytime starch feedings and nocturnal tube feedings is variable, and most abnormalities associated with GSD-I improve but are not corrected. Lactate, uric acid, and triglyceride levels continue to be mildly to moderately elevated in most patients.[19]

Nocturnal Tube Feedings.   Nighttime tube feedings need to provide exogenous glucose at a rate that minimizes the need for the liver to produce glucose, and thereby effectively take over the main function of the missing glucose-6-phosphatase.[20] Most normal infants and children produce glucose at the rate of 5 to 8 mg/kg of body weight/minute.[21] The major factor in controlling blood lactate levels of these patients may be the adjustment of the rate of feeding to be equal to or slightly greater than normal hepatic glucose production.[20] Glucose provided at the rate of 8 to 9 mg/kg of body weight/minute prevents hypoglycemia and minimizes organic acidemia in most GSD-I patients.[22] The infusion rate needs to be adjusted on an individualized basis and re-evaluated every 3 to 6 months. Infusion rates significantly greater than this may lead to daytime anorexia,[22] to difficulty in consuming adequate carbohydrate during the day, and to inadequate protein intake. Although glucose can be provided by a formula such as Tolerex™ or glucose polymers, the glucose (dextrose) obtained from wine-making shops or from bakery supply companies is usually less expensive.[22] After maximum adult growth is reached, the patient may be able to tolerate longer periods of time without starch.[18]

A combination of Tolerex™ and glucose polymers may also be used, with a fraction of the carbohydrate coming from each source. The protein in Tolerex™ tends to slow the absorption of carbohydrate and helps provide some of the child's protein needs.[18] For example, a patient requiring 9 mg/kg of body weight of carbohydrate/minute of infusion might receive 3 mg/kg of body weight/minute of Tolerex™ and 6 mg/kg of body weight/minute of glucose polymers. In order to calculate the amount that must be prepared each night, the following formula can be used:

$$\_\_\text{mg/kg/min} \times \text{Body Weight (kg)} \times \text{Infusion Time (min)} \times \frac{1\,\text{g}}{1{,}000\,\text{mg}} \times \frac{1.064\,\text{g of Glucose Polymers}}{1\,\text{g of Carbohydrate}} = \text{g of Glucose Polymers/Night}$$

$$\_\_\text{mg/kg/min} \times \text{Body Weight (kg)} \times \text{Infusion Time (min)} \times \frac{1\,\text{g}}{1{,}000\,\text{mg}} \times \frac{80\,\text{g of Tolerex}^{\text{TM}}}{68\,\text{g of Carbohydrate}} = \text{g of Tolerex}^{\text{TM}}/\text{Night}$$

These weight-based measures can then be calculated into volume-based measurements (e.g., cups, tablespoons) for ease of preparation.

It is essential to provide the formula by constant, even infusion using a feeding pump with an alarm system to warn of tube occlusion or power failure. Hypoglycemia occurs much more rapidly after the discontinuation of tube feedings than after a meal. Deaths have occurred from rapid and severe hypoglycemia in patients in whom the infusion was accidentally stopped.[20]

Most children can learn to insert their own nasogastric tubes nightly without difficulty. Parents and children need careful instruction in the use and care of the pump. If use of the nasogastric tube is unsuccessful, a gastrostomy tube may be inserted. However, with proper instruction most patients can be managed appropriately with nasogastric tubes.

Cornstarch Therapy.   In older children, adolescents, and adults, uncooked cornstarch can be used as an alternative form of effective therapy for GSD-I patients.[23,24]

Ingestion of 1.75 to 2.5 g of cornstarch per kilogram of body weight every 6 hours, which provides 5.3 to 7.6 mg of glucose per kilogram of body weight per minute, has been demonstrated to maintain a relatively constant blood glucose concentration if initial blood glucose concentration was normal. The long-term cornstarch regimen has been as effective as nocturnal nasogastric infusions at maintaining blood glucose levels and at promoting normal or catch-up growth.[23]

Cornstarch therapy originally was not recommended for infants or young children. Adult levels of pancreatic amylase, one of two enzymes needed for starch hydrolysis, are not reached until 2 to 4 years of age.[23] After 8 months of age, infants have been managed with a regimen of uncooked cornstarch in low fat (2%) milk every 4 hours plus 3 meals per day. A measured amount of cornstarch in an amount equal to the glucose production rate of 5 to 8 mg/kg of body weight/minute is added to 120 ml of low fat (2%) milk every 4 hours. In these infants, hypoglycemia was prevented and blood lactate levels were at near normal levels. Pancreatic amylase activity may be induced by the starch-milk mixture, or other factors may be involved.[25] Children 1 to 3 years of age have been managed with 2 g of cornstarch per kilogram of body weight 4 to 5 times per day with euglycemia and improved hyperlipidemia.[26]

Patients with Type Ia GSD can be safely managed in pregnancy under a tightly monitored and regulated protocol of uncooked cornstarch.[27]

Proper preparation of the cornstarch is imperative to proper management. The cornstarch must be prepared with tap water at *room temperature.* Cooked cornstarch, or cornstarch mixed with hot water or lemonade, results in a sharp rise in blood glucose followed by a rapid fall within 3 to 5 hours. Heating the cornstarch may disrupt the starch granules, thereby making them more accessible to hydrolysis by amylase. Side effects of transient diarrhea, abdominal distention, and increased flatulence are minor and resolve spontaneously. Cornstarch therapy is less effective when blood glucose concentrations are low.[23]

Patients should be provided with specific dosages of cornstarch in common household measurements. The following conversion should be used:

$$1 \text{ Tbsp} = 8.3 \text{ g of cornstarch}$$

For example, a child weighing 21 kg might require 2 g of cornstarch per kilogram of body weight (or 42 g cornstarch) every 6 hours. Since there are 8.3 g of cornstarch in 1 Tbsp, this would convert to 5 Tbsp of cornstarch every 6 hours. Most children prefer taking the cornstarch mixed with tap water or with a sugar-free fruit flavored beverage.

Oral Feedings. The child should consume small high starch feedings every $2^{1}/_{2}$ to $3^{1}/_{2}$ hours or as often as necessary to keep blood glucose levels above 70 mg/dl.[18] The first feeding of the day must be within approximately 30 minutes before, or *immediately* after, the child discontinues nocturnal tube feedings[28] due to the rapid onset of hypoglycemia after the cessation of intragastric feedings. From 5 to 6 oral feedings are given per day, depending upon the duration of the tube feeding schedule and the individual child's needs.[28] The last evening feeding should occur within the 2 to 3 hour period before nocturnal feeding begins.

TABLE 23-7   Food Exchanges for GSD-I Meal Planning

Exchange Groups	Protein (g)	Fat (g)	Carbohydrate (g)
Starch	2	0	15
Meat (½ oz)	3	2	0
Fat	0	5	0
Vegetables (free in small amounts)	—	—	—

From: Folk CC, Greene HL. Dietary management of type I glycogen storage disease. Copyright The American Dietetic Association. Reprinted with permission from J Am Diet Assoc 1984;84:293–301.

Oral feedings provide 60 to 70% of the kilocalories from carbohydrate, 25 to 35% of the kilocalories from fat, and 10 to 15% of the kilocalories from protein. The carbohydrate source should be primarily starch. Sucrose-, galactose-, and fructose-containing foods, such as fruits, table sugar, and milk, are limited or avoided because galactose and fructose are rapidly converted to lactate[19] and contribute little or nothing to a steady intake of adequate glucose.[18]

The child's meal plan provides guidelines for food intake and should be based on the child's food preferences and on family eating habits. Prime emphasis should be placed on the *frequency of feeding* and the *ingestion of the high starch feedings*. Carbohydrates other than starch, including that found in milk, fruit, and table sugar, are discouraged.

Food exchanges (Tables 23-7 and 23-8) that eliminate lactose, fructose, and sucrose are used in preparing a meal plan that provides small, equal-sized feedings at set intervals. Each feeding should contain, as much as possible, the same distribution of carbohydrate and of protein. Fat should be evenly distributed when possible. The incorporation of some protein and some fat in each high starch feeding seems to help prolong the period of absorption of the glucose.[28] Some school-aged children are able to meet their needs for glucose by eating cornstarch mixed with water or an unsweetened fruit flavored beverage.

The long-term prognosis for GSD-I patients is still unclear. Patients who survive past the second decade usually have less tendency toward hypoglycemia. Normal growth in height occurs when continuous overnight glucose feedings are started by 1.2 years of age. Normal growth is maintained with use of uncooked cornstarch, but excess body weight is common. When growth failure occurs before onset of overnight glucose feedings, however, genetic height potential is not reached.[29]

GLYCOGEN STORAGE DISEASE TYPES III AND VI

General Description

GSD-III is characterized by a deficiency in the hepatic debrancher enzyme (amylo-1,6-glucosidase), which is required for the release of glucose from all but the ter-

TABLE 23-8 Exchange Lists for Glycogen Storage Disease Type I

Starch Exchanges

Bagel	1/2 average	Crackers	
Bread	1 slice	Cheese Tid-bits‡	40
Bread crumbs, dry	1/4 cup	oyster	20
Bread stuffing, dry	1/3 cup	pretzels, very thin sticks	60
Buns		round, thin (1 1/2 in)	6
wiener	1/2	saltines (2 in square)	6
large hamburger	1/2	Wheat Thins‡	12
small hamburger	1	Starchy vegetables	
Cake, angel (1/2 in slice)	1	beans (lima, navy, pinto, white,	
Melba toast, oblong	4	lentils), dried, cooked	1/2 cup
Melba toast, round	8	corn	
Roll (2 in diameter)	1	hominy	1/2 cup
Rusk	2 slices	on the cob	1 small
Tortilla (6 in diameter)	1	whole kernel	1/3 cup
Zwieback	3 slices	mixed vegetables	1/2 cup
Cereals		peas (black-eyed, etc.)	1/2 cup
All-Bran*	1/3 cup	potato, white	
barley	1/2 cup	baked or boiled	1 small
bran flakes, raisin bran	1/2 cup	mashed	1/2 cup
cooked	1/2 cup	squash (acorn, butternut, or	
dry (flakes or puffed)	3/4 cup	winter)	3/4 cup
Cornmeal (dry)	2 Tbsp	sweet potatoes or yams	1/4 cup
Cornstarch	2 Tbsp	Prepared foods	
Flour	2 1/2 Tbsp	biscuit (2 in diameter)	1
Grape Nuts,† wheat germ	1/4 cup	cornbread (1 1/2 in cube)	1
Grits, cooked	1/2 cup	corn chips	1/3 cup
Macaroni, cooked	1/2 cup	corn muffin (2 in diameter)	1
Noodles, cooked	1/2 cup	French fries	8 or 1/2 cup
Popcorn (no fat added)	2 cups	pancake (5 in diameter)	1
Rice, cooked	1/2 cup	potato chips	15
Spaghetti, cooked	1/2 cup		

Meat Exchanges

Cooked meat, fish, poultry	1/2 oz	Peanut butter (no sugar)	1/2 oz
Canned fish	1/2 oz	Luncheon meat (avoid excessive	
Egg	1/2	sucrose)	1 oz
Cheese	1 oz		

Fat Exchanges

Avocado	1/8	Sunflower seeds	1 Tbsp
Cooking oil or shortening	1 tsp	Tartar sauce	2 tsp
Margarine, diet	2 tsp	Sour cream (commercial)	2 Tbsp
Margarine, regular	1 tsp	Sour cream substitutes	2 Tbsp
Mayonnaise	1 tsp	Bacon, crisp	1 slice
Nuts, pecans, or walnuts	4 large halves	Bacon drippings or grease	1 tsp
Olives	5 small	Butter	1 tsp
Peanuts, shelled	1 Tbsp	Chitterlings, boiled	1/8 cup
Salad dressings		Chocolate, unsweetened	1 tsp
French, Italian, oil/vinegar,		Coconut, shredded	2 Tbsp
Roquefort, Thousand Island	2 tsp	Cracklins	1 heaping tsp

TABLE 23-8 Exchange Lists for Glycogen Storage Disease Type I—cont'd

Fat Exchanges—cont'd

Cream cheese	1 Tbsp	Fatback (2 in × 1 in × ½ in)	1 slice
Cream		Gravy	2 Tbsp
heavy, unwhipped	1 Tbsp	Half and half	¼ cup
heavy, whipped	2 Tbsp	Lard	1 tsp
		Whipped topping (commercial)	3 Tbsp

Vegetables—½ cup cooked or 1 cup raw unless otherwise specified

Artichoke	Okra
Asparagus	Onions
Bamboo shoots	Parsley
Bean sprouts	Peppers, green
Broccoli	Pimiento
Brussels sprouts	Radishes
Cabbage	Rhubarb
Carrots	Romaine
Cauliflower	Rutabagas
Celery	Sauerkraut
Chicory	Squash, summer
Cucumber	String beans, young
Eggplant	Tomatoes
Endive	Tomato juice
Escarole	Tomato paste
Greens	Tomato puree
beet, chard, collard,	Tomato sauce
dandelion, kale, lettuce,	Turnips
mustard, poke, spinach,	Vegetable juice cocktail
turnip	Watercress
Mushrooms	Zucchini

Free Foods—in normal amounts unless otherwise specified

BEVERAGES

Kool-Aid,† artificially sweetened
lemonade, artificially sweetened
limeade, artificially sweetened
sugar-free carbonated drinks
    (avoid caffeine)

SAUCES

catsup	
chili sauce	1 Tbsp
hot sauce	1 Tbsp
seafood cocktail sauce	
soy sauce	
steak sauce	

SEASONINGS

artificial sweeteners
butter flavoring
butter-flavored salt

SEASONINGS—cont'd

garlic
herbs
lemon
liquid smoke
mint
onion
parsley
pepper
salt
seasoned salt
spices
tenderizers
vanilla and other flavorings
vinegar

SOUPS

bouillon
clear broth

Continued.

TABLE 23-8   Exchange Lists for Glycogen Storage Disease Type I—cont'd

Free Foods—cont'd

MISCELLANEOUS

Cranberries, fresh or frozen without sugar	Rennet tablets	
Gelatin, unsweetened or artificially sweetened	Salad dressing, calorie-free low calorie—up to 15 kcal	
Horseradish	Sugarless chewing gum	
Mustard, prepared or dry	Whipped topping	1 Tbsp
Pickles, sour or unsweetened dill	Corn syrup in small amounts	

Foods Restricted in Intake

Cakes, unless glucose is used	Ice Cream
Candy	Jam
Chewing gum, regular	Jelly
Cocoa	Marmalade or preserves
Coffee	Milk
Cookies, unless glucose is used	Milk shakes
Condensed milk	Molasses or sorghum
Custards or puddings	Pies
Doughnuts	Soft drinks containing sugar or caffeine
Fried foods, unless allowed fats are used	Sugar
Fruits	Sugar-coated cereals
Fruit juices	Sweet pickles
Fruit drink mixes, such as Tang† and Kool-Aid† (presweetened)	Sweet rolls
Honey	Syrups
	Tea

*Kellogg Co., Battle Creek, Mich.

†General Foods Corp, White Plains, NY.

‡Nabisco, East Hanover, NJ.

From: Folk CC, Greene HL. Dietary management of type I glycogen storage disease. Copyright The American Dietetic Association. Reprinted with permission from J Am Diet Assoc 1984;84:293–301.

minal portions of the glycogen polymer.[20] GSD-VI is characterized by a reduction of normal hepatic phosphorylase activity. The majority of patients have hepatomegaly, growth failure, and mild to moderate increases in serum lipids early in life. Fasting hypoglycemia develops because of diminished ability to mobilize glucose from hepatic glycogen stores.[20]

Nutritional Inadequacy

The meal plan and the nocturnal feedings provide adequate kilocalories for the child's age, size, and activity and adequate protein for growth. The diet needs to be evaluated for nutritional adequacy as compared with the RDA. Supplementation with a pediatric multiple vitamin and mineral supplement, including calcium, is required because of the limited intake of milk and fruit.

Indications and Rationale

These patients are distinguished from type I GSD by a normal or even exaggerated hyperglycemic response to galactose and usually also by a lower level of blood lactate and urate.[19] Patients can adapt to prolonged fasting by accelerated ketogenesis and can maintain normal blood glucose levels by gluconeogenesis when the onset of fasting is gradual. After a high carbohydrate meal, hypoglycemia occurs before the alternative sources of fuel can be mobilized. The increased demand for gluconeogenesis may result in increased protein catabolism and a decreased serum concentration of the potential gluconeogenic substrate alanine. The increased demand for alanine synthesis can deplete the branched-chain amino acids leucine, isoleucine, and valine, which are potential alanine precursors. A high protein diet has been used to provide sufficient substrate for gluconeogenesis. Prevention of hypoglycemia may also reduce protein catabolism and improve the amino acid abnormalities seen with GSD type III.[30]

Dietary Recommendations

Hypoglycemia and wide swings in plasma glucose levels can be averted by a diet that is high in protein,[20] that has small, frequent feedings, and that has a limited free sugar intake[20] (approximately 20 to 25% protein, 40 to 50% carbohydrate, and 25 to 35% fat).[31]

Frequent daytime feedings are usually sufficient to prevent hypoglycemia. However, some patients with GSD-III have more severe disease, with myopathy and growth failure. These abnormalities may result, in part, from muscle protein degradation that occurs in order to provide adequate amino acid as a gluconeogenic substrate to maintain hepatic glucose production.[31] A high protein nocturnal tube feeding combined with a high protein diet in one study demonstrated improved muscle strength, muscle mass, endurance, and growth rates and elimination of early morning hypoglycemia.[31]

Uncooked cornstarch is an alternative therapy. A diet of 3 meals with 2 snacks per day plus 1.75 g of cornstarch per kilogram of body weight every 6 hours is associated with maintenance of normoglycemia, increased growth velocity, and decreased serum aminotransferase concentrations.[30]

After puberty, the liver decreases in size,[31] symptomatic hypoglycemic episodes are rare, and there is a normal growth spurt.[31]

GLYCOGEN STORAGE DISEASE TYPE IV

General Description

GSD-IV is a disorder in which branching enzyme (α-1, 4-glycan 6-glycosyl transferase) activity in the liver or skin fibroblast cultures is deficient. Infants appear normal at birth, but progressive hepatic deterioration leads to failure to thrive, cirrhosis, portal hypertension, ascites, and esophageal varices, and usually results in death before the fourth year of life.[32]

Dietary Recommendations

Patients may benefit from nocturnal cornstarch or high carbohydrate continuous enteral feedings in order to prevent fasting-induced hypoglycemia.[32]

OTHER TYPES OF GLYCOGEN STORAGE DISEASE

General Description

Nutritional therapy has not proven beneficial with other types of GSD.

Physicians: How to Order Diets

The diet order should indicate:

GSD-I: Indicate *diet for GSD-I without cornstarch* or *diet for GSD-I with cornstarch*. The type and rate of nocturnal feeding must be specified.
GSD-III: Indicate *diet for GSD-III*. The type of nocturnal tube feeding (if any) must be specified.
GSD-IV: Indicate *diet for GSD-IV with* or *without cornstarch*. The type and amount of enteral feeding (if any) must be specified.
GSD-VI: Indicate *diet for GSD-VI*.
Other GSD: No diet therapy is indicated.

References

18. Folk C, Rarback S. Dietary management of glycogen storage disease type I. Top Clin Nutr 1988;3(4):77–81.
19. Hers H, Van Hoof F, de Barsy T. Glycogen storage diseases. In: Scriver CR, Beaudet AL, Sly WS, Valle D, eds. The metabolic basis of inherited disease, 6th ed. New York: McGraw-Hill, 1989:425–452.
20. Stanley CA. Intragastric feeding in glycogen storage disease and other disorders of fasting. In: Walker WA, Watkins JB, eds. Nutrition in pediatrics. Boston: Little, Brown, 1985:781–791.
21. Bier DM, Leake RD, Haymond MW, Arnold KJ, Gruenke LD, Sperling MA, Kipnis MK. Measurement of "true" glucose production rates in infancy and childhood with 6,6-dideuteroglucose. Diabetes 1977;26:1016–1023.
22. Haymond MW, Schwenk WF. Optimal rate of enteral glucose administration in children with glycogen storage disease type I. N Engl J Med 1986;314:682–685.
23. Chen UT, Cornblath M, Sidbury JB. Cornstarch therapy in type I glycogen-storage disease. N Engl J Med 1984;310:171–175.
24. Wolfsdorf JI, Plotkin RA, Laffel LMB, Crigler Jr JF. Continuous glucose for treatment of patients with type I glycogen-storage disease: comparison of the effects of dextrose and uncooked cornstarch on biochemical values. Am J Clin Nutr 1990;52:1043–1050.
25. Wolfsdorf JI, Keller RJ, Landy H, Crigler JF. Glucose therapy for glycogenosis type I in infants: comparison of intermittent uncooked cornstarch and continuous overnight glucose feedings. J Pediatr 1990;117:384–391.
26. Hayde M, Widhalm K. Effects of cornstarch treatment in very young children with type I glycogen storage disease. Eur J Pediatr 1990;149:630–633.
27. Johnson MP, Compton A, Drugan A, Evans MI. Metabolic control of Von Gierke disease (glycogen storage disease type IA) in pregnancy: maintenance of euglycemia with cornstarch. Obstet Gynecol 1990;75:507–510.
28. Folk CC, Greene HL. Dietary management of type I glycogen storage disease. J Am Diet Assoc 1984;84:293–301.

29. Wolfsdorf JI, Rudlin CR, Crigler JF. Physical growth and development of children with type I glycogen-storage disease: comparison of the effects of long-term use of dextrose and uncooked cornstarch. Am J Clin Nutr 1990;52:1051–1057.

30. Gremse DA, Bucuvalas JC, Balistreri WF. Efficacy of cornstarch therapy in type III glycogen storage disease. Am J Clin Nutr 1990;52:671–674.

31. Slonim AE, Coleman RA, Moses WS. Myopathy and growth failure in debrancher enzyme deficiency: improvement with high-protein nocturnal enteral therapy. J Pediatr 1984;105:906–911.

32. Greene HL, Gheshan FK, Brown B, McClenethen DT, Freese D. Hypoglycemia in type IV glucogenosis: hepatic improvement in two patients with nutritional management. J Pediatr 1988;112:55–58.

Family Resources

There is a support group for patients with GSD and their parents:

Association for Glycogen Storage Disease
RR #1, Box 46
Stockton, IA 52769

MAPLE SYRUP URINE DISEASE

General Description

In maple syrup urine disease (MSUD), dietary intake of the branched-chain amino acids (BCAA) leucine, isoleucine, and valine is controlled according to individual needs. A semisynthetic formula that is free of the BCCA provides most of the protein as well as calories, vitamins, and minerals. Food is added to the diet to provide some BCAA for ongoing protein synthesis, as well as additional calories.

Nutritional Inadequacy

The meal plan should provide adequate kilocalories for the child's age, size, and activity and adequate amino acid intake for growth. The diet should be evaluated for nutritional adequacy as compared with the RDA for age.

Indications and Rationale

Classic MSUD results from deficiency of an enzyme (branched-chain ketoacid decarboxylase) that catalyzes the oxidative decarboxylation of the BCAA leucine, isoleucine, and valine. The plasma concentration of leucine is significantly higher than that of the other two BCAA[33] in untreated children with MSUD. The disease is inherited as an autosomal recessive trait and is estimated to occur in 1 in 225,000 newborns.[33] Often, the first clue to diagnosis is the distinctive odor of the urine, perspiration, or ear wax toward the end of the first week of life. The substances responsible for the maple syrup odor are unknown at present; the odor is not attributable to the branched-chain ketoacids.[34] If untreated, MSUD leads to progressive hypoglycemia, seizures, metabolic acidosis, mental defects, neurological deterioration, coma, and death.[35] Delay in diagnosis or treatment beyond 6 days of life generally results in severe neurological damage and mental retardation in those

TABLE 23-9   Classification of MSUD by Branched-Chain Ketoacid Decarboxylase Activity

Classification	Decarboxylase Activity (% of Normal Level)	Dietary Protein Tolerance
Classic	0–2	Dietary restriction of leucine, isoleucine, and valine. Nitrogen provided as L-amino acids.
Mild (intermediate)	2–8	Moderate dietary restriction of leucine, isoleucine, and valine.
Intermittent	8–16	Unrestricted between attacks; same as classic during attacks.
Thiamine-responsive	Approximately 40	Thiamine supplementation (10–200 mg/day); possible mild restriction of leucine, isoleucine, and valine

who survive.[36] These problems may be minimized or averted with early diagnosis and proper therapy. Reportedly, normal growth and a mean IQ of 101 have been occasionally achieved in patients with MSUD.[37] However, mean IQs tend to be below average for these children. The age of diagnosis and control of leucine level are the most important factors affecting the outcome of the patient with MSUD.[36]

Variants of MSUD. Variants of MSUD are intermediate, intermittent, and thiamine-responsive, in addition to classic MSUD.[38] The severity and degree of protein tolerance are related to the amount of residual enzyme activity (Table 23-9).

Thiamine-responsive MSUD is a mild form characterized by a later onset of symptoms. There is only a partial deficiency of branched-chain ketoacid decarboxylase, and the administration of thiamine appears to stabilize this enzyme. A prolonged trial of high doses of thiamine in the range of 10 to 200 mg/day for at least 3 weeks may be needed to observe the effect of treatment.[39] Studies have shown that the chief error in treatment with thiamine is use of an inadequate dose for only a short period of time.

Responsivity to thiamine may not correlate with the clinical course because of other variables such as intercurrent infection. Therefore, it is recommended that the response be assessed by quantifying the concentration of BCAA in plasma before and after vitamin supplementation.[40]

Goals of Dietary Management

Depending on the severity of the child's clinical condition, the acute phase of treatment may consist of peritoneal dialysis or hemodialysis[41] to remove α-ketoacids, infusion of high rates of intravenous glucose (10 to 15 mg/kg of body weight/minute) to suppress proteolysis, and initiation of a BCAA-free diet. Oral feedings can be started after fluid and electrolyte imbalances are corrected. Anabolic requirements of the BCAA, including the requirement for growth, must be provided, yet must not permit the accumulation of metabolites proximal to the deficient enzyme (BCAA and their keto-acid derivatives).

Nutritional management involves assessment of growth, evaluation of nutritional adequacy of the diet, and careful monitoring of blood levels of the BCAA, especially leucine, and perhaps branched-chain α-ketoacids.[43] BCAA intake needs to be adjusted frequently to maintain plasma leucine levels between 2 to 5 mg/dl. Levels above 10 mg/dl are associated with α-ketoacidemia and neurologic symptoms.[44] During illness, BCAA intake must be decreased and carbohydrates increased to suppress proteolysis. Acute infections or catabolic illnesses may lead to encephalopathy and death despite treatment.

Dietary Recommendations

The diet for MSUD necessitates the use of a semisynthetic formula, such as MSUD™ diet powder (Mead Johnson) or Analog MSUD™ (Ross Laboratories). The formula contains crystalline L-amino acids except the BCAA, as well as appropriate amounts of carbohydrate, fat, minerals, and vitamins (Appendix 25). Small, carefully measured amounts of milk or regular infant formula need to be added to the MSUD formula to provide the BCAA needs of the infant. Occasionally, solutions of isoleucine and valine must be added to prevent these amino acids from becoming deficient while avoiding hyperleucinemia. Small amounts of low protein foods are used to provide the BCAA needs of the older child.

The child's daily requirements for kilocalories, protein, leucine, isoleucine, and valine should be individually assessed. Energy requirements are similar to those of normal children after the acutely ill child stabilizes and completes any catch-up growth needed after the initial illness.[39] Nutrient requirements of children and infants with MSUD are the same as those for normal children.[44] Little research has been done in MSUD to identify subclinical deficiencies of trace elements such as zinc, copper, and selenium, which have been seen in phenylketonuria. While nitrogen balance studies may be the most precise method of monitoring adequacy of the dietary protein intake, weight gain in infants is a fairly sensitive and easily monitored index of well-being and nutritional adequacy.[44]

The amount of MSUD diet powder to be used should be determined based on nutritional needs similar to those of normal children. Composition of the formulas is available from the manufacturer.

The amount of milk or regular infant formula to be added to meet the child's needs for BCAA is also estimated. The requirements for individual amino acids are difficult to determine since normal growth and development can be achieved over a wide range of intake. The guidelines in Table 23-10 are often used as the basis for amino acid requirements and the prescription for nutritional therapy.[42] This table should be used only as a guide. Tolerance to BCAA varies with individual patients.

The amount of water to be added to the MSUD diet powder is also determined. The total amount of fluid needed should be based on the child's age, weight, and hydration status.

The amount of solid foods to include in the diet, if any, should be considered in the nutritional plan. Table 23-11 provides a method of calculating daily intake of leucine, isoleucine, and valine to avoid either excessive or deficient amounts. Isoleucine and valine intakes may vary 10 to 30% from the prescription in the meal plan; leucine may vary 1 to 2%.[44] Supplementation of the diet with isoleucine and valine[44] is usually necessary in the newborn until the infant is on a mixed diet.

Exchange lists for MSUD are also available to aid in planning the diet.[45] It is useful to give serving portions in both household measurements and gram weights. High protein foods, ordinary breads and pasta, and foods for which the BCAA-containing ingredients cannot be determined are omitted from the diet. Even small amounts of high protein foods are excluded because imprecise measurements could result in a wide variation in intake of BCAA. Including these foods causes intake of fruits, vegetables, and cereals to be decreased and may further prove to be an undesirable temptation for the child.[33]

TABLE 23-10 Approximate Amino Acid Requirements for Infants and Children

	Nutrient		
Age	Isoleucine (mg/kg)	Leucine (mg/kg)	Valine (mg/kg)
0<6 mo	90–30	100–60	95–40
6<12 mo	90–30	75–40	60–30
1<4 yr	85–20	70–40	85–30
4<7 yr	80–20	65–35	50–30
7<11 yr	30–20	60–30	30–25
11<15 yr	30–20	50–30	30–20
15<19 yr	30–10	40–15	30–15

With permission from: Elsas LJ, Acosta PB. Amino acid requirements for infants and children. In: Shils MG, Young VR, eds. Modern nutrition in health and disease, 7th ed. Philadelphia: Lea & Febiger, 1988:1347.

TABLE 23-11 Average Nutrient Content of Equivalent Lists for Branched-Chain Amino Acid-Restricted Diets

Food List	Isoleucine (mg)	Leucine (mg)	Valine (mg)	Protein (g)	Fat (g)	Energy (kcal)
Breads/cereals	18	35	25	0.5	0	30
Fats	7	10	7	0.1	8	70
Fruits	17	25	22	0.6	0	75
Vegetables	22	30	24	0.6	0	15
Free foods A*	3	5	4	0.1	0	50
Free foods B†	0	0	0	0	varies	55

*Free foods A: very little protein–limit to recommended numbers of servings.

†Free foods B: no protein–may be used as desired if patient is not overweight and if they do not depress appetite for prescribed foods.

With permission from: Elsas LJ, Acosta PB. Amino acid requirements for infants and children. In: Shils MG, Young VR, eds. Modern nutrition in health and disease, 7th ed. Philadelphia: Lea & Febiger, 1988:1358.

Parents need frequent nutritional education and counseling. Food records kept by parents before each clinic visit are essential in assessing the consistency of intake and the adequacy of the home diet. Knowledge of the child's amino acid intake can be used to assess requirements for amino acids. Frequent adjustments in the child's meal plan are needed to meet changing needs for kilocalories, protein, and the BCAA. The diet needs to be continued indefinitely without liberalization.[42]

Physicians: How to Order Diets

The diet order should indicate *diet for MSUD*. Specify the amount of leucine, isoleucine, and valine to be allowed. The dietitian will determine the caloric level and adjust the nutritional care plan according to the preceding guidelines.

References

33. Bell L, Chas E, Milne J. Dietary management of maple syrup urine disease, extension of equivalency systems. J Am Diet Assoc 1979;74:357–361.
34. Tanaka K, Rosenberg LE. Disorders of branched chain amino acid and organic acid metabolism. In: Stansbury JB, Wyngaarden JB, Fredrickson DS, Goldstein JL, Brown MS, eds. The metabolic basis of inherited disease, 5th ed. New York: McGraw-Hill, 1983:451.
35. DiGeorge AM, Rezvanic I, Garebaldi LR, Schwartz M. Prospective study of maple syrup urine disease for the first four days of life. N Engl J Med 1982;307:1492–1495.
36. Kaplan P, Mazur A, Field M, Berlin JA, Benz GT, Heidenreich R, Yudkoff M, Segal S. Intellectual outcome in children with maple syrup urine disease. J Pediatr 1991;119:46–50.
37. Clow CL, Reade TM, Scriver CR. Outcome of early and long-term management of classical maple syrup urine disease. Pediatrics 1981;68:856–862.
38. Rohr FJ, Levy HL, Shih VE. Inborn errors of metabolism. In: Walker WA, Watkins JB, eds. Nutrition in pediatrics. Boston: Little, Brown, 1985:400.
39. Duran M, Wadman SK. Thiamine responsive inborn errors of metabolism. J Inher Metab Dis 1985;8(Supp I):70–75.
40. Fernhoff PM, Lubitz D, Danner DJ, Dembure PP, Schwartz HP, Hillman R, Bier DM, Elsas LJ. Thiamine response in maple syrup urine disease. Pediatr Res 1985;19:1011–1016.
41. Benz GT, Heidenreich R, Kaplan P, Levine F, Mazur A, Palmieri MJ, Yudkoff M, Segal S. Branched chain amino acid-free parenteral nutrition in the treatment of acute metabolic decompensation in patients with maple syrup urine disease. N Engl J Med 1991; 324:175–179.
42. Snyderman SE. Maple syrup urine disease. In: Wapnir PA, ed. Congenital metabolic diseases. New York: Marcel Dekker, 1985:153.
43. Krause MV, Mahan LK. Food, nutrition and diet therapy, 7th ed. Philadelphia: WB Saunders, 1984:818.
44. Acosta PB, Elas LJ. Dietary management of inherited metabolic disease: phenylketonuria, galactosemia, tyrosinemia, homocystinuria, maple syrup urine disease. Atlanta: Acelmu Publishers, 1976:65.
45. Acosta PB, Yannicelli S. Disorders of amino acid metabolism. In: Cameron AM, ed. The Ross metabolic formula system-nutrition support protocols. Columbus, OH: Ross Laboratories, 1993:91–252.

Additional References for Parents and/or Health Professionals

Cameron AM. The Ross Metabolic Formula System-Nutrition Support Protocols. Columbus, OH: Ross Laboratories, 1993.

Pennington JAT, Church HN. Bowes and Church's food values of portions commonly used, 14th ed. Philadelphia: JB Lippincott, 1985.

Bell L. Leucine equivalency system for dietary management of maple syrup urine disease. Nutrition Division, Clinical Investigation Unit, Room 815, The Hospital for Sick Children, 555 University Avenue, Toronto, Ontario, Canada, M5G 1X8. (Unpublished data available upon request.)

Family Resources

1. Maple Syrup Urine Disease Family Support Group. Contact:

   Bonnie Lou Koons
   7409 Moyer Road
   Harrisburg, PA 17112
   (717) 469-7167

Resources available include a newsletter, information for new families, cookbooks, and educational materials.

2. Nardella, M. A teacher's guide to MSUD. January 1988.

   Children's Rehabilitative Services Arizona Department of Health Services
   1740 W Adams, Room 208
   Phoenix, AZ 85007
   (602) 255-1890

NUTRITIONAL THERAPY FOR PHENYLKETONURIA (PKU)

General Description

Phenylalanine intake is controlled according to individual needs. The majority of the protein in the diet is provided by a product that is low in or free of phenylalanine. Foods that contain only small amounts of phenylalanine make up the rest of the diet.

Nutritional Inadequacy

Calorie, carbohydrate, fat, vitamin, and mineral requirements are the same as for children and infants without phenylketonuria (PKU). Total protein and amino acid requirements are also the same, with the exception of the need to restrict phenylalanine. In addition, tyrosine is an essential amino acid for individuals with PKU. Infants with PKU have been observed to have retarded growth, mental retardation, and impaired cognitive functioning. These conditions result from inadequate dietary intake, late initiation of the diet, and early diet termination.[46] Abnormalities of zinc, copper, iron, and selenium have been reported in children with PKU receiving semisynthetic diets.[46,47] The cause is thought to be inadequate intake (selenium, copper) or decreased bioavailability (iron, zinc).[48,49]

The adolescent is nutritionally vulnerable because of the rapidly changing needs of the adolescent growth spurt. The increased intake of calories and protein resulting from increased appetite and needs leads to a rapid change in body size and shape. Girls may gain weight because their formulas are too high in calories (see p. 527 for formula recommendations for adolescents). Calorie needs must be carefully monitored at this time. Another issue of concern with adolescents is that the diet they are eating is similar to a vegan diet. Consequently, iron and vitamin B_{12} may not be present in adequate amounts. Folacin needs are increased significantly during rapid growth, and this nutrient is not present in PKU formulas in amounts sufficient to meet needs. Several vitamins and minerals are needed in increased amounts for growth and development. Whether these needs are met depends on the type and amount of formula used.[46] These formulas do not contain fluoride. Supplements may be necessary.

Lofenalac™, Phenyl Free™, Maxamaid XP™, Analog XP™, Maxamum XP™, PKU-1™, and PKU-2™ contain recommended amounts of vitamins and minerals for the infant and child, as well as supplemental L-tyrosine. These products do not contain fluoride, which may need to be supplemented in the child's diet if the formula powders are not reconstituted with fluoridated water. See Pediatric Appendix 25, for formula compositions.

Indications and Rationale

PKU is an autosomal recessive genetic disorder seen in 1 in 11,000 births in the United States. PKU is a disease primarily of Caucasians. The phenylalanine hydroxylase activity in the liver of PKU patients is approximately 0.27% of normal.[50] This defect causes a block in the conversion of phenylalanine to tyrosine, thereby resulting in a markedly elevated level of blood phenylalanine and the excretion of phenylalanine and its metabolites, such as phenylpyruvic acid and phenylacetic acid, in the urine. Mutations leading to partial inactivity of phenylalanine hydroxylase result in less pronounced elevations of plasma phenylalanine, a condition called benign hyperphenylalaninemia.

Because tyrosine formation is blocked, the production of melanin is decreased. The affected children have blue eyes and are blonder than unaffected siblings if the disease has not been treated early and if retardation has occurred.[51] Untreated patients lose 50 IQ points the first year of life and 96 to 98% ultimately have an IQ of less than 50.[50] The most likely mechanism for retardation is that elevated phenylalanine competes with other amino acids for transport into the neurons and creates an amino acid imbalance that inhibits protein synthesis and synaptogenesis.[50]

Classic PKU can be defined as meeting these criteria: a plasma phenylalanine level consistently above 20 mg/dl; blood tyrosine levels less than about 3 mg/dl; the presence of phenylpyruvic acid and o-hydroxyphenylacetic acid in the urine; and inability to tolerate an oral challenge of phenylalanine. Patients with benign hyperphenylalaninemia usually have blood levels between 5 and 15 mg/dl. They have considerably higher tolerances for dietary phenylalanine and may require no or a shorter duration of therapy. Infants with phenylalanine levels consistently greater than 8 to 12 mg/dl should be treated.[52]

Atypical PKU is a less severe defect of phenylalanine hydroxylation in which blood phenylalanine is not as high as in classic PKU. Phenylketones may or may not be present in the urine. Untreated atypical PKU may cause central nervous system impairment. Diet therapy is usually initiated when blood phenylalanine levels exceed 12 mg/dl.[53]

The older untreated PKU patient who is difficult to manage due to hyperactivity and self-abuse may benefit from a trial of a low phenylalanine diet.[54]

Goals of Dietary Management

Nutritional therapy needs to provide sufficient amounts of the essential amino acid phenylalanine for proper growth and development but to restrict intake so that high blood phenylalanine levels are reduced and mental retardation is prevented. The optimal therapeutic range for blood phenylalanine levels in persons with PKU is between 2 and 10 mg/dl.[55] Values between 2 and 4 mg/dl are more desirable in the first year of life or while the infant is being strictly formula fed. Blood phenylalanine should be measured a minimum of once a week during the first year of life.[50] This interval can be reduced to once every 2 weeks when control is good in older infants. In children over 1 year of age, monthly determination of blood phenylalanine levels is sufficient during times of good control. Additional measurements should be obtained when the blood phenylalanine level is outside the desired therapeutic range. Excessive restriction of phenylalanine, resulting in phenylalanine deficiency, causes deficient growth, retarded bone age, hepatomegaly, repeated infections, hypoglycemia, neurological symptoms,[50] lethargy, anorexia, rashes, anemia, and diarrhea.[51]

Patients with hyperphenylalaninemia should be challenged with a phenylalanine load sometime in the first 1 to 2 years of life to identify classic PKU versus benign hyperphenylalaninemia.

Elevations in blood phenylalanine levels are generally caused by (1) intake of phenylalanine in excess of the child's need for growth, (2) insufficient caloric intake[54] or protein intake,[56] which promotes tissue catabolism resulting in an accumulation of phenylalanine in the blood, and (3) tissue catabolism during illness.[56]

Dietary Recommendations

Special dietary products used for treating PKU are either low in or free of phenylalanine. These products must be prescribed under the care of an experienced dietitian and physician. Infants reported as testing positive for PKU in the newborn screen should be started immediately on diet therapy while awaiting confirmatory testing. Infants can be fed either by breast or bottle. Lofenalac™ (Mead Johnson) is a casein hydrolysate formula from which most of the phenylalanine has been removed. Analog XP™ (Ross Laboratories) is a phenylalanine-free crystalline amino acid formula. These formulas have been optimally formulated for use in infants. Maxamum XP™ (Ross Laboratories), PKU-1™, and PKU-2™ (Milupa) are phenylalanine-free crystalline amino acid formulas most appropriate for use in older patients and in patients whose protein intake is inadequate. They contain a higher ratio of protein to calories than the other formulas. PKU-1™ and PKU-2™ are of relatively low caloric density and can be considered in patients with higher caloric intake from complete food sources or on caloric restriction. The use of these formulas can be considered for infants who are eating solid foods to allow for a more varied diet.[57] In order to meet the complete protein needs for growth in infancy and childhood, evaporated milk, cow milk, or standard infant formula must be added to the Lofenalac™ or Analog XP™. Lofenalac™ is also a good choice for the adolescent who is hungry, slender, and needs to consume the large volume of high calorie formula required to meet protein needs. Phenyl Free™ (Mead Johnson) and Maxamaid XP™ (Ross Laboratories) are crystalline amino acid formulas that contain no phenylalanine. They allow more flexibility in the diet of the older child by allowing all of the phenylalanine requirements to be supplied by foods other than formula. They are less calorically dense than their infant counterparts and are appropriate for the adolescent who is hungry but has a tendency to gain weight easily.[46]

The infant with PKU may be breast-fed, but modifications must be made to allow for excessive phenylalanine intake. Human milk contains approximately 13 mg/oz of phenylalanine, which is less than cow milk (52 mg/oz) or infant formulas (20 to 30 mg/oz). To limit phenylalanine intake to appropriate amounts, the diet for the infant with PKU must be supplemented at least partially with a low phenylalanine or a phenylalanine-free formula. Based on the average phenylalanine content of the mother's milk, the infant's estimated need for calories, and the infant's tolerance for phenylalanine, a quantity of low phenylalanine or phenylalanine-free formula is calculated to provide the appropriate phenylalanine intake. The infant is allowed to breast-feed, as desired, between scheduled formula feedings. Blood phenylalanine should be measured initially 2 to 3 times per week and adjustments made in the amount of formula and the frequency of breast feeding.[53]

Solid foods are substituted as the protein source for older infants and children within their dietary phenylalanine guidelines. Undue delay in the introduction of solid foods can result in problems with acceptance of such foods in the older child.

Phenylalanine-free formulas are usually introduced in the diet of the older child to allow greater flexibility in menu planning. This is especially important as the child enters school or other group settings. Criteria for introduction of these formulas include that the child accepts the meal plan and formula and consumes a wide variety of foods from the low phenylalanine food lists on a regular basis.[54] The low protein and phenylalanine-free products available are helpful for the adolescent who has a small appetite because they provide needed calories without excessive protein.[46] Care must also be taken to avoid excessive weight gain in adolescence since PKU formulas are relatively higher in calories than most standard beverages that might otherwise be consumed.

Parents of children with PKU need careful nutritional education with frequent follow-up. A meal plan (Table 23-12) provides parents with specific guidelines to follow. Phenylalanine intake can be determined directly by the parent and child, or phenylalanine exchange equivalents can be used to substitute foods within a prescribed phenylalanine intake level. Parents should be able to demonstrate the ability to prepare formula correctly, to plan accurate menus, and to plan replacements for foods not eaten. To avoid conflicts over food, children should be involved at an early age in choosing appropriate foods. Diet diaries should be kept by parents for the 3 days preceding each blood phenylalanine analysis. At each clinic visit the diet records should be evaluated for the variety of foods chosen and the adequacy of caloric, protein, phenylalanine, vitamin, and mineral intakes. These records are useful in adjusting intake if serum phenylalanine is above or below recommended values and for evaluating the accuracy and consistency of the home diet.

TABLE 23-12   Phenylalanine-Controlled Diet Meal Plan

Date _____ Age _____ Name _____

Weight _____ Height _____

Formula _____

Approximate total mg phenylalanine daily   _____

Approximate total g protein daily   _____

Approximate total energy (kcal) daily   _____

	Phenylalanine (mg)	Protein (g)	Energy (kcal)
____measures packed dry formula	_____	_____	_____
Add ____oz evaporated milk	_____	_____	_____
Add ____oz water	_____	_____	_____
1 oz contains	_____	_____	_____
BREAKFAST			
_____Formula			
____Servings fruit	_____	_____	_____
____Servings starch	_____	_____	_____
____Servings fat	_____	_____	_____
____Servings free food A	_____	_____	_____
____Servings free food B	_____	_____	_____
BETWEEN MEALS			
____Servings _____	_____	_____	_____
NOON			
_____Formula			
____Servings fruit	_____	_____	_____
____Servings vegetable	_____	_____	_____
____Servings starch	_____	_____	_____
____Servings fat	_____	_____	_____
____Servings free food A	_____	_____	_____
____Servings free food B	_____	_____	_____
BETWEEN MEALS			
____Servings _____	_____	_____	_____
EVENING MEAL			
_____Formula			
____Servings fruit	_____	_____	_____
____Servings vegetable	_____	_____	_____
____Servings starch	_____	_____	_____
____Servings fat	_____	_____	_____
____Servings free food A	_____	_____	_____
____Servings free food B	_____	_____	_____
BEDTIME			
____Servings _____	_____	_____	_____
Total	_____	_____	_____
Per kg	_____	_____	_____

COMMENTS:

The artificial sweetener aspartame (Equal™ or NutraSweet™) is a significant source of phenylalanine and should not be a part of the diet for the child with PKU. Foods containing aspartame have the statement "Phenylketonurics: Contains Phenylalanine" near the ingredient panel. Parents should be alerted to read labels for this statement and to look for the ingredients NutraSweet™, Equal™ or aspartame. In addition, some prescription and nonprescription medications contain aspartame as a sweetener. Patients and parents should always question a physician prior to taking medications.

Calculation of the Diet

The following are guidelines for determining the needed levels of phenylalanine, kilocalories, protein, and fluid. The diet should be adjusted frequently to meet the child's changing needs for kilocalories, protein, and phenylalanine and to accommodate changes in the child's eating habits.

1. Establish the child's daily requirements for kilocalories, protein, and phenylalanine. See Table 23-13 for suggested requirements. Infants with PKU have the same protein requirements as other infants but have a higher protein intake due to the high protein content of the phenylalanine-modified formulas. Phenylalanine intake needs to be adjusted frequently in response to blood levels.

2. Establish the amount of phenylalanine required each day. This is determined by the infant or child's protein requirement. Protein intake from formula is 85 to 90% of daily protein needs and must be met by a low phenylalanine formula in order to allow appropriate total protein and calorie consumption.[56] Phenylalanine-free formulas are generally used for the older child or adult. (See Table 23-14.)

3. Determine the amount of additional phenylalanine that needs to be consumed from complete food sources. For infants, cow milk or soy formula is added to the PKU formula to attain the desired phenylalanine intake. Milk should not be added to an older child's formula in order to allow addition of other solid foods.

TABLE 23-13   Suggestions for Daily Diet Prescription in Phenylketonuria

Age	Recommended Protein Intake (g/kg of body weight)	Recommended Phenylalanine Intake (mg/kg of body weight)	Recommended Caloric Intake*
0–2 mo	4.2	40–70	120
3–6 mo	3.0	25–55	115
6 mo–1 yr	2.5	25–50	110–115
1–3 yr	25	20–40	900–1,800
4–6 yr	30	10–40	1,300–2,300
7–10 yr	35	10–40	1,650–3,300

*Caloric intake for age 0 to 1 year is expressed as kcal/kg of body weight/day and caloric intake for age 1 to 10 years is expressed as total kcal/day.

With permission from: Koch R, et al. Phenylketonuria. A guide to dietary management. Evansville, IN: Mead Johnson Nutritional Group, 1981:16.

TABLE 23-14   Composition of Formulas Used in Phenylketonuria

Formula (Manufacturer)	Weight or Measure	Phenylalanine (mg)	Protein (g)	Kcal
Analog X-Phen™ (Ross Laboratories)	8.0 g or 1 Tbsp	0	1.04	38
Lofenalac™ (Mead Johnson)	9.5 g or 1 Tbsp	7	1.4	43
Phenyl Free™ (Mead Johnson)	9.8 g or 1 Tbsp	0	2.0	40
PKU-1™ (Milupa)	12 g or 1 Tbsp	0	6.0	34
PKU-2™ (Milupa)	12 g or 1 Tbsp	0	8.0	35
Maximaid XP™ (Ross Laboratories)	12 g or 1 Tbsp	0	2.5	35
Maxamum XP™ (Ross Laboratories)	12 g or 1 Tbsp	0	4.4	38

4. Calculate the amount of water to be added to the powder. The amount of water needed is determined by the child's weight, age, hydration status, preference for fluids, and taste for the formula. Higher fluid intakes may be needed because of the high protein content of the diet. Because the formula is a concentrated source of protein and carbohydrate, children taking this formula tend to have greater thirst than most children consuming regular milk or formulas.[56] The low phenylalanine formula can be made into a paste with water or apple juice and can be spoon-fed, particularly if the child rejects the formula when being weaned from the bottle. Additional phenylalanine-free fluids should be offered between feedings.[56]

5. Determine the amount and type of solid foods to be given. Solid foods are introduced at about 4 to 6 months of age as with non-PKU children. To calculate the amount and type of solid foods required, subtract the amount of phenylalanine, kilocalories, and protein provided by the low phenylalanine or hydrolyzed casein formula or phenylalanine-free mixture of crystalline amino acids from the diet prescription. Food lists are available that provide the phenylalanine, protein, and calorie content of foods per serving (see p. 538, Parent Resources, item 8). Such lists are used for calculating the diet as well as for parent instruction. Phenylalanine is 2.6% to 5.0% of the protein found in food.[56] A variety of foods similar to those normally eaten by infants should be given to ensure that these foods are accepted later in life, to meet increasing phenylalanine requirements and nutrient needs, to develop jaw

Text continued on p. 534.

TABLE 23-15   Phenylalanine Content of Infant Foods (Gerber)

	Phenylalanine Content mg/Tbsp
CEREALS AND BREADS	
Dry Cereals	
Barley cereal	22.2
High protein cereal	65.7
Mixed cereal	21.8
Mixed cereal with bananas	20.5
Oatmeal cereal	27.7
Oatmeal cereal with bananas	26.7
Rice cereal	13.2
Rice cereal with bananas	15.5
Wet Cereals with Fruit	
Strained mixed cereal with applesauce and bananas	9.0
Strained oatmeal cereal with applesauce and bananas	10.7
Strained rice cereal with applesauce and bananas	6.0
Jr. mixed cereal with applesauce and bananas	9.7
Jr. oatmeal cereal with applesauce and bananas	11.4
Jr. rice cereal with mixed fruit	8.7
Baked Goods	
Animal crackers (4 crackers or 11 g)	38 (4)
Arrowroot cookies (2 cookies or 11 g)	32 (2)
Toddler Biter biscuits (1 biscuit or 11 g)	26 (1)
Animal shaped cookies (2 cookies or 13 g)	44 (2)
Pretzels (2 pretzels or 12 g)	43 (2)
Zwieback toast (2 toasts or 14 g)	42 (2)
MEATS AND EGG YOLKS	
Strained Meats	
Beef	75.0
Chicken	86.1
Ham	85.0
Lamb	91.1
Pork	84.9
Turkey	84.6
Veal	78.1
Egg yolks	57.6
Junior Meats	
Beef	79.4
Chicken	92.4
Ham	90.0
Turkey	95.0
Veal	89.1
Chicken sticks	66.0
Meat sticks	58.0
Turkey sticks	62.0

Continued.

TABLE 23-17   Sample Calculation—Toddler (Lofenalac™ Formula with Table Foods)

Age: 21 mo
Weight: 12.5 kg

1. Approximate daily requirement for kcal: 1,190 kcal (basal + 70% using Table 23-13 on p. 529)
   Approximate daily requirement for protein: 25 g (from Table 23-13 on p. 529)
   Approximate daily requirement for phenylalanine: 375 mg (30 × 12.5)

2. Amount of protein from Lofenalac™ = 85–90% of total protein requirements: 25 × 0.85 = 21 g.
   Amount of Lofenalac™ to give: Divide the grams of protein required from Lofenalac™ by the amount of protein per measure of Lofenalac™ (1.4 g of protein/measure): 21 ÷ 1.4 = 15 measures Lofenalac™.

3. Amount of water to add to Lofenalac™: Water can be added to the child's taste; 2 oz of water/measure will prepare a 20 kcal/oz formula. Additional fluid given as water or juices.

4. Amount of table foods to give: Total phenylalanine requirements per day minus phenylalanine content of the day's prescription for Lofenalac™ equals amount of phenylalanine required from solid foods: 375 − 114 = 261 mg phenylalanine from table foods.

5. Divide phenylalanine allowance from table foods into exchange groups based on the child's eating preferences and caloric needs or specify the milligrams of phenylalanine allowed at each meal and snack.

Foods	Phenylalanine (mg)	Protein (g)	Energy (kcal)
2 vegetable servings	30	1.0	30
5 fruit servings	75	2.5	300
5 starch servings	150	3.0	150
1 fat serving	5	0.1	60
15 packed dry measures Lofenalac™ (add water to make 32 oz)	114	21.0	655
Total	**374**	**27.6**	**1,195**

lalanine-controlled diet after the diet has been discontinued is difficult and often unsuccessful. The PKU diet should not be discontinued under the assumption that it can easily be resumed whether undesirable effects of diet discontinuation occur. It is not clear if academic decline can be reversed by resumption of the diet.[61] Two-thirds of PKU clinics surveyed now reportedly recommend continuation of the PKU diet indefinitely.[62]

Maternal and Paternal PKU. Women with poorly treated or untreated classic PKU are at risk for bearing infants with mental retardation, microcephaly, low birth weight, and congenital heart disease. Miscarriage rates are also higher in these women. Fetal brain damage is correlated with maternal phenylalanine levels.[50] Apparently the infant is at high risk with classic maternal PKU (blood phenylalanine levels of 20 mg/dl or greater), while hypophenylalaninemia (blood phenylalanine level less than 10 mg/dl) carries little or no risk to the fetus. Toxicity to the fetus is uncertain with degrees of maternal hyperphenylalaninemia between these levels.[55]

Current recommendations are to maintain blood phenylalanine levels between 2 and 6 mg/dl. This therapy should be instituted prior to conception and continued during the pregnancy.[63] Diet and plasma phenylalanine levels should be monitored as carefully as during infancy. L-Tyrosine supplementation is needed to maintain the tyrosine intake at 110 mg/kg/day during pregnancy. Nutritional factors particularly important during pregnancy, such as kilocalories, protein, vitamins, and mineral intake, should be monitored.[54]

Compliance with the diet during pregnancy, even for the well-motivated woman, is usually difficult and requires support of family, physician, and dietitian.

The effect of high paternal levels of blood phenylalanine on pregnancy outcome has received less attention than for mothers. One large study has reported that no increase in birth defects and no adverse pregnancy outcome could be documented.[64] Long-term follow-up of such children has not yet been reported, so the question remains open. Regardless of which parent is affected with PKU, the offspring of such a pregnancy is at increased risk for inheriting PKU.

Physicians: How to Order Diet

The diet order should indicate *diet for PKU*. The level of phenylalanine should be specified.

PARENT RESOURCES

1. PKU Children's Network
   10525 Vista Sorrento Parkway #204
   San Diego, CA 92121
   Katie Andrews (619) 587-9421

   Resources available include information for new families, recommended reading list, product information and coupons, and letters from PKU parents.

2. *National PKU News*
   Virginia Schuett, Editor
   7760 Ridge Drive NE
   Seattle, WA 98115

3. Nardella, Maria. A teacher's guide to PKU, July 1985.
   Children's Rehabilitative Services
   Arizona Department of Health Services
   1740 W. Adams, Room 208
   Phoenix, AZ 85007
   (602) 255-1890

4. Castiglioni LL, Rouse BM. The young woman with PKU, 1986.
   PKU Treatment Center,
   University of Texas Medical Branch
   Galveston, TX 77550
   (409) 761-2355

5. Castiglioni LL, Rouse BM. The child with PKU, 1986.
   PKU Treatment Center,
   University of Texas Medical Branch
   Galveston, TX 77550
   (409) 761-2355

6. Michals K, Gleason L, Racster G, Hurtt L. PKU and teens: planning makes it easier, 1987.
   Illinois Department of Public Health
   Genetics Disease Program
   535 West Jefferson Street
   Springfield, IL 62761

7. Living with PKU, Evansville, IN: Mead Johnson, 1990.
   Inherited Metabolic Disease Clinic
   University of Colorado Health Science Center
   Denver, CO 80262

8. Schuett V. Low protein food list: for phenylketonuria and metabolic diseases requiring a low protein diet, 1991.
   University of Wisconsin Press
   114 North Murray Street
   Madison, WI 53715
   (608) 262-8782

9. Schuett V. Low protein cookery for phenylketonuria, 2nd ed. 1988.
   University of Wisconsin Press
   114 North Murray Street
   Madison, WI 53715
   (608) 262-8782

10. Dietary management of metabolic disorders, 1991.
    Mead Johnson & Co.
    Evansville, IN 47721
    (812) 429-5000

References

46. Hunt MM, Berry HK, White PP. Phenylketonuria, adolescence and diet. J Am Diet Assoc 1985;85:1328–1334.
47. Acosta PB, Farnhoff PM, Warshaw HS, Hambidge KM, Ernest A, MoCahe RB, Elsas LJ. Zinc and copper status of treated children with phenylketonuria. JPEN 1981;5:406–409.
48. Gropper SS, Acosta PB, Clark-Sheehan N, Wenz E, Cheng M, Kock R. Trace element status of children with PKU and normal children. J Am Diet Assoc 1988;88:459–465.
49. Reilly C, Barrett JE, Patterson CM, Tinggi U, Latham SL, Marrinan A. Trace element nutrition status and dietary intake of children with phenylketonuria. Am J Clin Nutr 1990;52:159–165.

50. Tourian A, Sidbury JB. Phenylketonuria and hyperphenylalaninemia. In: Stanbury JB, Wyngaarden JB, Fredrickson DS, Goldstein JL, Brown SB, eds. The metabolic basis of inherited disease, 5th ed. New York: McGraw-Hill, 1983:270.

51. Behrman RE, Vaughan VC III. Inborn errors of metabolism. In: Nelson WE, ed. Nelson textbook of pediatrics, 12th ed. Philadelphia: WB Saunders, 1983:424.

52. Scriver CR, Kaufman S, Woo SLC. Hyperphenylalaninemias. In: Scriver CR, Beaudet AL, Sly WS, Valle D, eds. The metabolic basis of inherited disease, 6th ed. New York: McGraw-Hill, 1989:495–546.

53. Rohr FJ, Levy HL, Shich VE. Inborn errors of metabolism. In: Walker WA, Watkins JB, eds. Nutrition in pediatrics. Boston: Little, Brown, 1985:384–391.

54. Trahms CM. Nutritional care for children with metabolic disorders. In: Krause MV, Mahan LK, eds. Food, nutrition, and diet therapy, 7th ed. Philadelphia: WB Saunders, 1984:802.

55. American Academy of Pediatrics Committee on Nutrition. Final report, Task Force on the Dietary Management of Metabolic Disorders. Dec 1985. Elk Grove Village, IL (unpublished report).

56. Acosta PB, Elsas LJ. Dietary management of inherited metabolic disease: phenylketonuria, galactosemia, tyrosinemia, homocystinuria, maple syrup urine disease. Atlanta: Acelmu Publishers, 1976:7.

57. Flannery DB, Hitchcock E, Mamunes P. Dietary management of phenylketonuria from birth using a phenylalanine-free product. J Pediatr 1983;103:247–249.

58. Koch R, Azan CG, Friedman EG, Williamson ML. Preliminary report of the effects of diet discontinuation in PKU. J Pediatr 1982;100:870–875.

59. Anon. Should dietary treatment of phenylketonuria be continued after infancy? Nutr Rev 1985;43:176–177.

60. Matthews WS, Barabas G, Cusack E, Ferrari M. Social quotients of children with phenylketonuria, before and after discontinuation of dietary therapy. Am J Ment Dis 1986;90:92–94.

61. Michals K, Dominck M, Schuett V, Brown E, Matalon R. Return to diet therapy in patients with phenylketonuria. J Pediatr 1985;106:933–936.

62. Schuett VE, Brown ES. Diet policies of PKU clinics in the United States. Am J Public Health 1984;74:501–503.

63. Matalon R, Michals K, Azen C, Friedman EG, Koch R, Wenz E, Levy H, Rohr F, Rouse B, Castiglioni L, Hanley W, Austin V, DeLaCruz F. Maternal PKU collaborative study: the effect of nutrient intake on pregnancy outcome. J Inherit Metab Dis 1991;14(3): 371–374.

64. Fisch RO, Matalon R, Weisber S, Michals K. Children of fathers with phenylketonuria: an international survey. J Pediatr 1991;118:739–741.

WEIGHT CONTROL

General Description

A weight control program for children and adolescents provides dietary guidelines that include sufficient energy to allow for weight stabilization or gradual weight reduction. Dietary guidelines allow for adequate nutrients so that growth and development are not compromised. The focus is on the identification of inappropriate eating and activity behaviors and modification to ones more appropriate for weight control.

Nutritional Inadequacy

This diet can be designed to meet the RDA for nutrients unless the child or adolescent has food dislikes or aversions that greatly limit the variety of foods eaten or unless the diet provides less than basal calories for weight-for-height and age. A multiple vitamin supplement may be indicated.

Indications and Rationale

From 25 to 30% of children and adolescents in the United States can be classified as overweight, depending on the criteria used.[65] Childhood obesity is associated with hyperinsulinemia, hyperlipidemia, hypertension, and carbohydrate intolerance. There is some evidence that obesity in children is an independent risk factor for later coronary heart disease and that many atherogenic serum lipid disorders originate in childhood. Even without primary medical implications, the psychological and social consequences of childhood and adolescent obesity are profound.

Obesity that begins during childhood is likely to persist into adulthood.[66-69] The chances are 1 to 4 against the achievement of normal body weight if a child enters adolescence being obese. The chances increase to 28 to 1 against achieving a normal body weight as an adult if a child is still obese at the end of adolescence.[70] Early intervention may help influence the development of eating and activity patterns and attitudes. Intervention may also result in satisfactory weight control during the critical years when body image is forming. Obesity among children continues in the vast majority of cases if no treatment is given.[65]

The problem of dietary control for obesity is more complicated in children and adolescents than in adults. In children, sufficient kilocalories and protein must be provided to allow for growth and development. If weight is stabilized, an increase in lean tissue and a decrease in depot fat will occur with growth. The extent to which diet is responsible for these changes depends on the age at which the diet is started. The period of adolescence includes a growth spurt, the intensity of which is exceeded only by the fetus and the infant during the first year. Since caloric and most nutritional needs parallel the growth rate, the adolescent's needs are higher in relation to body size than those of younger or older people. There is a considerable difference in nutritional needs between boys and girls during this time because growth begins earlier in girls and is less rapid than for boys. There is also considerable individual variation among adolescents with respect to the age of onset, the intensity, and the duration of the growth spurt. The growth period is more closely related to the stage of sexual maturation than to chronological age. The stages of growth and maturation need to be considered when formulating a kilocalorie-controlled diet for adolescents. Caution must be exercised when kilocalories are controlled in children[71] and in adolescents, and linear growth rates need to be monitored regularly. Energy expenditure from activity can safely enhance the effects of kilocalorie-controlled intake and result in better control of weight, better compliance, and fewer dropouts than diet without activity.[72]

Weight control measures in the young child are also directed toward the education of the family about the child's energy and nutrient needs and about the importance of regular exercise. In older children and adolescents, the success of weight control measures depends chiefly on the motivation of the individual.

Goals of Dietary Management

Rather than loss of body weight per se, the primary goal of weight management in children and adolescents is to aid the individual in becoming aware of inappropriate eating and activity patterns and to provide support for gradually modifying these behaviors to ones that result in achieving and maintaining an appropriate body weight. This concept needs to be described to the individual and the parents so that they have reasonable expectations for their efforts.

Dietary Recommendations

Assessment. Management of the obese child or adolescent initially involves an assessment of the current diet, both the amount and kind of foods eaten, and an inventory of family dietary patterns. Intake of school lunches, fast foods, snacks, convenience foods, and restaurant meals should be identified and discussed so that the diet plan can be tailored accordingly.

The primary goal is to achieve gradual changes in the child's caloric intake while maintaining nutritional adequacy for growth and development. Emphasis is placed on education for substitution and modification of current dietary practices rather than for significant change or complete elimination of favorite foods. The dietary modifications for calorie control and nutritional adequacy are to be made gradually over several months and at a pace identified as reasonable for each individual child or adolescent. The goal is longterm, with emphasis on gradually setting a lifestyle that can persist into adulthood. Modification should be flexible enough to accomodate a lifestyle that may include school lunch, fast foods, and other favorite foods.

A review of growth charts of children who become obese shows that weight gains in such children are rarely greater than 5 lb annually in excess of that expected for age. Such gains can be accounted for by an energy imbalance of approximately 50 kcal/day.[73] These observations suggest that the existing energy imbalance is generally small. Therefore, when designing the meal plan and counseling the child, even small deviations in caloric intake should be identified and addressed.

Identification of parental interest, individual interest, and potential for support within the family is helpful. Present activity level and activity preferences and availability also need to be assessed.

The dietary guidelines are individualized using Table 23-18 and Table 23-19 for determining calorie needs and the RDA for protein and nutrient needs (see also Chapter 2, Recommended Dietary Allowances).

Children. The degree of obesity needs to be considered when designing a kilocalorie-controlled diet for a child. This determination is most easily made by use of growth charts to identify percent of predicted weight (Pediatric Appendix 28, National Center for Health Statistics Growth Charts). A child who is 120 to 139% of the predicted weight for height and age would be considered mildly obese; a child who is 140 to 159% of the predicted weight for height and age would be considered moderately obese; and a child 160% or more of the predicted weight for height and age would be considered severely obese.[74]

The example at the top of the next page will help highlight this concept.

An 8 year old boy is referred for a weight control program.

Weight: 31 kg, 90th percentile

Height: 127 cm, 50th percentile

The weight expected for height and age is located using the growth chart and is 25 kg.

Present weight is 124% of predicted weight-for-height and age, so this boy is considered mildly obese:

$$\frac{31 \text{ kg}}{25 \text{ kg}} \times 100 = 124\%$$

If this boy were to maintain his present weight for approximately 2 years, his height and weight would be proportional (see Pediatric Appendix 28, National Center for Health Statistics Growth Charts).

Table 23-18 summarizes how caloric requirements are established according to degree of obesity. In our experience with mildly overweight children, basal calories that are determined from the Nomogram (Appendix 6) for present weight, height, and age are appropriate for weight control. This caloric level should result in stabilizing the child's weight and in achieving an appropriate weight with growth. (The calorie prescription for the mildly obese boy described above would be 1,275 daily.) In moderately or severely obese children, basal kilocalories, determined from the nomogram for predicted weight at present height and age deter-

TABLE 23-18   Suggested Caloric Allowances for Children by Degree of Obesity

	% of Predicted Weight for Height and Age*	Daily Kcal (Nomogram)†
Mildly obese	120–139	Basal for *present* weight, height, and age
Moderately obese	140–159	Basal for *predicted* weight at present height and age
Severely obese	> 160	Basal for *predicted* weight at present height and age

*See Appendix 28, National Center for Health Statistics Growth Charts.

†See Appendix 6, Nomogram for Estimating Caloric Requirements.

TABLE 23-19   Increase in Caloric Needs for Activity[75]

Activity	% Above Basal
Bed rest (eating and reading)	10
Very light (sitting, playing musical instrument, working with hands)	30
Light (playing, standing, walking, volleyball)	40–60
Moderate (cycling, fast walking, dancing)	60–80
Heavy (vigorous playing or working)	100

With permission from: Mahan LK, Rees JM. Nutrition in adolescence. St Louis: Mosby–Year Book, 1984:311.

mined from the growth charts, can be used to establish the caloric level of the weight control diet. Moderately and severely obese children have medically significant obesity, and gradual weight reduction is indicated. This caloric allowance results in gradual, yet consistent, weight loss.

Resting energy expenditure (basal calories) can be measured by indirect calorimetry and used as the calorie allowance for the mildly obese child. For moderately or severely obese children, one can choose a calorie level 200 to 300 calories less than basal calories, depending on activity level, to produce a gradual weight loss.

A caloric increment for habitual levels of activity (Table 23-19) may have to be added to the daily basal kilocalories to achieve the desired weight change goals if the child is more active. This need for change in the caloric prescription is most appropriately identified at follow-up visits when caloric intake and weight change can be assessed.

Efforts to bring about rapid weight reduction by strenuous diets are not justified and are rarely successful. Instead, a program of caloric control accompanied by an increase in activity and augmented by growth is encouraged.

Adolescents. During adolescence, the relatively uniform growth of childhood is suddenly altered by an increased velocity of development. This growth period is more closely related to the stage of sexual maturation than to chronological age. A scale for the stage of sexual maturation has been developed by Tanner[76] and is summarized in Table 23-20. (See also Appendix 37, Tanner Growth and Development Longitudinal Standards.)

In girls, peak height velocity occurs at approximately midpoint between stages III and IV, while peak height velocity for boys occurs just prior to stage IV. Therefore, adolescents in stages I, II, and III should have kilocalories identified for weight control that result in weight stabilization with sufficient kilocalories to cover the approaching growth spurt. Adolescents in stages IV and V can safely experience gradual weight loss[77] after having gone through the stage of peak

TABLE 23-20 Tanner Rating Stages of Maturity[76]

Stage	Boys	Girls
I	Prepubertal	Prepubertal
II	First visible signs of sexual maturation	Peak height velocity begins
III	Peak height velocity begins	Peak height velocity continues
IV	Peak height velocity continues; facial, axillary, and extremity hair growth; voice changes	Menarche
V	Adulthood	Axillary hair growth; adult distribution of breast tissue; adulthood

With permission from: Tanner JM. Growth at adolescence, 2nd ed. Oxford, England: Blackwell Scientific Publications, 1962.

demand for kilocalories and nutrients that is associated with height increase. In general, the weight control diet for adolescents in stages I, II, and III can be determined in a manner similar to that for the mildly obese child. Kilocalories prescribed for adolescents in stages IV and V are determined in a manner similar to that for the moderately or severely obese child (see Table 23-18).

Again, if the adolescent is more than normally active, additional kilocalories need to be prescribed to cover this activity. This need can best be determined by assessing the activity pattern and the weight response at follow-up sessions.

Activity.   A calorie-controlled diet and increased physical activity need to be employed for weight control. An activity program should be defined for the individual with self-improvement as the goal rather than some absolute duration or extent of exercise. The individual needs suggestions for ways of being active within the limits of the excess weight. Activities that the individual would enjoy, as well as those that are easily accessible, should be identified. Results reported by Huttunen and coworkers indicate that obese children and adolescents are in reality less fit than the nonobese subjects of the same age.[78] The reduction in fitness seems to be related to the degree of obesity. Successful weight reduction leads to increased maximum oxygen consumption, reflecting enhanced physical fitness in these children.[78]

Role of Family.   The role of the family in the genesis and treatment of obesity varies and is often difficult to assess. In younger obese children, difficulty in parental control or in the setting of limits for the child may contribute to the problem.[79] Assisting such parents with general techniques of behavior modification may help in modifying the child's eating behavior. The problem of obesity is frequently a source of disagreement and dissension between older obese children and their parents. In such instances, the dietitian and the physician may assume the role of enforcer to relieve intrafamily conflict. One should also inquire into television viewing and snacking habits and counsel the parents and child accordingly. Much television viewing obviously is conducive to inactivity, but it may also be strongly associated with increased snacking.[73]

Continuing Care.   Follow-up by return visits to the physician and dietitian is essential. Food and activity records are used at various times to help identify areas where the greatest attention should be directed. Discussions centered around the use of school lunches, favorite foods, fast foods, restaurant meals, convenience foods, and party and holiday foods are an important part of these follow-up sessions, with weight change being of secondary importance. Caloric intake and weight change should be assessed at these sessions so that the need for caloric revision can be identified. Height should also be monitored.

Guidelines for Long-Term Weight Control

When the patient has achieved a weight that is acceptable for height and age, dietary guidelines should be formulated, with the kilocalorie content adjusted for size, age, and activity. At this time, it is helpful to discuss with the child or adolescent how their weight will continue to change as growth and development proceed. The patient needs to understand that this weight change is normal as long as growth and development occur. The importance of an active lifestyle for successful weight control needs to be reinforced. The support and guidance that follow-up visits provide are also useful during this time.

Physicians: How to Order Diet

The diet order should indicate *diet for weight control*. The dietitian will determine the caloric level according to the preceding guidelines.

References

65. Spence SH. Behavioral treatment of childhood obesity. J Child Psychol Psychiatry 1986;27(4):447–453.
66. Leung AKC, Robson WLM. Childhood obesity. Postgrad Med 1990;87:123–131.
67. Story M, Alton I. Current perspectives on adolescent obesity. Top Clin Nutr 1991; 6:51–60.
68. Mellin LM. Managing child and adolescent obesity: the SHAPEDOWN program. Top Clin Nutr 1991;6:70–76.
69. Sorensen TIA, Sonne-Holm S. Risk in childhood of severe adult obesity: retrospective population-based case cohort study. Am J Epidemiol 1988;127:104–113.
70. Stunkard A, Burt V. Obesity and body image: II. Age at onset of disturbances in the body image. Am J Psychiatry 1967;123:1443–1447.
71. Epstein LH, McCurley J, Valoski A, Wing RR. Growth in obese children treated for obesity. Am J Dis Child 1990;144:1360–1364.
72. Reybrouck T, Vinckx J, Van Den Berghe G, Vanderschueren-Lodeweyckx M. Exercise therapy and hypocaloric diet in the treatment of obese children and adolescents. Acta Paediatr Scand 1990;79(1):84–89.
73. Dietz WH. Prevention of childhood obesity. Pediatr Clin North Am 1986;33(4):823–833.
74. Anon. Children and weight: changing perspectives. Berkeley: Nutr Communications Associates, 1985.
75. Mahan LK, Rees JM. Nutrition in adolescence. St. Louis: Mosby, 1984:311.
76. Tanner JM. Growth at adolescence, 2nd ed. Oxford, England: Blackwell Scientific Publications, 1962.
77. Carruth BR, Iszler J. Assessment and conservative management of the overfat adolescent. J Adolesc Health Care 1981;1:289–299.
78. Huttunen NP, Knip M, Paavilainen T. Physical activity and fitness in obese children. Int J Obes 1986;10(6):519–525.
79. Klesges RC, Stein RJ, Eck LH, Isbell TR, Klesges LM. Parental influence on food selection in young children and its relationship to childhood obesity. Am J Clin Nutr 1991;53:859–864.

24 / *Gastrointestinal Diseases and Disorders in Children*

CONSTIPATION AND ENCOPRESIS

General Description

Dietary recommendations emphasize the necessity of a varied and nutritionally balanced diet that provides adequate fiber and fluid to alleviate symptoms.

Nutritional Inadequacy

The diet is adequate in nutrients when compared to the Recommended Dietary Allowances (RDA). However, the diet for each child should be assessed for nutritional adequacy. On the basis of this assessment, vitamin or mineral supplementation may be necessary.

Indications and Rationale

Constipation is a common problem in infants and children, yet it is often ignored or incorrectly treated. Constipation is not a disease, but it can have many unpleasant consequences, such as abdominal pain, distention, flatulence, diarrhea by overflow, bedwetting, and nausea. This variety of symptoms can disrupt childhood activities and create parental anxiety. The spectrum of problems of fecal elimination ranges from simple constipation to chronic retention and may be either functional or organic in origin. Constipation can be associated with anal lesions, such as fissures and ulcers, and may also be a manifestation of more serious disorders, such as Hirschsprung's disease or even malabsorption. Table 24-1 lists the most common causes of constipation-encopresis.[1]

Constipation is defined as the passage of excessively dry stools, stools of insignificant size, or infrequent stools (less often than every other day).[2] In practice, parents may perceive constipation in a variety of ways, and inappropriate perceptions should be clarified. Encopresis is defined as fecal soiling of clothing that persists regularly beyond the usual age of completion of toilet training (between ages 4 to

TABLE 24-1   Causes of Constipation-Encopresis

Constipation without Encopresis	Encopresis without Constipation	Constipation with Encopresis
Lack of fecal bulk	Neurogenic	Anatomic obstruction
Unusually firm stools	Behavioral/psychogenic	Spinal cord lesion
Interference with contraction of the voluntary muscles of defecation		Behavioral/psychogenic
Anatomic obstruction		
Behavioral/psychogenic		

With permission from: Fitzgerald JF. Encopresis, soiling, constipation: what's to be done? Pediatrics 1975;56:348–349.

5 years).[3] It is often associated with chronic constipation because, eventually, watery content from the proximal colon may pass around hard retained stool and be eliminated through the rectum undetected by the child.[4]

One of the most common causes of simple constipation in infants is a change in feeding practices. These alterations can be as minor as a change from breast milk to formula, a change from one formula to another, or the introduction of new foods into the diet. Inappropriately chosen diets also cause constipation in children. Such diets are limited in variety and usually include only a few favorite foods. Fruits and vegetables are typically missing in most of these children's diets. Frequently, these children do not eat well-balanced meals at regular intervals.

There is historical evidence that the fiber intake of children in the United States is low. In a 1975 survey of 2,000 households, 75% of the children ate less than 4 servings per day of fruits and vegetables, and 62% ate less than 4 servings of breads and cereals.[4] The Health and Nutrition Examination Survey (HANES) data also revealed that a substantial number of children have low intakes of fiber-containing foods.[4]

Goals of Dietary Management

The goal of dietary management is to help the child establish a varied and nutritionally well-balanced diet, with high fiber meals and adequate fluid intake.

Dietary Recommendations

Recommendations for the child include the regular intake of a wide variety of foods that contain ample fiber, and adequate fluid. Management initially involves an assessment of food and fluid intake. This assessment helps the dietitian identify current problems and formulate dietary recommendations that also take into account growth, development, and activity needs (see Chapter 18, Pediatric Nutritional Assessment, and Chapter 19, Normal Nutrition). Dietary modification is indicated if an inappropriate diet is a major cause of the patient's constipation.

Fiber. The American Academy of Pediatrics Committee on Nutrition states that although no firm recommendations can be made at this time, a "substantial amount" of fiber probably should be eaten by all children (except those less than 1 year of age) to ensure normal laxation. Solid foods, when introduced, should include whole-grain breads and cereals, fruits, and vegetables. A diet for children that emphasizes high fiber foods (many of which are of low caloric density) to the exclusion of other common foods should not be advised.[5]

The diet should include enough fiber (vegetables, fruits, and whole-grain breads and cereals) so that the bulk left in the bowel after digestion encourages the movement of intestinal contents and stimulates periodic evacuation. In general, foods can be classified in order of increasing fecal bulk as follows: protein, fat, milk, digestible carbohydrate, and carbohydrate with nondigestible material. The fiber content of various foods is listed in Chapter 9, Fiber and Residue Modifications. Quantitative recommendations for fiber intake for children have not been established. However, data suggest that systematically increasing dietary fiber can be a useful treatment for constipation and encopresis.[6]

Two major areas of concern exist when the fiber intake of children is increased. The first concern is the small stomach capacity of children. Fiber-rich foods are bulky, filling, and have a low caloric density. Therefore, many children may be unable to consume sufficient kilocalories on a high fiber diet. The second area of concern is the influence that fiber can have on the absorption of essential minerals, such as calcium, iron, phosphorus, zinc, and magnesium.

Bran, the most concentrated source of food fiber, should be used in moderation. Large amounts may cause flatulence, abdominal pain, and discomfort. It is usually recommended that bran, when used, be added to foods typically eaten by the child and be given in at least 3 divided doses a day. Bran preparations usually are not well accepted by children. It is often possible to achieve an adequate fiber intake in the diet without bran supplements.

Fluid. Many children do not regularly drink an adequate amount of fluid. Fluid intake, essential to bowel function, is especially important with a higher fiber diet. There are several formulas for estimating water requirements. The minimum requirement of water approximates 60 ml/kg of body weight per day. An intake greater than this may be necessary. Excessive fluid intake is considered to be $2\frac{1}{2}$ times this amount.[7] Guidelines for maintenance water requirements are shown in Table 24-2.

Other Considerations. Although certain foods have been cited as causing constipation or as being inappropriate during treatment, there is no conclusive documented evidence. These foods include milk and cheese, apples in any form, and carrots. If the child's diet is limited in variety and includes these foods predominantly, one could expect that the child might become constipated, but the cause would be more related to the limited diet than to these specific foods.

Other components of the constipation-encopresis treatment program may include regular exercise; use of bulk agents, stool softeners, and lubricants; and behavior modification plans that include the encouragement of regular elimination.[6]

Follow-up is essential. Every 4 to 6 weeks, the patient or parent should keep a 3 to 5 day food record so that recommended changes can be monitored and modifications made if needed.

TABLE 24-2   Range of Average Water Requirements of Children at Different Ages under Ordinary Conditions[4]

Age	Average Body Weight (kg)	Total Water in 24 Hr (ml)	Water /kg of Body Weight in 24 Hr (ml)
3 days	3.0	250–300	80–100
10 days	3.2	400–500	125–150
3 mo	5.4	750–850	140–160
6 mo	7.3	950–1100	130–155
9 mo	8.6	1,100–1,250	125–145
1 yr	9.5	1,150–1,300	120–135
2 yr	11.8	1,350–1,500	115–125
4 yr	16.2	1,600–1,800	100–110
6 yr	20.0	1,800–2,000	90–100
10 yr	28.7	2,000–2,500	70–85
14 yr	45.0	2,200–2,700	50–60
18 yr	54.0	2,200–2,700	40–50

With permission from: Barness LA. Nutrition and nutritional disorders. In: Behrman RE, ed. Nelson textbook of pediatrics, 14th ed. Philadelphia: WB Saunders, 1992:107.

Physicians: How to Order Diet

The diet order should indicate *constipation-encopresis*.

References

1. Fitzgerald JF. Encopresis, soiling, constipation: what's to be done? Pediatrics 1975;56:348–349.
2. Devroede G. Constipation. In: Sleisenger MH, Fordtran JS, eds. Gastrointestinal disease. Philadelphia: WB Saunders, 1993:837–887.
3. Johns C. Encopresis. Am J Nurs 1985;85:153–156.
4. Hamilton JR. The digestive system. In: Behrman RE, ed. Nelson textbook of pediatrics, 14th ed. Philadelphia: WB Saunders, 1992:937–938.
5. American Academy of Pediatrics. Plant fiber intake in the pediatric diet. Pediatrics 1981; 67:572–575.
6. Houts AC, Mellen MW, Whelan JP. Use of dietary fiber and stimulus control to treat retentive encopresis: a multiple baseline investigation. J Pediatr Psychol 1988;13:435–445.
7. Greene HL, Ghishan FK. Excessive fluid intake as a cause of chronic diarrhea in young children. J Pediatr 1983;102:836–840.

DIARRHEA

General Description

Diarrhea has been defined as a change in stool consistency, an excessive intestinal loss of fluid and electrolytes, or a significant increase in frequency or volume of stool to the degree that the child feels ill. For a child, daily fecal losses exceeding

$200 \text{ ml}/\text{m}^2$ of body surface are considered excessive. Acute diarrhea in children is caused by various viral, bacterial, or parasitic intestinal tract infections. The most common cause is infection with rotavirus.[8] Secondary disaccharidase deficiency may prolong the diarrhea.

Chronic diarrhea is the presence of diarrhea for a period of more than 2 weeks.[9] Chronic diarrhea may result from cystic fibrosis, celiac disease, Crohn's disease, and ulcerative colitis.[9] Chronic diarrhea is often associated with weight loss and with growth failure. Delayed growth is chiefly related to an inadequate supply of dietary protein and kilocalories, although poor zinc status may also play a role.[10] Inadequate intake of food because of anorexia, defective digestion and absorption of ingested food, and increased metabolic demands may contribute to nutritional deficiencies, even in the absence of malabsorption. If diarrhea and malabsorption are severe and persistent, malnutrition may result, with complications such as loss of immunocompetence and further impairment of gastrointestinal function. Chronic nonspecific diarrhea (often called toddler's diarrhea) has also been found to be associated with inappropriately low fat diets, with excessive ingestion of apple juice, and with excessive fluid intake.[9]

Nutritional Inadequacy

Nutritional recommendations for acute and chronic diarrhea are aimed at replacing fluid and electrolyte losses and provision of sufficient quantities of nutrients to meet the patient's requirements and increased needs imposed by infection and malabsorption. Oral intake should be assessed and supplemental vitamins, minerals, and electrolytes provided either enterally or parenterally if the patient is not eating.

Indications and Rationale

Treatment of acute diarrhea is aimed at replacing fluid and electrolyte losses as well as preventing a state of starvation. Unless treated aggressively, progressive dehydration and deterioration of health can occur. The infant is at high risk for dehydration because of its high insensible losses, high daily intestinal fluid turnover, and increased sensitivity to enterotoxins. The infant's high metabolic rate results in rapid depletion of nutrient stores since intake is usually decreased or some degree of malabsorption is present with diarrhea.[8]

Treatment of chronic diarrhea is more complex. In addition to replacing fluids and electrolytes and promoting adequate nutrient intake, treatment focuses on the underlying disease or nutrient intolerance causing the diarrhea.

Goals of Dietary Management

Oral Rehydration Solutions. Terminology used in the literature varies, but generally the solutions available to treat dehydration are referred to as oral rehydration solutions (ORS). Two types of ORS are then referred to, based on sodium content: a rehydration solution contains 75 to 90 mEq/L of sodium, and a maintenance solution contains 40 to 60 mEq/L of sodium. To treat dehydration, a solution containing 75 to 90 mEq/L of sodium, 20 mEq/L of potassium, 20 to 30% anions as base (acetate, citrate, lactate, or bicarbonate) and the remainder as chloride, and 2 to 2.5% glucose is recommended.[11] The World Health Organization's formula and Rehydralyte™ (Ross Laboratories) meet these specifications. These rehydration solutions should be used under medical supervision.

A solution with similar composition (except that sodium content is reduced to 40 to 60 mEq/L) is recommended to prevent dehydration or maintain hydration after dehydration treatment.[11] Pedialyte™ (Ross Laboratories) and Ricelyte™ (Mead Johnson Nutrition) meet these specifications and are examples of maintenance solutions. Compositions of these solutions are shown in Appendix 22.

Although ORS replace fluid and electrolyte losses, the actual volume and duration of diarrhea does not decrease significantly.[12] Studies indicate that solutions containing glucose polymers, such as rice starch, have the advantage of slightly reducing volume and duration of diarrhea.[12] The glucose polymers improve sodium and water absorption; therefore cereal-based ORS are being researched. Cereal proteins provide small peptides and amino acids that also

---

TABLE 24-3 Diarrhea Treatment Chart[11]

Degree of Dehydration	Signs* and Symptoms	Rehydration Therapy (within 4 hr)	Replacement of Stool Losses	Maintenance Therapy
Mild	Slightly dry buccal mucous membranes, increased thirst (Decreased urination 5% weight loss)†	ORS 50 ml/kg	10 ml/kg or ½–1 cup of ORS for each diarrheal stool	Human milk feeding, half-strength lactose-containing milk or formula, undiluted lactose-free formula, juices
Moderate	Sunken eyes, sunken fontanelle, loss of skin turgor, dry buccal mucous membranes 10% weight loss	ORS 100 ml/kg	Same as above	Same as above
Severe	Signs of moderate dehydration plus one of following: rapid thready pulse, (hypotension)†, cyanosis, rapid breathing, lethargy, coma (No urination 15% weight loss)†	Intravenous fluids (Ringer's lactate), 40 ml/kg/hr until pulse, blood pressure, and state of consciousness return to normal and urination is reestablished; then 50–100 ml/kg of ORS	Same as above	Same as above

ORS = Oral rehydration solutions.

*If no signs of dehydration are present, rehydration therapy is not required. Proceed with maintenance therapy and replacement of stool losses. Infants and children who receive solid food may continue their usual diet.

†Additional Mayo Clinic criteria.

With permission from: Santosham M, Greenough WB. Oral rehydration therapy: a global perspective. J Pediatr 1991;118:S44–S51.

facilitate absorption of sodium. Further research will focus on the optimal mix of amino acids in ORS.

Fluid and Electrolyte Therapy.   Whenever possible, the oral route should be used, but intravenous fluid and electrolyte therapy is indicated for patients who are severely dehydrated and in shock. Once stabilized, the oral route should be used. Therapy consists of three components: the rehydration phase, ongoing replacement of stool losses, and the maintenance phase. Therapy also depends on the degree of dehydration. Table 24-3 describes signs and symptoms of mild, moderate, and severe dehydration and suggests solutions and volumes to provide during the treatment phases.

During the rehydration phase, usually about 4 hours, a higher sodium ORS is given. Vomiting may interfere with retention of the ORS. However when the ORS is given by spooning rather than through a nipple or from a cup, successful retention is usually obtained, despite small amounts being vomited.[11]

Nutritional Therapy.   Once dehydration is corrected, the *maintenance phase* consists of providing a normal diet. Human milk or formula feeding should continue. Switching to a lactose-free formula remains controversial. Study results varied when lactose-free and lactose-containing formulas were compared when fed to children with diarrhea.[13] If a lactose-containing formula is not tolerated (vomiting or worsening diarrhea), the formula may be diluted to half strength or a lactose-free formula can be used. A maintenance solution should also be used to replace additional fluid losses. A rehydration solution of higher sodium content may be used during this (maintenance) phase but should be alternated (on a one-to-one basis) with low sodium or sodium-free fluids such as water, human milk, or low carbohydrate juices. Children who have advanced to solid foods should resume their normal diet.[11,13] Solid food has the advantage of slowing gastric emptying in the breast-fed or milk-based formula-fed infant, thus reducing the amount of lactose in the small intestine per unit of time. More frequent, smaller feedings have the same benefit on lactose digestion and on absorption.[13]

The patient should receive an adequate, balanced nutrient intake as soon as possible. Considerable absorption of nutrients can take place in spite of malabsorption, and feeding will assist in the repair of intestinal absorptive surfaces. The Subcommittee on Nutrition and Diarrheal Disease Control of the Food and Nutrition Board reviewed the nutritional consequences of diarrhea and concluded that "continued feeding" is both safe and beneficial. In order to promote catch-up growth, the subcommittee recommended frequent feeding of small amounts of high caloric, nutrient-dense foods at levels that provide at least 25% more energy than the estimated mean requirement for healthy children and that provide 100% more protein than the RDA.[14]

The recommendations of the World Health Organization's Program for Control of Diarrheal Diseases[15] for feeding during diarrhea are as follows:

1. Breast-feeding should be continued once rehydration, if needed, is complete.
2. Children who are fully weaned should eat their regular diet; if they are not fully weaned and are under 9 months, milk and milk-based formulas should be diluted to at least half strength for 1 to 2 days, or a lactose-free formula should be offered for 1 to 2 days.

3. Children who are 4 months of age or older should be encouraged to eat solid foods if they cannot satisfy their energy needs by breast-feeding or by formula alone.

4. Children should be allowed to determine the amount of food they need. Anorexic children should not be forced to eat. However, fluids should be encouraged.

5. Children should be allowed to have extra food when the diarrhea has subsided in order to recover from any nutritional deficit caused by the illness.

6. Foods high in carbohydrate content, particularly those containing disaccharides and monosaccharides (fruits, sweet desserts), should be avoided or limited during convalescence since they tend to overwhelm damaged absorptive mechanisms.

Use of the BRAT diet (consisting of bananas, rice, applesauce, and tea or toast) for exclusive treatment of diarrhea is not recommended. This diet is deficient in protein, fat, and energy. Traditionally the BRAT diet excluded the use of any formula and led to further nutritional decline.[16] This diet may also be referred to as the BRATTY diet (bananas, rice, applesauce, tea, toast, and yogurt).

Chronic Diarrhea. Therapy for chronic diarrhea should first be focused on treatment of the underlying disease. Chronic intractable diarrhea, a rare cause of chronic diarrhea, requires parenteral nutrition. Several reports show benefits from continuing minimal oral feeding. The introduction of one new food at a time in small amounts helps to re-establish food tolerance because of the trophic effect on the small intestine. Intravenous feeding is continued until a satisfactory weight gain has been achieved and is sustained by oral intake.[10]

In rare situations, intestinal sucrase is decreased. This decrease requires the use of elemental formulas containing glucose or its polymers [Pregestimil™ (Mead Johnson Nutrition), Nutramigen™ (Mead Johnson Nutrition), or Carbohydrate-Free™ formula (Ross Laboratories)] to which monosaccharides can be added in sequential increments (see Pediatric Appendix 25, for composition). Those few children who are unable to absorb monosaccharides require parenteral nutrition.

Physicians: How To Order Diet

The diet order should indicate *acute or chronic diarrhea*. The individual patient's situation will be assessed, and dietary restrictions (e.g., lactose) will be implemented.

References

8. Cohen MB. Etiology and mechanisms of acute infectious diarrhea in infants in the United States. J Pediatr 1991;118:S34–S39.

9. American Academy of Pediatrics Committee on Nutrition. Chronic diarrhea and malabsorption. In: Barness LA, ed. Pediatric nutrition handbook. Elk Grove Village, IL: AAP, 1993:209–219.

10. Meadows NJ, Walker-Smith JA. Chronic diarrhea. In: Walker WA, Watkins WA, eds. Nutrition in pediatrics. Boston: Little, Brown, 1985:529.

11. Santosham M, Greenough WB. Oral rehydration therapy: a global perspective. J Pediatr 1991;118:S44–S51.

12. Lebenthal E, Rong-Bao L. Glucose polymers as an alternative to glucose in oral rehydration solutions. J Pediatr 1991;118:S62–S69.

13. Brown KH. Dietary management of acute childhood diarrhea: optimal timing of feeding and appropriate use of milks and mixed diets. J Pediatr 1991;118:S92–S96.

14. American Academy of Pediatrics Committee on Nutrition. Use of oral fluid therapy and post-treatment feeding following enteritis in children in a developed country. Pediatrics 1985;75:358–361.

15. Anon. Feeding during diarrhea. Nutr Rev 1986;44:102.

16. Self TW. Pitfalls of the "BRAT" diet. Nutr and the M.D. 1986;12:1–3.

GLUTEN-SENSITIVE ENTEROPATHY: CELIAC DISEASE

General Description

Wheat, rye, oats, barley, and products containing these grains are omitted from the diet in order to eliminate the intake of gluten, the protein found in these grains. Corn, rice, and products made from them may be used as substitutes. Other substitutes include wheat starch, tapioca, and soybean, buckwheat, arrowroot, and potato flours.

Transient lactose intolerance is commonly seen, and temporary fat intolerance sometimes occurs. Initially, lactose and fat restriction should be considered, usually for less than 2 weeks.

Nutritional Inadequacy

The gluten-controlled diet is adequate in nutrients when compared to the RDA. However, prior to the initiation of dietary treatment, nutrient deficiencies may be seen as a result of fat malabsorption and inadequate dietary intake. Water-miscible preparations of fat-soluble vitamins and a daily vitamin supplement may be indicated to correct these deficiencies. Increased absorption of nutrients occurs with dietary treatment, even if the recovery of intestinal mucosa may not be seen for a few months, so supplements may not be needed for more than a few months. Therefore, ongoing supplementation should be assessed for each patient individually.

If diarrhea has been severe, electolyte supplements might be needed for the first few days of therapy. With severe malabsorption, calcium and magnesium blood levels may be low and thus may need to be corrected by supplementation.

Indications and Rationale

Celiac disease is one of the most common chronic intestinal diseases to cause malabsorption in childhood.[17] Symptoms often begin during the second 6 months of life after wheat-containing foods are added to the diet. The affected child gradually becomes irritable and unwell, experiences loss of appetite, and begins to pass frequent, foul, bulky stools. Vomiting is also common. Weight gain slows during this time. Small bowel biopsy shows atrophy of intestinal mucosa, and the typical clinical findings are those of malnutrition. Diminished body weight is seen in almost all patients, especially in those with prolonged active disease; short stature is also common. These growth problems are related more closely to inadequate caloric and protein intake than to the severity of the malabsorption. Studies have shown that in infants and children with celiac disease who follow a diet controlled in gluten, complete recovery in weight, height, and bone age occurs.[18]

If gluten is eliminated from the diet, patients may become asymptomatic within 2 weeks, even though regeneration of the small bowel mucosa may extend over a period of several months. If the disease is associated with exacerbations, one must suspect the inadvertent intake of gluten-containing foods. In only a few patients, the disease is reported to be transient and is possibly related to an infection or to another inflammatory process. The patient and the parents must be cautioned against resuming the use of gluten-containing foods in the diet when symptoms subside, because mucosal damage usually recurs with the reintroduction of dietary gluten.[19] Since the diet must be continued for life, it is important to confirm the diagnosis of celiac disease by biopsy of the small intestine before diet therapy begins.

Goals of Dietary Management

For the infant or child with celiac disease, the goals of dietary management are to control gluten intake while providing all nutrients in quantities adequate to ensure that needs are met for growth, development, and activity. The infant or child's dietary intake should be assessed for adequacy, as well as for the presence of food intolerances. Dietary guidelines should be designed using catch-up growth energy and protein recommendations (see Chapter 20, Failure to Thrive). When catch-up growth has occurred, a gluten-controlled diet that reflects normal energy and nutrient needs should be recommended.

Dietary Recommendations

Dietary management requires the use of a gluten-controlled diet (see Chapter 9, Gluten Sensitivity: Celiac Sprue and Dermatitis Herpetiformis, Table 9-13). Temporary intolerance to lactose is common, and temporary intolerance to fat is sometimes seen. Therefore, the recommended diet should not only be controlled in gluten but initially should contain milk only if it is well tolerated.[20] See Chapter 9, Lactose Intolerance. Some control of dietary fat content should be considered because unabsorbed long-chain fatty acids may be converted to hydroxy-fatty acids, which may produce diarrhea. See Chapter 9, Fat Malabsorption. With control of symptoms, milk and milk products should again be added to the diet, and the level of fat can be increased.[21]

Manufacturers may be contacted for information regarding the gluten content of infant foods when planning the diet for infants.

Physicians: How to Order Diet

The diet order should indicate *gluten-restricted diet* for a child with celiac disease.

References

17. Hamilton JR. Gastrointestinal disease: an important cause of malnutrition in childhood. In: Suskind RM, ed. Textbook of pediatric nutrition. New York: Raven Press, 1981:465–474.

18. DeLuca F, Astori M, Pandullo E, Medazzu G. Effects of a gluten-free diet on catch up growth and height prognosis in coeliac children with growth retardation recognized after the age of 5 years. Eur J Pediatr 1988;147:188–191.

19. Anson O, Weizman A, Zeevi N. Celiac disease: parental knowledge and attitudes of dietary compliance. Pediatrics 1990;85(1):98–103.
20. Roggero M, Ceccatelli C, Volpe C, Donattini T, Giuliani G, Lambri A, Tavani E, Careddu P. Extent of lactose absorption in children with active celiac disease. J Pediatr Gastroenterol Nutr 1989;9:290–294.
21. Trier JS. Celiac sprue. N Engl J Med 1991;325(24):1709–1719.

INFLAMMATORY BOWEL DISEASE

General Description

The primary nutritional emphasis for patients with inflammatory bowel disease should be on recommendations for a well-balanced diet that meets protein and caloric needs to restore normal growth and to promote catch-up growth. Dietary restrictions are not recommended unless there is a specific food intolerance or symptoms of intestinal obstruction. Nutritional support via enteral or parenteral routes may be indicated.[22]

Nutritional Inadequacy

Multiple vitamin and mineral supplementation is frequently needed to prevent or correct nutrient deficiencies. Folic acid, vitamin D, iron, calcium, vitamin B_{12}, magnesium, and zinc should be provided when their need is indicated by the dietary assessment or when laboratory findings are consistent with a deficiency state.[22] Drug therapy may also contribute to nutrient deficiencies. Examples are sulfasalazine, which interferes with folate absorption; corticosteroids, which suppress calcium absorption; and cholestyramine, which impairs the absorption of fat and fat-soluble vitamins.[23] A daily multiple vitamin-mineral combination that meets 100 to 150% of the RDA is recommended when the child is following a low residue diet since the diet is not nutritionally adequate.[22]

Indications and Rationale

Ulcerative colitis and Crohn's disease are the two chronic idiopathic inflammatory bowel diseases. Ulcerative colitis is an inflammatory process that is limited to the colon. In contrast, Crohn's disease may occur in any portion of the gastrointestinal tract, although the majority of patients have disease that involves primarily the terminal ileum and the colon.[24] Major symptoms commonly associated with ulcerative colitis and with Crohn's disease include diarrhea (often bloody), abdominal pain, and fever. Inflammatory bowel disease in children, especially Crohn's disease, is associated with a lack of weight gain, the cessation of linear growth, delayed bone maturation, and delayed sexual maturation.[23]

Growth failure represents one of the most serious complications of inflammatory bowel disease in children and is one of the most difficult to treat. The cause of the growth failure is multifactorial, including inadequate dietary intake, excessive gastrointestinal losses, malabsorption, and increased nutritional requirements for growth.[22,23] Inadequate intake of energy and protein largely account for the poor growth and lack of weight gain in these patients.[24] Inadequate food intake often results from anorexia and from fear of postprandial abdominal pain and diarrhea. Intestinal malabsorption and enteric losses of protein, blood, vitamins, and minerals may occur. The most common nutritional deficiencies are of folate, vitamin B_{12}, vitamin D, zinc, iron, calcium, and magnesium.[22-25]

The need for nutritional assessment in the routine management of children with inflammatory bowel disease is now apparent as the influence of early nutritional intervention on malnutrition and delayed growth is being seen.[24] Although nutritional consideration should be given to all patients with inflammatory bowel disease, nutritional therapy has its primary impact in the treatment of Crohn's disease, particularly in individuals with small bowel involvement.

Goals of Dietary Management

The goals of nutritional therapy are to replace the nutrient losses associated with the inflammatory processes, to correct body deficits, to provide sufficient nutrients to promote energy and nitrogen balance, to restore normal growth, and to promote catch-up growth.

Dietary Recommendations

For children, a balanced diet that meets energy and protein needs is recommended for catch-up growth. Estimates of energy and protein requirements should be based on ideal weight for actual height rather than actual weight,[26] 75 to 100 kcal/kg and 2 to 3 g of protein per kilogram have also been suggested.[27]

The limitation of dietary choices is discouraged because this limitation usually results in further nutritional deficiencies and creates stress associated with eating for the child. There is no clear evidence that the consumption or avoidance of specific foods induces a remission or influences the severity of the disease or the frequency of relapses.[23] However, the diet should be modified accordingly when the disease is active, when specific foods exacerbate symptoms, or when laboratory tests suggest specific abnormalities, such as steatorrhea or lactose intolerance.[25] A low fat diet supplemented with medium-chain triglyceride oil may be helpful in the control of symptoms in children with steatorrhea or diarrhea. Some patients may have secondary lymphangiectasia owing to chronic inflammation or to previous surgery and may also benefit from the use of medium-chain triglyceride oil as a source of kilocalories. A low residue diet in small, frequent feedings is recommended when severe postprandial pain or partial bowel obstruction is present. Renal oxalate stones have been seen in patients with Crohn's disease who also have steatorrhea. When fat malabsorption is present, excess oxalate is absorbed by the colon and results in hyperoxaluria. Restriction of dietary oxalate (see Chapter 14, Oxalate Restriction) may be indicated in these patients. This would only apply to those patients who still have the colon in place.[28]

Nutritional supplementation with a liquid formula may be necessary when the child is unable to increase dietary protein and energy intakes with ordinary foods. Dietary intake supplementation may be achieved with these formulas, but sometimes children experience satiety when taking these formulas and therefore cannot increase their total nutrient intake significantly. Nasogastric infusions of an enteral formula, either continuously or intermittently, have been effective in improving the nutritional status, growth rates, and well-being of selected patients with inflammatory bowel disease.[27] Nocturnal nasogastric feedings permit these children to go to school during the day. A program of nocturnal nasogastric feedings for 1 out of every 4 months for a year produced significant height and weight gain.[28]

Patients with inflammatory bowel disease who are unable to tolerate sufficient amounts of enteral feeding because of active inflammatory disease or diarrhea, obstruction, or short bowel syndrome may receive substantial benefit from parenteral nutrition.[22,29]

Physicians: How to Order Diet

The diet order should indicate a diet for a child with *inflammatory bowel disease.*

References

22. Michener WM, Wyllie R. Management of children and adolescents with inflammatory bowel disease. Med Clin North Am 1990;74:103–117.
23. Seidman E, LeLeiko N, Ament M, Berman W, Caplan D, Evans J, Kocoshis S, Lake A, Motil K, Sutphen J, Thomas D. Nutritional issues in pediatric inflammatory bowel disease. J Pediatr Gastroenterol Nutr 1991;12:424–438.
24. Afonso JJ, Rombeau JL. Nutritional care for patients with Crohn's disease. Hepato-gastroenterology 1990;37:32–41.
25. Sabbah SJ, Seidman EG. Dietary management of Crohn's disease in children and adolescents. In: Bayless TM, ed. Current management of inflammatory bowel disease. Philadelphia, BC Decker; 1989:236.
26. Sanderson IR, Udeen S, Davies PS, Savage MO, Walker-Smith JA. Remission induced by an elemental diet in small bowel Crohn's disease. Arch Dis Child 1987;62:123–127.
27. Belli DC, Seidman E, Bouthillier L, Weber AM, Roy CC, Pletinex M, Beaulieu M, Morin CL. Chronic intermittent elemental diet improves growth failure in children with Crohn's disease. Gastroenterology 1988;94:603–610.
28. Seftel A, Resnick MI. Metabolic evaluation of urolithiasis. In: Barry JM, Resnick MI, eds. The urologic clinics of North America. Philadelphia: WB Saunders, 1990:159–169.
29. Fleming CR. Enteral and parenteral nutrition. In: Peppercorn MA, ed. Therapy of inflammatory bowel disease. New York: Marcel Dekker, 1990:145–157.

FAT ABSORPTION TEST DIET

General Description

The diet is generally planned to provide 100 grams of fat in adults, but in children estimates of actual fat intake are made since many children are not able to consume this amount of fat. Interpretation of the test results according to actual fat intake is possible by using the formula given below.

Indications and Rationale

The test diet is used to determine if steatorrhea is present. Steatorrhea is an indication of gastrointestinal maldigestion or malabsorption.

Stools are collected during a 24, 48, or 72 hour period while the patient's dietary intake is being recorded. Ordinarily, the test is done in the hospital or in a facility that allows outpatients to be served accurately measured diets. With children, however, the estimates of actual fat intake are based on a food record, so the test can be done at home. The patient and parents are instructed to keep a food record during the time of the stool collection. The actual amount of fat ingested can be determined from the food record, and this information can be used to interpret results of the stool fat collection by the following formula:

$$(0.021 \times \text{g of dietary fat } /24 \text{ hr}) + 2.93 = \text{g of fecal fat}/24 \text{ hr}$$

According to this formula, a stool fat of about 3.98 g would be expected after a dietary fat intake of 50 g. Values greater than those obtained by use of this formula indicate the presence of maldigestion or malabsorption.

25 / *Neurological Disease in Children*

KETOGENIC DIET

General Description

The ketogenic diet was suggested in 1921 by Wilder[1] for the prophylactic treatment of some types of epilepsy in children. It has been used since then and in the recent past has received further review and application.[2,3]

The intent of the ketogenic diet is seizure control with minimal medication, thus minimizing drug side effects. The diet is high in fat and low in carbohydrate and is planned to produce ketosis by reversing the usual ratio of dietary carbohydrate to fat. The diet may be planned with or without medium-chain triglyceride (MCT) oil.

Nutritional Inadequacy

A multivitamin, a calcium supplement, and an iron supplement should be prescribed since this diet does not meet the Recommended Dietary Allowances (RDA) for these nutrients for children.

Indications and Rationale

When children are being selected for the diet, type of seizure disorder, response to medication, age, and probable compliance should be considered. Myoclonic seizures, which resist drug therapy, respond best; tonicoclonic seizures are less responsive; and others rarely respond.[2] The diet is designed to produce ketone bodies as a result of the incomplete oxidation of fat, although the exact mechanism of its anticonvulsant effects is not known. Ketone bodies (acetone, acetoacetic acid, and β-hydroxybutyric acid) are thought to have an anticonvulsant action.

The diet is planned to provide adequate calories for normal growth, development, and activity. The amount of fat in the diet is gradually increased, and the carbohydrate content is decreased. The amount of protein stays at the level recom-

561

mended for the individual (see Chapter 2, RDA). The diet is thought to be most effective in children aged 2 to 5 years. Under age 2, maintenance of ketosis is difficult. Above age 5, and especially over the age of 8, noncompliance is a major problem, primarily because of the diet's unpalatability.[3] There is usually a period of 10 to 21 days after initiation of the diet before complete seizure control is achieved.[4] Some data suggest that the diet is an ineffective treatment; if the diet does not control seizures within 3 months, it should be discontinued.[5]

This dietary program is used when drug therapy is not fully effective in controlling seizures.[6] Although several new and useful anticonvulsant drugs have become available in recent years, some patients have incomplete control of seizures or have unpleasant side effects with drug therapy but obtain a therapeutic effect from the diet. The drugs are ordinarily continued with the diet, but the dose can often be reduced, and sometimes the drugs can be discontinued.

Goals of Dietary Management

The goal of the ketogenic diet is to produce and maintain a ketotic state in a child by gradually reversing the usual proportions of dietary fat and carbohydrate while meeting the child's kilocalorie and protein needs.

Dietary Recommendations

A 3:1 ratio of ketogenic to antiketogenic substances should be achieved* to produce ketosis of sufficient degree for beneficial control of seizures. The time usually required to reverse the usual ratio (1:3) to the 3:1 ratio is 4 days. A further increase in the amount of fat and a decrease in the amount of carbohydrate may be necessary if this diet does not produce ketosis.

Tests of the urine should show the presence of ketones consistently and definitely when the desired state of ketosis has been achieved. Children on a ketogenic diet tend to excrete ketones at a maximal rate in the midafternoon and at a minimal rate in the early morning hours. Hence, it is usually sufficient to test the urine only on arising.

An abrupt change in a ketogenic diet may cause nausea or even vomiting. The practice is to alter the ratio of ketogenic to antiketogenic substances over a 4 day period in order to avoid these symptoms. If nausea or vomiting occurs, 1 or 2 meals should be omitted and small amounts of fruit juice should be given before the ketogenic diet is resumed. No significant changes have been seen in blood cholesterol, blood triglycerides, electrolytes, or blood pressure in the classic or MCT oil-based ketogenic diets. An increase in plasma uric acid is seen consistently, however. Uric acid levels should be monitored regularly.[7] Prolonged elevation of serum uric acid levels results in a high rate of renal stone formation. Although this is largely unex-

---

*For the purpose of calculating this ratio, it is assumed that glucose is antiketogenic and fatty acids are ketogenic and that 100 g of dietary carbohydrate yield 100 g of glucose; 100 g of dietary fat yield 10 g of glucose and 90 g of fatty acids; and 100 g of dietary protein produce 58 g of glucose and 46 g of fatty acids. Then the ketogenic-to-antiketogenic ratio may be calculated by dividing the sum of 90% of dietary fat and 46% of dietary protein by the sum of 100% of dietary carbohydrate, 10% of fat and 58% of protein. All terms in this calculation are in grams of carbohydrate, protein, or fat.

plained in individuals on a ketogenic diet, it may be associated with ketonuria and subsequent acidic urine pH as well as chronic fluid restriction.[8] Abnormalities in neutrophil function develop in patients with ketosis. Consideration should be given to discontinuing the ketogenic diet if bacterial infections occur.[9]

A diet containing MCT oil can be used to produce ketosis, instead of the classic ketogenic diet (see Table 25-7). Because MCTs are said to be more ketogenic than other dietary fats, the diet can include a greater proportion of foods containing carbohydrate and protein while maintaining adequate levels of ketosis. This dietary regime is usually more effective in controlling seizures than is the classic ketogenic diet. However, the diet is often not as well accepted by the patient and the family.[6]

Calculation of Ketogenic Diet without MCT Oil

Ratio of Ketogenesis to Antiketogenesis. In 4 days, the ratio of protein and carbohydrate to fat can be reversed. The ratio of ketogenic (K) to antiketogenic (AK) materials can be altered as suggested in Table 25-1. The physician may indicate a different rate of progression and ratio if desired.

The 4 day dietary regimen of fat, protein and carbohydrate can be calculated as shown in Table 25-2.

Kilocalories, Protein, Fat, and Carbohydrates. Protein, fat, and carbohydrate can be calculated as follows (also see example below).

1. Determine the total kilocalorie requirement of the child. The kilocalorie needs of the child are determined primarily from current dietary intake obtained by a thorough dietary history. RDA and caloric requirements determined by the Nomogram for Estimating Caloric Requirements (Appendix 6) and the estimated level of activity are additional sources of data for calculating kilocalorie needs.

2. Divide total kilocalories by kilocalories per unit:

$$\frac{\text{Total kcal}}{\text{kcal/unit}} = \text{total units/day}$$

3. For grams of fat, multiply the number of units by the K value in the K:AK ratio:

$$\text{No. of units} \times K = \text{g of fat}$$

TABLE 25-1 Alteration of Ketogenic to Antiketogenic (A:AK) Ratio

Day	K:AK
First	1.1:1
Second	1.6:1
Third	2.2:1
Fourth	2.8:1

TABLE 25-2 Calculation of the 4 Day Dietary Regimes

Day	K:AK	Calculation		
First	1.1:1	1 g F	= 9 kcal × 1.1 =	9.9 kcal
		1 g P + C	= 4 kcal × 1.0 =	4.0 kcal
				13.9 kcal/unit
Second	1.6:1	1 g F	= 9 kcal × 1.6 =	14.4 kcal
		1 g P + C	= 4 kcal × 1.0 =	4.0 kcal
				18.4/per unit
Third	2.2:1	1 g F	= 9 kcal × 2.2 =	19.8 kcal
		1 g P + C	= 4 kcal × 1.0 =	4.0 kcal
				23.8 kcal/unit
Fourth	2.8:1	1 g F	= 9 kcal × 2.8 =	25.2 kcal
		1 g P + C	= 4 kcal × 1.0 =	4.0 kcal
				29.2 kcal/unit

K:AK = Ketogenic to antiketogenic; F = fat; P = protein; C = carbohydrate.

4. For grams of protein and carbohydrate, multiply the number of units by the AK value in the K:AK ratio:[10]

$$\text{No. of units} \times \text{AK} = \text{g of protein} + \text{carbohydrate}$$

5. For grams of protein, a patient 3 years of age or younger needs 1.5 g of protein per kilogram of weight for height and age. A patient older than 3 years needs 1 g of protein per kilogram of weight for height and age.
6. For grams of carbohydrate, subtract the grams of protein in the diet from the total units per day:

$$\text{Total units/day} - \text{g of protein} = \text{g of carbohydrate}$$

The carbohydrate level should not be reduced below 10 g. For some patients, it may be necessary to decrease the carbohydrate content at a slower rate if an intolerance to fat is exhibited.

The diet may be planned with 3 meals or 3 meals and snacks as desired by the patient. Each meal and snack *must* have fat exchanges and/or cream to maintain the ratio. Each meal should consist of one-third of the total fat in the diet. If snacks are planned, each meal is planned with the remaining fat divided into thirds. All foods should be weighed.

Sample Determination of the Ketogenic Diet without MCT Oil

Calculation of the diet, composition of the diet (Table 25-3), sample daily food exchanges (Table 25-4), and a sample menu pattern (Table 25-5) are given for the following child.

Age: 5 year old male
Height: 110 cm
Weight: 18 kg
Kilocalories: 1,530 (18 kg × 85 kcal)

The values for the 4 day dietary regimen are calculated as follows:

First Day	
1,530 kcal ÷ 13.9 kcal	= 110 units
F 110 × 1.1	= 121 g
P + C = 110 × 1.0	= 110 g
P (1 g/kg)	= 18 g
C (110 − 18)	= 92 g

Second Day	
1,530 kcal ÷ 18.4 kcal	= 83 units
F 83 × 1.6	= 133 g
P + C = 83 × 1.0	= 83 g
P (1 g/kg)	= 18 g
C (83 − 18)	= 65 g

Third Day	
1,530 kcal ÷ 23.8 kcal	= 64 units
F 64 × 2.2	= 141 g
P + C = 64 X 1.0	= 64 g
P (1 g/kg)	= 18 g
C (64 − 18)	= 46 g

Fourth Day	
1,530 kcal ÷ 29.2 kcal	= 52 units
F 52 × 2.8	= 146 g
P + C = 52 × 1.0	= 52 g
P (1 g/kg)	= 18 g
C (52 − 18)	= 34 g

F = Fat; P = protein; C = carbohydrate.

TABLE 25-3 Calculated Values of the Dietary Program

Day	Protein (g)	Fat (g)	Carbohydrate (g)	Kcal	K:AK Ratio	Kcal/unit*
First	18	121	92	1,529	1.1:1	13.9
Second	18	133	65	1,529	1.6:1	18.4
Third	18	141	46	1,525	2.2:1	23.8
Fourth	18	146	34	1,522	2.8:1	29.2

K = Ketogenic; AK = antiketogenic.

*The procedure for calculation is on p. 563.

TABLE 25-4 Sample Daily Food Exchanges

Day	Meat	Fat	Whipping Cream	Bread	Bread Product	Vegetable	Fruit
First	1½	14	3	1	5	1	10
Second	1½	12	4	—	4	1	8
Third	1½	14	4	—	4	1	5
Fourth and subsequent	1½	15	4	—	3	1	3

TABLE 25-5   Sample Meal Plan

| Foods | Number of Servings* | | | |
	First Day	Second Day	Third Day	Fourth Day
Breakfast				
Starch	1	—	—	—
Bread product	2	2	2	1
Fat	5	2	2	4
Whipping cream	1	2	2	2
Fruit	3	1	1	—
Noon Meal				
Meat	$^1/_2$	$^1/_2$	$^1/_2$	$^1/_2$
Starch	—	—	—	—
Bread product	1	1	1	1
Vegetable	$^1/_2$	$^1/_2$	$^1/_2$	$^1/_2$
Fat	5	5	6	5
Whipping cream	1	1	1	1
Fruit	4	4	2	$1^1/_2$
Evening Meal				
Meat	1	1	1	1
Starch	—	—	—	—
Bread product	2	1	1	1
Vegetable	$^1/_2$	$^1/_2$	$^1/_2$	$^1/_2$
Fat	4	5	6	6
Whipping cream	1	1	1	1
Fruit	3	3	2	$1^1/_2$

*All food is weighed.

The composition of the diet varies slightly from the calculated values depending on the foods included in the diet.

Alternative Method of Calculation

Instead of calculating each diet individually, Table 25-6 may be used. Proceed as follows:

1. Determine the kilocalorie and the protein requirement.
2. Check the ratio to be used.
3. Grams of fat are given under the heading F.
4. Grams of carbohydrate and protein are given under the heading C + P.
5. Subtract the number of grams of protein required by the patient from the total number of grams of carbohydrate plus protein. The remainder equals the number of grams of carbohydrate.

TABLE 25-6 Ketogenic Calculation Table

Kcal	Ketogenic to Antiketogenic (K:AK) Ratio							
	1.1:1		1.6:1		2.2:1		2.8:1	
	F	C + P	F	C + P	F	C + P	F	C + P
800	64	58	69	43	73	33	76	27
900	72	65	78	49	84	38	87	31
1,000	79	72	87	54	92	42	96	32
1,100	87	79	96	60	102	46	105	38
1,200	95	86	104	65	111	50	115	41
1,300	103	94	113	71	120	55	125	45
1,400	111	101	122	76	129	59	134	48
1,500	119	108	130	82	139	63	144	51
1,600	127	115	139	87	148	67	153	55
1,700	135	122	148	92	158	71	163	58
1,800	143	130	157	98	167	76	173	62
1,900	151	137	165	103	176	80	182	65
2,000	159	144	174	109	185	84	192	68
2,100	166	151	183	114	194	88	201	72
2,200	174	159	191	120	203	92	211	75

F = Fat; C + P = carbohydrate plus protein.

Calculation of Ketogenic Diet with MCT Oil

The diet containing MCT oil can include a greater proportion of foods containing carbohydrate and protein. Because MCTs are said to be more ketogenic, this diet may be more effective in controlling seizures. Table 25-7 presents information helpful for calculating a ketogenic diet with MCT oil.

The MCT oil should be introduced slowly, beginning with approximately 10 or 15 ml/day and increasing by 10 or 20 ml daily.

The patient may have diarrhea, vomiting, and abdominal pain during the introduction of the MCT oil. These symptoms usually begin when one-half the oil has been introduced. The gradual increase of MCT oil can be continued if the symptoms are not distressing. If the patient becomes ill, reduce the MCT oil by one-half and slowly begin to increase to the required amount again. The full allowance of food should not be given until the required amount of MCT oil has been reached.

Each of 3 meals should consist of one-third of the MCT oil planned in the diet. The equal distribution of MCT oil and its slow ingestion may be helpful in alleviating side effects. All foods should be weighed.

Physicians: How to Order Diet

The diet order should indicate *ketogenic diet* or *ketogenic diet with MCT*. The diet will be planned without MCT oil unless it is requested. The dietitian will determine content and kilocalorie level according to the preceding principles.

TABLE 25-7 Calculation of Ketogenic Diet with MCT Oil[11]

Component	Comments
Kilocalories	Determined primarily from current dietary intake obtained by a thorough diet history. RDA for calories and basal caloric requirement determined by Nomogram and the estimated level of activity are additional sources for estimating caloric needs.

Protein	Approximately 10% of kcal
	  Children ≤ 3 years: 1.5 g/kg*
	  Children > 3 years: 1.0 g/kg*

Carbohydrate	18% of kcal
Fat	12% of kcal Include a source of linoleic acid, such as corn or safflower oil.
MCT oil	60% of kcal MCT oil contains 8.3 kcal/g.

MCT = Medium-chain triglycerides.

*Weight for height and age.

EXCHANGE LIST FOR KETOGENIC DIET

Foods to Avoid

The following foods contain a substantial and variable amount of carbohydrate and should be *avoided*.

All breads, bread products, and cereals, unless they are calculated into the meal plan	Ice cream, commercial
Cake	Jam
Candy	Jelly
Carbonated beverages	Marmalade
Catsup	Molasses
Chewing gum	Pastries
Cookies	Pies
Cough drops or syrups that contain sugar	Pudding
Granola bars	Sherbet
Honey	Sugar
	Sweet rolls
	Sweetened condensed milk
	Syrup

Foods to Use as Desired

The following foods contain negligible amounts of protein, fat, and carbohydrate and may be used as desired without calculation into the meal plan.

Bouillon, broth, or consommé	Flavoring extracts	Parsley
Chives	Gelatin, unsweetened,	Pepper
Cocoa powder, unsweetened	unflavored	Salt
(limit to 1 tsp/day)	Herbs	Tea
Coffee	Horseradish, without sugar	Vinegar
Decaffeinated coffee	Mustard, dry	

Use of Products Prepared with Artificial Sweeteners

Products made with non-nutritive artificial sweeteners contain minimal (less than 0.5 g/serving) or no carbohydrate. Products made with nutritive artificial sweeteners may contain from 0.5 g to 12 g of carbohydrate per serving.

The ketogenic diet should not include more than 1 g of carbohydrate or 1 g of protein (4 kcal) from artificially sweetened products. A choice of *one* product in the *amount* given is allowed each day (Table 25-8).

TABLE 25-8   Caloric Content of Artificially Sweetened Products

Artificially Sweetened Products	Amount	Kcal/Serving
Carbonated beverage	6 oz	1
Lemonade prepared from dry mix	6 oz	3
Gelatin dessert prepared from mix	¼ cup	4
Granulated tabletop artificial sweetener	2 tsp	4

FOOD EXCHANGE LIST FOR KETOGENIC DIET WITHOUT MCT OIL

This exchange list differs from the other exchange lists in the manual. This exchange list should be used in planning menus for a ketogenic diet. Accuracy in portion sizes is important; foods should be weighed. Table 25-9 summarizes the composition of each of the food exchange lists.

TABLE 25-9

Food Exchange List	Weight (g)	Kcal	Protein (g)	Fat (g)	Carbohydrate (g)
Meat	30	73	7	5	—
Starch	Varies	68	2	—	15
Bread products	2	7	—	—	1.6
Vegetable					
Group 1	100	16	1	—	3
Group 2	50	16	1	—	3
Fat	5	36	—	4	—
Whipping cream	60	187	2	19	2
Fruit	Varies	24	—	—	6

Meat Exchange

One meat exchange is equivalent to the weight listed and contains 7 g of protein, 5 g of fat, and 73 kcal.

Medium Fat Meat

Bacon (omit 2 fat exchanges)	30 g
Beef, lamb, pork, veal	30 g
Cold cuts: bologna, luncheon meat, minced ham, liverwurst (all meat, no cereal)	45 g
Dried beef (add 1 fat exchange)	20 g
Frankfurters or wieners (all meat, no cereal) (omit 1 fat exchange)	50 g
Liver (add 1 fat exchange and omit 50 g of group 1 vegetable)	30 g
Pork sausage (omit 2 fat exchanges)	40 g
Salami (omit 1 fat exchange)	30 g

Fowl

Chicken, duck, goose, turkey	30 g

Egg   1

Fish

Clams (add 1 fat exchange and omit 100 g of group 1 vegetable)	50 g
Lobster (add 1 fat exchange)	40 g
Oysters (add 1 fat exchange and omit 100 g of group 1 vegetable)	70 g
Salmon or tuna, canned	30 g
Sardines	35 g
Scallops (add 1 fat exchange)	50 g
Shrimp (add 1 fat exchange)	30 g

Cheese

American, brick, cheddar, processed, Roquefort, or Swiss cheese (omit 1 fat exchange)	30 g
Cottage cheese, creamed (add 1 fat exchange and omit 50 g of group 1 vegetable)	50 g

Starch Exchange

One starch exchange is equivalent to the weight listed and contains 2 g of protein, 15 g of carbohydrate, and 68 kcal.

Bread	25 g
Melba toast	20 g
Saltines	20 g
White potato	100 g

Bread Products

One bread product contains 1.6 g of carbohydrate and 7 kcal.

Low calorie rice wafer	2 g

Vegetable Exchange

One serving of group 1 or group 2 vegetable contains 1 g of protein, 3 g of carbohydrate, and 16 kcal.

Group 1 Vegetable (100 g)

Asparagus	Chard, Swiss	Garden cress	Spinach
Bean sprouts	Chinese cabbage	Lettuce	Summer squash
Beans, green or wax	Collards	Mushrooms	Tomato juice
Beet greens	Cucumber	Mustard greens	Tomatoes
Broccoli	Dill pickle	Peppers, green or red	Turnip greens
Cabbage	Eggplant	Radishes	Turnips
Cauliflower	Endive	Sauerkraut	Watercress
Celery			

Group 2 Vegetable (50 g)

Artichokes	Dandelion greens	Leeks	Pumpkin
Beets	Kale	Okra	Rutabaga
Brussels sprouts	Kohlrabi	Onions	Winter squash
Carrots			

Fat Exchange

One fat exchange is equivalent to the weight listed and contains 4 g of fat and 36 kcal.

Almonds, slivered	5 g	Mayonnaise	5 g
Avocado		Olives, green or ripe	30 g
(omit 50 g of group 1 vegetable)	30 g	Pecans, shelled	5 g
Bacon	5 g	Salad oils	5 g
Butter or margarine	5 g	Walnuts, shelled	5 g
Cooking fats	5 g		

Whipping Cream Exchange

One whipping cream exchange is 60 g and contains 2 g of protein, 19 g of fat, 2 g of carbohydrate, and 187 kcal. Whipping cream that is at least 32% fat should be used. One whipping cream exchange (60 g) may be exchanged for 65 g of group 1 vegetable and 5 fat exchanges.

Whipping cream (32% fat)   60 g

Fruit Exchange

One fruit exchange is equivalent to the weight listed and contains 6 g of carbohydrate and 24 kcal.

Apple		Apricots	
Fresh	40 g	Canned	60 g
Juice	60 g	Dried	10 g
Sauce	60 g	Fresh	60 g
		Nectar	40 g

Banana
  Whole   30 g

Berries, fresh
    Blackberries   50 g
    Blueberries   40 g
    Boysenberries   60 g
    Cranberries   50 g
    Gooseberries   60 g
    Loganberries   50 g
    Raspberries   50 g
    Strawberries   75 g

Cherries
  Canned   60 g
  Fresh   40 g

Dates
  Pitted   8 g

Figs
  Canned   60 g
  Dried   8 g
  Fresh   30 g

Fruit cocktail
  Canned   60 g

Grapefruit
  Fresh   60 g
  Juice   60 g
  Nectar   40 g
  Sections, canned   75 g

Grapes
  Canned   40 g
  Fresh   40 g
  Juice, bottled   30 g
  Juice, frozen   40 g

Lemon juice   75 g

Lime juice   65 g

Mandarin orange
  Canned   100 g

Mango
  Fresh   35 g

Melon
  Cantaloupe   100 g
  Honeydew   100 g
  Watermelon   100 g

Nectarine
  Fresh   40 g

Orange
  Fresh, whole   50 g
  Juice   60 g
  Sections, fresh or canned   50 g

Papaya
  Fresh   60 g

Peach
  Canned   60 g
  Dried   10 g
  Fresh   60 g

Pear
  Canned   60 g
  Dried   10 g
  Fresh   40 g

Pineapple
  Canned   60 g
  Fresh   40 g
  Juice   40 g

Plums
  Canned   60 g
  Fresh   40 g

Prunes
  Juice   30 g
  Whole   8 g

Raisins   8 g

Rhubarb
  Raw   160 g

Tangerine
  Fresh, whole   50 g
  Juice   60 g
  Sections   50 g

FOOD EXCHANGE LIST FOR KETOGENIC DIET WITH MCT OIL

These additional food exchange lists are needed when planning the diet with MCT oil. Use these lists in addition to the previous ketogenic exchange lists.

Skim Milk Exchanges

One milk exchange is equivalent to 120 g of milk and contains 4 g of protein, 6 g of carbohydrate, and 40 kcal.

Buttermilk, fat-free	120 g
Skim milk, fat-free	120 g

MCT Oil Exchange

MCT oil contains 8.3 kcal/g (ml). MCT oil can be combined with the allowance of skim milk. The two ingredients can be mixed in a blender. Chipped ice, non-caloric carbonated beverages, fruit allowance, or tomato juice from the vegetable A allowance may be added for flavor. The beverage with MCT oil should be sipped slowly.

Starch Exchange

One starch exchange is equivalent to the weight listed and contains 2 g of protein, 1 g of fat, 15 g of carbohydrate, and 77 kcal.

Breads

Bread	25 g
Bun, hamburger or frankfurter	30 g
Cornbread	35 g
Pancake	45 g
Roll	25 g

Cereals

Cooked	140 g
Dry, flake	20 g
Dry, puffed	20 g
Shredded wheat	20 g

Crackers

Graham	20 g
Melba toast	20 g
Oyster	20 g
Ritz, plain or cheese	20 g
Ry-Krisp	30 g
Saltines	20 g
Soda	20 g

Desserts

Commercial flavored gelatin	100 g
Sherbet	50 g
Sponge or angel food cake	25 g
Vanilla wafers	15 g

Grain Products

Macaroni, cooked	50 g
Noodles, cooked	50 g
Rice, cooked	50 g
Spaghetti, cooked	50 g

Starchy Vegetables

Beans	
Baked (no pork), cooked	90 g
Kidney, cooked	90 g
Lima, cooked	90 g
Navy, cooked	90 g
Pinto, cooked	90 g
White marrow, cooked	90 g
Corn	
Canned or frozen	80 g
Fresh on cob	50 g
Hominy	100 g
Parsnips	100 g
Peas	
Canned, fresh or frozen	100 g
Dry, split, cooked	90 g
Popcorn (without butter)	15 g
Potatoes	
Sweet or yams	50 g
White, baked or boiled	100 g
White, mashed	100 g

References

1. Wilder RM. The effects of ketonemia on the course of epilepsy. Mayo Clin Bull 1921:307–314.
2. Gasch AT. Use of the traditional ketogenic diet for treatment of intractable epilepsy. J Am Diet Assoc 1990;90(10):1433–1434.
3. Livingston S. Comprehensive management of epilepsy in infancy, childhood, and adolescence. Springfield, IL: Charles C Thomas, 1972.
4. Dodson WE, Prensky AL, DeVivo DC, Goldring S, Dodge PR. Management of seizure disorders: selected aspects. J Pediatr 1976;89:695–703.
5. Huttenlocher PR. Ketonemia and seizures: metabolic and anticonvulsant effects of two ketogenic diets in childhood epilepsy. Pediatr Res 1976;10:536–540.
6. Signore JM. Ketogenic diet containing medium-chain triglycerides. J Am Diet Assoc 1973;62:285–290.
7. Schwartz RM, Boyes S, Aynsley-Green A. Metabolic effects of three ketogenic diets in the treatment of severe epilepsy. Dev Med Child Neurol 1989;31(2):152–160.
8. Herzberg GZ, Fivush BA, Kinsman SL, Gearhart JP. Urolithiasis association with the ketogenic diet. J Pediatr 1990;117(5):743–745.
9. Woody RC, Steele RW, Knapple WL, Pilkington NS Jr. Impaired neutrophil function in children with seizures treated with the ketogenic diet. J Pediatr 1989;115(3):427–430.
10. Keith HM. Convulsive disorders in children with reference to treatment with ketogenic diet. Boston: Little, Brown, 1963.
11. Clark BJ, House FM. Medium-chain triglyceride oil ketogenic diets in the treatment of childhood epilepsy. J Hum Nutr 1978;32:111–116.

26 / *Oncologic Disease in Children*

CANCER

Introduction

The prevalence of malnutrition in children with cancer is related to diagnosis, stage of disease, age, and therapy.[1] In general, children with advanced stages of solid tumors are more likely to have malnutrition than children with localized disease or leukemias.[2] Approximately 10% of newly diagnosed patients and 40% of those with advanced disease are undernourished.[1] Malnutrition may not be present at diagnosis but frequently occurs during treatment.[2] Children especially at risk for malnutrition are those with malignant gastrointestinal tumors, neuroblastomas, Ewing's sarcoma, gliomas, and metastatic Wilms tumor. Malnutrition is associated with an increased incidence of infections and a decreased tolerance to treatment.[1-3] Children who are malnourished at diagnosis have a significantly poorer outcome than those who are well nourished.[3]

Causes of Malnutrition

The weight loss and growth delay seen in children with cancer results from metabolic changes due to the disease itself[1-3] and from food intake inadequate to meet energy and nutrient demands. This discussion will focus on the reasons for decreased intake.

   Anorexia. It is not clear how cancer causes anorexia. Some studies suggest that serotonin levels are increased, which leads to a feeling of satiety.[1] Metabolic by-products of tumor metabolism may cause anorexia directly or secondarily. Both interlukin I and tumor necrosis factor (cachectin), products of activated macrophages, enhance triglyceride release from adiposities and amino acids from muscle cells. Tumor necrosis factor suppresses appetite, which is probably the major factor in producing cancer cachexia.

Anorexia is also related to the nausea and vomiting caused by chemotherapy and radiation therapy. Children may develop aversions for foods consumed immediately before or during treatments that result in nausea or vomiting.

Chemotherapy. The use of most chemotherapeutic agents results in anorexia. Most also cause nausea and vomiting, but this may be limited or prevented with the use of antiemetics. Mucosal injury from chemotherapeutic agents presents as stomatitis, glossitis, cheilosis, and esophagitis and significantly interferes with intake. Chemotherapeutic damage to intestinal mucosa also results in diarrhea and malabsorption.[1,3] Ileus is a frequent side effect of the periwinkle alkaloids: vincristine, vinblastine, and vindesine.[3] Chemotherapy may also cause renal damage resulting in significant protein, mineral, and magnesium losses. The latter is especially likely to occur with the use of platinum derivatives.[3]

Radiation. Damage to mucosa of the head, neck, and gastrointestinal tract may also occur in patients undergoing radiation therapy. Mucositis, stomatitis, dysphagia, alterations in taste and smell, and changes in the saliva may impair nutrient intake.[1] Anorexia, nausea, vomiting, and diarrhea may also be present in patients receiving radiation to the stomach and small and large intestines. Some degree of lactose intolerance may develop with chronic radiation therapy.

Nutritional Assessment

Nutritional assessment should include review of the disease type and duration, type of treatment, and presence of complications. A thorough diet and weight history is most useful in assessing the impact of cancer on nutritional intake. Weight-for-height measurement is the first parameter to be affected.[2] Laboratory data can be difficult to interpret because they may be affected by the disease process itself as well as by poor nutrition. Criteria have been identified that can be used when assessing nutritional status. These appear in Table 26-1. In practice, however, current weight, recent weight change, and current ability to eat are usually the deciding factors in planning nutritional intervention.

TABLE 26-1 Criteria Suggesting Need for Nutritional Intervention[3]

1. There is an interval or total weight loss of greater than 5% of the preillness body weight.
2. The relative weight for height is less than or equal to 90%; weight/height percentile determined from the National Center for Health Statistics (NCHS) growth charts is less than or equal to the 10th percentile channel.
3. Serum albumin is less than 3.2 mg/dl.
4. The energy reserves as estimated by arm fat area or subcapsular skinfold (less than 1 year old) is less than the 5th percentile for age and sex.
5. The current percentile for weight and/or height has fallen 2 percentile channels (e.g., preillness height 75th to 90th percentile for age and sex, currently 25th to 50th percentile for age and sex).

With permission from: Maurer AM, Burgess JB, Donaldson SS, Rickard KA, Stallings VA, van Eyes J, Winick M. Special nutritional needs of children with malignancies: a review. JPEN 1990;14(3):315–324.

Intervention

Nutritional counseling by the dietitian should provide the patient and the patient's parents with practical suggestions that can help improve the intake, in spite of the side effects of cancer treatment (see Chapter 12, Cancer, for specific examples). Emphasis should be placed on adequate calorie and protein intake to ensure normal growth and development.[1-3] Parents may express interest in self-prescribed special diets, megavitamin therapy, and health food supplements. These should be discussed during nutritional education.[3] There is no evidence that individual nutrient supplements improve outcome. Macrobiotic diets are discouraged because they are not nutritionally adequate to support growth and development.[3]

Parents should be encouraged to be with their children at meal times when a child is hospitalized for cancer treatment. An effort should be made to avoid interrupting meal times with tests, treatments, or discussions of upsetting topics. If nausea is present after a treatment, meals should be planned to avoid this time. A calm, positive attitude can help a child increase his or her intake more effectively than trying to force the child to eat. Some children eat better in a room other than the hospital room where treatment has taken place. A pleasant distraction during meal time, such as watching a favorite television program or the promise of a small reward, may be helpful. Small quantities of food should be encouraged at frequent intervals, and nutritious snacks can be small meals in themselves. Nutritional supplements, such as "instant breakfast drinks," Ensure™ (Ross Laboratories), or Polycose™ (Ross Laboratories), are well tolerated but not always well accepted. Children should be able to take part in the planning of their diets. New foods can be offered if the child's sense of taste has been altered and if old favorite foods no longer appeal.

Enteral or parenteral nutritional support should be considered when the child is unable to maintain adequate oral intake. The child's intake can be supplemented by night-time tube feedings (see Chapter 29, Enteral Nutritional Support of Children) if he or she is not able to consume adequate kilocalories. Caution should be exercised when nasogastric tube feeding is considered. Aspiration pneumonia may be potentiated in patients with neutropenia. When platelet count is low or if other clotting factors are deficient, there may also be a risk for bleeding. A gastrostomy feeding tube may be placed if long-term nutritional support is anticipated. Peripheral parenteral nutrition can supplement oral intake if the child can tolerate a limited amount of food, but cannot be used as the sole access for nutritional support because of the limited tolerance of small veins for hypertonic solutions. Central parenteral nutrition (CPN) is needed if the child is unable to tolerate enteral feedings owing to severe gastrointestinal disturbances, such as obstructions, fistulas, ileus, malabsorption, or protracted vomiting.[1,2] Patients may need to be continued on CPN until the end of the intense treatment period in order to reverse and prevent recurrence of the protein energy malnutrition associated with treatment.[3,4] However, CPN may not be sufficient in itself to restore lost weight for all cancer patients.

Data on long-term nutritional status of children who have had cancer are limited. A survey of the effects of treatment in children with acute lymphocytic leukemia revealed that growth was slower than normal during the 2.3 to 3 year period of treatment. However, 5 years after diagnosis, 19 of 22 children had weights within 1 SD of normal average children. Therefore, all but two of 22 resumed normal growth after cessation of therapy.[5] In general, the well-nourished child has an improved prognosis and lower morbidity and mortality, provided effective antitumor therapy is also available.[2]

References

1. Jaffe N. Nutrition in cancer patients. In: Grand RJ, Stephen JL, Dietz WH, eds. Pediatric nutrition: theory and practice. Boston: Butterworth, 1987:571–578.
2. Holcomb GW, Ziegler MM. Nutrition and cancer in children. In: Nyhus LM, Judge C, eds. Surgery Annual. Vol. 22. Connecticut: Appleton & Lange, 1990:129–142.
3. Mauer AM, Burgess JB, Donaldson SS, Rickard KA, Stallings VA, van Eyes J, Winick M. Special nutritional needs of children with malignancies: a review. JPEN 1990;14(3):315–324.
4. Rickard KA, Kirksey A, Baehner RL, Grosfeld JL, Provisor A, Weetman RM, Boxer LA, Ballantine TVN. Effectiveness of enteral and parenteral nutrition in the nutritional management of children with Wilms' tumors. Am J Clin Nutr 1980;33:2622–2629.
5. Donaldson SS. Effects of therapy on nutritional status of the pediatric cancer patient. Cancer Res 1982;42(2 suppl):729s–736s.

27 / *Pulmonary Disease in Children*

CYSTIC FIBROSIS

General Description

The diet for cystic fibrosis should meet the patient's nutritional needs with an emphasis on increased kilocalorie and protein intake. Impairment of the digestive and absorptive process results in maldigestion and malabsorption of energy and nutrient substrates. In the past, fat was restricted in the diets of some patients in order to minimize steatorrhea. Currently, use of pancreatic enzymes given orally to control steatorrhea allows for more liberal use of fat in the diet.

Nutritional Inadequacy

The diet for patients with cystic fibrosis is planned to exceed the Recommended Dietary Allowance (RDA) for kilocalories and for all other nutrients. Nutritional deficiencies in cystic fibrosis are most likely to occur when growth rates are greatest. However, many variables influence the nutritional status of cystic fibrosis patients. Nutritional deficiencies may occur at any time and with a varying degree of severity, depending on the degree of steatorrhea (level of pancreatic enzyme supplementation),[1] the degree of azotorrhea, the growth rate, the presence or severity of chronic respiratory disease and infection, and the quantity and quality of the foods consumed.

Supplemental vitamins should be prescribed for all cystic fibrosis patients. Multiple vitamin capsules, tablets, or drops that contain C and B complex should be given daily to meet the RDA. Every patient with cystic fibrosis and pancreatic insufficiency will eventually require supplemental fat-soluble vitamins. For patients who do not maintain adequate serum vitamin concentrations, water miscible forms of fat-soluble vitamin preparations are available. Table 27-1 presents recommended levels of vitamin supplementation from the Cystic Fibrosis Foundation.[1] If needed, iron should also be given.

579

TABLE 27-1   Recommended Levels of Vitamin Supplementation[1]

Age	Vitamins	Dose/Day
MULTIPLE VITAMIN—Recommended for all patients with cystic fibrosis		
≤ 2 yr	Polyvisol™ or similar (liquid)	1 ml
2–8 yr	Standard multiple vitamin with 400 IU of vitamin D 5000 IU of vitamin A	1 tablet
Adolescents and adults	Standard adult-type multiple vitamin	1–2 tablets
VITAMIN E*—In addition to the above		
≤ 6 mo	Aquasol E™ or Liqui-E™	25 IU
6–12 mo		50 IU
1–4 yr	(After age 1–2, capsules of α-tocopherol or d-α-tocopherol may be used)	100 IU
4–10 yr		100–200 IU
> 10 yr		200–400 IU
VITAMIN K†—In addition to the above		
≤ 12 mo	Phytonadione™ or similar product	2.5 mg (twice weekly if taking antibiotics)
> 1 yr		5.0 mg (twice weekly if taking antibiotics or if cholestatic liver disease present)
VITAMIN A—Patients with low serum vitamin A may need in addition to the above a water miscible vitamin A preparation		
	Aquasol A™ or similar product	Varies
VITAMIN D—Patients not exposed to sunlight may need in addition to the above		
	Drisdol™ or similar product	400 IU

*More than 1,000 IU of vitamin E may exacerbate coagulopathy associated with vitamin K deficiency.

†These reflect prudent recommendations. More research is required to define optimal supplementation.

Caloric supplements, such as medium-chain triglyceride oil and commercial formulas, are generally not well accepted by the patient. In our experience, a beverage such as an "instant breakfast" can be used to increase calories and protein without the patient's experiencing aversion or flavor fatigue. An adjunct to the oral route may be sought in some patients where supplements have failed to prevent or correct malnutrition. An overnight nasogastric tube feeding that provides a portion of the patient's recommended intake may be helpful for some patients.[2,3]

Indications and Rationale

Cystic fibrosis is a hereditary disease of the exocrine glands that affects infants, children, adolescents, and adults. This disorder is found predominately in Caucasians and occurs in about 1 of every 2,000 live births.[1] People with cystic fibrosis are now commonly living to adulthood. A number of physical signs, such as growth retardation, failure to gain weight, abdominal protuberance, lack of subcutaneous fat, and poor muscle tone, are seen in individuals with the disease.

Cystic fibrosis is characterized by excessively viscid exocrine gland secretions that may obstruct the pancreatic and bile ducts, the intestine, and the bronchi. The major criteria for diagnosing cystic fibrosis include elevated concentration of electrolytes in the sweat of the patient, pulmonary involvement, pancreatic insufficiency, and a family history of the disorder.[1] Pancreatic insufficiency, gastrointestinal malabsorption, and frequent pulmonary infections predispose individuals with cystic fibrosis to undernutrition. Inadequate lipase activity accounts for the most profound clinical effects, although all three pancreatic enzymes (amylase, protease, and lipase) are either insufficient or missing.[4] The resulting steatorrhea leads to significant energy loss and to malabsorption of fat-soluble vitamins, essential fatty acids, some minerals, and bile salts.

The importance of nutritional status in long-term survival is well documented. There are multiple factors that affect the nutritional status of cystic fibrosis patients, some of which are not fully understood. Genetic factors have an influence on the presence or absence of pancreatic insufficiency. Patients with pancreatic insufficiency, steatorrhea, and undernutrition have a poorer prognosis in terms of growth, pulmonary function, and long-term survival than patients with pancreatic sufficiency.

Variables affecting nutritional status are maldigestion and/or malabsorption of fat, losses of bile salts and bile acids associated with steatorrhea (which can exacerbate maldigestion and malabsorption), intestinal resection secondary to bowel obstruction, and factors that reduce appetite and consumption, such as recurrent vomiting from coughing, gastroesophageal reflux, chronic respiratory infections, and psychosocial stresses. There is also a clear association between deteriorating lung function and malnutrition. Chronic pulmonary infections are associated with anorexia and increased metabolic rate resulting in increased energy needs.

Nutritional deficiency ranges from mildly depleted fat stores to frank signs and symptoms of protein and energy malnutrition. Deficiencies are most likely to occur at times of rapid growth or pulmonary exacerbations.[1]

Treatment for cystic fibrosis is aimed at control of the pulmonary obstructive process, prevention of pulmonary infection, and correction of pancreatic and nutritional deficiencies. Treatment consists of chest physical therapy, aerosol inhalation, antibiotics, pancreatic enzyme replacement, vitamin and mineral supplementation, and a nutritionally adequate diet. Nutrition is of prime importance in the treatment of individuals with cystic fibrosis. Undernutrition contributes to pulmonary complications, susceptibility to infection, poor growth, and decreased energy and motivation. Nutritional support is needed to offset (1) nutrient losses that are secondary to pancreatic insufficiency and malabsorption, and (2) an increase in metabolic rate due to labored respiration and periods of infection and fever.

Goals of Dietary Management

The primary goal of nutritional therapy for the cystic fibrosis patient is to encourage caloric, protein, vitamin, and mineral intakes in sufficient quantities to achieve consistent growth and weight gain. Dietary prescriptions providing an intake of

150% of the RDA do not seem unreasonable, since studies have shown that children with cystic fibrosis do not grow until the percentage of energy intake that is absorbed exceeds 100 to 110% of the RDA.[4] Patients often consume much less than this, however.[5]

Normal ranges on the growth curves are used as guidelines for determining energy and nutrient needs for the infant and young child; ideal weights for height are the guidelines used for the older child. Children with cystic fibrosis are often remarkably underweight for height and age. Current research suggests strongly that growth failure in cystic fibrosis is nutritional in origin. Therefore it should be possible to restore normal growth in growth-retarded patients through adequate enzyme and nutritional supplementation.[6] Adequate pancreatic enzyme supplementation has allowed liberalization of the diet to include more fat as a high energy source for growth.[4]

Dietary Recommendations

A consensus on nutritional recommendations for infants and children with cystic fibrosis has been outlined for the Cystic Fibrosis Foundation.[1]

TABLE 27-2   Estimating Energy Requirements[1]

Energy Need = [BMR × (Activity Level + Disease Coefficient)] × Fat Absorption

BMR

Equations for predicting BMR (in kcal) from body weight (in kg)

Age Range (yr)	Females	Males
0–3	61.0 (wt) − 51	60.9 (wt) − 54
3–10	22.5 (wt) + 499	22.7 (wt) + 495
10–18	12.2 (wt) + 746	17.5 (wt) + 651
18–30	14.7 (wt) + 496	15.3 (wt) + 679
30–60	8.7 (wt) + 829	11.6 (wt) + 879

Activity Level

Confined to bed	= 1.3
Sedentary	= 1.5
Active	= 1.7

Disease Coefficient

Normal lung function (≥ 80%)	0
Moderate lung function (40–79%)	0.2
Severe lung function (< 40%)	0.3–0.5

Fat Absorption

0.93 ÷ % of fat absorbed[*]

BMR = Basal metabolic rate.

[*]100 − Stool Fat (g)/24 hours = % absorbed while subject is on a 100 g fat test diet.

Energy.   For patients with cystic fibrosis who are growing normally and whose steatorrhea is under good control, the total daily energy requirement is consistent with the RDA for age and sex. If a patient fails to grow while receiving caloric intake based on the RDA, energy needs can be estimated (see Table 27-2).

Protein.   The infant, child, or adolescent with cystic fibrosis has the same protein needs as the otherwise healthy person. Protein deficiency may be seen in the first year of life when average requirements are highest.

Fat.   The traditional practice of restricting fat may aggravate energy deficiency. Whenever possible, a normal diet pattern with no specific restrictions should be followed.[7] Pancreatic enzyme replacement therapy should be adjusted according to the individual's intake, with the aim of minimizing maldigestion and malabsorption.

In our experience, it may be helpful to aim for fat to provide 30 to 40% of caloric needs. The diet and its fat content can be liberalized, as tolerated, by gradually introducing new foods and noting any signs of distress caused by these foods. Any food that persistently causes distress should be omitted from the diet. The patient learns how much fat and what combination of foods cause gastrointestinal distress. These patients, especially adolescents, should be free to adjust their diets instead of being bound to a strict regimen. Some patients would rather experience some discomfort and occasionally enjoy foods they might not eat routinely. Others prefer to be more restrictive with their diets in order to avoid discomfort and inconvenience. The patient should be permitted to make these decisions.[8] Behavior modification approaches have been helpful in shaping intake patterns.

Sodium.   Most, if not all, children with cystic fibrosis lose excessive amounts of sodium and chloride in their sweat; therefore, additional salt is needed in the diet. The child needs more salt during periods of extremely hot weather, febrile illness, and strenuous physical exertion than during times of sedentary activity. This salt can be provided by liberal use of table salt.[9]

Infants.   In the past, predigested formulas with medium-chain triglycerides provided the main nutritional source for infants with cystic fibrosis. Current guidelines encourage use of pancreatic enzyme replacement therapy along with all types of milk products, including human breast milk.[1] Because the first 2 years of life incur the highest growth rate and relative energy needs, frequent evaluation is recommended, including assessment of pancreatic function.

Breast-fed infants should be monitored for hypoproteinemia and hyponatremic alkalosis and impaired growth velocity. Supplemental sodium chloride is generally required.

Cows' milk-based infant formulas and milk products provide the predominant nutrients for infants during the first 2 years of life. Lactose intolerance is not more common in patients with cystic fibrosis. In some instances supplemental fat or carbohydrate may be needed to increase caloric density to over 20 kcal/oz. Pancreatic enzyme replacement adjustment may also be indicated. It is prudent to continue formula for up to 24 months.

Introduction of other foods is no different for infants with cystic fibrosis.[1]

Children and Adolescents.   Toddlers, preschoolers, and school age children develop self-feeding behaviors and individual food preferences (see Chapter 19, Normal Nutrition of Children). Continued monitoring of nutritional adequacy of the diet, compliance with pancreatic enzyme prescriptions, and growth patterns are important. As the child becomes older and more independent, compliance with diet and prescribed medications may become an issue.[10] Adolescence and puberty are characterized by accelerated growth, development, and physical activity. Because of this, nutrient needs are high. Caloric needs may be increased further by pulmonary infections, which are common during this period.[1] Growth failure and pubertal delay are also observed. Nutritional counseling is directed toward the individual rather than the parents.

Assessment of the Diet.   A food record of at least 3 days should be completed for the initial nutritional consultation. This food record helps the dietitian formulate initial dietary recommendations. Re-evaluation is needed at regular intervals to determine whether the original recommendations were adequate to support growth and to evaluate the foods that are being added back to the diet. Re-evaluation is also needed because growth and the disease process change the child's nutritional needs.

Weight gain, linear growth, and level of pancreatic enzyme replacement therapy must be assessed when the adequacy of nutritional intake is evaluated.

Physicians: How to Order Diet

The diet order should indicate *diet for cystic fibrosis.* The dietitian determines the content and the caloric level according to the preceding principles.

References

1. Ramsey BS, Farrell PM, Pincharz P. Nutritional assessment and management in cystic fibrosis: a consensus report. Am J Clin Nutr 1992;55:108–116.
2. Gaskin KJ, Waters DL, Baur LA, Soutter VL, Gruca MA. Nutritional status, growth and development in children undergoing intensive treatment for cystic fibrosis. Acta Paediatr Scand 1990;366:106–110.
3. Laing SC. The nutritional management of children with cystic fibrosis. Hum Nutr 1986; 40A:24–31.
4. George DE, Mangos JA. Nutritional management and pancreatic enzyme therapy in cystic fibrosis patients: state of the art in 1987 and projections into the future. J Pediatr Gastroenterol Nutr 1988;7(Suppl 1):S549–S557.
5. Dodge JA. Nutritional requirements in cystic fibrosis: a review. J Pediatr Gastroenterol Nutr 1988;7(Suppl 1):S8–S11.
6. Gaskin KJ. The impact of nutrition in cystic fibrosis: a review. J Pediatr Gastroenterol Nutr 1988;7(Suppl 1):S512–S517.
7. Daniels L, Davidson GP, Martin AJ. Comparison of the macronutrient intake of healthy controls and children with cystic fibrosis on low fat or nonrestricted fat diets. J Pediatr Gastroenterol Nutr 1987;6(3):381–386.
8. Stark, LJ, Bowen AM, Tyc VL, Evans S, Passero MA. A behavioral approach to increasing calorie consumption in children with cystic fibrosis. J Pediatr Psychol 1990;15(3):309–326.
9. Daniels LA, Davidson GP. Current issues in the nutritional management of children with cystic fibrosis. Aust Paediatr J 1989;25:261–266.
10. Wilson-Goodman V, Taylor ML, Mueller D, Palmer J. Factors affecting the dietary habits of adolescents with cystic fibrosis. J Am Diet Assoc 1990;90:429–431.

28 / *Renal Disease and Disorders in Children*

CHRONIC RENAL FAILURE

General Description

The diet for the child with chronic renal failure is controlled in protein, sodium, potassium, and phosphorus. The primary goals of treatment include (1) adequate kilocalories for growth, (2) protein control to minimize uremic symptoms that might result from an accumulation of nitrogenous waste products, while providing adequate protein to promote growth, (3) control of sodium to regulate blood pressure and fluid balance (edema or dehydration), (4) moderation of dietary phosphorus intake in order to minimize secondary hyperparathyroidism, and (5) moderation of dietary potassium when hyperkalemia is present. Current data suggest that an overall improvement in general health and a reduction in the rate of decline of renal function can be achieved by long-term dietary management of children with chronic renal failure.[1]

Nutritional Inadequacy

Potential deficiencies of pyridoxine, niacin, B_{12} folic acid, iron, and zinc exist with the renal failure diet. A pediatric multiple vitamin and folic acid are recommended for diets providing less than two thirds of the Recommended Dietary Allowances (RDA) for age (see Chapter 2, Recommended Dietary Allowances and Table 28-1).[2] The diet is low in calcium because of the need to restrict protein and phosphorus. Therefore, calcium supplements will be needed to provide the RDA for age.

Indications and Rationale

Growth retardation is common in children with renal failure. Its cause is multifactorial and is related to inadequate energy intake, secondary hyperparathyroidism, abnormal vitamin D metabolism, acidosis, and disorders of electrolyte, enzyme, and hormone metabolism.[3] The use of National Center for Health Statistics charts

TABLE 28-1   Guidelines for Dietary Management of Infants, Children, and Adolescents in Chronic Renal Failure (Recommendations Based on Height-Age)*

Component	Comments	
Kcal	Infants:	105–115 kcal/kg
	1–3 yr:	100 kcal/kg
	4–10 yr:	85 kcal/kg
	11–14 yr, male:	60 kcal/kg
	11–14 yr, female:	48 kcal/kg
	15–18 yr, male:	42 kcal/kg
	15–18 yr, female:	38 kcal/kg
Protein[6]	Birth–1 yr:	2–3 g/kg of actual body weight
	1–2 yr:	2 g/kg of actual body weight
	2 yr–adolescence:	1–2 g/kg of actual body weight
	Adolescent:	1 g/kg of actual body weight
Sodium	Infants: 2–4 mEq/kg/day, if needed to control blood pressure and edema Children and adolescents: No extra salt (actual intake varies with caloric intake)	
Fluid	Not restricted unless severe edema present. Increased fluid may be necessary for children with a renal concentrating defect.	
Potassium	Infants: 2–4 mEq/kg/day Children and adolescents: 2–4 mEq per 100 kcal expended, if needed. Potassium binder may be necessary.	
Calcium and phosphorus	Calcium supplements generally prescribed to meet RDA. Restrict high phosphorus foods or use phosphate binders if serum phosphorus elevated.	
Vitamins and minerals	Pediatric one–a-day type multivitamin recommended daily 50 µg folic acid recommended for infants receiving a liquid multivitamin	

*Height-age: Age for which child's height is equal to the 50th percentile of National Center for Health Statistics Growth Chart (see Pediatric Appendix 28).

for assessment of growth prior to and during nutritional therapy is essential (see Pediatric Appendix 28).[4]

Weight-to-height ratio is frequently a more accurate measure of nutritional state than either weight or height alone. Care must be taken to correct for altered body water content.[5] Bone age, when available, should be used as a basis for estimating and evaluating caloric and nutritional needs.[6] However, when bone age is not available, use height-age for assessment purposes. An adequate caloric intake is essential to maximize growth, to reduce alterations in body composition, and to promote a sense of well-being.[3] Patients and parents must be reminded that it is essential to maintain an adequate caloric intake. Nasogastric feedings may be necessary if appetite or growth do not improve.

Dietary Management

The rationale and indications for dietary management of renal failure are similar for children and adults (see Chapter 14, Renal Disease).

Energy.   Growth retardation occurs when the caloric intake of children with chronic renal failure falls below 70 to 80% of the RDA for height-age.[7] Caloric recommendations should be equal to the RDA for the child's height-age as shown in Table 28-1. The greater the amount of energy over and above maintenance requirements, the more energy there is available for growth. The average caloric cost for growth is about 5 kcal per gram of weight gain.[7] When protein is restricted, kilocalories must be provided from other sources. Fats, low protein products, and carbohydrate supplements provide nonprotein caloric sources for such children.

Protein.   Protein restriction is used to decrease the accumulation of nitrogenous products and to minimize, and even decrease, uremic symptoms. Protein restriction may also delay the progression of renal insufficiency. Severe protein restriction is not recommended, because it may limit the variety of foods allowed, resulting in decreased caloric intake, which can lead to body tissue catabolism and poor growth. The protein requirement for children with chronic renal failure has not been established.[8] Generally, the protein intake should provide the RDA and not be reduced below 1 g/kg of body weight per day. Current recommendations are summarized in Table 28-1. The majority of the protein (approximately 70%) in the diet should be of high biological value.[6,9] Preparations of essential amino acids or ketoacid mixtures are not recommended.

Sodium.   Sodium control in children is individualized according to the cause of renal failure. In children with renal dysplasia, tubulointerstitial diseases, or obstructive uropathy, there may be excessive sodium losses in the urine, and the child may crave salt. Chronic sodium depletion may also adversely affect growth. Salt depletion may occur as a result of vomiting. In such circumstances, a more generous allowance of sodium, rather than a restriction, may be needed. Measurements of 24 hour urinary sodium excretion can aid in deciding how much sodium should be provided. The amount of sodium needed for growth must also be considered. Infants from birth to 3 months require an additional 0.5 mEq/kg/day, which tapers to 0.2 mEq/kg/day by 6 months of age.[10]

If hypertension and/or edema are present, a no-extra-salt restriction is recommended. The actual amount of sodium in the diet varies with the caloric intake of the child. A more limited sodium intake may be necessary if the edema or hypertension is severe. For infants, a sodium intake of 2 to 4 mEq/kg/day is usually recommended.

Fluid.   During the predialysis period, fluid restriction is imposed only if edema is severe or if dilutional hyponatremia is a major clinical problem. Children with renal concentration defects, as with nephrogenic diabetes insipidus, may require large daily oral fluid volumes. In order to monitor fluid balance, weighing the child daily is encouraged.

Potassium.   Children and adolescents who are approaching end-stage renal disease may have hyperkalemia. Generally, as the dietary protein decreases, the potassium content of the diet decreases. Recommendations for potassium control can range from the avoidance of foods containing high amounts of potassium to the specification of a range of 2 to 4 mEq of potassium per kilogram per day. An ion exchange resin may be prescribed rather than a more rigid dietary potassium restriction, if necessary.

Calcium and Phosphorus. One should seek to achieve as nearly normal serum calcium and serum phosphorus levels as possible during the time prior to dialysis and/or transplantation. Secondary hyperparathyroidism is frequently seen in children with chronic renal failure and may cause serious bone disease and interfere with normal statural growth (see Chapter 14, Chronic Renal Failure). Generally, the phosphorus content of the diet is low because of the protein restriction, but milk and milk products may also need to be strictly controlled in order to avoid excessive phosphorus intake. The need for further restriction of high phosphorus foods is determined by careful monitoring of laboratory tests. Phosphate binders may be necessary to prevent high serum levels of phosphorus. Calcium carbonate or calcium acetate is strongly preferred over aluminum-based phosphate binders[11] since infants and young children may be at particular risk of aluminum accumulation. In addition, the calcium carbonate improves calcium intake. Calcium intake is frequently inadequate and should be supplemented if the total intake from diet and medications is less than the RDA.

Vitamins and Minerals. A one-a-day type of pediatric multiple vitamin is recommended for children whose current intake and diet limit the variety of food choices, with subsequent potential for nutritional inadequacy. Infants who receive a liquid multiple vitamin should also be supplemented with 50 μg of folic acid daily. Iron supplementation is given when indicated, especially to children receiving recombinant erythropoietin.

Table 28-1 summarizes the guidelines for dietary management of renal failure in infants, children, and adolescents. For infants, the use of whole cows' milk is not recommended owing to its high renal solute load. Generally, breast milk or a formula that is low in sodium and phosphorus (such as Similac PM 60/40™ or SMA™) is recommended until at least 1 year of age. The caloric density of the formula may need to be increased by the addition of carbohydrate and fat in order to achieve adequate caloric intake. Solid foods should be introduced as for a normal infant. For children and adolescents, the diet is planned using the dietary exchanges for renal diets in Chapter 14.

Physicians: How to Order Diet

The diet order should indicate specific *levels of protein, sodium, fluid, potassium, calcium, and phosphorus.*

References

1. Jureidni KF, Hogg RJ, Van Renen MJ, Southwood TR, Henning PH, Cobiac L, Daniels L, Harris S. Evaluation of long-term aggressive dietary management of chronic renal failure in children. Pediatr Nephrol 1990;4:1–10.
2. Raymond NG, Dwyer JT, Nevins P, Kurtin P. An approach to protein restriction in children with renal insufficiency. Pediatr Nephrol 1990;4:145–151.
3. Wassner SJ. The role of nutrition in the care of children with renal insufficiency: symposium on pediatric nephrology. Pediatr Clin North Am 1982;29:973–990.

TABLE 28-2

Component
Kcal
Protein[6]
Sodium
Potassium
Calcium and ph
Fluid
Vitamins and m

*Height-age: Age for wh
Appendix 28).

†Dry Weight: The weigh

4. National Center for Health Statistics. NCHS growth curves for children 0–18 years. U.S. Vital and Health Statistics, Series 11, No. 165. Washington, DC: U.S. Government Printing Office, 1977.
5. Sharer K, Guilio G. Growth in children with chronic renal insufficiency. In: Fine RN, Gruskin AB, eds. End stage renal disease in children. Philadelphia: WB Saunders, 1984:271.
6. Nelson P, Stover J. Principles of nutritional assessment and management of the child with ESRD. In: Fine RN, Gruskin AB, eds. End stage renal disease in children. Philadelphia: WB Saunders, 1984:209.
7. Chantler C. Nutritional assessment and management of children with renal insufficiency. In: Fine RN, Gruskin AB, eds. End stage renal disease in children. Philadelphia: WB Saunders, 1984:193.
8. Chantler C, El Bishti M, Counaham R. Nutritional therapy in children with chronic renal failure. Am J Clin Nutr 1984;33:1682–1689.
9. Spinozzi NS, Grupe WE. Nutritional implications of renal disease. J Am Diet Assoc 1977; 70:493–497.
10. National Research Council. Recommended Dietary Allowances, 10th ed Washington, DC: National Academy Press, 1989:254.
11. Committee on Nutrition. Aluminum toxicity in infants and children. Pediatrics 1986;78: 1150–1154.

HEMODIALYSIS AND CONTINUOUS AMBULATORY PERITONEAL DIALYSIS

General Description

The goal of the diet for both dialysis modalities is provision of adequate calories, protein, and other nutrients for growth and to replace any nutrient losses in the dialysate. Additionally, unnecessary loads of substances such as urea, sodium, and phosphorus that must be excreted in the urine or removed by dialysis should be avoided. The diet for hemodialysis (HD) is controlled in protein, sodium, potassium, phosphorus, and fluid to minimize biochemical fluctuations and weight changes that may occur between dialysis sessions. The diet for peritoneal dialysis (PD) emphasizes an adequate protein intake to offset loss of protein in the dialysate, along with a mild sodium and potassium restriction and possible limitation of high phosphorus foods.

Nutritional Inadequacy

The pediatric dialysis patient is at risk for deficiencies of amino acids, water-soluble vitamins, and minerals. The extent of the losses of vitamins is unknown, and recommendations for blood levels of vitamins and minerals for children have not been established.[12] Therefore, an age-appropriate one-a-day type multiple vitamin and 1 mg of folic acid are recommended. Iron is not routinely supplemented, unless serum ferritin levels are low,[13] or if the child is receiving human recombinant erythropoietin. Calcium will need to be supplemented if intake is less than two-thirds of RDA.

The potential also exists for amino acid deficiencies since they are lost in the dialysate. Adequate protein intake is essential, but may be difficult because of taste

If the appetite is poor, liberalization of dietary sodium may help increase food intake and improve adherence to diet. For certain patients, foods with greater amounts of sodium may be allowed during the 8 to 10 hours before HD to encourage greater caloric and protein consumption. However, a high sodium intake just prior to HD causes excess fluid weight gain and elevated blood pressure, and this practice is discouraged for the majority of patients.

Potassium.   Potassium intake is determined by the frequency of HD, the concentration of potassium in the dialysate, and the urinary potassium losses. The size of the child also determines intake. In our experience, for the small child weighing less than 20 kg, a restriction of 40 to 60 mEq of potassium per day has maintained serum potassium levels within acceptable ranges. For the child and adolescent weighing more than 20 kg, 60 to 70 mEq of potassium per day are typically provided.

Kayexalate™, an ion-exchange resin, may be used to improve overall dietary intake by permitting the incorporation of certain high potassium foods in limited quantities.[13] Kayexalate™ can be taken as a candy, baked into cookies, or mixed with sweetened beverages. Kayexalate™ is a prescription item, thus it must be ordered by the patient's physician.

Calcium and phosphorus.   Dietary management of calcium and phosphorus for infants, children, and adolescents on HD is the same as for predialysis (see Chapter 28, Chronic Renal Failure). Phosphorus intake and the use of phosphate binders should be distributed throughout the day.[13]

Fluid.   The fluid allowance is based on insensible losses plus urine output. Insensible losses in children are approximately 30 to 35 ml per 100 calories expended each day. Interdialytic weight gain of not more than 5% of estimated dry weight is acceptable and can be used to adjust the fluid allowance.[13] Those foods that are liquid at room temperature are included in the fluid allowance.

Vitamins.   Children receiving HD require vitamin supplementation owing to dietary restrictions that may prevent adequate intake of all vitamins; poor appetite; iatrogenic dysgeusia, which may limit or eliminate certain groups of foods from the diet; and loss of water-soluble vitamins in the dialysate. Supplements of 1.2 to 2 mg of pyridoxine, 50 to 100 mg of ascorbic acid, and 1 mg of folic acid are recommended daily, plus supplements of other B-complex vitamins.[13] An age-appropriate one-a-day multiple vitamin plus 1 mg of folic acid is recommended daily for all infants and children under 11 years of age. Adolescents should be given the same multiple vitamin as adults. (See Chapter 14, Chronic Renal Failure and Hemodialysis.)

Cholesterol and triglycerides.   Serum lipids are monitored, but dietary treatment of hypercholesterolemia and hypertriglyceridemia is a lower priority since fats and simple carbohydrates are essential in the diet as caloric sources. Therefore, tight restriction is not possible. The use of unsaturated fats should be encouraged, but a high total fat intake is unavoidable in the diet.

Peritoneal Dialysis.   The goals for the nutritional management of the pediatric patient on PD are summarized in Table 28-3.

Energy.   Caloric requirements are based upon the RDA for patients' height-age, although actual requirements may be higher.[13] Early satiety and inadequate energy intake are common problems. Small, frequent meals are recommended to overcome a sense of fullness. Unlike the adult patient on PD, the pediatric patient

TABLE 28-3   Guidelines for Dietary Management of Infants, Children, and Adolescents on Peritoneal Dialysis (PD) (Recommendations Based on Height-Age* and Dry-Weight†)

Component	Comments	
Kcal	Infants:	105–115 kcal/kg
	1–3 yr:	100 kcal/kg
	4–10 yr:	85 kcal/kg
	11–14 yr, male:	60 kcal/kg
	11–14 yr, female:	48 kcal/kg
	15–18 yr, male:	42 kcal/kg
	15–18 yr, female:	38 kcal/kg
	Dietary kcal = total caloric requirement (above) − kcal from dialysate	
Protein[6]	Birth–1 yr:	3–4 g/kg
	1–5 yr:	3 g/kg
	5–10 yr:	2.5 g/kg
	10–12 yr:	2 g/kg
	> 12 yr:	1.5 g/kg
	70% of total protein should be of high biological value.	
Sodium	Infants: May require sodium supplementation	
	Children and adolescents: No extra salt (actual intake varies with caloric intake)	
Potassium	Use high potassium foods in moderation.	
	If serum potassium elevated, restrict potassium as appropriate.	
Calcium and phosphorus	Calcium supplements generally prescribed to meet RDA.	
	Avoid very high phosphorus foods, except meat; limit milk and milk products to ½ to 1 cup/day.	
Vitamins and minerals	Infant or pediatric one-a-day type multiple vitamin plus 1 mg of folic acid for patients up to 11 yr	
	Adolescents: Adult multiple vitamin supplement that contains 1 mg folic acid and calcium to equal the RDA	
Fluid	Generally not restricted	
Carbohydrates	Emphasize more complex carbohydrate (versus simple) sources if hypertriglyceridemia exists.	
Saturated fat	Use unsaturated fats rather than saturated fats if hypercholesterolemia exists.	
Cholesterol	If hypercholesterolemia exists, restrict only if able to consume adequate protein from low cholesterol sources.	

*Height-age: Age for which child's height is equal to the 50th percentile of National Center for Health Statistics Growth Chart (see Pediatric Appendix 28).

†Dry Weight: The weight at which no edema is present.

is seldom obese.[13] In some cases, fat and carbohydrate supplements may be necessary to increase total caloric intake.[16]

Theoretically, the total dietary kilocalories required can be determined by subtracting the kilocalories contributed by the dialysate from the total caloric requirements based on height-age (see Chapter 14, Peritoneal Dialysis). However, it is not known precisely what percentage of the dialysate is absorbed per individual, nor what effect the smaller volume of infused dialysate has on the number of kilocalories actually contributed by the dialysate in children.

Protein.   Currently, absolute protein requirements of children or adolescents on PD have not been determined. However, protein intake should be higher than predialysis. Losses in dialysate can average 0.3 g/kg/day in infants and young children up to 6 years of age.[13] It is suggested that 3 to 4 g of protein per kg/day for infants and children up to age 5 years is required for growth and to replace amino acids lost in the dialysate. However, protein intake should be individualized. Dialysate losses of protein can average 4 to 8 g/day for children over 5 years of age. Current recommendations for protein are adapted from adult recommendations and are summarized in Table 28-3.

About 70% of the dietary protein must be from high biological value sources such as meat, egg, fowl, and fish.

Calcium and phosphorus.   Dietary management of phosphorus is similar to that for adults on PD. Generally, milk or milk products are limited to 1 cup/day. However, the amount of dairy products may be increased if appetite is poor and if the child or the adolescent is unable to increase protein intake from other food sources.

Calcium supplements are often necessary to provide the RDA for age. Phosphate binders are also typically needed to maintain a proper serum calcium and phosphorus balance (see Chapter 14, Peritoneal Dialysis, for additional information).

Vitamins and minerals.   Vitamin and mineral needs of the pediatric population on PD have not been established.[12,13] Generally, guidelines used for adult patients on PD are followed. The loss of water-soluble vitamins in the dialysate may result in deficiencies. Currently, a pediatric one-a-day type multiple vitamin and 1 mg of folic acid are recommended daily.

Recent literature suggests that infants receiving chronic PD are at risk for developing significantly elevated plasma fluoride levels. The tolerance of these elevated levels and the effect on tooth and bone development in infants with end-stage renal disease (ESRD) have not yet been determined. Therefore, it is recommended that fluoride not be used in addition to a daily vitamin supplement for infants with ESRD.[17]

Fluid.   A fluid restriction should not be necessary, unless edema, intravascular volume excess, or hypertension is considered a clinical problem.

Cholesterol and triglycerides.   An elevation in serum lipids occurs in children receiving PD, as it occurs in adults. The emphasis in the diet is to decrease simple dietary carbohydrates and to increase food sources of complex carbohydrates. Use of more unsaturated fats, rather than saturated fats, is also recommended.

Physicians: How to Order Diet

For HD, the diet should indicate the specific levels of protein, sodium, potassium, phosphorus, and fluid. The dietitian will establish the caloric level.

For PD, the diet should indicate the specific levels of protein, sodium, and potassium, the number of dialysis exchanges, and the concentrations of the dialysate.

References

12. Kriley M, Warady BA. Vitamin status of pediatric patients receiving long-term peritoneal dialysis. Am J Clin Nutr 1991;53:1476–1479.

13. Nelson P, Stover J. Principles of nutritional management of the child with ESRD. In: Fine RN, Gruskin AB. End-stage renal disease in children. Philadelphia: WB Saunders, 1984:209–226.

14. Milliner DS. Pediatric nephrologist, Mayo Clinic. Personal communication.

15. Harmon WE, Spinozzi N, Meyer A, Grupe WE. Use of protein catabolic rate to monitor pediatric hemodialysis. Proc Eur Dial Transplant Assoc 1981;10:324–330.

16. Salvsky IB, Lucullo L, Nelson P, Fine RN. Continuous ambulatory peritoneal dialysis in children. Pediatr Clin North Am 1982;29:1005–1012.

17. Warady BA, Koch M, O'Neal DW, Higginbotham M, Harris DJ, Hellerstein S. Plasma fluoride concentration in infants receiving long-term peritoneal dialysis. J Pediatr 115; 1989:436–439.

NEPHROTIC SYNDROME

General Description

Nephrotic syndrome in children is characterized by proteinuria, hypoproteinemia, hyperlipidemia, edema, and disordered fluid and electrolyte metabolism. Typically, the diet is restricted in sodium, but depending upon the extent of the hyperlipidemia, it may also be restricted in fat, cholesterol, and simple carbohydrates. The primary goals of dietary treatment include (1) adequate calories to promote growth yet prevent obesity for children receiving corticosteroid therapy, (2) restricted sodium if needed to manage blood pressure and fluid balance, and (3) control of fat, cholesterol, and simple carbohydrates if needed to minimize severity of hyperlipidemia.

Nutritional Inadequacy

When dietary intervention includes restriction of sodium and/or fat, cholesterol, and simple carbohydrates, the diet is not inherently lacking in nutrients when compared to the RDA for age. However, if the child has many food dislikes or intolerances that greatly limit the variety of foods eaten, a multiple vitamin supplement should be recommended.

Indications and Rationale

Childhood nephrotic syndrome may evolve into chronic renal failure but will often resolve after a few months or years, without residual renal injury. Sometimes symptoms will resolve and reappear in cycles of several months, a condition designated as relapsing nephrotic syndrome. Generally, if a child is not experiencing any complications, it is important to encourage continuation of normal activities both at home and away from home because this is important for the child's physical and emotional development.

Corticosteroid therapy is the treatment of choice in childhood nephrotic syndrome. Quite often, the therapy is limited in duration; however, in relapsing nephrotic syndrome, a repeated or prolonged course of steroids may be necessary to establish control of the syndrome.[18] In such circumstances, the child will be maintained on a smaller dose just sufficient to control manifestations of the disorder in order to minimize the typical steroid-induced problems such as cushingoid appearance, growth retardation, and obesity. If the syndrome requires large doses of steroids or is unresponsive to steroid therapy, a second agent such as cyclophosphamide, chlorambucil, or cyclosporine is introduced. Unfortunately, some children are not responsive to the above-mentioned regimens and develop progressive renal failure. If this occurs, the child is then treated with a protein-controlled diet as outlined in Chapter 28, Pediatric Chronic Renal Failure.

When assessing the nutritional status of the child, refer to Table 18-1 of Chapter 18, Pediatric Nutritional Assessment, which offers guidelines for a thorough review of all parameters to be considered. Height-age should be used as a basis to estimate and evaluate caloric and nutritional needs. Care must be taken to correct for altered body water content.

Dietary Management

Energy.   Growth in children with nephrotic syndrome is variable and dependent upon the dose of corticosteroid required and the degree to which the syndrome is controlled. For example, children experiencing unrelenting nephrotic syndrome are quite often experiencing anorexia, dyspepsia, and sometimes diarrhea, which have been attributed to bowel edema. Thus, to attain normal growth, calories must be encouraged, which often requires oral supplementation. On the other hand, a child on high dose corticosteroids should receive no more than the RDA for calories and may even require some restriction if the child's intake is excessive and obesity seems imminent. Therefore, when assessing energy requirements, the progression of the illness, nutritional status, activity level, and age of the child must all be carefully considered.[19,20]

Protein.   Traditionally, high protein diets were advocated as a means of compensating for protein losses in the urine and correcting hypoproteinemia. These diets were not effective and were difficult for patients to follow. Recent investigations show that ordinary dietary protein intakes such as specified by the RDA will result in levels of proteinuria less than those on large intakes of protein. Total albumin mass and albumin synthesis rates are no greater with higher protein dietary regimens than with dietary protein set at the RDA.[19]

Even though some literature suggests that use of a protein-restricted diet in nephrotic syndrome patients can decrease protein losses in the urine, it is felt that the absolute benefit of this therapy for children is minimal when compared to possible disadvantages incurred while following a highly restricted diet (i.e., malnutrition resulting in growth retardation or failure to thrive). Therefore, continuation of the child's normal protein intake is recommended, keeping in mind that it must be adequate according to the RDA for age. Forced protein intake with the intent of compensating for urinary losses is discouraged.

Sodium. A "no added salt" diet (usually 2 to 4 mEq/kg of body weight) is recommended to prevent water retention and high blood pressure. The child should avoid added salt at the table. Typically, salt may be used in moderation while cooking, but use of processed foods that are high in sodium should be avoided. However, if this restriction does not result in adequate control, further restriction of sodium may be necessary. These restrictions are necessary only during the acute phase of the syndrome. Typically, once control of proteinuria is established via medications, and the edema has subsided, no dietary restriction is required.

Hyperlipidemia. Children with nephrotic syndrome usually present with an increase in total cholesterol, triglycerides and various lipoproteins such as very low-density lipoproteins, low-density lipoproteins, and apo-protein B. Neither the pathogenesis nor the best approach to the management of hyperlipidemia resulting from nephrotic syndrome has been clearly established.[21] Most evidence suggests that an increased hepatic synthesis of lipoproteins is the principal cause.

The degree of hyperlipidemia can be quite variable from one patient to the next. Factors influencing this variation include severity of proteinuria, age, diet, obesity, family history, nutritional status, degree of renal function, use of corticosteroids, diuretics, and beta-blockers. Hyperlipidemia may place the patient at increased risk for heart disease, may influence the progression of the nephrotic syndrome to a sclerotic form of the disease, and has been associated with increased platelet aggregation. Currently proposed management of hyperlipidemia includes a diet that contains less than 30% of the calories from fat, less than 250 mg of cholesterol, and no more than one-half of the carbohydrate as simple carbohydrate, along with regular aerobic exercise.[19] However, it should be noted that this form of hyperlipidemia is not particularly responsive to diet, because it is a result of increased hepatic synthesis. Therefore, care should be taken to avoid an overrestrictive diet that could lead to an inadequate intake resulting in growth retardation.

Physicians: How to Order Diet

This diet may be ordered as *nephrotic syndrome diet*. The dietitian will follow the preceding guidelines for restriction of sodium, fat, cholesterol, and simple carbohydrates.

References

18. Elzouki A, Jaiswal OP. Long-term, small dose prednisone therapy in frequently relapsing nephrotic syndrome of childhood: effect on remission, statural growth, obesity and infection rate. Clin Pediatr 1988;27:387–392.
19. Strauss J, Zilleruelo G, Freundlich M, Abitol C. Less commonly recognized features of childhood nephrotic syndrome. Pediatr Clin North Am 1987;34:591–607.
20. Merritt R, Hack SL, Kalsch M, Olson D. Corticosteroid therapy-induced obesity in children. Clin Pediatr 1986;25:149–152.
21. Grundy SM. Management of hyperlipidemia of kidney disease. Kidney Int 1990;37:847–853.

29 / *Nutritional Support in Pediatrics*

ENTERAL NUTRITION

Enteral alimentation is the most acceptable and effective method for maintaining or repleting nutrition in the compromised pediatric patient who has a functional gastrointestinal tract. Tube feedings are also indicated for patients unable to take oral feedings due to neurological disorders. Nocturnal tube feedings can be useful in patients with certain inborn errors of metabolism, including type I glycogen storage disease. Patients unable to achieve adequate oral intake due to anorexia or chronic disease warrant consideration of tube feeding also.[1,3,4] Enteral feedings are accompanied by fewer complications, are easier to administer, and are lower in cost when compared with parenteral nutrition.[1,2] Nasogastric feedings are manageable for short-term therapy; however, in patients requiring long-term support, a feeding gastrostomy can offer several advantages.[1] Whenever tube feeding is utilized, growth and biochemical status must be monitored carefully.

Criteria for Selection of Tube Feeding Formulas

Selection of tube feeding formulas for infants, children, and adolescents should be based on a careful assessment of the patient's energy, nutrient, and fluid needs. Also, careful assessment of the patient's medical and nutritional status, gastrointestinal tract function, renal function, and the site of tube placement is essential. Feeding formula concentration and volume can then be tailored to meet the patient's individual needs.

The composition of infant and pediatric formulas is described in Appendix 25. Infant formulas are most suitable for those less than 1 year old. These types of formulas include modified cows' milk formulas, soy-protein formulas, formulas for premature infants, predigested or "elemental" formulas, and formulas for infants with inborn errors of metabolism. These formulas are used for oral feeding and are also suitable for tube feeding. Table 29-1 lists formula types appropriate for different patient conditions.[4]

TABLE 29-1   Formula Selection for Infants Younger Than 1 Year

Patient Condition	Formula Type
< 34 wk gestation	Premature infant formula
Healthy term infant	60:40 whey: casein or casein formula
Primary or secondary lactose intolerance Casein-sensitive	Lactose-free soy protein Isolate formula (Sucrose- and corn-free also available)
Organ dysfunction (e.g., renal, cardiac)	Low electrolyte Low renal solute load
Severe steatorrhea associated with bile acid deficiency; ileal resection or lymphatic anomalies	Infant formula with MCT oil
Sensitive to casein and soy protein	Hypoallergenic casein hydrolysate
Abnormal nutrient absorption, digestion, and transport; severe intractable diarrhea; protein calorie malnutrition	Hydrolyzed casein with part of fat from MCT oil (lactose-free and sucrose- free are available)

MCT = Medium-chain triglycerides.

Adapted from: Warman KY. Enteral nutrition: support of the pediatric patient. In: Walker WA, Hendricks KM, eds. Manual of pediatric nutrition, 2nd ed. Philadelphia: BC Decker, 1990:79.

PediaSure™ (Ross Laboratories), a formula designed to meet the needs of the 1 to 6 year old, is available with and without added fiber. The volume of adult formula that meets the caloric needs of a young pediatric patient will usually not provide adequate vitamins and minerals, especially vitamin D, calcium, phosphorus, and iron are inadequate.[5] Whatever formula is utilized, the desired volume of formula should be assessed for vitamin and mineral content and supplemented accordingly.

The selection of a particular formula should be based on nutrient composition, renal solute load, and the patient's ability to concentrate urine.[6] At times, diarrhea can be a limiting factor in the use of formulas, and close attention should be given to the osmolality and carbohydrate content of the formulas. Stools can be tested for reducing substance to determine if carbohydrate malabsorption is present. In older children, the test for reducing substance may be negative because of metabolism of carbohydrate by colonic bacteria. In this case, stool pH is often acid (pH < 4).[3] The application of tube feeding for infants and children with short bowel syndrome has recently received much attention, and in these cases not only the osmolality and carbohydrate content but also the volume should be watched carefully. A combination of enteral and parenteral feeding is often initially necessary.[6]

Administration

Feedings may be administered by constant drip or by intermittent gavage. The choice of method depends on the child's age, the length of time without adequate food intake, the severity of the illness, and the type of feeding being used. In general, tube feeding is best tolerated and most effective if initiated slowly and continuously. However, intermittent feedings have been claimed to be more "physiological." The volume of intermittent feedings may be large, and since children require more nutrients per kilogram of body weight than adults, the risk of inducing cramping and diarrhea may be greater. Pump administration improves the tolerance of many tube-fed patients and is essential for patients who do not tolerate fluctuations in volume of intake or for patients who undergo continuous nocturnal feedings (see Chapter 16, Enteral Nutritional Support of Adults). When selecting a pump, it is important to choose one that enables the infusion rate to be adjusted in small increments.

The institution of tube feeding should proceed cautiously, and tolerance should be monitored carefully. Individual tolerance determines how rapidly feedings can be advanced. Following are guidelines for initiating tube feeding. Figure 29-1, p. 602 and 603, shows an order form for pediatric tube feedings.

Guidelines for Initiating Tube Feeding

1. Begin with 1 to 2 ml of formula per kg of body weight per hour by constant drip or by frequent intermittent feedings. Intermittent feedings should be administered by slow drip or by gravity over 15 to 30 minutes and never forced by syringe.
2. Initially, use isotonic formulas (less than 350 mOsm). Initial feedings should have a concentration no greater than 0.5 kcal/ml for patients who have not been fed for more than 7 days or who are critically ill.
3. Increase volume and concentration separately. Increase to one-third to one-half of desired total volume, and then begin to increase feeding to desired concentration. Gradually increase to full volume.
4. Changes are usually made every 24 hours, depending on tolerance, but may be made as frequently as every 6 to 8 hours.
5. Regress to the most recent administration schedule that was tolerated if signs of intolerance (vomiting, diarrhea, or excessive residual volume) develop. Later, advance the administration schedule more slowly.
6. Supplemental fluid and electrolyte sources may be needed when these guidelines are used.

There are several equations for estimating water requirements (see Chapter 18, Pediatric Nutritional Assessment). Most give similar results. Patients receiving enteral nutrition usually tolerate additional water, but parenteral supplementation may be needed if the patient takes less than the recommended amount (Table 29-2).

Monitoring

Monitoring of nutritional status and of tolerance to tube feeding is mandatory and should include (1) the daily evaluation and documentation of caloric, protein, and fluid intake, (2) the use of vitamin and mineral supplements, (3) the daily weight of the infant or child, (4) a review of intake and output for indications of intolerance (aspiration, vomiting, diarrhea, constipation) and of fluid balance,

PHYSICIAN'S PEDIATRIC ENTERAL NUTRITION ORDER SHEET

See next page for Guidelines for Ordering Enteral Nutrition

YES NO	Pediatric Nutrition Consult
YES NO	Patient likely to leave hospital on tube feedings.

FORMULA _____ **VOLUME GOAL** _____ **cc/day**

TUBE POSITION _____ **TYPE** _____ **SIZE** _____

P.O. INTAKE   **YES**   **NO**   IF YES, SPECIFY: _____

DELIVERY

_____

☐   **CONTINOUS (pump)**

Starting rate____cc/hr. over____hr./day

   Optional: If feeding is tolerated for____hours,
   increase rate by____cc/hour every____hours
   up to____cc per hour.

Water____cc/24 hours.   Flushes with medications and at
                             least qid for tube patency

Gastric residual   Check q_____hours

   If greater than____cc, hold feeding for one hour and recheck.

   Call service if _____

DATE_____TIME _____DR. _____

☐   **INTERMITTENT (gravity)**

Start with____cc over____minutes.

____**times/day.**

   Optional: If feeding is tolerated for____hours, increase rate
   by____cc/feeding every____hours up to____cc per feeding.

Water____cc/24 hours.   Flushes with medication and after
                             each feeding.

Gastric residual   Check before each feeding.

   If greater than____cc, hold feeding for one hour and recheck.

   Call service if _____

DATE_____TIME _____DR _____

_____

Changes in enteral nutrition order:

DATE_____TIME _____DR. _____

_____

Changes in enteral nutrition order:

DATE_____TIME _____DR. _____

_____

Changes in enteral nutrition order:

DATE_____TIME _____DR. _____

_____

FIGURE 29-1   Physician's pediatric enteral nutrition order sheet.

Enteral Nutrition Recommendations for Infants and Children
(Guidelines only; individual patients may have different requirements)

		Children	
NUTRIENT	**Full term neonate and infants (> 3 kg)**	**1-6 years**	**7-12 years**	**12-18 years**
Calories (RDA for age)	98-108 kcal/kg	90-102 kcal/kg	55-70 kcal/kg	45-55 kcal/kg
Formula selection	Milk based infant formula	Pediatric lactose free formula	Pediatric or adult lactose free formula	Adult lactose free formula
Tube flushes—warm water (qid for tube patency)[1]	5-10 ml/flush	15-30 ml/flush	30 ml/flush	30 ml/flush

INITIATION OF FEEDING — CONTINUOUS

Rate	1-2 ml/kg/hour	1-2 ml/kg/hour	1ml/kg/hour	0.5 ml/kg/hour
Concentration	1/2 to full strength[2,3,4]	1/2 to full strength[2,3,4]	1/2 to full strength[2,3,4]	1/2 to full strength[2,3,4]
Increases in volume	1ml/kg/hour increments	1ml/kg/hour increments	0.5 ml/kg/hour increments	0.5 ml/kg/hour increments

FOOTNOTES

1. Additional free water flushes will be needed if fluid needs are not met by tube patency flushes and/or IV hydration.
2. Begin with an isotonic formula (< 350 mOsm/kg water). *Either the strength or the volume delivered may be increased, but not both at once, every 8-12 hours as tolerated.*
3. During transition from parenteral to enteral feedings, increase concentration of enteral feedings so calorie content of enteral feedings is not lower in calories than the parenteral feedings being replaced.
4. Begin with 1/2 to full strength if the patient has not been fed enterally for < 6 days.
   Begin with 1/2 to 2/3 strength formula if a hypertonic solution is used.
   Begin with 1/4 to 1/2 strength if the patient has not been fed enterally > 7 days.

GASTRIC RESIDUAL CHECK

Continuous feeding: Check at least every 4 hours. If residual is equal to the previous hourly rate, hold feedings for 1 hour and recheck. Residual checks are usually not indicated when the tube is placed past the pylorus, but frequent abdominal girth measurements and/or abdominal examinations are recommended.
Intermittent feeding: Check prior to each feeding. In general, hold the feeding if the amount is 1/2 the volume of the previous feeding.

POINTERS

1. Intermittent feedings may be appropriate when the patient has been on an established intermittent program at home or when continuous feedings in the hospital have been well tolerated. Discharge planning for enterally fed patients should consider the appropriateness of intermittent feedings.
2. Medication should be ordered in a liquid form.
3. Anti-aspiration procedures include:
   Head of bed elevated to 30-45° angle.
   Gastric residual checks q4h unless ordered otherwise.
   Hold gastric feeding 1/2 to 1 hour prior to recumbent position (such as CPT).

FIGURE 29-1, cont'd   Enteral nutrition recommendations for infants and children.

TABLE 29-2   General Guidelines for Maintenance Water Requirements[1]

Patient Weight (kg)	Water Requirement
< 2.5 kg	120 ml/kg/day
2.5–10 kg	100 ml/kg/day
10–20 kg	1,000 ml + 50 × (weight in kg − 10) ml/day
> 20 kg	1,500 ml + 20 × (weight in kg − 20) ml/day

With permission from: Wilson SE. Pediatric enteral feeding. In: Grand RJ, Stephen JL, Dietz WH, eds. Pediatric nutrition theory and practice. Boston: Butterworth, 1987:772.

TABLE 29-3   Common Tube Feeding Problems and Causes

Problem	Cause
Vomiting	Improper tube placement
	Tube too large
	Rate of feeding too fast
	Residual volume from previous feeding too great
	Osmolality of feeding too high
	Medication given with feeding
Diarrhea	Rate of feeding too fast
	Osmolality of feeding too high
	Intolerance to formula ingredients (e.g., lactose)
	Medications (e.g., antibiotics)
	Severe protein and caloric malnutrition
	Malabsorption
	Bacterial overgrowth
Constipation	Lack of fiber in the formula
	Inadequate fluid
	Lack of activity

and (5) a review of serum electrolytes, glucose, albumin, urea, hematocrit, and other biochemical parameters specific to the patient's medical condition.

Common complications of tube feeding include vomiting, diarrhea, and constipation. See Table 29-3 for possible causes.

References

1. Wilson SE. Pediatric enteral feeding. In: Grand RJ, Stephen JL, Dietz WH, eds. Pediatric nutrition theory and practice. Boston: Butterworth, 1987:771–786.
2. Wilson SE, Dietz WH, Grand RJ. An algorithm for pediatric enteral alimentation. Pediatr Ann 1987;16:233–240.

3. Moore MC, Greene HL. Tube feeding of infants and children. In: Pencharz PB, ed. Pediatric clinics of North America. Philadelphia: WB Saunders, 1985:32(2):401–417.

4. Warman KY. Enteral nutrition: support of the pediatric patient. In: Walker WA, Hendricks KM, eds. Manual of pediatric nutrition, 2nd ed. Philadelphia: BC Decker, 1990:72–109.

5. Brammer EM. Shortcomings of current formulae for long-term enteral feeding in pediatrics. Nutr Clin Pract 1990;5:160–162.

6. Kennedy-Caldwell C, Caldwell MD, Zitarelli ME. Pediatric enteral nutrition. In: Rambeau JL, Caldwell MD, eds. Clinical nutrition: enteral and tube feeding. Philadelphia: WB Saunders, 1990:325–360.

PARENTERAL NUTRITION

General Description

When a pediatric patient cannot or should not eat by mouth and is unable to absorb nutrients through the gastrointestinal tract, parenteral nutrition is indicated. Providing nutritional support to children, especially in early life, is essential because of their limited body stores of essential nutrients.[7] In the pediatric patient, parenteral nutrition must be modified to meet anabolic needs and support normal growth and development.

A peripheral access is used if intravenous nutrition is anticipated for less than 1 to 2 weeks; a central access is required if parenteral nutrition is needed for longer periods of time. The umbilical artery may be used for short-term parenteral nutrition in the neonate.

Indications and Rationale

Pediatric patients who become candidates for parenteral nutrition usually have complex illnesses and/or structural gastrointestinal abnormalities. Parenteral nutrition is indicated when oral intake or tube feeding is limited or impossible for prolonged periods of time or when metabolic needs exceed that which can be delivered to and assimilated by the gut.[7] Indications for pediatric parenteral nutrition include but are not necessarily limited to surgical gastrointestinal disorders such as gastroschisis or omphalocele; intractable diarrhea of infancy; low birth weight; short bowel syndrome; inflammatory bowel disease; chylothorax; or intensive cancer therapy.

Components of Parenteral Nutrition

Parenteral nutritional solutions are formulated by the hospital pharmacy department on a daily basis. Calorie, protein, fat, fluid, electrolyte, and vitamin and mineral needs are evaluated and reordered daily. See Table 29-4 and Chapter 20, Nutritional Requirements of Sick Infants, Children, and Adolescents for recommended intakes.

Components of pediatric parenteral nutrition include the following.

Fluid. Fluid requirements depend on hydration status, size of the child, environmental factors (i.e., radiant warmers, ultraviolet light therapy), and disease state. Infants and children have a higher metabolic rate when this is expressed as per unit of body weight than adults so they have greater fluid (and caloric) needs per kilogram. A common method for determining fluid requirements is as follows:

Body Weight	Fluid Requirements per Day
3–10 kg	100 ml/kg
11–20 kg	1,000 ml + 50 ml/kg over 10 kg
> 20 kg	1,500 ml + 20 ml/kg over 20 kg

Maintaining desired fluid balance is essential because dehydration, hypernatremia, and hyperosmolarity may occur with inadequate administration of fluids. On the other hand, administration of excessive amounts of water may result in hyponatremia and water intoxication with symptoms of tremulousness and even seizures. If excessive water is administered in conjunction with excessive amounts of sodium, symptoms of fluid overload with peripheral edema, pulmonary edema, and congestive heart failure may result.

Amino Acids.   Recommendations for protein appear in Table 29-4. Protein needs are assessed on an individual basis since requirements vary with the patient's age, stage of development, and disease. Premature infants require sufficient protein to match normal intrauterine growth rates, although intakes in excess of 3 g of protein per kg of body weight per day have not been shown to increase body protein gain and may be associated with complications.[8] Older children need adequate protein to maintain normal growth.[9]

Standard synthetic crystalline L-amino acid solutions, which were developed to meet the essential and nonessential amino acid requirements for adults, are also used for children. Specialized amino acid solutions for low-birth-weight infants have been developed, which are high in histidine and tyrosine, have added taurine and glutamic and aspartic acids, and contain less phenylalanine, methionine, and glycine than adult formulations. Cysteine is not present in the solution due to instability but may be added at the time of preparation. Use of these solutions has been shown to result in a plasma amino acid profile that is closer to that of the breast-fed infant.[10] With all parenteral amino acid solutions, careful attention must be paid to calcium and phosphorus solubility, and particularly when using these solutions with infants, whose calcium and phosphorus needs are increased.

Dextrose.   Dextrose monohydrate provides 3.4 kcal/g and is used in parenteral solutions. When mixed with amino acids to reach final desired concentration, it provides the major calorie source for most parenteral nutrition patients. Dextrose calories from intravenous medications also need to be taken into account when determining carbohydrate calories. To reduce glucose intolerance, glucose is often provided at an initial concentration of 10% and slowly increased to the goal concentration (usually 20 to 25%) over several days.[11] Peripheral solutions are usually limited to 5 to 10% dextrose or as needed to keep the osmolality of the solution around 800 mOsm/kg of water (maximum of 1,000 mOsm) in order to limit the risk of phlebitis.

Fat Emulsions.   Intravenous fat emulsion is a dense isotonic calorie source available in either 10 or 20% concentration of soybean or safflower oil. Essential fatty acid deficiency is prevented by providing a minimum of 0.5 to 1.0 g of fat per kg of body weight per day.[11] High lipid infusion rates, decreased lipid clearance, or both have been associated with impaired neutrophil and reticuloendothelial function, increased rate of infection, defective platelet function, hypoxia, and increased pulmonary artery pressure.[12] The premature and small-for-gestational-age infant have a decreased ability to clear both free fatty acids and triglycerides from their serum. Ability to tolerate fat increases with postnatal age.[8] Recommendations for parenteral fat appear in Table 29-4.

TABLE 29-4 Intravenous Nutrient Recommendations for Neonates, Infants, and Children*

Nutrient	Pre-Term Neonate (< 3 kg)	Full-Term Neonates and Infants (> 3 kg)	Children
Total kcal†	Start at 60–80 kcal/kg/day (maintenance), increase progressively as glucose and/or fat tolerance permits to 100–120 kcal/kg/day	100–120 kcal/kg/day	1–7 yr: 75–90 kcal/kg/day 7–12 yr: 60–75 kcal/kg/day 12–18 yr: 30–60 kcal/kg/day
Protein‡	0.5 g/kg/day, increase to 2.5 g/kg/day with increase in nonprotein kcal	2.0–2.5 g/kg/day	1.5–2.5 g/kg/day
Fat§	For kcal: 0.5–1.0 g/kg/day, increase by 0.5 g/kg/day to a maximum of 2.5 g/kg/day For EFA supplementation only: 0.5 g/kg/day	For kcal: 1.5 g/kg/day, increase by 0.5–1.0 g/kg/day to a maximum of 3 g/kg/day For EFA supplementation only: 0.5–1.0 g/kg/day or 2.0 g/kg twice a week	For kcal: 1.5 g/kg/day, increase by 0.5–1.0 g/kg/day to a maximum of 3 g/kg/day For EFA supplementation only: 0.5–1.0 g/kg/day or 2.0 g/kg twice a week
Sodium and chlorine	3–4 mEq/kg/day or slightly higher when newborn	3–4 mEq/kg/day	3–4 mEq/kg/day
Potassium	2–3 mEq/kg/day or slightly lower when newborn	2–3 mEq/kg/day	2–3 mEq/kg/day
Calcium	1–2 mEq/kg/day, increase to 2–4 mEq (425–850 mg Ca gluconate)/kg/day as protein and kcal are increased	1–2 mEq (212–425 mg Ca gluconate)/kg/day	0.5–1.0 mEq (106–212 mg Ca gluconate)/kg/day
Phosphorus	0.5 mmol/kg/day, increase to 1.0–1.3 mmol/kg/day as protein and kcal are increased	1.0 mmol/kg/day	1.0–1.3 mmol/kg/day
Magnesium	0.5 mEq/kg/day	0.5 mEq/kg/day	0.25–0.5 mEq/kg/day

EFA = Essential fatty acid.

*The recommendations represent intakes appropriate for the metabolically stable patient. Other patients may require alterations of the above intakes.

†Caloric values: amino acids: 4 kcal/g; 10% fat emulsion: 1.1 kcal/ml; IV dextrose: 3.4 kcal/g; 20% fat emulsion: 2.0 kcal/ml.

‡A ratio of 160–200 nonprotein kcal/g of nitrogen (or 25–32 nonprotein kcal/g of protein) is needed for protein anabolism.

§Do not begin until bilirubin is less than 3 mg/dl.

Continued.

TABLE 29-4   Intravenous Nutrient Recommendations for Neonates, Infants, and Children*—cont'd

| Nutrients | Standard Daily Dose | | | |
	(< 1 kg)	(≥ 1 kg and < 3 kg)	(≥ 3 kg and < 11 years)	(≥ 11 years)
VITAMINS				
A	690 IU	1,495 IU	2,300 IU	3300 IU
D	120 IU	260 IU	400 IU	200 IU
E	2.1 IU	4.55 IU	7 IU	10 IU
C	24 mg	52 mg	80 mg	100 mg
Folic acid	42 µg	91 µg	140 µg	400 µg
Thiamine	0.36 mg	0.78 mg	1.2 mg	3 mg
Riboflavin	0.42 mg	0.91 mg	1.4 mg	3.6 mg
Pyridoxine	0.3 mg	0.65 mg	1.0 mg	4 mg
Niacin	5.1 mg	11.05 mg	17 mg	40 mg
B_{12}	0.3 µg	0.65 µg	1 µg	5 µg
Dexpanthenol	1.5 mg	3.25 mg	5 mg	15 mg
Biotin	6 µg	13 µg	20 µg	60 µg
K_1	0.06 mg	0.13 mg	0.2 mg	0.2 mg

	Standard Daily Dose	Maximum Daily Dose
TRACE ELEMENTS		
Zinc	100 µg/kg (≥ 3 kg) or 300 µg/kg (< 3 kg)	4,000 µg
Copper	20 µg/kg	800 µg
Manganese	5 µg/kg	200 µg
Chromium	0.17 µg/kg	6.8 µg

Electrolytes.   Guidelines for electrolyte requirements are stated in Table 29-4, but requirements will vary with the individual patient. Patients with excessive losses of body fluids need replacement electrolytes in addition to daily maintenance requirements due to vomiting, diarrhea, or need for diuretics (such as furosemide). If deficits are severe, a separate intravenous solution may be needed.

Vitamins.   MIV-Pediatric™ is the only parenteral multiple vitamin marketed for infants and children in the United States. Composition is based on recommendations of the Food and Drug Administration and approved by the Nutrition Advisory Group of the American Medical Association. Dosage is based on the weight and/or age of the infant or child and is designed to provide maintenance requirements (Table 29-4). Some children may require additional supplementation.[13]

Trace Elements.   Trace elements appropriate for pediatric use are available in a solution containing a combination of zinc, copper, manganese, and chromium. Composition is based on amounts suggested by the American Medical Association. Recommendations are calculated based on requirements for growth together with the need to replace endogenous losses.[13] Deficiencies of individual trace elements may require targeted therapy. For instance, zinc deficiency may result from persistent diarrhea, and additional amounts of that element may need to be given. At the present time, the standard trace element solutions designed for children do not contain selenium. If the child is going to receive parenteral nutrition for more than 1 month, our practice is to add 2 µg of selenium per kg of body weight (maximum of 30 µg/day) to the solution. Because selenium is excreted primarily by the kidneys, a lower dosage should be given to patients with impaired renal function. Caution is required in administration of copper and manganese when cholestatic liver disease is present.[13]

Iron may be added to the parenteral solution or provided by intramuscular injection. Iron tolerance should be determined with caution due to the risk of allergic reaction (anaphylaxis), iron overload, increased demand for vitamin E, and potential for gram-negative septicemia. Iron intake from transfusions must be considered. An intravenous requirement of 100 µg of iron per kg of body weight per day has been recommended for the term infant over 3 months of age, or 1 to 2 mg of iron per liter of parenteral nutrition for infants and children after an initial test dose.[13]

Patient Monitoring

All pediatric parenteral nutrition patients should be monitored. Criteria monitored include initial weight, length or height, head circumference, growth, urine diastix for glucose, temperature, and laboratory data. Fluid status is monitored by following daily weight, intake, and output. A growth chart is helpful in longer term treatment.

Baseline laboratory data should include tests for liver function, uric acid, albumin, total protein, blood glucose, calcium, phosphorus, triglycerides, sodium, potassium, acid-base balance, and renal function. Trace elements are measured when indicated by the patient's disease state. Normal serum levels of zinc and copper, however, do not guarantee positive nutrient balance, and bacterial endotoxin may cause a decrease in serum zinc concentrations. Corticosteroids can do the same to serum copper values.[14]

Daily monitoring of glucose and electrolytes is recommended until the patient is stable and then 1 to 2 times per week. Other tests are performed 1 to 2 times per week or more frequently as needed until the patient is stable and then once a week. Trace elements are usually checked monthly.

Complications

Complications of parenteral nutrition can be classified as related to the IV catheter, infection, or metabolic response to the nutrients delivered.

Technical complications that occur at the time of catheter insertion include pneumothorax, hemothorax, injury to arteries and veins, air embolism, and cardiac perforation. After catheter placement, there is the possibility of thrombus formation, dislodgement of the catheter, fibrin clots in the catheter tip, and precipitates in the catheter.[9]

Sepsis can occur due to bacteria and fungi carried along the catheter or through the infusate. The major cause of infection is improper care of the catheter, especially infrequent dressing changes. The likelihood of sepsis appears related to the duration of therapy. Early indications of infection are fever, leukocytosis, and/or unexplained glycosuria; these should be responded to immediately.[11]

FIGURE 29-2 Physician's pediatric parenteral nutrition order sheet.

PHYSICIAN'S PEDIATRIC PARENTERAL NUTRITION ORDER SHEET

(use a new sheet for each daily order)

CLINIC NUMBER
NAME
ROOM NUMBER

For more detailed information, see Pediatric Parenteral Nutrition guidelines (see Table 29-4)

PATIENT'S WEIGHT _____ KG.

PATIENT'S AGE _____

PARENTERAL NUTRITION SOLUTION COMPOSITION

Dextrose	_____ %
Amino acids	_____ g/kg/day
Others _____	_____ g/kg/day
Sodium	_____ mEq/kg/day
Potassium	_____ mEq/kg/day
Calcium	_____ mEq/kg/day
Magnesium	_____ mEq/kg/day
Phosphorus	_____ mmol/kg/day

Chloride (select one)

☐ Sodium = Chloride (anions are added as chloride to equal the amount of sodium)

☐ Minimal Chloride (Anions are added as acetate to minimize amount of chloride)

☐ Minimal Acetate (Anions are added as chloride to minimize amount of acetate)

☐ Chloride _____ mEq/kg/day

Heparin Sodium _____ Units/ml (Final Conc.)

INTRAVENOUS FAT EMULSION

☐ 10% Fat Emulsion (1.1 kcal/ml)

☐ 20% Fat Emulsion (2.0 kcal/ml)

_____ g/kg/day

or _____ ml/day

at _____ ml/hr

OTHER FLUIDS
Oral or NG

_____ ml/kg/day

or _____ ml/day

☐ Standard pediatric multivitamin injection to one bottle daily

☐ Patient on warfarin (no vitamin K)

☐ Standard pediatric trace element injection to one bottle daily

> **VOLUME** (specify one)
> _____ ml/kg/day
> _____ ml/day

NOTE: The parenteral nutrition solution ordered above is the amount the patient will receive daily. All other forms of fluid intake will be in addition to these amounts.

ROUTE OF ADMINISTRATION (select one)

☐ Central   ☐ Umbilical   ☐ Peripheral

Estimated kilocalories from parenteral nutrition:

_____ kcal/kg/day or _____ kcal/day

TIME NEEDED (Nurse)

_____

Date _____   Time _____   Dr. _____

Meds Solution

_____
_____
at _____ ml/hr

Other IV #1

_____
_____
at _____ ml/hr

Other IV #2

_____
_____
at _____ ml/hr

SPECIAL INSTRUCTIONS

_____
_____

Metabolic complications can occur and can be difficult to manage. Table 16-8 in Chapter 16, Adult Parenteral Nutrition, describes common complications, signs, treatments, and prevention. Excessive amino acid administration can result in azotemia as evidenced by increased plasma urea levels but must be differentiated from other causes of increased urea levels. Rickets has been seen in infants on long-term parenteral nutrition. Causes of these complications include inadequate ability of premature infants to convert vitamin D_3 to its active form, inadequate amounts of calcium and phosphorus and excessive urinary losses of these two minerals. Although calcium and phosphorus, should be provided to premature neonates in amounts that approximate intrauterine accretion rates, calcium and phosphorus precipitation can occur when they are in solution together. Guidelines are available for each amino acid solution to help determine whether calcium phosphate precipitation is likely at different concentrations of calcium and phosphorus.

Hyperglycemia occurs in 45 to 80% of premature infants and may improve with a controlled continuous insulin infusion.[15,16] Cholestasis can occur, usually after 2 weeks of parenteral nutrition, but should be differentiated from other causes of abnormal liver function.[9]

Physicians: How to Order

Before parenteral nutrition is ordered, the physician should consider if the patient could instead be a candidate for enteral nutrition support. If so, enteral nutrition should be utilized rather than parenteral nutrition. The type of parenteral access device to use needs to be determined and baseline laboratory data ordered.

At the Mayo Medical Center, solutions are ordered on a daily basis, using the Physician's Pediatric Parenteral Nutrition Order Sheet (Fig. 29-2). Dextrose is ordered by percentage of final composition; electrolytes and amino acids are ordered on a per kilogram basis; and fat is ordered either by volume or on a per kilogram basis. The multiple vitamin, with or without vitamin K, and trace elements are ordered separately. All fluids should be taken into account, including intravenous fluids with medications, oral intake, or enteral feedings. The Adult Parenteral Nutrition Order Sheet (Appendix 13) may be used for adolescents, particularly those past their peak growth spurt. Guidelines for calories, fat, protein, and electrolytes are shown in Table 29-4.

References

7. Testerman EJ. Current trends in pediatric total parenteral nutrition. J Intravenous Nurs 1989;12(3):152–162.
8. Pereira GR, Glassman M. Parenteral nutrition in the neonate. In: Rombeau JL, ed. Parenteral nutrition. Vol 2. Philadelphia: WB Saunders, 1986:702–720.
9. Cochran EB, Phelps SJ, Helms RA. Parenteral nutrition in pediatric patients. Clin Pharm 1988;7:351–366.
10. Heird WC, Hay W, Helms RA, Storm MC, Sudha K, Dell RB. Pediatric parenteral amino acid mixture in low birth weight infants. Pediatrics 1988;81:41–50.
11. Varms RN, Suskind RM. Parenteral nutrition in the pediatric patient. In: Rombeau JL, ed. Parenteral nutrition. Vol 2. Philadelphia: WB Saunders, 1986:721–730.

12. Miles JM. Intravenous fat emulsions in nutrition support. Curr Opin Gastroenterol 1991;7:306–311.

13. Greene HL, Hambridge KM, Schanler R. Guidelines for the use of vitamins, trace elements, calcium, magnesium and phosphorus in infants and children receiving total parenteral nutrition. Am J Clin Nutr 1988;48:1324–1342; rev reprint 1990.

14. Shulman RJ. Zinc and copper balance studies in infants receiving total parenteral nutrition. Am J Clin Nutr 1989;49:879–83.

15. Collins JW, Hoppe M, Brown K, Edidin DV, Padbury J, Ogata ES. A controlled trial of insulin infusion and parenteral nutrition in extremely low birth weight infants with glucose intolerance. J Pediatr 1991;118:921–927.

16. Kanarek KS, Santeiro ML, Malone JI. Continuous infusion of insulin in hyperglycemic low–birth weight infants receiving parenteral nutrition with and without lipid emulsion. JPEN 1991;15:417–420.

A. GENERAL APPENDICES

Standards of Practice for Nutrition Support Dietitians*

These Standards of Practice for Nutrition Support Dietitians should be used in conjunction with the following A.S.P.E.N. publications:

Definitions of terms used in A.S.P.E.N. guidelines and standards. Nutr Clin Pract 1988;3(1):26–27.

Guidelines for the use of total parenteral nutrition in the hospitalized adult patient. JPEN 1986;10(5):441–445.

Guidelines for the use of home parenteral nutrition in adults. JPEN 1987; 11(4):342–344.

Guidelines for the use of enteral nutrition in the adult patient. JPEN 1987; 11(5):435–439.

Standards for nutrition support: hospitalized patients. Nutr Clin Pract 1988; 3(1):28–31.

Standards for nutrition support: home patients. Nutr Clin Pract 1988; 3(5):202–205.

Standards for nutrition support: hospitalized pediatric patients. Nutr Clin Pract 1989;4(1):33–37.

Standards for nutrition support for residents of long-term care facilities. Nutr Clin Pract 1989;4(4):148–153.

Standards of practice: nutrition support pharmacist. Nutr Clin Pract 1987; 2(4):166–169.

Standards of practice: nutrition support nurse. Nutr Clin Pract 1988;3(2):78–80.

Standards of practice: nutrition support physician. Nutr Clin Pract 1988; 3(4):154–156.

---

*Developed under the aegis of a multidisciplinary task force of the American Society for Parenteral and Enteral Nutrition (A.S.P.E.N.). With permission from the American Society for Parenteral and Enteral Nutrition, 8630 Fenton Street, Suite 412, Silver Springs, MD 20910-3805 (301) 587-6315. Originally printed in: Nutr Clin Pract 1990; 5(2):74–78.

These Standards of Practice for Nutrition Support Dietitians should also be used in conjunction with the following American Dietetic Association publication:

Standards of Practice for the Profession of Dietetics. ADA Council on Practice, Feb 1984.

A.S.P.E.N. has developed these standards as general guidelines for health professionals. Their application in any individual case should be determined by the best judgment of the professional. The standards represent a consensus of A.S.P.E.N.'s members as to that minimal level of practice necessary to assure safe and effective enteral and parenteral nutrition care. A.S.P.E.N. disclaims any liability to any health care provider, patient, or other persons affected by these standards.

These standards have been developed, reviewed, and approved by the following A.S.P.E.N. groups: Standards Committee, Dietitians' Committee, Executive Committee, and Board of Directors.

SCOPE OF PRACTICE

Background.   The advent and sophistication of specialized nutrition support—enteral and parenteral therapies—have allowed the health care professional to ensure that even patients who are unable to eat will receive adequate nutrition. As the importance of specialized nutrition support has become recognized and techniques for the delivery of enteral and parenteral therapies have evolved, specialized nutrition support has become an established area of dietetic practice.

Role.   The Nutrition Support Dietitian, in conjunction with other health care professionals including a physician, registered nurse, and registered pharmacist, shall participate in the provision of specialized nutrition support. If a formal nutrition support service has not been established, the Nutrition Support Dietitian shall function, along with other appropriate health care professionals, as a member of the nutrition support committee or subcommittee.

The Nutrition Support Dietitian is a registered dietitian with clinical expertise in specialized nutrition support obtained through education and specialized training or experience in this field. The Nutrition Support Dietitian works specifically with assessment of nutritional status and with oral, enteral, parenteral, and transitional therapies. The role of the dietitian includes nutritional assessment, therapeutic plan, implementation, monitoring, and documentation of the patient's response to specialized nutrition support. Other activities include facilitating a smooth transition to an oral diet and the termination of enteral and parenteral therapies when appropriate. The Nutrition Support Dietitian should also be involved in research activities and with the education of patients, families, and other health care professionals concerning principles of nutrition therapy.

GOALS

Using current knowledge of nutrition therapy and scientific theory, the Nutrition Support Dietitian strives to provide optimal nutrition support for all patients. Specific functions include:

1. Identifying patients at nutritional risk.

2. Performing periodic nutritional assessments of patients receiving nutrition support.
3. Participating in design, implementation, and monitoring of parenteral and enteral nutrition regimens.
4. Participating in design, implementation, and monitoring of home enteral and home parenteral nutrition programs.
5. Assuring trouble-free and nutritionally complete transitional feedings.
6. Documenting nutrition care plans.
7. Providing education to patients, families, and health care professionals.

The Nutrition Support Dietitian should actively pursue new knowledge in nutrition support. When appropriate, the Nutrition Support Dietitian should assist in and/or initiate nutrition support, as appropriate, and be an active participant in local, regional, and national education and research programs. Through these endeavors, the Nutrition Support Dietitian may share expertise, knowledge, and investigational findings with other health care professionals.

CHAPTER A. ASSESSMENT

A.1. Criteria shall be established for identifying a patient who is, or may become, malnourished.

A.1.1. All patients admitted to the hospital should undergo a screening assessment of nutrition status, documented in the medical record, which may include: age, gender, diagnosis, weight history and growth history (when appropriate), history of nutrient intake, and drug-nutrient interactions.

A.1.2. All patients who are considered to be "nutritionally at risk" should undergo an in-depth review of nutrition history and an evaluation of: anthropometric indices (when appropriate), biochemical indices of nutrition status, and clinical factors (mechanical, physiological or psychological, economic, and/or social) that may interfere with ingestion, digestion, absorption, or metabolism of nutrients.

A.1.3. Results of the nutritional assessment and nutrient recommendations should be documented in the medical record.

A.2. Individual plans for the use of specialized nutrition support should be appropriate for the patient's clinical status.

A.2.1. Guidelines for the use of parenteral nutrition (peripheral and central), enteral nutrition, oral supplements, and transitional feedings will be developed and should include:

A.2.1.1. Indications and contraindications;

A.2.1.2. Constraints on nutrient and fluid administration imposed by delivery system and/or clinical conditions;

A.2.1.3. Criteria for use of disease-specific solutions/formulas.

A.2.2. Guidelines for the use of specialized nutrition support will be reviewed and updated at regular intervals.

A.2.3. Response to nutrition therapy should be evaluated and documented. Recommendations for a change in the therapeutic plan will be based upon changes in clinical status and biochemical indices (see D.1.6.).

A.2.4. Education/information will be given to the patient and/or family members to assist them in making informed decisions concerning nutrition support.

A.3. A quantitative and qualitative evaluation of nutrient needs shall precede initiation of nutrition support.

A.3.1. Determination of nutrient needs should be based upon the patient's resting energy expenditure, activity, disease, treatment, nutritional status, metabolic demands, medications, and goals of nutrition therapy.

A.3.2. Modifications of nutrient delivery to the patient will be based upon the specific disease state, medical/surgical therapy, nutritional status, and the duration of anticipated inadequate intake.

CHAPTER B. THERAPEUTIC PLAN

B.1. A nutrition care plan will be established based on the results of the comprehensive nutritional assessment.

B.1.1. The therapeutic plan should be modified when changes in clinical status are identified.

B.2. The objectives and indications for nutrition support shall be determined and documented prior to initiating therapy.

B.2.1. Immediate, intermediate, and long-term goals of nutrition therapy should be established.

B.2.2. Educational needs of the patient and/or significant other should be evaluated.

B.2.3. The objectives and indications for use of home nutrition support will be provided to the patient in preparation for home training if appropriate.

B.2.4. The patient's progress toward achieving nutrition goals will be detailed in the medical record.

B.3. The route recommended to provide nutrition support should be appropriate to the medical condition, should provide the assessed nutrient requirements, and should achieve therapeutic objectives safely and effectively.

B.3.1. The gastrointestinal tract should be used when there is no contraindication.

B.3.2. Parenteral nutrition or parenteral supplementation should be initiated when nutrient needs cannot be met by the enteral route.

B.3.3. The method of nutrition support will be reassessed periodically during the course of therapy.

B.4 The feeding formulation recommended/selected should be appropriate for the disease process and estimated nutrient needs, and compatible with the route of access.

B.4.1. The nutrition care plan should include recommendations for oral diets, enteral tube feedings, and parenteral formulations as appropriate.

B.4.2. Feeding formulations should be tailored for disease-specific constraints and clinical status that may affect tolerance and nutrient utilization.

B.4.3. When similarly effective preparations that meet patient nutrient requirements are available, the most cost-effective product should be selected.

CHAPTER C. IMPLEMENTATION

C.1. There shall be verification that enteral formulations are prepared according to established guidelines for safe and effective nutrition therapy.

   C.1.1. Enteral feeding formulations will be prepared accurately, with attention to the feeding prescription, the prevention of contamination, the compatibility of ingredients, and the appropriateness of packaging and labeling.

   C.1.2. Written guidelines for the preparation of enteral feeding formulations will be maintained. Policies and procedures shall specify allowable hang time for enteral formulations.

   C.1.3. There shall be written policies specifying that the components of compounded formulations are labeled accurately.

   C.1.4. Quality assurance monitoring will be performed to ensure that guidelines are being met.

C.2. There shall be verification that specialized nutrition support is administered in accordance with the prescribed therapeutic plan and consistent with patient tolerance.

   C.2.1. Administration of enteral and parenteral feeding should be monitored to ensure safe and effective delivery of nutrition support.

   C.2.2. Proper placement of enteral feeding tubes should be confirmed prior to initiating enteral nutrition support.

   C.2.3. Patient identification on feeding formulations will be verified. Discrepancies shall be reported to appropriate personnel.

   C.2.4. Errors in feeding formulation administration will be minimized by verifying accuracy in cooperation with other health care disciplines.

   C.2.5 Progression of the feeding formulation (concentration and/or volume) will be based on patient tolerance. There will be documentation that the feeding formulation progresses toward or meets the nutrient needs of the patient.

   C.2.6. The rate of administration and concentrations for initiation of the feeding formulation will be recommended.

   C.2.7. Signs and symptoms of intolerance to feeding formulations will be identified and modifications of the formulation and/or formulation administration will be recommended as needed to minimize intolerance.

C.3. Protocols for implementing nutrition support shall be established to ensure safe and effective delivery.

   C.3.1. Protocols will be established and should include guidelines for administration, monitoring, and infection control.

   C.3.2. Protocols will be reviewed regularly to ensure that they are consistent with current knowledge of feeding formulations and access devices.

CHAPTER D. PATIENT MONITORING

D.1. The clinical and metabolic response to nutrition support shall be monitored to provide a basis for modifying nutrition support therapy.

    D.1.1. Protocols should be developed for timely review and documentation of the patient's clinical, metabolic, and nutritional status.

    D.1.2. Nutrient intake by oral, enteral tube, and parenteral routes should be monitored and recorded during the administration of feeding formulations.

    D.1.3. Anthropometric measurements and nutritionally relevant biochemical parameters should be documented and assessed serially to evaluate response to nutrition therapy.

    D.1.4. Gastrointestinal intolerance (including diarrhea, gastric residuals, abdominal distention, aspiration, nausea, vomiting, and malabsorption) to the advancing or restarting of tube feedings should be evaluated. Recommendations for alteration in the feeding plan (route, type, amount) based on gastrointestinal intolerance should be made as appropriate.

    D.1.5. Clinical tolerance (including fluid and electrolyte balance and nutritionally relevant biochemical parameters) to nutrient formulations should be evaluated.

    D.1.6. Changes in nutrient needs according to clinical/nutritional status (e.g., sepsis, hypermetabolism, hypometabolism, repletion, depletion) should be identified; corresponding alternations in nutrient formulations (route, type, amount) to meet patient requirements should be recommended.

    D.1.7. Alterations in nutrition therapy to manage organ failure, if present, should be recommended.

    D.1.8. Transitional feeding should be initiated, modified, and discontinued according to established criteria (see E.1.).

    D.1.9. Drug-nutrient and nutrient-nutrient interactions should be evaluated in order to minimize adverse side effects.

D.2. Patients should be monitored for physical, social, psychological, cognitive, and environmental factors that may influence the response to nutrition support.

    D.2.1. Protocols should be developed for timely review and documentation of pertinent physical, social, psychological, cognitive, and environmental patient factors.

    D.2.2. Adjunctive services for optimization of nutrition care (e.g., physical, occupational, or speech therapy, social services, psychology, or dental services) should be recommended.

    D.2.3. Compliance of patient, family, and health care professionals with nutrition care criteria, protocols, or therapeutic plans should be evaluated.

CHAPTER E. TRANSITIONAL FEEDING

E.1. Criteria shall be established for transitional feeding from parenteral to enteral nutrition and from enteral tube feedings to oral diet.

E.1.1. Parenteral nutrition should not be discontinued until estimated nutrient and fluid requirements are met by enteral intake.

E.1.2. Enteral tube feedings should not be discontinued until estimated nutrient and fluid requirements are met by oral intake.

E.1.3. Recommendations should be made for gradual decrease and/or cycling of parenteral, tube, or enteral feeding in order to maintain adequate nutrient delivery.

E.2. Adequacy of intake shall be documented prior to discontinuing parenteral or enteral nutrition support.

E.2.1. A quantitative and qualitative estimate of intake should be determined.

E.2.2. Tolerance of adequate enteral intake should include assessment of gastrointestinal status (e.g., diarrhea, abdominal distention, nausea, vomiting, malabsorption, constipation, and aspiration), nutrient intake, and metabolic status (e.g., hyperglycemia, hypoproteinemia, and mineral imbalances).

E.2.3. Tolerance of adequate oral intake and of individual foods should include assessment of chewing or swallowing difficulties, gag reflex, pain with eating, changes in elimination patterns, and status of gastrointestinal function.

E.2.4. Oral diet prescriptions should be verified for appropriateness before implementation.

E.2.5. Oral nutrition supplements should be recommended/provided when necessary and appropriate to increase inadequate oral nutrient intake.

DEFINITIONS

Nutrition Support Service: A multidisciplinary group of health care professionals who aid in the provision of specialized nutrition support.

Nutritional assessment: A comprehensive approach to defining nutritional status that employs clinical and dietary histories, physical examination, anthropometric measurements, and laboratory data.

Nutritionally at risk: Any patient who demonstrates clinical signs of malnutrition and/or mechanical, physiological, psychological, economic, and/or social constraints that interfere with the ingestion, digestion, absorption, or metabolism of nutrients.

Malnutrition: Any disorder of nutrition, including a deficiency of nutrient intake, impaired nutrient metabolism, or overnutrition.

Diet: A prescribed allowance of food or nutrients provided via the oral route.

Nutrients: Protein, carbohydrate, fat, vitamins, electrolytes, minerals, and water.

Specialized nutrition support: Provision of tube enteral or parenteral nutrients to maintain or restore optimal nutritional status.

Enteral nutrition: Nutrition provided via the gastrointestinal tract. Oral enteral nutrition is taken through the mouth. Tube enteral nutrition is provided through a tube or catheter that delivers nutrients distal to the oral cavity.

Feeding formulation: A ready-to-administer mixture of nutrients.

Modular enteral feeding: The combination of individual sources of nutrients so that an existing formula is modified or a new formula is created to meet the patient's individual nutritional requirements.

Parenteral nutrition: Provision of nutrients intravenously. Central parenteral nutrition is delivered through a large-diameter vein, usually the superior vena cava, the subclavian, or the jugular vein. Peripheral parenteral nutrition is delivered through a peripheral vein, usually of the hand or forearm.

Transitional feeding: Progression from one mode of feeding to another, while attempting to maintain/achieve estimated nutrient requirements.

Standard: The benchmark representing the minimum level of care that should be given in order to assure sound and efficient enteral or parenteral nutrition.

Interactions between Drugs, Nutrients, and Nutritional Status*

The interactions between drugs and nutrient intake and the nutritional status of the individual is becoming more appreciated. Drugs can influence nutrient absorption, metabolism, or excretion; the effects may alter nutritional status. On the other hand, specific nutrients, foods, or beverages interact with drug metabolism, action, or excretion. The dietitian must be attentive to the interactions of drugs and nutrients and to the effect on nutritional status.

*Adapted from Smith CH, Bidlack WR. Dietary concerns associated with the use of medications. Copyright The American Dietetic Association. Reprinted by permission from JOURNAL OF THE AMERICAN DIETETIC ASSOCIATION 1984;84(8):901–914.

Dietary Suggestions Associated with Drugs That Alter Nutrient Absorption

| Drug (Usage) | Nutritional Implications | | Dietary Suggestions |
	Gastrointestinal Side/Adverse Effects	Other Reactions	
Aluminum hydroxide gel (antacid, phosphate binder)	Bloating, constipation, fecal impaction, nausea or vomiting, stomach cramps	Phosphate malabsorption, hypophosphatemia, vitamin A malabsorption, thiamin destruction, loss of appetite, unpalatable (chalky)	*Ulcer therapy—Drug:* Take between meals, chew chewable tablets until thoroughly wetted, then follow with 125 ml water. *Diet Rx:* Teach dietary principles associated with treatment of ulcer disease. *Phospate-binding therapy—Drug:* Take at mealtime with 250 ml water or fluids indicated for patients with renal disease. *Diet Rx:* Dietary phosphate restriction may be prescribed. If permissable, include a high-bulk diet to counter constipation. *Other:* Prolonged usage or large doses, especially with a low-phosphate diet, may result in hypophosphatemic osteomalacia. Decreased absorption of fat-soluble vitamins (especially vitamin A) may be due to precipitated bile acids.
Bisacodyl (laxative)	Belching, mild cramping, diarrhea, nausea	Fluid and electrolyte loss, hypokalemia (long use)	*Drug:* Take on empty stomach with at least 250 ml water and at least 1 hr away from milk. (Milk may dissolve enteric coating, causing gastric irritation.) Swallow tablet whole (do not chew or crush). *Diet Rx:* Drink at least 6 to 8 glasses of 250 ml fluid/day to aid stool softening. Teach the importance of diet, increased fluid intake, and exercise. See table on pp. 641-643. *Other:* Prolonged usage or large doses may result in nutrient loss, fluid and electrolyte disturbances, and dependence on drug for bowel function.

Continued.

Cholestyramine (antihyperlipemic, bile acid sequestrant)	Belching, bloating, constipation, flatulence, heartburn, nausea or vomiting, steatorrhea, stomach pain	Malabsorption of fat, iron, carotene, vitamins A, D, and K, and folacin; hypoprothrombinemia; gritty texture; unpalatable taste	*Drug:* Thoroughly hydrate drug with at least 120 to 180 ml water, milk, fruit juice, or noncarbonated or other beverages prior to ingestion; disguise gritty texture and unpalatable taste by mixing with highly flavored liquids, thin soups, milk in cereals, or pulpy fruits (applesauce, crushed pineapple). *Diet Rx:* If permissible, include a high bulk diet with increased fluid intake to counter constipation. During long-term therapy, supplementation with a water-soluble (or parenteral) form of vitamins A and D may be prescribed. Parenteral or oral administration of vitamin K may also be considered if hypoprothrombinemia occurs. Folacin supplementation may be prescribed for patients with reduced serum or red cell folacin. *Other:* Evaluate for drug-drug interactions. Prior to drug therapy, control of serum cholesterol is attempted by diet therapy. During drug therapy, advise patient of the importance of following a prescribed diet.
Colchicine (antigout)	Diarrhea (may be severe), nausea or vomiting, abdominal pain	Malabsorption of sodium, potassium, fat, carotene, and vitamin B_{12} due to altered mucosal function; decreased lactase activity; loss of appetite	*Drug:* Take with water immediately before, with, or after meals to reduce gastric irritation. *Diet Rx:* May indicate increased intake of alkaline ash foods or beverages and low purine foods, no alcoholic beverages, and a high fluid intake of > 2,000 ml/day. *Other:* Gradual weight reduction may be suggested. Alert physician if patient reports any gastrointestinal side/adverse effects.

Dietary Suggestions Associated with Drugs That Alter Nutrient Absorption—cont'd

| Drug (Usage) | Nutritional Implications | | Dietary Suggestions |
	Gastrointestinal Side/Adverse Effects	Other Reactions	
Mineral oil (laxative)	Flatulence, indigestion, nausea or vomiting (with long use)	Malabsorption of carotene, vitamins A, D, E, and K, calcium, and phosphorus; tasteless and odorless (when cold); disagreeable consistency; loss of appetite and of weight; hypokalemia (with long use)	*Drug:* Take at least 2 hr away from food (to avoid delayed digestion and movement of chyme from stomach). May mix with or follow by orange juice to counter consistency. *Diet Rx:* See bisacodyl. Concurrent use with fat-soluble vitamins may interfere with vitamin absorption. Do not use in the preparation of low calorie salad dressings. *Other:* See bisacodyl.
Phenolphthalein (laxative)	(See bisacodyl)	Malabsorption of vitamin D, calcium, and other minerals; hypokalemia (long use); may be excreted in breast milk	*Drug:* Take on empty stomach. Chew chewable tablets or wafers well before swallowing. Chew gum well. (Do not swallow gum.) *Diet Rx:* See bisacodyl. *Other:* See bisacodyl.
Sulfasalazine (anti-inflammatory)	Diarrhea, gastric distress, nausea or vomiting	Impaired folacin absorption, loss of appetite, excreted in breast milk	*Drug:* Take with 250 ml water or after meals or with food to minimize gastric irritation. *Diet Rx:* Ensure adequate fluid intake to maintain at least 1,200 to 1,500 ml urine output/day. Encourage the intake of foods high in folacin.

Dietary Suggestions Associated with Drugs That Alter Nutrient Metabolism

| Drug (Usage) | Nutritional Implications | | Dietary Suggestions |
	Gastrointestinal Side/Adverse Effects	Other Reactions	
Hydralazine (antihypertensive)	Diarrhea, nausea or vomiting, constipation (rare)	Vitamin B_6 antagonism (may result in peripheral neuropathy), sodium and water retention (long-term therapy), loss of appetite	*Drug:* Intake with food may increase bioavailability of drug. Consistently take with food. *Diet Rx:* If appropriate, teach and emphasize the importance of dietary modifications associated with treatment of hypertension. May also indicate a sodium-restricted diet, weight reduction and monitoring, and alcoholic beverage restriction. Vitamin B_6 supplementation may be prescribed if symptoms of peripheral neuropathy develop. *Other:* Avoid over the counter (OTC) preparations that contain indirect acting sympathomimetics, especially those advertised for weight control, unless discussed with physician.
Isoniazid (antitubercular)	Epigastric distress, nausea or vomiting (may be signs of hepatotoxicity)	Vitamin B_6 antagonism (may result in peripheral neuropahty), tyramine-type reactions with certain foods, dry mouth, loss of appetite, excreted in breast milk	*Drug:* Take with 250 ml water on an empty stomach, as food decreases drug absorption. If gastrointestinal irritation occurs, drug may be taken with food to lessen that effect. *Diet Rx:* May indicate avoidance of alcoholic beverages and foods high in pressor amines. Vitamin B_6 supplementation may be prescribed for the malnourished or for those patients predisposed to vitamin B_6 deficiency or exhibiting signs of peripheral neuropathy. *Other:* Alert physician if patient reports loss of appetite, nausea, or vomiting.

Continued.

Dietary Suggestions Associated with Drugs That Alter Nutrient Metabolism—cont'd

| | Nutritional Implications | | |
Drug (Usage)	Gastrointestinal Side/Adverse Effects	Other Reactions	Dietary Suggestions
Methotrexate (antineoplastic, antipsoriatic)	Abdominal distress, diarrhea, GI ulceration and bleeding, nausea or vomiting	Folacin antagonist (irreversibly binds with dihydrofolate reductase); malabsorption of folacin, vitamin B_{12}, and fat; hyperuricemia; loss of appetite; altered taste acuity; sore mouth and lips	*Drug:* To reduce nausea and to help foster compliance. See table on pp. 641-643. Absorption may be decreased by milky meals. See table on p. 638. *Diet Rx:* May indicate increased intake of alkaline ash foods and beverages and the ingestion of 2,000 ml water/day to aid in excretion of uric acid. Patients should avoid the use of alcoholic beverages. Caution patient against self-medication with OTC preparations, especially the use of supplements that contain para-aminobenzoic acid and folacin. See table on p. 640. *Other:* Alert physician if patient reports diarrhea, abdominal distress, bloody vomit, or black tarry stools.
Penicillamine (chelating agent, antiarthritic, antiurolithic, heavy metal antagonist)	Diarrhea, epigastric pain, nausea or vomiting	Inhibits pyridoxal-dependent enzymes; chelates copper, iron, and zinc; unpleasant taste; decreased taste acuity (salt, sweet); loss of appetite	*Wilson's disease—Drug:* Take on an empty stomach 30 min to 1 hr before and at least 2 hr after meals. *Diet Rx:* A low copper diet (< 2 mg/day) may be prescribed. Advise patient to drink demineralized drinking water if local supply contains > 100 μg copper/L. *Cystinuria—Diet Rx:* May indicate a low methionine diet (not for children) and a high fluid intake (3 to 4 L/day), with some intake during the night. *Rheumatoid arthritis—Drug:* Take with water on an empty stomach at least 1 hr apart from any meals, food, milk, or snacks. *Lead poisoning—Drug:* Take with water on an empty stomach 2 hr before and at least 3 hr after meals.

| Phenobarbital (anticonvulsant, sedative-hypnotic) | Nausea or vomiting | Hepatic microsomal enzyme induction increases inactivation of 25-OH vitamin D and may result in rickets or osteomalacia; may decrease serum folacin, vitamin B$_{12}$, pyridoxine, calcium, and magnesium; appetite changes; excreted in breast milk | *Other:* Diet Rx may include pyridoxine supplementation for patients with rheumatoid arthritis, cystinuria, and Wilson's disease. Drug should be taken away from iron and other mineral supplements. See table on p. 640. *Drug:* Swallow extended-release tablet whole. Take oral solution straight or mix with water, milk, or juice. *Diet Rx:* Emphasize the importance of good dietary habits with adequate intake of vitamin D-containing foods. Serum folacin, calcium, or 25-OH vitamin D levels as well as indexes of bone resorption may be monitored in patients on prolonged therapy (especially children and those concomitantly prescribed phenytoin) prior to vitamin D supplementation. Avoid alcoholic beverages. |
| Phenytoin (anticonvulsant, antiarrhythmic) | Constipation, nausea or vomiting | Hepatic microsomal enzyme induction increases inactivation of 25-OH vitamin D and may result in rickets or osteomalacia; may decrease serum folacin levels and result in megaloblastic anemia; decreased taste acuity; possible weight changes; serum levels of minerals and vitamins may be altered; excreted in breast milk | *Drug:* Take with food or immediately after meals to minimize gastric irritation. *Diet Rx:* May include information that concerns hydration status, alcoholic beverage restriction, and the importance of consistent caloric intake. Emphasize the importance of good dietary and health habits, especially the intake of vitamin D-containing foods. If folacin or pyridoxine supplementation is indicated, vitamins must be administered cautiously. See table on p. 640. *Other:* Enteral tube feedings have been associated with reduced phenytoin blood levels. Monitor blood levels closely. |

Continued.

Dietary Suggestions Associated with Drugs That Alter Nutrient Metabolism—cont'd

| Drug (Usage) | Nutritional Implications | | Dietary Suggestions |
	Gastrointestinal Side/Adverse Effects	Other Reactions	
Pyrimethamine (antimalarial)	Vomiting (dose related)	Inhibits dihydrofolate reductase (inhibitory potential greater on the intact microorganisms than on host); megaloblastic anemia (large doses); loss of appetite (large doses); excreted in breast milk	*Drug:* Take with meals or snacks to minimize gastric irritation. *Diet Rx:* May indicate concomitant administration of preformed folic acid (folinic acid) to prevent anemia; caution against the use of para-aminobenzoic acid supplements. See table on p. 640.
Triamterene (potassium-sparing diuretic)	Diarrhea, gastric upset, nausea or vomiting	Weak folacin antagonist, electrolyte imbalance (possible hyperkalemia), dry mouth, increased thirst, excreted in breast milk	*Drug:* Take with or after meals to minimize gastric irritation. Dosing information may indicate to take drug with or after breakfast or no later than 6 P.M. *Diet Rx:* If appropriate, teach and emphasize the importance of dietary modifications associated with treatment of hypertension. May also indicate allowable fluid and sodium intake and caution against the use of potassium-containing salt substitutes, low salt foods with high potassium content, and intake of potassium-rich foods or potassium supplements. *Other:* Drug should be cautiously used in patients with poor nutritional status. May decrease serum folacin. Alert physician if patient reports dry mouth, increased thirst, or severe nausea, vomiting, or diarrhea (may indicate or contribute to fluid and electrolyte imbalance).

Dietary Suggestions Associated with Drugs That Alter Nutrient Excretion

Drug (Usage)	Nutritional Implications		Dietary Suggestions
	Gastrointestinal Side/Adverse Effects	**Other Reactions**	
Aspirin (analgesic, antipyretic, anti-inflammatory)	Gastric pain or bleeding, heartburn, nausea or vomiting	Increased ascorbic acid excretion and potassium depletion (large doses), iron-deficiency anemia (long use or over-use), salicylate excreted in breast milk	*Drug:* Take with 250 ml water (for rapid analgesia) or food to reduce gastric irritation. (However, drug absorption may be delayed when aspirin is taken with food.) Swallow enteric tablets whole. Some buffered preparations contain sodium and may be contraindicated for patients on sodium-restricted diets. *Diet Rx:* May caution against concomitant intake with alcoholic beverages; may indicate the need for adequate fluid intake and emphasize the intake of foods rich in ascorbic acid. Ascorbic acid supplementation may be prescribed for ascorbic acid-depleted patients who receive large doses of the drug. *Other:* Drug should be cautiously used in patients prone to vitamin K deficiency. Drug-induced gastric bleeding may contribute to or aggravate iron-deficiency anemia.
Furosemide (potassium-depleting diuretic)	Constipation (or diarrhea), nausea or vomiting, stomach distress	Enhances the excretion of potassium, calcium, magnesium, sodium, chloride, and water; fluid and electrolyte disturbances; dry mouth; increased thirst; loss of appetite; excreted in breast milk	*Drug:* Intake with food may slow the rate of drug absorption without altering the bioavailability of drug. To minimize the effect of increased urinary output at night, take single daily dose early in the morning.

Continued.

Dietary Suggestions Associated with Drugs That Alter Nutrient Excretion—cont'd

Drug (Usage)	Nutritional Implications		Dietary Suggestions
	Gastrointestinal Side/Adverse Effects	Other Reactions	
Furosemide—cont'd			*Diet Rx:* If appropriate, teach and emphasize the importance of dietary modifications associated with treatment of hypertension. May also indicate the need for a sodium-restricted diet, a high intake of potassium and magesium-rich foods (especially in patients taking digitalis), weight reduction and monitoring, and alcoholic beverage restriction. Limit the intake of natural licorice. See table on p. 639. *Other:* See hydralazine (table on pp. 629-632). Alert physician if patient reports dry mouth, increased thirst, or severe nausea, vomiting, or diarrhea (may indicate or contribute to fluid and electrolyte imbalance).
Spironolactone (potassium-sparing diuretic)	Abdominal cramps, diarrhea, nausea or vomiting	Enhances the excretion of sodium, chloride, and water; fluid and electrolyte disturbances; dry mouth; increased thirst; loss of appetite; canrenone (metabolite) in breast milk	*Drug:* Take with food to minimize gastric irritation. *Diet Rx:* See triamterene (table on pp. 629-632). *Other:* See hydralazine (table on pp. 629-632). Alert physician if patient reports dry mouth, increased thirst, or severe nausea, vomiting, or diarrhea (may indicate or contribute to fluid and electrolyte imbalance).
Thiazide (potassium-depleting diuretic)	Constipation (or diarrhea), nausea or vomiting, upset stomach or cramping	Enhances the excretion of potassium, magnesium, sodium, and water; fluid and electrolyte disturbances; decreased urinary calcium excretion; dry mouth; increased thirst; loss of appetite; excreted in breast milk	*Drug:* Take after food to lessen gastric irritation. To minimize the effect of increased urinary output at night, take single dose early in the morning. *Diet Rx:* If appropriate, teach and emphasize the importance of dietary modifications associated with treatment of hypertension. May also indicate the need for a sodium-restricted diet, a high intake of potassium- and magnesium-rich foods, weight reduction and monitoring, alcoholic beverage restriction, and limited intake of natural licorice. See table on p. 639. *Other:* See furosemide.

Dietary Suggestions Associated with Selected Drugs That May Produce Fluid or Electrolyte Disturbances

| Drug (Usage) | Nutritional Implications | | Dietary Suggestions |
	Gastrointestinal Side/Adverse Effects	Other Reactions	
Adrenal corticosteroids	Bloating, indigestion, nausea or vomiting, ulcerogenic potential	Fluid and electrolyte disturbances; negative nitrogen balance; protein catabolism; lipolysis with possible redistribution of body fat; anti-vitamin D activity (inhibits calcium absorption); appetite stimulation; weight gain; excreted in breast milk	*Diet Rx:* May include the need for a sodium-restricted diet, a diet high in potassium and protein, and caloric restriction or weight monitoring (especially during long-term therapy). Adequate intake of vitamin D-containing foods may be indicated. Advise patient that alcohol may enhance ulcerogenic potential of drug.
Anabolic steroids	Abdominal fullness, nausea or vomiting, stomach pain	Fluid and electrolyte retention, edema, weight gain (large doses), burning tongue, possible appetite stimulation	*Diet Rx:* Drug effectiveness (improved nitrogen balance) may depend on a diet high in calories and protein. May indicate the need for weight monitoring and a sodium-restricted diet to control edema. (Concurrent diuretic therapy may be prescribed.) *Other:* Drugs may exert a placebo effect in athletes. Enlargement of muscles is believed to be caused by cells retaining water, thus adding bulk but not fiber. Risk of various side or adverse effects may outweigh beneficial effects.
Clonidine (antihypertensive)	Constipation, nausea or vomiting	Salt and fluid retention, dry mouth (common), loss of appetite, weight gain (edema)	*Diet Rx:* If appropriate, teach and emphasize the importance of dietary modifications associated with treatment of hypertension. May also indicate the need for a sodium-restricted diet, weight reduction and monitoring, and alcoholic beverage restriction. (Concurrent diuretic therapy may be prescribed.) *Other:* See hydralazine (table on pp. 629-632).

Continued.

Dietary Suggestions Associated with Selected Drugs That May Produce Fluid or Electrolyte Disturbances—cont'd

| Drug (Usage) | Nutritional Implications | | Dietary Suggestions |
	Gastrointestinal Side/Adverse Effects	Other Reactions	
Estrogens	Abdominal cramping, diarrhea (mild), nausea or vomiting	Salt and fluid retention, loss of appetite, weight gain (edema), excreted in breast milk (inhibits lactation)	*Drug:* Take with or immediately after food to lessen peak blood levels thereby lessening chance for nausea. *Diet Rx:* May indicate the need for a sodium-restricted diet and weight monitoring. Probable effectiveness in the treatment of estrogen-deficient osteoporosis may also depend on diet, calcium balance, and good health habits.
Guanethidine (antihypertensive)	Diarrhea, nausea or vomiting	Sodium and fluid retention (with continuing use), dry mouth, taste disturbances, weight gain (edema)	*Diet Rx:* See clonidine. *Other:* See hydralazine (table on pp. 629-632).
Indomethacin (anti-inflammatory, analgesic)	Bloating, constipation (or diarrhea), heartburn or indigestion, nausea or vomiting, stomach pain, ulcerogenic potential	Sodium and fluid retention, (mild) weight gain (edema), excreted in breast milk	*Drug:* Even though food may slightly delay or reduce drug absorption, take drug after meals or with food to reduce gastric irritation. (An antacid may be prescribed.) *Diet Rx:* Inform patient to avoid alcoholic beverages. Even though salt and fluid retention effects are less pronounced than with phenylbutazone, a sodium-restricted diet may be indicated. *Other:* Drug-induced gastric bleeding may contribute to or aggravate iron-deficiency anemia.

Methyldopa (anti-hypertensive)	Diarrhea, nausea or vomiting	*Diet Rx:* See clonidine. *Other:* See hydralazine (table on pp. 629-632). Also see tables on pp. 638 and 640 with regard to protein and amino acid effects on drug action.
Phenylbutazone (anti-inflammatory)	Salt and fluid retention, dry mouth, weight gain (edema), excreted in breast milk	*Drug:* Take with meals to minimize gastric irritation. *Diet Rx:* May indicate the need for a sodium-restricted diet. Instruct patient to avoid alcoholic beverages. *Other:* See indomethacin.
Sodium polystyrene sulfonate (antihyperkalemic, cation-exchange resin)	Constipation (or diarrhea), heartburn or indigestion; nausea or vomiting, ulcerogenic potential	*Drug:* Mix oral dose with food or suspend in water or other fluids appropriate for patients with renal disease. May be mixed with sorbitol. *Diet Rx:* May indicate sodium restriction, as drug contains about 100 mg sodium/g. (Drug is usually administered with sorbitol to hasten elimination of potassium, prevent constipation, and reduce tendency toward fecal impaction.)
	Sodium retention, hypokalemia, hypocalcemia, hypomagnesemia, loss of appetite	
	Constipation, fecal impaction, nausea or vomiting	

Effects of Various Foods and Beverages on Drug Absorption

Food or Beverage	Drug	Effect
Coffee and tea	Neuroleptic agents (fluphenazine, haloperidol)	Mixing drug with coffee or tea can precipitate the drug, prevent absorption, and impede its therapeutic effects.
Fiber		
bran	Digoxin	May reduce drug absorption.
pectin(?) or high carbohydrate meal	Acetaminophen	May depress rate of drug absorption.
Food (in general)	Chlorothiazide	May increase drug absorption.
	Propranolol	May increase drug absorption.
	Nitrofurantoin	Increases bioavailability of the drug.
	Cimetidine	Delayed absorption may benefit patient by maintaining blood concentration of drug between meals.
	Aspirin	May decrease drug absorption and absorptive rate.
	Antimicrobial agents (cephalexin, penicillin G, erythromycin stearate, penicillin V, tetracycline)	May reduce drug absorption.
High fat meal	Griseofulvin	Increases drug absorption.
High protein diets	Levodopa, methyldopa	Amino acids from dietary protein inhibit absorption of drugs.
Milk and milk products	Tetracycline	Calcium inhibits drug absorption.
Milky meal*	Methotrexate	May inhibit drug absorption.

*Milky meal contained milk, corn flakes, white bread, butter, and sugar.

Effects of Various Foods and Beverages on Drug Action

Food or Beverage	Drug	Effect
Beverages		
coffee, tea, and other caffeine-containing beverages	Theophylline	Increased intake may enhance drug side effects (nervousness, insomnia).
	Neuroleptic agents	Increased intake may result in a large variation in plasma concentration of drug and may reduce its clinical effectiveness.
citrus juices	Quinidine	Excessive intake may increase blood levels of drug (alkalinization of urine).
Licorice	Antihypertensive agents, diuretics	Glycyrrhizic acid in natural licorice tends to induce hypokalemia and sodium retention; ingestion in large amounts may complicate antihypertensive drug therapy.
	Digoxin	Licorice-induced hypokalemia may enhance the action of digitalis and result in drug toxicity.
Protein or charcoal-broiled meats	Theophylline	High protein or low carbohydrate diet or ingestion of charcoal-broiled meats may decrease plasma half-life of drug.
Salty foods, sodium (salt)	Lithium	Increased intake of sodium may reduce therapeutic response to drug. Low-salt diets may enhance drug activity.
Vegetables		
boiled or fried onions	Warfarin	May increase fibrinolytic activity of drug.
broccoli, turnip greens, lettuce, cabbage	Warfarin	Vegetables rich in vitamin K may inhibit hypoprothrombinemic response to oral anticoagulants.

Vitamins, Minerals, and Other Supplements That Affect Drug Action

Supplement	Drug	Effect
Vitamins		
vitamin A	Alcohol	Hypervitaminosis A may enhance hepato-toxicity of alcohol.
	Isotretinoin	Additive toxic effects may result from combination therapy with vitamin A or other supplements containing vitamin A.
	Tetracycline	Combination therapy may enhance drug-induced intracranial hypertension (severe headache).
vitamin D	Digoxin	Vitamin D-induced hypercalcemia may potentiate the effects of the drug and result in cardiac arrhythmias.
vitamin E	Warfarin	May enhance anticoagulant response to warfarin.
vitamin K	Warfarin	Vitamin K in liquid food supplements may inhibit the hypoprothrombic effect of drug.
ascorbic acid	Fluphenazine	Large doses may interfere with drug absorption and result in a return of manic behavior.
	Warfarin	Megadoses may decrease prothrombin time.
folacin	Methotrexate	Folacin or its derivatives in vitamin preparations may alter responses to drug.
	Phenytoin	May decrease anticonvulsant action of drug.
pyridoxine	Levodopa	Reverses the antiparkinsonism effect of drug.
	Phenytoin	Large doses may reduce phenytoin levels.
	Hydralazine, isoniazid, penicillamine	May correct drug-induced peripheral neuropathy.
Minerals		
calcium, iron, magnesium, zinc	Tetracycline	Concurrent use may decrease drug absorption.
iron	Penicillamine	Concurrent use may decrease drug effectiveness.
Other supplements		
para-aminobenzoic acid	Methotrexate	?May increase toxicity by displacing drug from plasma protein binding (*in vitro study*).
	Pyrimethamine	?May interfere with drug action against toxoplasmosis.
protein or amino acids	Levodopa, methyldopa, theophylline	?May inhibit drug absorption. ?May decrease plasma half-life of drug.
tryptophan	Monoamine oxidase inhibitors	May cause a deterioration in mental status.
yeast extracts	Monoamine oxidase inhibitors	Concomitant intake may produce significant hypertension.

Dietary and Other Suggestions to Aid in the Relief of Unpleasant Side Effects of Drugs

Drug-induced Side Effects	Suggestions*
Loss of appetite	Question patient regarding factors contributing to appetite loss.
	Determine food likes and dislikes.
	Serve favorite or special snack foods.
	Inform patient that food interests tend to diminish as the day progresses (breakfast may be an important first meal).
	Provide variety in color, texture, and temperature of food at each meal or snack.
	Offer small, frequent, attractive meals or snacks in a pleasant environment.
	Enhance food flavors by using various seasonings.
	Marinate meats in sauces, wines, or fruit juices.
	Advise patient to maintain adequate fluid intake.
	Instruct patient to avoid excessive alcohol intake.
Appetite stimulation or weight gain	Encourage the intake of low calorie foods, beverages, and snacks.
	Evaluate the intake of various beverages used to counter dry mouth.
	Alert patients that certain drugs may increase desire for sweets and other foods.
	Instruct patient or food provider to control access to various foods, snacks, or beverages.
Altered taste perception, bitter taste, or aftertaste	If permissable, advise patients to mask taste of drug with food, pulpy fruits (applesauce, crushed pineapple), fruit juices, or milk.
	Unless otherwise indicated, urge patient to take medication with adequate fluid.
	To improve taste, suggest the use of sugarless gum or water or lemon juice as mouth rinses.
	Encourage good oral hygiene.
Dry or sore mouth	Counsel patient to moisten (dunk) dry foods in beverages or to swallow foods or snacks with a beverage.
	Decrease the use of dry (or salty) foods or snacks.
	Offer moist, soft-textured foods (mashed potatoes or pureed vegetables, milk toast without crust, custards or puddings, fruit whips, creamed ground meat, or fish).
	Advise patient to avoid spicy, rough textured, or highly acidic foods or snacks.
	Add milk-flavored sauces, gravies, or syrups to food.
	Suggest the patient lick or suck on ice chips.
	Incorporate cold foods or beverages into meals or snacks (sherbets, ice or cold milk, ice cream, melons, fruit ices).
	Avoid overuse of calorie-containing fluids (weight gain may occur).
	Suggest the use of sugarless gum.
	Caution patient that the use of hard candies may increase the incidence of dental caries.
	Advise patient to maintain adequate fluid intake.
	Encourage good oral hygiene.
	Inquire about the use of artificial saliva.

*Suggestions are intended to reinforce rather than replace any information in the diet prescription provided by the physician.

Continued.

Dietary and Other Suggestions to Aid in the Relief of Unpleasant Side Effects
of Drugs—cont'd

Drug-induced Side Effects	Suggestions
Nausea	Offer small quantities of easily digestible foods at frequent intervals.
	Reduce food volume at meals; serve beverages after meals or limit beverage intake with meals.
	Suggest the intake of toasted or dry enriched white bread, crackers, or cooked or dry ready-to-eat cereals.
	Serve cold, clear beverages or juices.
	Instruct the patient to avoid any fried, greasy, or fatty foods.
	Inform the patient or food provider that aromas from hot food may aggravate nausea.
	Reschedule mealtimes if nausea occurs at consistent times each day.
	Evaluate discomfort as a possible side effect of drug (nausea in a digitalized patient may be a possible indication of drug toxicity, especially in the elderly).
	Suggest that patient take deep breaths or find other distractions to relieve nausea.
Heartburn	Question patient regarding factors that may contribute to heartburn.
	Offer small quantities of food at frequent intervals. Advise patient to avoid overeating.
	Instruct the patient not to homogenize, mince, or puree food (may stimulate acid secretion).
	Control the use of alcohol; coffee, tea, and other caffeine-containing beverages; decaffeinated coffee; chocolate or peppermint; and pepper.
	Avoid serving orange and citric juices, tomato products and other highly acidic foods, and concentrated fruit beverages if they are found to cause heartburn.
	Advise patient to avoid spicy, greasy, fried, or fatty foods.
	Evaluate the intake of milk or cream (may stimulate acid secretion).
	Urge patient to avoid eating before bedtime.
	If patient is overweight, advise patient to decrease food intake sensibly to lose weight.
Constipation	Question patient about the prolonged use or overuse of cathartics or laxatives.
	Incorporate sources of bulk or fiber in diet (include raw vegetables and fruits high in fiber, whole grain breads and cereals, bran or pulpy fruit, and vegetable juices).
	Advise patient to maintain adequate fluid or water intake.
	Encourage a daily program of exercise, if permissible.
	Inform patient about the importance of good health habits—regular meals, defecation reflex recognition (usually active after meals), and regularity in defecation time.
Diarrhea	Focus on fluid and electrolyte replacement. Maintain adequate fluid intake and encourage the intake of juices high in postassium.
	Urge patient to drink a variety of beverages between meals to counter dehydration.

Dietary and Other Suggestions to Aid in the Relief of Unpleasant Side Effects
of Drugs—cont'd

Drug-induced Side Effects	Suggestions
	Serve small quantities of food at frequent intervals.
	Suggest the incorporation of pectin-containing foods in the diet (applesauce, grated raw apple).
	Let hot foods cool slightly before eating; cold foods or beverages may also aggravate diarrhea.
	Evaluate the intake (and amount) of foods high in fiber, caffeine-containing beverages, alcohol, milk products, or other foods that may be contributing to the diarrhea.
Flatulence	Question patient regarding factors that may contribute to flatulence.
	Encourage patient to avoid gas-forming foods (a matter of individual response).
	Advise patient to chew food slowly with mouth closed.

3 / *Nutritive Values for Alcoholic Beverages and Mixes*

Beverage	Serving (oz)	Alcohol (g)	Carbohydrate (g)	Calories	Exchanges for Calorie Control
Beer					
Regular	12	13	13	150	1 Starch, 2 Fat
Light	12	11	5	100	2 Fat
Near beer	12	1.5	12	60	1 Starch
Distilled spirits					
80 proof (gin, rum, vodka, whiskey, scotch)	1.5	14	Trace	100	2 Fat
Dry brandy, cognac	1	11	Trace	75	1.5 Fat
Table wine					
Dry white	4	11	Trace	80	2 Fat
Red or rosé	4	12	2	85	2 Fat
Sweet wine	4	12	5	105	$\frac{1}{3}$ Starch, 2 Fat
Light wine	4	6	1	50	1 Fat
Wine cooler	12	13	30	215	2 Fruit, 2 Fat
Dealcoholized wines	4	Trace	6–7	25–35	0.5 Fruit
Sparkling wines					
Champagne	4	12	4	100	2 Fat
Sweet kosher wine	4	12	12	132	1 Starch, 2 Fat
Appetizer/dessert wines					
Sherry	2	9	2	74	1.5 Fat
Sweet sherry, port, muscatel	2	9	7	90	0.5 Starch, 1.5 Fat
Cordials, liqueurs	1.5	13	18	160	1 Starch, 2 Fat
Vermouth					
Dry	3	13	4	105	2 Fat
Sweet	3	13	14	140	1 Starch, 2 Fat

Continued.

Beverage	Serving (oz)	Alcohol (g)	Carbohydrate (g)	Calories	Exchanges for Calorie Control
Cocktails					
Bloody Mary	5	14	5	116	1 Vegetable, 2 Fat
Daiquiri	2	14	2	111	2 Fat
Manhattan	2	17	2	178	2.5 Fat
Martini	2.5	22	Trace	156	3.5 Fat
Old-fashioned	4	26	Trace	180	4 Fat
Tom Collins	7.5	16	3	120	2.5 Fat
Mixes					
Mineral water	Any	0	0	0	Free
Sugar-free tonic	Any	0	0	0	Free
Club soda	Any	0	0	0	Free
Diet soda	Any	0	0	0	Free
Tomato juice	4	0	5	25	1 Vegetable
Bloody Mary mix	4	0	5	25	1 Vegetable
Orange juice	4	0	15	60	1 Fruit
Grapefruit juice	4	0	15	60	1 Fruit
Pineapple juice	4	0	15	60	1 Fruit

With permission from: Franz MJ. Alcohol and diabetes: its metabolism and guidelines for its occasional use. Part II Diabetes Spectrum 1990; 3(4):210–216.

CALORIC VALUE OF ALCOHOLIC BEVERAGES

The caloric contribution from alcohol of an alcoholic beverage can be estimated by multiplying the number of ounces by the proof and then again by the factor 0.8. For beers and wines, kilocalories from alcohol can be estimated by multiplying ounces by percentage of alcohol (by volume) and then by the factor 1.6.

4

Adult Weight for Height Tables

Metropolitan Weight* and Height† Tables (1983)

Height		Women Weight				Men Weight			
		Pounds		Kilograms		Pounds		Kilograms	
Feet	Centimeters	Average	Range	Average	Range	Average	Range	Average	Range
4'9"	145	117	102–131	53.2	46.4–59.5	—	—	—	—
4'10"	147	119	103–134	54.1	46.8–60.9	—	—	—	—
4'11"	150	121	104–137	55.0	47.3–62.3	—	—	—	—
5'0"	152	123	106–140	56.0	48.2–63.6	—	—	—	—
5'1"	155	126	108–143	57.3	49.1–65.0	139	128–150	63.2	58.2–68.2
5'2"	158	129	111–147	58.6	50.5–66.8	142	130–153	64.5	59.1–69.5
5'3"	160	133	114–151	60.5	51.8–68.6	144	132–156	65.5	60.0–70.1
5'4"	163	136	117–155	61.8	53.2–70.4	147	134–160	66.8	60.1–72.7
5'5"	165	140	120–159	63.6	54.5–72.3	150	136–164	68.2	61.8–74.5
5'6"	168	143	123–163	65.0	55.9–74.1	153	138–168	69.5	62.3–76.4
5'7"	170	147	126–167	66.8	57.3–75.9	156	140–172	70.9	63.6–78.2
5'8"	173	150	129–170	68.2	58.6–77.3	159	142–176	72.3	64.5–80.0
5'9"	175	153	132–173	69.5	60.0–78.6	162	144–180	73.6	65.4–81.8
5'10"	178	156	135–176	70.9	61.4–80.0	165	146–184	75.0	66.4–83.4
5'11"	180	159	138–179	72.3	62.7–81.4	169	149–188	76.8	67.7–85.4
6'0"	183	—	—	—	—	172	152–192	78.2	69.1–87.3
6'1"	185	—	—	—	—	176	155–197	80.0	70.4–89.5
6'2"	188	—	—	—	—	180	158–202	81.8	71.8–91.8
6'3"	191	—	—	—	—	185	162–207	84.1	73.6–94.1

*Weights are at ages 25 to 59 yr based on lowest mortality. Weight is in pounds (indoor clothing weighing 3 lb for women, 5 lb for men).

†The table is adjusted to reflect subject *without shoes* for height measurement.

Adapted from 1979 Build Study Society of Actuaries and Association of Life Insurance Medical Directors of America, 1980, Metropolitan Life Insurance Company; with permission.

U.S. Department of Agriculture, U.S. Department of Health and Human Services Acceptable Weights for Adults

| Height* | Weight in Pounds†‡ | |
	19 to 34 Years	35 Years and Over
5'0"	97–128	108–138
5'1"	101–132	111–143
5'2"	104–137	115–148
5'3"	107–141	119–152
5'4"	111–146	122–157
5'5"	114–150	126–162
5'6"	118–155	130–167
5'7"	121–160	134–172
5'8"	125–164	138–178
5'9"	129–169	142–183
5'10"	132–174	146–188
5'11"	136–179	151–194
6'0"	140–184	155–199
6'1"	144–189	159–205
6'2"	148–195	164–210
6'3"	152–200	168–216
6'4"	156–205	173–222
6'5"	160–211	177–228
6'6"	164–216	182–234

*Without shoes.

†Without clothes.

‡The higher weights in the ranges generally apply to men, who tend to have more muscle and bone; the lower weights more often apply to women, who have less muscle and bone.

From Human Nutrition Information Service. U.S. Department of Agriculture. Report of the Dietary Guidelines Advisory Committee on the dietary guidelines for Americans—1990. Hyattsville, MD: U.S. Government Printing Office, June, 1990:8.

The table above shows higher weights for people 35 years and above than for younger adults. This is because recent research suggests that people can be a little heavier as they grow older without added risk to health. Just how much heavier is not yet clear. The weight ranges given in the table are likely to change based on research under way.

Ranges of weights are given in the table because people of the same height may have equal amounts of body fat but differ in muscle and bone. The higher weights in the ranges are suggested for people with more muscle and bone.

Weights above the range are believed to be unhealthy for most people. Weights slightly below the range may be healthy for some small-boned people but are sometimes linked to health problems, especially if sudden weight loss has occurred.

Research also suggests that, for adults, body shape as well as weight is important to health. Excess fat in the abdomen is believed to be of greater health risk than that in the hips and thighs. There are several ways to check body shape. Some require the help of a doctor; others can be done by the patient.

A look at one's profile in the mirror may be enough to make it clear that there is too much fat in the abdomen. Or one can check body shape this way:

- Measure around the waist near the navel while standing relaxed, not pulling in the stomach.
- Measure around the hips, over the buttocks, where they are largest.
- Divide the waist measure by the hips measure to get the waist-to-hip ratio. Research in adults suggests that ratios close to or above 1.0 (0.80 for women and 0.95 for men) are linked with greater risk for several diseases. However, ratios have not been defined for all populations or age groups.

If one's weight is within the range in the table, if the waist-to-hip ratio does not place one at risk, and if there is no medical problem for which the doctor advises weight gain or loss, there appears to be no health advantage to changing body weight. If one does not meet all of these conditions, or if one is not sure, one may want to talk to a doctor about how one's weight might affect one's health and what should be done about it.

Heredity plays a role in body size and shape, as do exercise and what is eaten. Some people seem to be able to eat more than others and still maintain a good body size and shape.

Reference

U.S. Department of Agriculture, U.S. Department of Health and Human Services. Nutrition and your health: dietary guidelines for Americans, 3rd ed. Home and Garden Bulletin No. 232. Washington, DC: U.S. Government Printing Office, 1990.

Mayo Clinic Normal Physiological Values

Blood or Serum Values	Normal Ranges
Ascorbic acid (vitamin C)	0.6–2.0 mg/dl
Bleeding time—Surgicutt	1.5–8.0 min
Calcium, total	8.9–10.1 mg/dl
Carotene	48–200 μg/dl
Chloride	100–112 mEq/L
Copper	0.75–1.45 μg/ml
Erythrocyte count (adults)	M: 4.44–5.51 × 10^{12} L
	F: 3.89–5.03 × 10^{12}/L
Ferritin	Newborn: 25–200 μg/L
	1 mo: 200–600 μg/L
	2–5 mo: 50–200 μg/L
	6 mo–15 yr: 7–142 μg/L
	M: 20–300 μg/L
	F: 20–120 μg/L
Folate (serum)	3.5–25.0 μg/ml
Glucose, fasting (>1 yr)	70–100 mg/dl
Glycosylated hemoglobin	4.0–7.0%
Hematocrit	M: 38.8–50%
	F: 34.9–44.5%
Hemoglobin	M: 13.5–17.5 g/dl
	F: 12.0–15.5 g/dl
Iron	M: 50–150 μg/dl
	F: 35–145 μg/dl
Iron binding capacity, total	250–400 μg/dl
Iron binding capacity, % saturation	14–50%

*Surface area is a standard measure of body surface area: 1.73 m².

Continued.

Blood or Serum Values	Normal Ranges			

Lipids—cholesterol and triglycerides

	Male (mg/dL)		Female (mg/dL)	
Age (Yr)	Cholesterol Upper 75th Percentile	Triglyceride Upper 95th Percentile	Cholesterol Upper 75th Percentile	Triglyceride Upper 95th Percentile
6	172	102	173	76
10	179	103	174	121
15	167	124	175	122
20	185	137	181	97
25	202	157	190	100
30	216	171	199	106
35	226	182	209	110
40	235	189	219	117
45	242	193	229	122
50	246	195	241	128
55	250	197	253	134
60	253	198	265	140

HDL cholesterol

(for males and females > 20 yr, values 30–37 mg/dl are considered "marginally low")	<20 yr: 30–65	30–70
	20–29 yr: 30–70	30–75
	30–39 yr: 30–70	35–80
	40–49 yr: 30–70	35–85
	50–59 yr: 30–70	35–85
	>60 yr: 30–70	35–85

Magnesium	1.7–2.1 mg/dl
Osmolality	275–295 mOsm/kg
Phosphorus	2.5–4.5 mg/dl
Potassium	3.6–4.8 mEq/L
Prealbumin	18–36 mg/dl
Protein, total	6.3–7.9 g/dl
Protein electrophoresis	
Albumin	3.1–4.3 g/dl
Alpha-1 globulin	0.1–0.3 g/dl
Alpha-2 globulin	0.6–1.0 g/dl
Beta-globulin g/dl	0.7–1.4 g/dl
Gamma globulin	0.7–1.6 g/dl
Prothrombin time	8.4–12.0 sec
Sodium	135–145 mEq/L
Urea	M: 17–51 mg/dl
	F: 13–45 mg/dl
Uric acid	M: 4.3–8.0 mg/dl
	F: 2.3–6.0 mg/dl
Vitamin A, free retinol	360–1,200 μg/L
Vitamin B$_{12}$	190–900 ng/L

Blood or Serum Values	Normal Ranges
Vitamin E	5.5–17.0 mg/L
1, 25 dihydroxy vitamin D	15–60 pg/ml
25-hydroxy vitamin D	Winter: 14–42 ng/ml
	Summer: 15–80 ng/ml
Zinc	0.66–1.10 μg/ml

Urine Values	Normal Ranges
Ammonia	36–86 mEq/24 hr
Calcium	M: 25–300 mg/24 hr
	F: 20–275 mg/24 hr
Chromium	<8 μg/24 hr specimen
Creatinine clearance	M: (20 yr): 90 ml/min/SA
	F: (20 yr): 84 ml/min/SA
	(decreased by 6 ml/min/ decade)
Osmolality	300-800 mOsm/kg
	<100 mOsm/kg overhydrated
	>800 mOsm/kg dehydrated
Oxalate	0.11–0.46 mmol/24 hr specimen
Potassium	30–90 mEq/24 hr
Protein, total	M: 0–150 mg/24 hr
	F: 27–93 mg/24 hr
Renal clearance—standard	
Glomerular filtration rate (inulin or iothalamate.I[125])	90-130 ml/min/surface area* at age 20 (decreased by 4 ml/min/decade)
Effective renal plasma flow (PAH)	400-700 ml/min/surface area* at age 20 (decreased by 17 ml/min/decade)
Filtration fraction	18–22%

Renal clearance—short
  Glomerular filtration rate (iothalamate.I[125])

Age (yr)	Males and Females (ml/min/surface area*)
18–22	>90
23–27	>88
28–32	>86
33–37	>84
38–42	>82
43–47	>80
48–52	>78
53–57	>75
58–62	>73
63+	>70

*Surface area is a standard measure of body surface area: 1.73 m².

Continued.

Urine Values	Normal Ranges	
Glomerular filtration rate (creatinine)		
Age (yr)	Males	Females
	(ml/min/surface area*)	
20	>92	>84
21–25	>88	>82
26–30	>85	>78
31–35	>82	>75
36–40	>78	>72
41–45	>74	>69
46–50	>72	>67
51–55	>68	>64
56–60	>65	>61
61–65	>62	>58
66–70	>58	>55
71–75	>55	>52
76–80	>52	>50
Sodium	40–217 mEq/24 hr	
Uric acid	<750 mg/24 hr	
Zinc	300–600 μg/24 hr	

Miscellaneous Values	Normal Ranges
Basal metabolism rate	-10 to +10%
Stool examination	
Fat, quantitative	2–7 g/24 hr
Fat, percent	0–20%
Nitrogen	1–2 g/24 hr
Vitamin B_{12} absorption (Schilling test)	>8%

*Surface area is a standard measure of body surface area: 1.73 m^2.

APPENDIX

6 / *Nomogram for Estimating Caloric Requirements*

DIRECTIONS FOR ESTIMATING CALORIC REQUIREMENT

To determine the desired allowance of kilocalories, proceed as follows:
1. Locate the ideal weight on Column I by means of a common pin.
2. Bring edge of one end of a 12- or 15-inch ruler against the pin.
3. Swing the other end of the ruler to the patient's height on Column II.
4. Transfer the pin to the point where the ruler crosses Column III.
5. Hold the ruler against the pin in Column III.
6. Swing the left-hand end of the ruler to the patient's sex and age (measured from last birthday) given in Column IV (these positions correspond to the Mayo Clinic's metabolism standards for age and sex).
7. Transfer the pin to the point where the ruler crosses Column V. This gives the basal kilocaloric requirement (basal kilocalories) of the patient for 24 hours and represents the kilocalories required by the fasting patient when resting in bed.
8. To provide the extra kilocalories for activity and work, the basal kilocalories are increased by a percentage. To the basal kilocalories for adults, add 50 to 80% for manual laborers, 30 to 40% for light work, or 10 to 20% for restricted activity such as resting in a room or in bed. To the basal kilocalories for children, add 50 to 100% for children ages 5 to 15 years. This computation may be done by simple arithmetic or by the use of Columns VI and VII. If the latter method is chosen, locate the "per cent above or below basal" desired in Column VI. By means of the ruler, connect this point with the pin on Column V. Transfer the pin to the point where the ruler crosses Column VII. This represents the kilocalories estimated to be required by the patient.

W. M. Boothby and J. Berkson
October, 1933
Copyright, 1959
Mayo Association

MC-702 Rev. 10-59

655

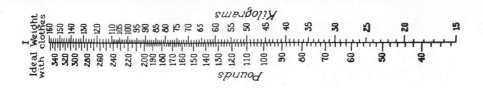

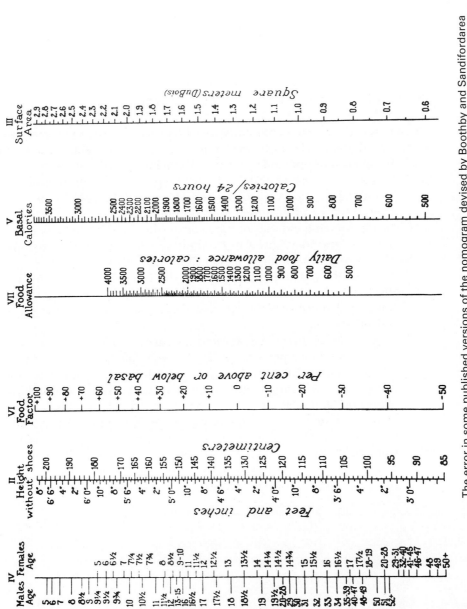

The error in some published versions of the nomogram devised by Boothby and Sandifordarea (N Engl J Med 1979;300:1339 [letter to the editor]) does not occur in this nomogram.

7 / *Nomogram for Body Mass Index*

The nomogram on the next page shows body mass index (BMI) (body weight in kilograms/height in meters^2) for specified height and weight, barefoot and unclothed. A woman with a BMI over 27.3, or a man with a BMI over 27.8, is at increased risk of the health complications of obesity. (Reproduced with permission from the Portland Health Institute, Portland, Oregon, and Frankel HM. Determination of body mass index. JAMA 1986;255:1292.)

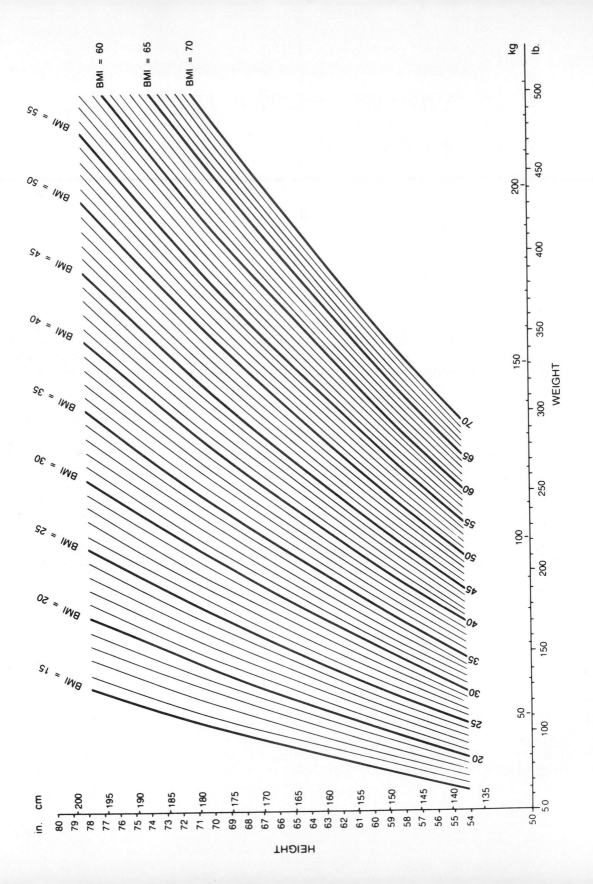

NUTRIENT CONTENT CLAIMS

Food Labels

Under regulations from the Food and Drug Administration of the Department of Health and Human Services and the Food Safety and Inspection Service of the U.S. Department of Agriculture, food labels have been revised. These regulations meet the provisions of the Nutrition Labeling and Education Act of 1990. Manufacturers have until May 1994 to comply with the new labeling requirements, although regulations pertaining to health claims and some parts of ingredient labeling became effective in May 1993.

"High," "Rich In," or "Excellent Source Of"—contains 20% or more of the (RDI) or (DRV) per reference amount customarily consumed.

"Good Source," "Contains," or "Provides"—contains 10 to 19% of the (RDI) or (DRV) per reference amount customarily consumed.

"More," "Fortified," "Enriched," and "Added"—contains at least 10% or more of the RDI for protein, vitamins, or minerals or of the DRV for dietary fiber or potassium per reference amount customarily consumed; based upon nutrients added to the food.

"Light" or "Lite"—the food derives 50% or more of its calories from fat and its fat content is reduced by 50% or more per reference amount customarily consumed.

- The food derives less than 50% of its calories from fat and its total calories are reduced by at least one-third.
- Its fat content is reduced by 50% or more.
- Its sodium content is reduced by 50% or more.

"Calorie Free," "Free of Calories," "No Calories," etc.—contains less than 5 kcal per reference amount customarily consumed.

"Low Calorie," "Few Calories," "Low in Calories"—contains less than 40 cal per 30 g.

"Reduced Calorie," "Fewer Calories," "Lower in Calories"—contains at least 25% fewer calories per reference amount customarily consumed.

"Sugar Free," "No Sugar," "Sugarless," etc.—contains less than 0.5 g of sugar per reference amount customarily consumed.

"No Added Sugar"—no sugar or ingredient containing sugar is added during processing and packaging.

"Reduced Sugar," "Less Sugar," etc.—contains at least 25% less sugar per reference amount customarily consumed.

"Sodium Free," "No Sodium," etc.—contains less than 5 mg of sodium per reference amount customarily consumed.

"Very Low Sodium"—contains 35 mg or less of sodium per 30 g.

"Low Sodium"—contains 140 mg or less of sodium per 30 g.

"Reduced Sodium," "Less Sodium," "Lower in Sodium," etc.—contains at least 25% less sodium per reference amount customarily consumed.

"Salt Free"—food is sodium-free.

"Unsalted," "Without Added Salt," "No Salt Added," etc.—no salt is added during processing (if the food is not sodium-free, the label must indicate "not a sodium-free food").

"Fat Free," "Nonfat," "No Fat," etc.—contains less than 0.5 g of fat per reference amount customarily consumed.

"Low Fat," "Low in Fat," "Little Fat," etc.—contains 3 g or less of fat per 30 g.

"Reduced Fat," "Less Fat," "Lower in Fat"—contains at least 25% less fat per reference amount customarily consumed.

"Cholesterol Free," "No Cholesterol," etc.—contains less than 2 mg of cholesterol per reference amount. It must also be labeled to disclose that cholesterol is not usually present in the food.

"Low Cholesterol," "Low in Cholesterol," "Little Cholesterol"—contains 20 mg or less of cholesterol per 30 g.

"Reduced Cholesterol," "Less Cholesterol," "Lower in Cholesterol"—contains at least 25% less cholesterol per reference amount customarily consumed.

"Lean"—contains less than 10 g of total fat, less than 4 g of saturated fat, and less than 95 mg of cholesterol per reference amount customarily consumed and per 100 g.

"Extra Lean"—contains less than 5 g of total fat, less than 2 g of saturated fat, and less than 95 mg of cholesterol per reference amount customarily consumed and per 100 g.

Reference

Superintendent of Documents. Federal Register 1993;58(3):2413–2426.

Characteristics of Nutritive and Nonnutritive Sweeteners

Nutritive Sweeteners

Sweetener	Derivation	Sweetness Compared to Sucrose	Kcal/g	Considerations	Cariogenic	Uses
Sucrose	Disaccharide* (fructose and glucose)	1†	4		Yes	Tabletop sweetener, foods, beverages, drugs
Fructose‡ or levulose	Monosaccharide	1.1–1.8	4		Yes	Tabletop sweetener, foods, beverages, drugs
Sorbitol or mannitol	Monosaccharide, reduction of polyalcohol	0.5–0.7	4	Osmotic diarrhea can occur with ingestion of 30–50 g of sorbitol or 20 g of mannitol	No	Sugarless gum and candies
Dextrose	Starch hydrolysate	0.7	4		Yes	Liquid base foods
Polydextrose	Polymer dextrose	<1	1	Osmotic diarrhea can occur with ingestion of 15 g	Preliminary no	Foods, beverages, drugs
High fructose corn syrup	Fructose and dextrose		4		Yes	Foods, beverages, drugs
Extraction 55%		1				
Extraction 90%		1.5				
NOT AVAILABLE IN THE UNITED STATES						
Maltitol	Reduction of maltose polyalcohol	0.8	NA		No	
Xylitol	Reduction of xylose polyalcohol	1	4	Osmotic diarrhea can occur with ingestion of 30–40 g	No	

*Derived from sugar cane and beets.

†Used as standard for sweeteners; therefore is assigned the number 1.

‡Occurs naturally in fruit.

NA = Information not available.

Nonnutritive Sweeteners

FDA APPROVED

Aspartame (Equal,™ Nutrasweet™)	Dipeptide (phenylalanine and aspartic acid)	180–200	4	Unstable when heated Sweet, bitterless taste Questions of safety; therefore moderate ingestion recommended People with phenylketonuria (PKU) must avoid	No	Foods, beverages, drugs, tabletop sweetener
Saccharin	Phthalic anhydrice derivative	300–400	0	Bitter aftertaste Stable at physiological pH and temperature Questions of safety; therefore moderate ingestion recommended	No	Foods, beverages, drugs, tabletop sweetener
Acesulfame-K (Sweet One,™ Sunette™)	Acetoacetic acid derivative	200	4	Does not lose sweetness in cooking Questions of safety; therefore moderate ingestion recommended	No	Foods, beverages, tabletop sweetener

Continued.

Nonnutritive Sweeteners—cont'd

Sweetener	Derivation	Sweetness Compared to Sucrose	Kcal/g	Considerations	Cariogenic	Uses
NOT FDA APPROVED						
Cyclamates	Organic acid derivative	30	0	No aftertaste Stable in heat and cold Long shelf life Possible cocarcinogen (cancer promoting)	No	
Stevioside	Extract from leaves of stevia rebalciana plant	200–400	0	Strong aftertaste Possible cause of infertility in women	NA	Baked goods
Aspartame encapsulate	Dipeptide with polymer coating and fat layer	180	0	Retains sweet flavor due to an outer fat layer as an initial moisture barrier When fat melts during baking, aspartame is released from core	No	Foods, beverages
Alitame	Protein	2,000	2	No aftertaste Synergistic sweetening effect Stable at high temperature	NA	Foods, beverages, table-top sweeteners
Sucralose	Sucrose derivative	600	0	Soluble Stable in heat and cold	NA	
L-sugars (left-handed sugars)	Optical isomer of glucose	1	0	Bulking and browning agent	NA	

NA = Information not available.

10 / *Enteral Nutrition Formulas*

Polymeric Formulas—Blended Foodstuffs*

		Nutrients per 1,000 ml					
Formula	Caloric Density (kcal/ml)	Protein (g) (% kcal)	Fat (g) (% kcal)	Carbohydrate (g) (% kcal)	Dietary Fiber (g)	Non-protein kcal:N	mOsm/kg
Compleat Regular (Sandoz)	1.07	43 (16%)	43 (36%)	130 (48%)	4.2	131:1	450
Compleat Modified (Sandoz)	1.07	43 (16%)	37 (31%)	140 (53%)	4.2	131:1	300
Vitaneed (Sherwood Medical)	1.0	40 (16%)	40 (36%)	128 (48%)	8	134:1	300

*Characteristics: contain nondigestible residue; ± lactose; require intact bowel function; protein, fat, and carbohydrate are based on blended mix of food; not intended for oral use

Polymeric Formulas—Lactose Containing*

		Nutrients per 1,000 ml					
Formula	Caloric Density (kcal/ml)	Protein (g) (% kcal)	Fat (g) (% kcal)	Carbohydrate (g) (% kcal)	Dietary Fiber (g)	Non-protein kcal:N	mOsm/kg
Carnation Instant Breakfast (Clintec)—made with 2% milk	0.93	44 (19%)	19 (18%)	148 (63%)	0	107:1	590–646
Carnation Diet Instant Breakfast (Clintec)—made with 2% milk	0.7	44 (25%)	19 (23%)	92 (52%)	0	76:1	500–524
Meritene Powder (Sandoz) made with whole milk	1.06	69 (26%)	34 (29%)	120 (45%)	0	71:1	690
Sustacal Powder (Mead Johnson) made with skim milk	1.07	78 (30%)	3 (3%)	178 (67%)	0	63:1	1,000
Sustagen (Mead Johnson)	1.86	98 (25%)	14 (8%)	270 (67%)	0	78:1	1,130

*Characteristics: Moderate to low residue; milk base
Protein—intact: semipurified isolates; high molecular weight
Carbohydrate—lactose, sucrose, corn syrup solids
Hyperosmolar
Palatable, designed as oral supplement

Nutrients per 1,000 ml

Sodium (mg/mEq)	Potassium (mg/mEq)	Volume to Meet Vitamin Requirements (ml)	Protein Sources	Fat Sources	Carbohydrate Sources
1,300/57	1,400/36	1,500	Beef, nonfat milk	Beef, corn oil	Maltodextrin, vegetables, fruits, lactose
1,000/44	1,400/36	1,500	Beef, calcium caseinate	Beef, canola oil	Maltodextrin, vegetables, fruits
680/30	1,250/32	1,500	Beef, calcium, and sodium caseinates	Beef, corn oil	Maltodextrin, vegetables, fruits, soy fiber

Nutrients per 1,000 ml

Sodium (mg/mEq)	Potassium (mg/mEq)	Volume to Meet Vitamin Requirements (ml)	Protein Sources	Fat Sources	Carbohydrate Sources
815/35	2,222/57	—	Nonfat milk, lowfat milk,	Milk fat	Maltodextrin, sucrose, lactose
778/34	2,222/57	—	Nonfat milk, whey protein, lowfat milk	Milk fat	Maltodextrin, lactose (contains aspartamine)
1,100/48	2,800/72	1,040	Nonfat milk, whole milk	Milk fat	Lactose, sucrose, hydrolyzed cornstarch
1,185/51	3,592/93	810	Nonfat milk	Milk fat	Lactose, sucrose, corn syrup solids
901/39	2,883/74	1,030	Nonfat milk, whole milk, calcium caseinate	Milk fat	Corn syrup solids, lactose, dextrose

Polymeric Formulas—Lactose-Free*

Formula	Caloric Density (kcal/ml)	Nutrients per 1,000 ml					
		Protein (g) (% kcal)	Fat (g) (% kcal)	Carbohydrate (g) (% kcal)	Dietary Fiber (g)	Non-protein kcal:N	mOsm/kg
HYPERCALORIC							
Isosource (Sandoz)	1.2	43 (14%)	41 (30%)	170 (56%)	0	148:1	360
Comply (Sherwood Medical)	1.5	60 (16%)	60 (36%)	180 (48%)	0	134:1	410–600
Ensure Plus (Ross)	1.5	55 (15%)	53 (32%)	200 (53%)	0	146:1	690
Nutren 1.5 Diet (Clintec)	1.5	60 (16%)	68 (39%)	169 (45%)	0	131:1	410–590
Resource Plus (Sandoz)	1.5	55 (15%)	53 (32%)	200 (53%)	0	146:1	600
Sustacal Plus (Mead Johnson)	1.5	61 (16%)	58 (34%)	190 (50%)	0	134:1	650
Ultralan (Elan Pharma)	1.5	60 (16%)	50 (30%)	202 (54%)	0	131:1	610
Isocal HCN (Mead Johnson)	2.0	75 (15%)	102 (45%)	200 (40%)	0	145:1	640
Magnacal (Sherwood Medical)	2.0	70 (14%)	80 (36%)	250 (50%)	0	157:1	590
Nutren 2.0 Diet (Clintec)	2.0	80 (16%)	106 (45%)	196 (39%)	0	131:1	710
HYPERCALORIC—HIGH NITROGEN							
Isosource HN (Sandoz)	1.2	53 (18%)	41 (30%)	160 (52%)	0	116:1	330
Isotein HN (Sandoz)	1.2	68 (23%)	34 (25%)	160 (52%)	0	86:1	300

*Characteristics: Moderate to low residue. Protein—intact: semipurified isolates; high molecular weight; derived from casein salts or egg white solids. Carbohydrate—starches, maltodextrins; glucose oligosaccharides; corn syrup solids. Fat—contributes balanced percentage of calories; corn oil, soy oil, safflower oil, and canola oil, as well as MCT. Isosmolar or hyperosmolar. Palatable.

| Nutrients per 1,000 ml | | | | | |
Sodium (mg/mEq)	Potassium (mg/mEq)	Volume to Meet Vitamin Requirements (ml)	Protein Sources	Fat Sources	Carbohydrate Sources
1,200/52	1,700/43	1,500	Sodium and calcium caseinates, soy protein isolate	MCT, canola oil	Hydrolyzed cornstarch
1,100/48	1,850/47	1,000	Sodium and calcium caseinates	Corn oil	Hydrolyzed cornstarch
1,050/46	1,940/50	1,420	Sodium and calcium caseinates, soy protein isolate	Corn oil	Corn syrup, sucrose
752/33	1,875/48	1,000	Casein	MCT, canola oil corn oil	Maltodextrin
1,300/57	2,100/54	1,400	Sodium and calcium caseinates, soy protein isolate	Corn oil	Hydrolyzed cornstarch, sucrose
850/37	1,480/38	1,185	Calcium and sodium caseinates	Corn oil	Corn syrup solids, sucrose
1,035/45	1,755/45	1,000	Sodium and calcium caseinates, soy protein isolate	MCT, corn oil	Maltodextrin
800/35	1,700/43	1,000	Calcium and sodium caseinates	Soy oil, MCT	Corn syrup
1,000/44	1,250/32	1,000	Sodium and calcium caseinates	Partially hydrogenated soy oil	Maltodextrin, sucrose
1,000/44	2,500/64	750	Casein	MCT, canola oil	Corn syrup solids, maltodextrin, sucrose
1,100/48	1,700/43	1,500	Sodium and calcium caseinates, soy protein isolate	MCT, canola oil	Hydrolyzed cornstarch
620/27	1,100/28	1,770	Delactosed lactalbumin	Partially hydrogenated soybean oil, MCT	Hydrolyzed cornstarch, fructose

Continued.

Polymeric Formulas—Lactose-Free—cont'd

Formula	Caloric Density (kcal/ml)	Nutrients per 1,000 ml					
		Protein (g) (% kcal)	Fat (g) (% kcal)	Carbohydrate (g) (% kcal)	Dietary Fiber (g)	Non-protein kcal:N	mOsm/kg
HYPERCALORIC—HIGH NITROGEN—cont'd							
Nitrolan (Elan Pharma)	1.24	60 (19%)	40 (29%)	160 (52%)	0	104:1	310
Ensure Plus HN (Ross)	1.5	63 (17%)	50 (30%)	200 (53%)	0	125:1	650
TwoCal HN (Ross)	2.0	84 (17%)	91 (40%)	217 (43%)	0	125:1	690
NORMOCALORIC							
Attain (Sherwood Medical)	1.0	40 (16%)	35 (30%)	135 (54%)	0	134:1	300
Ensure (Ross)	1.06	37 (14%)	37 (32%)	145 (55%)	0	153:1	470
Isocal (Mead Johnson)	1.06	34 (13%)	44 (37%)	135 (50%)	0	167:1	270
Isolan (Elan Pharma)	1.06	40 (15%)	36 (31%)	144 (54%)	0	141:6	300
Nutren 1.0 Diet (Clintec)	1.0	40 (16%)	38 (33%)	127 (51%)	0	131:1	300–390
Nutrilan (Elan Pharma)	1.06	38 (14%)	37 (31%)	143 (54%)	0	149.1	320
Osmolite (Ross)	1.06	37 (14%)	38 (31%)	145 (55%)	0	153:1	300
Precision Isotonic (Sandoz)	0.96	29 (12%)	30 (28%)	140 (60%)	0	184:1	300
Resource (Sandoz)	1.06	37 (14%)	37 (32%)	140 (54%)	0	154:1	430
NORMOCALORIC—HIGH NITROGEN							
Ensure HN (Ross)	1.06	44 (17%)	36 (30%)	141 (53%)	0	125:1	470
Entrition HN Diet (Clintec)	1.0	44 (18%)	41 (37%)	114 (46%)	0	117:1	300

Nutrients per 1,000 ml		Volume to Meet Vitamin Requirements (ml)	Protein Sources	Fat Sources	Carbohydrate Sources
Sodium (mg/mEq)	Potassium (mg/mEq)				
690/30	1,170/30	1,250	Sodium and calcium caseinates	MCT, corn oil	Maltodextrin
1,180/51	1,820/47	947	Sodium and calcium caseinates, soy protein isolate	Corn oil	Hydrolyzed cornstarch, sucrose
1,310/57	2,456/63	947	Sodium and calcium caseinates	Corn oil, MCT	Hydrolyzed cornstarch, sucrose
805/35	1,600/41	1,250	Sodium and calcium caseinates	MCT, soy oil	Maltodextrin
846/37	1,564/40	1,887	Sodium and calcium caseinates, soy protein isolate	Corn oil	Corn syrup, sucrose
530/23	1,320/34	1,887	Calcium and sodium caseinates, soy protein isolate	Soy oil, MCT	Maltodextrin
690/30	1,170/30	1,250	Caseinates	MCT, corn oil	Maltodextrin
500/22	1,252/32	1,500	Casein	Corn oil, MCT, canola oil	Maltodextrin, corn syrup solids
640/28	1,057/27	1,585	Caseinates	Corn oil, MCT	Maltodextrin
640/28	1,020/26	1,887	Sodium and calcium caseinates, soy protein isolate	Safflower oil, canola oil, MCT	Hydrolyzed cornstarch
770/33	960/25	1,560	Egg white solids	Partially hydrogenated soy oil	Hydrolyzed cornstarch, sucrose
890/39	1,600/41	1,890	Sodium and calcium caseinates, soy protein isolate	Corn oil	Hydrolyzed cornstarch, sucrose
802/35	1,564/40	1,321	Sodium and calcium caseinates, soy protein isolate	Corn oil	Corn syrup, sucrose
845/37	1,579/41	1,300	Casein, soy	Corn oil	Maltodextrin

Continued.

Polymeric Formulas—Lactose-Free—cont'd

Formula	Caloric Density (kcal/ml)	Nutrients per 1,000 ml					
		Protein (g) (% kcal)	Fat (g) (% kcal)	Carbohydrate (g) (% kcal)	Dietary Fiber (g)	Non-protein kcal:N	mOsm/kg
NORMOCALORIC—HIGH NITROGEN—cont'd							
Isocal HN (Mead Johnson)	1.06	44 (17%)	45 (37%)	124 (46%)	0	125:1	270
Osmolite HN (Ross)	1.06	44 (17%)	36 (38%)	141 (53%)	0	125:1	300
Promote (Ross)	1.0	63 (25%)	26 (23%)	130 (52%)	0	75:1	330
Replete Diet (Clintec)	1.0	63 (25%)	34 (30%)	113 (45%)	0	75:1	290
Replete Oral (Clintec)	1.0	63 (25%)	34 (30%)	113 (45%)	0	75:1	350
Sustacal Liquid (Mead Johnson)	1.01	61 (24%)	23 (21%)	140 (55%)	0	78:1	670
Travasorb MCT (Clintec)	1.0	50 (20%)	33 (30%)	123 (50%)	0	101:1	250

Polymeric Formulas—with Fiber*

Formula	Caloric Density (kcal/ml)	Nutrients per 1,000 ml					
		Protein (g) (% kcal)	Fat (g) (% kcal)	Carbohydrate (g) (% kcal)	Dietary Fiber (g)	Non-protein kcal:N	mOsm/kg
Ensure with Fiber	1.1	40 (15%)	37 (31%)	162 (55%)	14.4	148:1	480
Fiberlan (Elan Pharma)	1.2	50 (17%)	40 (30%)	160 (53%)	14	122:1	310

*Characteristics: Fiber—containing soy polysaccharides or oat fiber; lactose-free. Protein—intact; semipurified isolates; high molecular weight; derived from casein salts. Carbohydrate—starches, maltodextrins, sucrose, corn syrup solids. Fat—contributes balanced percentage of calories; corn oil, soy oil, safflower oil, and canola oil, as well as MCT. Isosmolar or hyperosmolar. Palatable.

| Nutrients per 1,000 ml | | | | | |
Sodium (mg/mEq)	Potassium (mg/mEq)	Volume to Meet Vitamin Requirements (ml)	Protein Sources	Fat Sources	Carbohydrate Sources
930/40	1,610/41	1,180	Calcium and sodium caseinates, soy protein isolate	Soy oil, MCT	Maltodextrin
930/41	1,570/40	1,321	Calcium and sodium caseinates, soy protein isolate	Safflower and canola oil, MCT	Hydrolyzed cornstarch
930/40	1,980/51	1,250	Sodium and calcium caseinates, soy protein isolate	Safflower and canola oil, MCT	Hydrolyzed cornstarch, sucrose
500/22	1,560/40	1,000	Casein	Canola oil, MCT	Maltodextrin, corn syrup solids
500/22	1,560/40	1,500	Casein	Corn oil	Sucrose, maltodextrin
930/40	2,100/54	1,069	Calcium and sodium caseinates, soy protein isolate	Soy oil	Sucrose, corn syrup
350/15	1,000/26	2,000	Lactalbumin, sodium and potassium caseinates	MCT, sunflower oil	Corn syrup solids

| Nutrients per 1,000 ml | | | | | |
Sodium (mg/mEq)	Potassium (mg/mEq)	Volume to Meet Vitamin Requirements (ml)	Protein Sources	Fat Sources	Carbohydrate Sources
846/37	1,693/43	1,391	Sodium and calcium caseinates, soy protein isolate	Corn oil	Hydrolyzed cornstarch, sucrose, soy polysaccharides
1,100/48	1,800/46	1,500	Sodium and calcium caseinates	Canola oil, MCT	Hydrolyzed cornstarch, soy polysaccharides

Continued.

Special Formulas—cont'd

Formula	Caloric Density (kcal/ml)	Nutrients per 1,000 ml					
		Protein (g) (% kcal)	Fat (g) (% kcal)	Carbohydrate (g) (% kcal)	Dietary Fiber (g)	Non-protein kcal:N	mOsm/kg
RENAL—cont'd							
Suplena (Ross)	2.0	30 (6%)	96 (43%)	255 (51%)	0	393:1	600
Travasorb Renal Diet (Clintec)	1.35	23 (7%)	18 (12%)	271 (81%)	0	339:1	590
STRESS/IMPAIRED GI FUNCTION							
Advera (Ross)	1.28	60 (18%)	23 (15%)	216 (67%)	8.9	133:1	680
Alitraq (Ross)	1.0	53 (218%)	16 (13%)	165 (66%)	0	94:1	575
Impact (Sandoz)	1.0	56 (22%)	28 (25%)	130 (53%)	0	71:1	375
Impact with Fiber (Sandoz)	1.0	56 (22%)	28 (25%)	140 (53%)	10	71:1	375
Lipisorb Liquid (Mead Johnson)	1.35	57 (17%)	57 (35%)	161 (48%)	0	125:1	630
Perative (Ross)	1.3	67 (20.5%)	37 (25%)	177 (54.5%)	0	97:1	385
Stresstein (Sandoz)	1.2	70 (23%)	28 (20%)	170 (57%)	0	83:1	910
TraumaCal (Mead Johnson)	1.5	83 (22%)	68 (40%)	145 (38%)	0	91:1	490
Traum-Aid HBC (Kendall McGaw)	1.0	56 (22%)	12 (11%)	166 (67%)	0	102:1	760

Nutrients per 1,000 ml					
Sodium (mg/mEq)	Potassium (mg/mEq)	Volume to Meet Vitamin Requirements (ml)	Protein Sources	Fat Sources	Carbohydrate Sources
783/34	1,116/29	947	Sodium and calcium caseinates	Safflower oil, soy oil	Hydrolyzed cornstarch, sucrose
0/0	0/0	—	Essential L-amino acids, selected nonessential amino acids	MCT, sunflower oil	Glucose oligosaccharides, sucrose
1,012/44	2,531/65	1,184	Soy protein hydrolysate, sodium caseinate	Canola oil, MCT, sardine oil	Hydrolyzed cornstarch, sucrose, soy fiber
1,000/44	1,200/31	1,500	Peptides and amino acids from soy hydrolysate, whey, lactalbumin	MCT, safflower oil	Hydrolyzed cornstarch, sucrose, fructose
1,100/48	1,300/33	1,500	Sodium and calcium caseinates, L-arginine	Structured lipid, menhaden oil	Hydrolyzed cornstarch
1,100/48	1,300/33	1,500	Sodium and calcium caseinates, L-arginine	Structured lipid, menhaden oil	Hydrolyzed cornstarch, soy polysaccharide
1,350/59	1690/43	1,600	Sodium and calcium-caseinate	MCT, corn oil	Maltodextrin, sucrose
1,040/45	1,730/44	1,155	Partially hydrolyzed sodium caseinate, lactalbumin hydrolysate, L-arginine	Canola oil, MCT, corn oil	Hydrolyzed cornstarch
650/28	1,100/28	2,000	Free amino acids (44% branched-chain)	MCT, soy oil	Hydrolyzed cornstarch
1,200/52	1,400/36	2,000	Sodium and calcium caseinates	Soy oil, MCT	Corn syrup, sucrose
533/23	1,170/30	3,000	High branched-chain amino acids (50%), essential and nonessential amino acids	MCT, soy oil	Maltodextrin

Supplemental Nutrient Sources*

| Formula | Caloric Density (kcal/ml) | Nutrients per 1,000 ml | | | | | |
		Protein (g) (% kcal)	Fat (g) (% kcal)	Carbohydrate (g) (% kcal)	Dietary Fiber (g)	Non-protein kcal:N	mOsm/kg
CARBOHYDRATE							
Moducal (Mead Johnson)	3.8 kcal/g			95† (100%)	0		
Polycose Liquid (Ross)	2.0			500 (100%)	0		900
Polycose Powder (Ross)	3.8 kcal/g			94† (100%)	0		
Sumacal (Sherwood Medical)	3.8 kcal/g			95 (100%)	0		
FAT							
MCT Oil (Mead Johnson)	7.7 8.3 kcal/g		933 (100%)		0		
Microlipid (Sherwood Medical)	4.5		500 (100%)		0		80
PROTEIN							
Casec (Mead Johnson)	3.7 kcal/g	88† (98%)	2† (2%)	0† (0%)	0		
Elementra (Clintec)	3.8 kcal/g	79† (85%)	5† (12%)	2† (3%)	0		
ProMod (Ross)	4.2 kcal/g	76† (72%)	<9.1† (19%)	<10† (9%)	0		
Propac (Sherwood Medical)	4.0 kcal/g	75† (76%)	20† (18%)	15† (6%)	0		

*Characteristics: Specific nutrients to be added
                Not nutritionally complete
                Contents per 1,000 ml unless otherwise specified
†Nutrients per 100 g of powder

| Nutrients per 1,000 ml | | | | | |
Sodium (mg/mEq)	Potassium (mg/mEq)	Volume to Meet Vitamin Requirements (ml)	Protein Sources	Fat Sources	Carbohydrate Sources
70/3†	<10/<0.26†				Maltodextrin (hydrolyzed cornstarch)
700/30	60/1.5				Hydrolyzed cornstarch (glucose polymers)
110/<5†	<10/<0.3†				Hydrolyzed cornstarch (glucose polymers)
100/4.3	—			Fractionated coconut oil	Maltodextrin
				Safflower oil	
120/5†	10/0.3†		Calcium caseinate		
39/1.7†	1,515/39†		Whey protein		
227/10†	1,000/26†		Whey protein		
225/10†	500/13†		Whey protein		

11 / *Physician's Adult Enteral Nutrition Order Sheet*

Enteral Nutrition Order Sheet—Adults

- Please check appropriate boxes and write specific orders.
- Complete a new form for any change in orders.
- See reverse side for ordering considerations.

Clinic Number: _____
Name: _____
Room Number: _____

☐ Standard formula at full strength   ☐ Other _____

☐ CONTINUOUS (pump)

Flow rate: ☐ 20 ml/hour
            ☐ Other: _____ ml/hr

Duration: ☐ 24 hours
            ☐ Nocturnal
            _____ ml/hour from
            _____ PM to _____ AM
            ☐ Other: _____
            _____

Progression: ☐ Do not advance
            ☐ Standard: Increase by 10 ml q 12
              hours to goal of _____ ml/hour
            ☐ Other: Increase by _____ ml/hour
              q _____ hours to goal of _____
              ml/hour

*Water for tube patency:
            ☐ Standard: 30 ml Q 6 hours

☐ INTERMITTENT (gravity)

Initial rate: ½ can (120 ml) per feeding over 60
minutes 5 times per day during the first day
☐ Other: _____
_____

Progression   ☐ Do not advance
on   ☐ Standard: If tube feedings are
Following   tolerated during the first day, increase
Days: volume of feeding to 1 can (240 ml)
              over 60-90 minutes. Infusion rate and
              frequency will be adjusted as tolerated
              to goal of _____ ml/day.
            ☐ Other: _____
              _____
              _____

*Water for tube patency:
            ☐ Standard: 30 ml before and 30 ml
              after each gravity feeding

Total daily water required: the daily requirement should be determined for each patient. The order should be written on the Physician's Order Sheet.

*Per nursing policy, additional water is required pre/post administration of medications via feeding tube.

Supplemental protein: Occasionally it is necessary to add supplemental protein to feeding in order to provide adequate protein without giving excessive calories (see reverse side).

☐ Add _____ g/day supplemental protein to feeding (1 scoop of Promod is 5 g of protein; order in multiples of 5 g)

Tube Position   ☐ Prepyloric   ☐ Postpyloric

Aspiration precautions will be instituted. The head of the bed should be elevated 30°-45° during feeding.

For *prepyloric continuous* feedings, gastric residual volume should be checked q 4-6 hours. If the residual volume exceeds twice the hourly feeding infusion rate or is greater than 100 ml, hold feeding for 1 hour and recheck residual volume. If the repeat residual volume still exceeds these values, the primary service should be notified.

For *prepyloric gravity* feeding, the residual volume should be checked prior to the feeding. If the residual volume exceeds 100 ml, hold the feeding for 1 hour and recheck residual volume. If the residual volume still exceeds 100 ml, the primary service should be notified.

For *postpyloric* feedings, residual volume need not be checked. Patient should be examined at regular intervals for abdominal distention.

Additional Recommendations:
1. Please obtain an X-ray to verify nasal feeding tube position.
2. Please notify the floor dietitian if you anticipate the patient to be dismissed from the hospital on tube feedings.
3. Please contact the Nutrition Support Service if you wish assistance in the management of tube feedings.

Date _____   Time _____   Physician _____

CONSIDERATIONS FOR ORDERING ADULT ENTERAL NUTRITION FORMULAS*

CALORIES

Energy requirements may be estimated from a formula or measured by indirect calorimetry.

Estimated Energy Requirements

The Harris Benedict equation may be used to estimate daily caloric requirements:

For Females,
$$BEE = 665 + 9.6(W) + 1.9(H) - 4.7(A)$$
For Males,
$$BEE = 66.5 + 13.8(W) + 5.0(H) - 6.8(A)$$

Where BEE is *basal* energy expenditure, W is weight in kilograms, H is height in centimeters, and A is age in years.

Measured Resting Energy Expenditure (REE)

Indirect calorimetry calculates energy expenditure by the measurement of respiratory gas exchange. The actual measurements made during indirect calorimetry are oxygen consumption, carbon dioxide production, and minute ventilation. From these variables, REE and respiratory quotient can be calculated. Indirect calorimetry provides measurements of individual energy requirements. It is recommended for patients who are suspected of having greatly increased or decreased energy requirements, those for whom accurate weight is not possible, and those who will be fed for long periods of time enterally. REEs are ordered on the Respiratory Order Sheet.

PROTEIN

The Recommended Dietary Allowance (RDA) for protein for healthy normal adults is 0.8 g/kg/day. Protein needs may be increased with significant stress. Most hospitalized patients can be adequately maintained on protein intakes between 1.0 and 1.5 g/kg of actual body weight. If necessary, supplemental protein can be provided in the form of Promod.

WATER FOR TUBE PATENCY

Tube should be flushed with 30 ml of water 4 times per day to maintain tube patency.

VITAMINS

The volume of each formula required to provide 100% of the RDA for adults is listed in the Enteral Product Handout. A standard multivitamin should be ordered if this volume is not met.

MEDICATIONS

Medications should be given in liquid form when possible.

INITIATION AND PROGRESSION OF ENTERAL FEEDING

- Isotonic (approximately 300 mOsm) formulas may be initiated at full strength.
- Hypertonic formulas may be initiated at half strength and advanced to full strength as tolerated.

---

*These considerations may not be applicable to some patients.

Adjustments to Energy Requirements

It seems prudent at this time to provide caloric intakes of 0-20% above *basal* energy requirements for most hospitalized patients. The complications of caloric excess include hyperglycemia, excessive fluid retention, electrolyte disturbances (especially hypokalemia and hypophosphatemia), and an increased susceptibility to fatty liver. In addition, the provision of glucose (and calories in general) in excessive amounts increases the production of carbon dioxide and therefore may be contraindicated in patients with pulmonary insufficiency.

LABORATORY MONITORING

Baseline laboratory tests should include a chemistry group, hematology group, and electrolyte panel. An essential element screen may be useful in patients with malabsorption or with significant renal or gastrointestinal losses. The frequency and extent of additional laboratory monitoring tests should be individualized.

12 / *Parenteral Nutrition Solutions*

General Parenteral Amino Acid Products*

Amino Acids (grams per 100 g)	10% Aminosyn	10% Aminosyn II	10% Freamine III	11.4% Novamine	15% Novamine	10% Travasol
Isoleucine	7.20	6.60	6.90	5.00	5.00	6.00
Leucine	9.40	10.00	9.10	6.93	6.93	7.30
Lysine	7.20	10.50	7.30	7.89	7.87	5.80
Methionine	4.00	1.72	5.30	5.00	5.00	4.00
Phenylalanine	4.40	2.98	5.60	6.93	6.93	5.60
Threonine	5.20	4.00	4.00	5.00	5.00	4.20
Tryptophan	1.60	2.00	1.50	1.67	1.67	1.80
Valine	8.00	5.00	6.60	6.40	6.40	5.80
	47.00	42.8	46.30	44.82	44.80	40.50
Alanine	12.80	9.93	7.10	14.47	14.47	20.70
Arginine	9.80	10.18	9.50	9.82	9.80	11.50
Histidine	3.00	3.00	2.80	5.97	5.96	4.80
Proline	8.60	7.22	11.20	5.97	5.96	6.80
Serine	4.20	5.30	5.90	3.95	3.95	5.00
Tyrosine	0.44	2.70	—	0.26	0.26	0.40
Glycine	12.80	5.00	14.00	6.93	6.93	10.30
Cysteine	—	—	0.24	—	—	—
Glutamate	—	7.38	—	2.90	2.89	—
Aspartate	—	7.00	—	11.4 g	15.0 g	10.0 g
Total amino acids per 100 ml	10.0 g	10.0 g	10.0 g	1.80 g	2.37 g	1.65 g
Total nitrogen per 100 ml	1.57 g	1.53 g	1.53 g	18.33%	18.33%	19.10%
% BCAA	24.6%	21.6%	22.6%	1.6	1.6	3

ELECTROLYTES (mEq/L)

Na	—	45.3	—	—	—	—
K	5.4	—	3	—	—	40
Cl	—	—	89	114	151	87
Acetate	148	71.8	10	—	—	—
P (mmol/L)	—	—	—	—	—	—
mOsm/L	1,000	873	950	1,057	1,388	1,000
Bottle volume (ml)	500 / 1,000	500 / 1,000	500 / 1,000	250 / 500 / 1,000	500	200 / 500 / 1,000 / 2,000
Manufacturer	Abbott	Abbott	McGaw	Clintec	Clintec	Clintec

*10% or greater concentration for general adult or pediatric patients.

Pediatric Parenteral Amino Acid Products

Amino Acids (grams per 100 g)	10% Trophamine™	10% Aminosyn-PF™
Isoleucine	8.2	7.6
Leucine	14.0	12.0
Lysine	8.2	6.77
Methionine	3.4	1.8
Phenylalanine	4.8	4.27
Threonine	4.2	5.12
Tryptophan	2.0	1.8
Valine	7.8	6.73
	52.6	46.09
Alanine	5.4	6.98
Arginine	12.0	12.27
Histidine	4.8	3.12
Proline	6.8	8.12
Serine	3.8	4.95
Taurine	0.25	0.70
Tyrosine	2.4	0.40
Glycine	3.6	3.85
Cysteine	<0.16	—
Glutamate	5	6.2
Aspartate	3.2	5.27
Total amino acids per 100 ml	10 g	10 g
Total nitrogen per 100 ml	1.55 g	1.52 g
ELECTROLYTES (mEq/L)		
Na	5	3.4
K	—	—
Cl	<3	—
Acetate	97	46.3
Mg	—	—
P (mM/L)	—	—
mOsm/L	875	829
Bottle volume (ml)	500	1,000
Other AA (%)	6	7
Manufacturer	McGaw	Abbott

Amino Acid Products for Renal or Hepatic Diseases

Amino Acids (grams per 100 g)	6.5% Ren Amin™	5.2% Aminosyn-RF™	5.2% Aminess™	5.4% Nephramine™	8% Hepat Amine™
Isoleucine	7.69	8.88	10.14	10.37	11.25
Leucine	9.23	13.96	15.93	16.30	13.75
Lysine	6.92	10.29	11.58	11.85	7.63
Methionine	7.69	13.96	15.93	16.30	1.25
Phenylalanine	7.54	13.96	15.93	16.30	1.25
Threonine	5.85	6.35	7.24	7.41	5.63
Tryptophan	2.46	3.17	3.63	3.70	0.83
Valine	12.62	10.15	11.58	11.58	10.50
	60.00	80.72	91.96	94.08	52.09
Alanine	8.62	—	—	—	9.63
Arginine	9.69	11.54	—	—	7.50
Histidine	6.46	8.25	7.95	4.63	3.00
Proline	5.38	—	—	—	10.00
Serine	4.62	—	—	—	6.25
Tyrosine	0.62	—	—	—	—
Glycine	4.62	—	—	—	11.25
Cysteine	—	—	—	<0.37	<0.25
Total amino acids per 100 ml	6.5 g	5.2 g	5.18 g	5.4 g	8.0 g
% BCAA	30	33	38	38	36
Total nitrogen per 100 ml	1.0 g	0.79 g	0.66 g	0.65 g	1.2 g
ELECTROLYTES (mEq/L)					
Na	3	—	—	5	10
K	—	5.4	—	—	<3
Cl	31	—	—	<3	<3
Acetate	60	105	50	44	62
P (mmol/L)	—	—	—	—	10
mOsm/L	600	475	416	435	785
Bottle volume (ml)	250 and 500	300	400	250	500
Manufacturer	Clintec	Abbott	Clintec	McGaw	McGaw

Amino Acid Products for Stress or Trauma

Amino Acids (grams per 100 g)	6.9% Freamine HBC™	7.0% Aminosyn-HBC™	4.0% Branchamine™
Isoleucine	11.01	11.27	34.5
Leucine	19.86	22.51	34.5
Lysine	8.41	3.79	
Methionine	3.62	2.94	
Phenylalanine	4.64	3.26	
Threonine	2.90	3.89	
Tryptophan	1.30	1.26	
Valine	12.75	11.27	31.0
	64.49	60.19	100.0
Alanine	5.80	9.43	
Arginine	8.41	7.24	
Histidine	2.32	2.20	
Proline	9.13	4.48	
Serine	4.78	3.16	
Tyrosine	—	0.47	
Glycine	4.78	9.43	
Cysteine	<0.29	—	
% BCAA	44	45	100
Total amino acids per 100 ml	6.9 g	7.0 g	4.0 g
Total nitrogen per 100 ml	0.973 g	1.12 g	0.433 g
ELECTROLYTES (mEq/L)			
Na	10	7	
K	—	—	
Cl	<3	—	
Acetate	57	72	
mOsm/L	620	665	316
Bottle volume (ml)	750	500 and 1,000	500
Manufacturer	McGaw	Abbott	Clintec

Electrolyte Products Used in Parenteral Nutrition

	Per Milliliter
Sodium chloride	2.5 or 4.0 mEq
Sodium acetate	2.0 or 4.0 mEq
Sodium phosphate	4.0 mEq of Na and 3.0 mmol of P
Sodium lactate	2.5 mEq
Potassium chloride	2.0 mEq
Potassium acetate	2.0 or 4.0 mEq
Potassium phosphate	4.4 mEq of K and 3.0 mmol of P
Magnesium sulfate	50%, 8.1 mEq/2 ml
Calcium gluconate	10%, 4.7 mEq/10 ml
Calcium chloride	10%, 13.6 mEq/10 ml

Combined Electrolyte Combinations

Electrolytes mEq/dose	Hyperlyte[1] Lypholyte[2] Multilyte-40[2]	Lypholyte II[2] TPN Electrolytes[3]	Hyperlyte R[1] Multilyte-20[2]
Sodium	25	35	25
Potassium	40.5	20	20
Calcium	5	4.5	5
Magnesium	8	5	5
Chloride	33.5	35	30
Acetate	40.6	29.5	25
Gluconate	5		
mOsm/L	Hyperlyte—6,015 Lypholyte—7,562 Multilyte-40—6,050	Lympholyte II—6,200 TPN Electrolytes—6,200	Hyperlyte R—4,205 Multilyte-20—4,200

Manufacturers: [1]McGaw
[2]Lyphomed
[3]Abbott

Intravenous Multivitamins

Vitamins	Total Contents per Vial: *AMA/NAG*	
	Adult*	Pediatric†
A (IU)	3,300	2,300
D (IU)	200	400
E (IU)	10	7
C (mg)	100	80
Folic acid (μg)	400	140
B_1 (mg)	3	1.2
B_2 (mg)	3.6	1.4
B_6 (mg)	4	1.0
Niacin (mg)	40	17
B_{12} (μg)	5	1
Dexpanthenol (mg)	15	5
Biotin (μg)	60	20
K_1 (mg)	—	0.2
Dose:	1 vial per day for 11 yr of age or over	1 vial per day (under 11 yr of age and 3 kg of body weight or over) 65% vial per day (for 1 kg of body weight and less than 3 kg of body weight) 30% vial per day (under 1 kg of body weight)

AMA/NAG = American Medical Association and Nutrition Advisory Group

*MVI-12, MVC 9 + 3

†MVI Pediatric, MVC 9 + 4

Intravenous Fat Emulsions

	Intralipid™		Liposyn II™		Liposyn III™	
Fat content (%)	10	20	10	20	10	20
Oil source	Soybean oil		Safflower oil, soybean oil		Soybean oil	
Egg phospholipids (%)	1.2		1.2		1.2	
Glycerin (%)	2.25		2.5		2.5	
Osmolarity (mOsm/L)	260	260	276	258	292	292
pH	6–8.9		8.0	8.3	6–9	
Particle size (μm)	0.5		0.4		0.4	
Caloric value (per ml)	1.1	2.0	1.1	2.0	1.1	2.0
FATTY ACIDS (%)						
Linoleic acid	50		65.8		54.5	
Linolenic acid	9		4.2		8.3	
Oleic acid	26		17.7		22.4	
Palmitic acid	10		8.8		10.5	
Stearic acid	3.5		3.4		4.2	
Container volumes (ml)	50,100, 250,500		100, 200,500		100,200, 500	200, 500
Manufacturer	Clintec		Abbott		Abbott	

Composition of Intralipid™ (per 1,000 ml)

Component	10%	20%
Triglycerides (g)	100	200
Phospholipid (g)	12	12
Glycerol (g)	22.5	22.5
Water (ml)	867	766
Polyunsaturated fatty acids (PUFA) (g)	62	121
Saturated fat (g)	21	37
P/S ratio	3.0	3.3
Tocopherol (mg)		
Total tocopherol	71 (41–111)	148 (107–203)
Alpha tocopherol	6 (2–19)	12 (6–24)
Gamma tocopherol	40 (15–72)	92 (63–130)
Delta tocopherol	24 (11–58)	44 (26–67)
Vitamin E activity*	15 (22 IU)	31 (47 IU)
Vitamin E activity/PUFA (min reg = 0.4)	0.24	0.24
Sterols (mg)		
Cholesterol	304 (85–409)	304 (85–409)
Total plant sterols	370	740
Campesterol	84	168
Stigmasterol	76	152
Sitosterol	210	410
Electrolytes and trace minerals (mEq)		
Mg^{++}	0.011	0.008
Ca^{++}	0.027	0.014
Na^+	3.4	3.5
K^+	0.82	0.87
Zn^{++}	0.002	0.001
Cu^{++}	0.001	<0.001
Cl^-	3.0	3.1
Phosphorus (from phospholipids) (mmol)	15	15
Kcal (total)	1,100	2,000
Triglycerides (9.3 cal/g)	930	1,860
Phospholipid (6.0 cal/g)	72	72
Glycerol (4.2 cal/g)	94.5	94.5
Osmolarity (mOsm/L of emulsion)	260	268
Osmolality (mOsm/kg of water)	300	350

*Vitamin E activity is the same as α-tocopherol equivalent and is based on α:γ:δ- 1.0:0.2:0.01.
1 mg of α-tocopherol = 1 IU

Parenteral Nutrition Order Form (Adults)

PARENTERAL NUTRITION ORDER FORM (ADULTS)

PHYSICIAN'S ADULT PARENTERAL NUTRITION ORDER SHEET
  (Use a new sheet for each daily order)

CLINIC NUMBER:

NAME:

PLEASE WRITE SPECIFIC ORDERS. See hospital procedure guide
and parenteral nutrition monograph (pharmacy bulletin) for
information on parenteral nutrition orders. Unless otherwise
specified, these orders will begin upon completion of any currently
existing parenteral nutrition orders.

ROOM NUMBER:

STANDARD FORMULAS—ORDER ALL VITAMINS AND TRACE ELEMENTS BELOW

☐ Central parenteral nutrition (CPN-D)
  with standard electrolytes

☐ Peripheral parenteral nutrition (PPN-A)
  with standard electrolytes

	Final Conc.			
Dextrose	☐10%	☐15%	☐20%	☐25%
Amino acids	4.25%			
Sodium	36.5 mEq/L			
Potassium	30.0 mEq/L			
Calcium	4.7 mEq/L			
Magnesium	5.0 mEq/L			
Chloride	35.0 mEq/L			
Phosphorus	15.0 mmol/L			
Acetate	70.5 mEq/L			

	Final Conc.
Dextrose	5%
Amino acids	4.25%
Sodium	36.5 mEq/L
Potassium	30.0 mEq/L
Calcium	4.7 mEq/L
Magnesium	5.0 mEq/L
Chloride	35.0 mEq/L
Phosphorus	15.0 mmol/L
Acetate	70.5 mEq/L

Grams nitrogen	7.15 g/L				
Total kilocalories	510	680	850	1020 kcal/L	
Approx. osmolarity	1090	1340	1595	1845 mOsm/L	
Approx. volume	1000 ml				

Grams nitrogen	7.15 g/L
Total kilocalories	340 kcal/L
Approx. osmolarity	835 mOsm/L
Approx. volume	1000 mL

Optional additives to standard electrolytes
☐ Increase total sodium to ____ mEq/L
    as: (check one) ☐ Chloride ☐ Acetate ☐ Phosphate
☐ Increase total potassium to ____ mEq/L
    as: (check one) ☐ Chloride ☐ Acetate ☐ Phosphate
☐ Regular insulin _____ units/L
☐ Other _____
Formulas for less than standard electrolyte concentrations
must be ordered in nonstandard formula section.

Flow rate (specify one)

_____ mL/hr

_____ L/day

To be completed by nurse
        Time needed _____

PARENTERAL NUTRITION ORDER FORM (ADULTS)—cont'd

NONSTANDARD FORMULA   ☐ CENTRAL   ☐ PERIPHERAL

Dextrose   _____ % (Final Conc.)
Amino Acids   _____ % (Final Conc.)
  Other _____   _____ % (Final Conc.)
Sodium   _____ mEq/L
Potassium   _____ mEq/L
Calcium   _____ mEq/L
Magnesium   _____ mEq/L
Chloride   _____ mEq/L
Phosphorus   _____ mmol/L

_____   _____

_____   _____

Unless specified otherwise, Pharmacy will compound such that the
Na:Cl ratio is approximately 1:1; the balance of anions to be provided primarily as acetate.

DAILY VITAMIN AND TRACE ELEMENTS

☐ Standard Adult Multivitamin Injection to
   one bottle daily (See Hospital Formulary for contents).
☐ Standard Adult Trace Element Injection to
   one bottle daily (see reverse side for contents).

☐ Other _____

_____

INTRAVENOUS FAT EMULSION
☐ 10% Fat Emulsion (1.1 kcal/mL)
☐ 20% Fat Emulsion (2.0 kcal/mL)

Volume _____   ☐ Central
Flow Rate _____   ☐ Peripheral

COMPLETE THIS SECTION WHEN INITIATING PARENTERAL NUTRITION AND CHECK EACH APPLICABLE BOX
BELOW _____

Indication for Parenteral Nutrition   NO   YES
                                                       ☐   ☐   Initiate Laboratory Monitoring-   ⎛NO HMSR ⎞
                                                                   see back of form   ⎝REQUIRED⎠

  ☐ Bowel obstruction due to: _____   ☐   Enteral feeding was considered before parenteral
  ☐ Ileus   nutrition initiated.
  ☐ Malabsorption/Maldigestion due to: _____   ☐   Anticipated duration of therapy greater than 7 days
  ☐ Fistula/Abscess
  ☐ Pancreatitis   ☐   X-ray verification of central catheter position com-
  ☐ Inflammatory Bowel Disease   pleted.
  ☐ Short Bowel
  ☐ Bone Marrow Transplant   ☐   Order Nutrition Consult ⎛ordering physician must   ⎞
  ☐ Other: _____   ⎜complete Consultation Request⎟
                                                                                     ⎝Card MC 1376   ⎠

SPECIAL INSTRUCTIONS _____
Date _____ Time _____ Dr. _____

GUIDELINES FOR ORDERING ADULT PARENTERAL NUTRITION SOLUTIONS*

CALORIES

Energy requirements may be estimated from a formula or measured by indirect calorimetry.

Estimated Energy Requirements

A formula commonly used is that of Harris and Benedict:

$$\text{For Females:} \quad \text{BEE} = 655 + 9.6(W) + 1.8(H) - 4.7(A)$$
$$\text{For Males:} \quad \text{BEE} = 66.4 + 13.7(W) + 5(H) - 6.8(A)$$

Where BEE is basal energy expenditure, W is weight in kilograms, H is height in centimeters, and A is age in years.

Measured Resting Energy Expenditure (REE)

Measurement of energy expenditure is particularly useful in critically ill (i.e., intensive care unit) patients because the ability of standard equations to predict energy expenditure in these individuals is poor. Indirect calorimetry calculates energy expenditure by the measurement of respiratory gas exchange. The actual measurements made during indirect calorimetry are VO_2, VCO_2, and minute ventilation (VE). From these variables, REE and respiratory quotient (RQ) can be calculated. Indirect calorimetry provides measurements of individual energy requirements. It is recommended for patients who are suspected of having greatly increased or decreased energy requirements, those for whom accurate weight is not possible, and those who will be fed for long periods of time enterally or parenterally. REEs are ordered on the Respiratory Order Sheet.

Adjustments to Energy Requirements

It seems prudent at this time to provide caloric intakes of 0–20% above energy requirements for most hospitalized patients. Patients receiving below 10% or above 20% of their estimated/measured resting energy needs will be reviewed by the Nutrition Support Team.

The complications of caloric excess include hyperglycemia, excessive fluid retention, electrolyte disturbances (especially hypokalemia and hypophosphatemia), and an increased susceptibility to fatty liver. In addition, the provision of glucose (and calories in general) in excessive amounts increases the production of carbon dioxide and therefore may be contraindicated in patients with pulmonary insufficiency.

PROTEIN

The recommended dietary allowance (RDA) for protein for normal healthy adults is 0.8 g/kg. The minimum requirement for maintenance of nitrogen balance in otherwise healthy adults is between 0.4 and 0.5 g/kg. Fever, sepsis, surgery, trauma, and burns increase protein catabolism and therefore the amount of amino acids and/or

---

*These guidelines may not be applicable to some patients.

protein that must be supplied in order to achieve nitrogen balance. The most direct way of assessing nitrogen requirements in acutely ill patients is to measure 24 hour urinary nitrogen. Multiplying urinary nitrogen (plus an allowance of 1–2 g for fecal and other losses) by 6.25 yields an estimate of the grams of protein catabolized.

Most hospitalized patients can be adequately maintained on protein intakes between 1.0 and 1.5 g/kg of actual body weight. Intakes greater than 2 g/kg should not be ordered in the absence of documentation of the rate of protein catabolism by 24 hour urinary nitrogen. When such orders are received, they will be discussed with the primary service.

VITAMINS

A standard adult multiple vitamin supplement can be ordered on the Physician's Adult Parenteral Nutrition Order Sheet. In nearly all circumstances, this supplement is adequate to prevent the development of vitamin deficiency. Vitamin K is not included in the standard adult supplement to avoid complications with warfarin therapy. Patients not receiving anticoagulants should receive 5 mg IM once weekly. If a vitamin deficiency has already occurred, it may be necessary to supplement individual vitamins as indicated.

TRACE ELEMENTS

The standard adult trace element injection contains zinc 4 mg, copper 0.8 mg, manganese 0.4 mg, chromium 8 μg, and selenium 48 μg. Patients who are severely malnourished may need additional supplementation. The decision regarding trace element supplementation should be made after obtaining the baseline Essential Element Screen, as indicated in the Laboratory Monitoring Guidelines.

USES OF INTRAVENOUS FAT

In the past, intravenous fat has been used primarily to prevent essential fatty acid deficiency. However, recent studies have provided strong evidence that a combination of glucose and fat is optimal for good nutrition in most patients. Current recommendations are that fat be administered on a daily basis to provide between 25 and 50% of total calories. CPN orders that provide no fat on a daily basis or provide fat at more than 60% of total calories will be discussed with the primary service. Daily intravenous fat (10% or 20%) should be infused over a minimum of 12 hours and may be given as a continuous 24 hour infusion. As noted in the Laboratory Monitoring Guidelines, serum triglycerides should be checked prior to initiating fat infusion and again immediately prior to the second day's infusion of intravenous fat.

CENTRAL VERSUS PERIPHERAL PARENTERAL NUTRITION

Parenteral nutrition via central venous access (CPN) is necessary when the volume and osmolarity of the solution preclude peripheral administration and the anticipated duration of therapy is greater than 2 weeks.

Parenteral nutrition via peripheral venous access (PPN) is appropriate when the solution osmolarity required to meet the patient's needs is less than 1,000 mOsm/L and the anticipated duration of therapy is less than 2 weeks.

14 / *Conversion of Milligrams to Milliequivalents*

To convert milligrams to milliequivalents:

$$\text{Milliequivalents} = \frac{\text{Milligrams}}{\text{Atomic Weight}} \times \text{Valence}$$

To convert milliequivalents to milligrams:

$$\text{Milligrams} = \frac{\text{Milliequivalents} \times \text{Atomic Weight}}{\text{Valence}}$$

Mineral Element	Chemical Symbol	Atomic Weight	Valence
Calcium	Ca	40	2
Chlorine	Cl	35.4	1
Magnesium	Mg	24.3	2
Phosphorus	P	31	2
Potassium	K	39	1
Sodium	Na	23	1
Sulfate	SO_4	96	2
Sulfur	S	32	2

To convert specific weight of sodium to sodium chloride:

Milligrams of Sodium $\times$ 2.54 = Milligrams of Sodium Chloride

To convert specific weight of sodium chloride to sodium:

Milligrams of Sodium Chloride $\times$ 0.393 = Milligrams of Sodium

Sodium (mg)	Sodium (mEq)	Sodium Chloride (g)
500	21.8	1.3
1,000	43.5	2.5
1,500	75.3	3.8
2,000	87.0	5.0

15 / *Approximate Conversions to and from Metric Measures*

Approximate Conversions to Metric Measures

When You Know	Multiply By	To Find
LENGTH		
Inches	2.5	Centimeters
Feet	30	Centimeters
Yards	0.9	Meters
Miles	1.6	Kilometers
AREA		
Square inches	6.5	Square centimeters
Square feet	9.09	Square meters
Square yards	0.8	Square meters
Square miles	2.6	Square kilometers
Acres	0.4	Hectares
MASS (WEIGHT)		
Ounces	28	Grams
Pounds	0.45	Kilograms
Short tons (2,000 lb)	0.9	Metric tons (1,000 kg)
VOLUME		
Teaspoons	5	Milliliters
Tablespoons	15	Milliliters
Fluid ounces	30	Milliliters
Cups	0.24	Liters
Pints	0.47	Liters
Quarts	0.95	Liters
Gallons	3.8	Liters
Cubic feet	0.03	Cubic meters
Cubic yards	0.76	Cubic meters
TEMPERATURE (EXACT)		
Fahrenheit temperature	$\frac{5}{9}$ (after subtracting 32)	Celsius temperature

Approximate Conversions From Metric Measures

When You Know	Multiply By	To Find
LENGTH		
Millimeters	0.04	Inches
Centimeters	0.4	Inches
Meters	3.3	Feet
Meters	1.1	Yards
Kilometers	0.6	Miles
AREA		
Square centimeters	0.16	Square inches
Square meters	1.2	Square yards
Square kilometers	0.4	Square miles
Hectares (10,000 m²)	2.5	Acres
MASS (WEIGHT)		
Grams	0.035	Ounces
Kilograms	2.2	Pounds
Metric tons (1,000 kg)	1.1	Short tons (2,000 lb)
VOLUME		
Milliliters	0.03	Fluid ounces
Liters	2.1	Pints
Liters	1.06	Quarts
Liters	0.26	Gallons
Cubic meters	35	Cubic feet
Cubic meters	1.3	Cubic yards
TEMPERATURE (EXACT)		
Celsius temperature	$\frac{9}{5}$ (then add 32)	Fahrenheit temperature

Prefixes for Metric Units

10^{6}	mega-	M
10^{3}	kilo-	k
10^{-1}	deci-	d
10^{-2}	centi-	c
10^{-3}	milli-	m
10^{-6}	micro-	μ
10^{-9}	nano-	n
10^{-12}	pico-	p

16 / Medical Abbreviations, Prefixes, and Suffixes

AAA—aortic abdominal aneurysm
ABGs—arterial blood gases
ADL—activities of daily living
AIDS—acquired immune deficiency syndrome
ALL—acute lymphoblastic leukemia
ALS—amyotrophic lateral sclerosis
AML—acute myelocytic leukemia
AODM—adult onset diabetes mellitus
AP—angina pectoris
ARC—aids-related complex
ARDS—adult respiratory distress syndrome
ARF—acute renal failure
ASA—aspirin (acetylsalicylic acid)
ASHD—atherosclerotic heart disease
ASO—atherosclerosis obliterans
ATN—acute tubular necrosis
AVM—arteriovenous malformation
BKA—below knee amputation
BMR—basal metabolic rate
BMT—bone marrow transplantation
BPH—benign prostatic hypertrophy
Bx—biopsy
CA—cancer
CAD—coronary artery disease
CAH—chronic active hepatitis; congenital adrenal hyperplasia
CALD—chronic active liver disease
CAPD—continuous ambulatory peritoneal dialysis
CAT—computed axial tomography
CBC—complete blood count
CBD—common bile duct
CC—chief complaint
CCK—cholecystokinin

CCU—coronary care unit
CDE—common duct exploration
CHD—coronary heart disease
CHF—congestive heart failure
CHI—closed head injury
CIIP—chronic idiopathic intestinal obstruction
CMV—chronic cytomegalovirus infection
CNS—central nervous system
C/O—complains of
COPD—chronic obstructive pulmonary disease
CPN—central parenteral nutrition
CRF—chronic renal failure
CSF—cerebrospinal fluid
CT—collagenous/connective tissue (disease)
CVA—cerebral vascular accident
CVI—cerebral vascular insufficiency
CVP—central venous pressure
D&C—dilatation and curettage
D/C—discontinue
DIC—disseminated intravascular coagulopathy
DIP—distal interphalangeal (joint)
DJD—degenerative joint disease
DKA—diabetic ketoacidosis
DM—diabetes mellitus
DOA—dead on arrival
DOE—dyspnea on exertion
DU—duodenal ulcer
DVT—deep vein thrombosis
Dx—diagnosis
ECG, EKG—electrocardiogram
ECT—electric convulsive therapy
EEG—electroencephalogram
EENT—eye, ear, nose, and throat
ERCP—endoscopic retrograde cholangiopancreatography
ESR—erythrocyte sedimentation rate
ESRD—end-stage renal disease
FBG—fasting blood glucose
FBS—fasting blood sugar
FFA—free fatty acid
FTT—failure to thrive
FUO—fever of unknown origin
Fx—fracture
GB—gallbladder
GE—gastroenteritis; gastroenterology
GI—gastrointestinal
GSE—gluten-sensitive enteropathy

GTT—glucose tolerance test
GU—genitourinary
GYN—gynecology
HA—headache
Hb, Hgb—hemoglobin
HBP—high blood pressure
HCM—hypertrophic cardiomyopathy
HEN—home enteral nutrition
HPI—history of present illness
HPN—home parenteral nutrition
HPT—hyperparathyroidism
HTN—hypertension
Hx—history
ICU—intensive care unit
IDA—iron deficiency anemia
IDDM—insulin dependent diabetes mellitus
IHD—ischemic heart disease
IHSS—idiopathic hypertrophic subaortic stenosis
IM—intramuscular
IMP—impression
IPJ—interphalangeal joint
IPPB—intermittent positive pressure breathing
IV—intravenous
IVC—inferior vena cava
J—joule
KUB—kidney, ureter, bladder
LBP—low back pain
LFT—liver function tests
LLQ—left lower quadrant
LMD—local medical doctor
LOC—loss of consciousness
LUQ—left upper quadrant
MCA—middle cerebral artery
MCT—medium-chain triglyceride
MCTD—mixed convertive tissue disease
MI—myocardial infarction; mitral insufficiency
MOM—milk of magnesia
MS—multiple sclerosis; mitral stenosis
MUGA—multiple-graded acquisition study
NAD—no apparent distress
NG—nasogastric
NIDDM—noninsulin dependent diabetes mellitus
NPN—nonprotein nitrogen
NPO—nothing by mouth
NTS—nontropical sprue
N&V—nausea and vomiting

OBS—organic brain syndrome
OHD—organic heart disease
OR—operating room
ORIF—open reduction (surgical alignment) internal fixation
OT—occupational therapy
PA—pulmonary atresia; pernicious anemia
PAME—preanesthesia medical exam
PAN—para-arteritis nodosa
PAT—paroxysmal atrial tachycardia
PBI—protein-bound iodine
PCM—protein calorie malnutrition
PEG—percutaneous endoscopic gastrostomy
PID—pelvic inflammatory disease
PND—paroxysmal nocturnal dyspnea
PNH—paroxysmal nocturnal hemoglobinuria
PPN—peripheral parenteral nutrition
PS—pulmonary stenosis
PSE—portal systemic encephalopathy
Pt—patient
PT—physical therapy; prothrombin time
PTA—prior to admission
PTCA—percutaneous transluminal coronary angiography
PTT—partial thromboplastin time
PVC—premature ventricular contractions
PVD—peripheral vascular disease
PU—peptic ulcer
RE—reticuloendothelial system
REE—resting energy expenditure
RHD—rheumatic heart disease
RIND—reversible ischemic neurological deficit
RLQ—right lower quadrant
R/O—rule out
RōRx—radiation therapy
ROS—review of systems
RUQ—right upper quadrant
SAH—subarachnoid hemorrhage
SBE—subacute bacterial endocarditis
SBO—small bowel obstruction
SCI—spinal cord injury
SCUF—slow continuous ultrafiltration
SIADH—syndrome of inappropriate antidiuretic hormone
SLE—systemic lupus erythematosis
SMAS—superior mesenteric artery syndrome
SOB—shortness of breath
S/P—status postop
STA—superior temporal artery

STSG—split-thickness skin graft
SVC obst—superior vena cava obstruction
Sx—symptoms
T&A—tonsillectomy and adenoidectomy
TCE—transitional cell epithelioma
TE—tracheoesophageal fistula
TG—triglycerides
THA—total hip arthroplasty
THC—transhepatic cholangiogram
TI—tricuspid insufficiency
TIA—transient ischemic attacks
TKA—total knee arthroplasty
TLA—translumbar aortogram
TPN—total parenteral nutrition
TUR—transurethral resection
U/A—urinary analysis
UGI—upper gastrointestinal
URI—upper respiratory infection
UTI—urinary tract infection
V&P—vagotomy and pyloroplasty
VH—vaginal hysterectomy
VIP—vasoactive intestinal peptides
VS—vital signs
WDHA—watery diarrhea, hypokalemia, achlorhydria (pancreatic chlorea)
WNL—within normal limits
ZE—Zollinger-Ellison (syndrome)

Other Abbreviations

Abbreviation	Derivation	Meaning
aa	ana	of each
ac	ante cibum	before meals
ad lib	ad libitum	as needed or desired
alt dieb	alternis diebus	every other day
alt hor	alternis horis	every other hour
alt noc	alternis noctibus	every other night
bid	bis in die	twice a day
c	cum	with
contin	continuetur	let it be continued
dil	dilutus	dilute
div	divide	divide
fl	fluidus	fluid
h	hora	hour
hd	hora decubitus	at bedtime
hs	hora somni	at sleeping time
m et n	mane et nocte	morning and night
nb	nota bene	note well
od	omni die	daily
om	omni mane	every morning
on	omni nocte	every night
part vic	partibus vicibus	in divided doses
pc	post cibum	after food
prn	pro re nata	as required
pulv	pulvis	powder
qd	quaque die	every day
qh	quaque hora	every hour
q2h	quaque secunda hora	every 2 hours
q3h	quaque tertia hora	every 3 hours
qid	quater in die	4 times a day
qs	quantum sufficit	as much as is sufficient
Rx	recipe	take
S or sig	signa	give the following directions
s	sine	without
sos	si opus sit	if necessary
ss	semis	one-half
stat	statim	at once
tid	ter in die	3 times a day

Common Prefixes

Prefix	Meaning
a- or an-	without
cardi-	heart
chol-	bile
col-	colon
cyst-	bladder
enter-	intestine
gastr-	stomach
hepat-	liver
hydr-	water
hyper-	too much
hypo-	too little
myel-	marrow
nephr-	kidney
neur-	nerve
oste-	bone
poly-	many
proct-	anus, rectum
pseud-	false
pulm-	lung
pyel-	pelvis

Common Suffixes

Suffix	Meaning
-algia	pain
-clysis	drenching
-cyte	cell
-ectomy	excision
-emia	presence in blood (usually implies excess)
-genic or -genesis	formation
-gnosis	knowledge
-itis	inflammation
-lytic or -lysis	destruction
-malacia	softening
-opia	vision
-pathy	disease of
-phagia	eating
-phobia	fear of
-pnea	breath
-privia or -penia	poverty of: without
-ptosis	fallen
-sclerosis	hardening
-scopy	inspection
-stenosis	narrowing
-stomy	mouth (new opening)
-tomy	cutting operation
-trophy	nutrition or growth
-uria	urine

17 / *Cholesterol, Triglyceride, and Lipoprotein Levels in the United States*

U.S. Male Serum Total Cholesterol Levels (mg/dl)*

Age (yr)	Overall Mean	Percentiles						
		5	10	25	50	75	90	95
0–4	159	117	129	141	156	176	192	209
5–9	165	125	134	147	164	180	197	209
10–14	162	123	131	144	160	178	196	208
15–19	154	116	124	136	150	170	188	203
20–24	172	128	134	150	170	189	210	225
25–29	188	137	147	164	183	208	224	251
30–34	198	142	152	172	196	219	246	262
35–39	207	150	162	181	203	230	257	278
40–44	213	156	168	187	209	235	258	276
45–49	219	163	174	194	216	241	266	284
50–54	219	163	174	193	216	242	269	285
55–59	220	161	172	195	218	242	270	284
60–64	219	164	176	194	216	242	267	284
65–69	219	163	175	196	216	240	266	282
70+	213	156	167	187	211	236	260	278

*All values have been converted from plasma to serum (Plasma Value × 1.03 = Serum Value).

From The Lipid Research Clinics population studies data book, Vol 1: The prevalence study. NIH Publication No. 80-1527. U.S. Department of Health and Human Services, Public Health Service, July 1980.

U.S. Female Serum Total Cholesterol Levels (mg/dl)*

Age (yr)	Overall Mean	Percentiles						
		5	10	25	50	75	90	95
0–4	161	115	124	143	161	177	195	206
5–9	169	130	138	150	168	184	201	211
10–14	164	128	135	148	163	179	196	207
15–19	162	124	131	144	160	177	197	209
20–24	177	129	138	153	175	196	220	235
25–29	181	134	144	160	178	199	223	236
30–34	184	135	145	163	181	202	229	245
35–39	192	145	152	169	189	211	235	252
40–44	201	151	160	176	198	222	244	261
45–49	211	157	166	183	207	233	259	276
50–54	224	168	178	198	222	247	274	294
55–59	233	174	186	206	230	255	284	303
60–64	235	178	189	208	223	260	286	305
65–69	237	176	189	211	233	260	285	306
70+	233	172	186	205	231	259	284	297

U.S. Male Serum Triglyceride Levels (mg/dl)*

Age (yr)	Overall Mean	Percentiles						
		5	10	25	50	75	90	95
0–4	58	30	34	41	53	69	87	102
5–9	30	31	34	41	53	67	88	104
10–14	68	33	38	46	61	80	105	129
15–19	80	38	44	56	71	94	124	152
20–24	103	45	52	65	89	123	170	207
25–29	120	47	56	72	98	140	205	257
30–34	132	52	60	77	107	153	219	274
35–39	149	56	64	83	116	175	259	331
40–44	156	57	66	89	126	179	255	330
45–49	156	60	70	92	128	179	261	337
50–54	156	60	70	90	128	185	258	330
55–59	146	60	69	90	123	175	242	266
60–64	147	60	70	90	123	174	242	300
65–69	141	59	66	85	115	153	214	275
70+	134	60	69	85	114	153	218	266

*All values have been converted from plasma to serum (Plasma Value × 1.03 = Serum Value).

From The Lipid Research Clinics population studies data book, Vol 1: The prevalence study. NIH Publication No. 80-1527. U.S. Department of Health and Human Services, Public Health Service, July 1980.

U.S. Female Serum Triglyceride Levels (mg/dl)*

Age (yr)	Overall Mean	Percentiles						
		5	10	25	50	75	90	95
0–4	66	35	39	46	61	79	99	115
5–9	30	33	37	45	57	73	93	108
10–14	78	38	45	56	72	93	117	135
15–19	78	40	45	55	70	90	117	136
20–24	92	41	48	62	83	111	145	170
25–29	91	41	47	60	80	110	146	177
30–34	91	42	47	60	78	109	150	181
35–39	97	42	48	62	82	116	165	200
40–44	108	48	56	67	91	126	175	215
45–49	115	48	56	71	97	136	190	235
50–54	124	56	63	79	104	145	198	245
55–59	129	58	60	83	111	152	209	265
60–64	130	59	66	83	111	152	207	247
65–69	135	62	68	85	115	162	209	248
70+	135	62	71	88	114	155	209	242

U.S. Male Serum High-Density Lipoprotein Levels (mg/dl)*

Age (yr)	Overall Mean	Percentiles						
		5	10	25	50	75	90	95
5–9	57	39	43	50	56	65	72	76
10–14	57	38	41	47	57	63	73	76
15–19	48	31	35	40	47	54	61	65
20–24	47	31	33	39	46	53	59	65
25–29	46	32	33	38	45	52	60	65
30–34	47	29	33	39	46	54	61	65
35–39	45	30	32	37	44	50	60	64
40–44	46	28	32	37	44	53	62	69
45–49	47	31	34	39	46	54	62	66
50–54	45	29	32	37	45	53	60	65
55–59	49	29	32	39	47	57	66	73
60–64	53	31	35	42	50	63	71	76
65–69	53	31	34	40	50	64	76	80
70+	52	32	34	41	49	58	72	77

*All values have been converted from plasma to serum (Plasma Value × 1.03 = Serum Value).

From The Lipid Research Clinics population studies data book, Vol 1: The prevalence study. NIH Publication No. 80-1527. U.S. Department of Health and Human Services, Public Health Service, July 1980.

U.S. Female Serum High-Density Lipoprotein Levels (mg/dl)*

Age (yr)	Overall Mean	Percentiles						
		5	10	25	50	75	90	95
5–9	57	39	43	50	56	65	72	76
10–14	57	38	41	47	57	63	73	76
15–19	48	31	35	40	47	54	61	65
20–24	55	34	38	45	53	64	74	81
25–29	58	38	40	48	57	65	76	85
30–34	58	37	41	47	57	66	75	79
35–39	57	35	39	45	55	66	76	84
40–44	60	35	40	49	58	67	81	91
45–49	61	35	42	48	60	70	84	90
50–54	64	38	42	52	64	73	87	95
55–59	64	38	42	52	62	75	88	94
60–64	66	39	45	53	63	77	90	95
65–69	65	36	39	50	64	75	88	101
70+	63	34	39	49	62	73	84	95

U.S. Male Serum Low-Density Lipoprotein Cholesterol Levels (mg/dl)*

Age (yr)	Overall Mean	Percentiles						
		5	10	25	50	75	90	95
5–9	95	65	71	82	93	106	121	133
10–14	99	66	74	83	97	112	126	136
15–19	97	64	70	82	96	112	127	134
20–24	106	68	75	88	104	122	142	151
25–29	120	72	77	99	119	142	162	170
30–34	130	80	91	110	128	148	171	191
35–39	137	83	95	113	135	159	181	195
40–44	140	90	101	118	139	162	178	192
45–49	148	101	109	124	145	168	192	208
50–54	147	92	105	122	147	167	191	203
55–59	150	91	106	127	149	173	197	209
60–64	151	85	109	125	147	170	194	216
65–69	155	101	107	129	150	175	205	216
70+	147	91	103	123	146	169	187	192

*All values have been converted from plasma to serum (Plasma Value × 1.03 = Serum Value).

From The Lipid Research Clinics population studies data book, Vol 1: The prevalence study. NIH Publication No. 80-1527. U.S. Department of Health and Human Services, Public Health Service, July 1980.

U.S. Female Serum Low-Density Lipoprotein Cholesterol Levels (mg/dl)*

Age (yr)	Overall Mean	Percentiles						
		5	10	25	50	75	90	95
5–9	103	70	75	91	101	118	129	144
10–14	100	70	75	83	97	113	130	140
15–19	99	61	67	80	96	114	133	141
20–24	107	59	67	84	105	122	145	164
25–29	114	73	77	93	111	130	152	169
30–34	115	72	79	94	112	132	151	161
35–39	123	77	83	99	119	143	166	177
40–44	129	76	87	107	126	150	170	179
45–49	133	81	92	108	131	155	178	192
50–54	142	91	97	114	138	165	192	207
55–59	150	92	100	124	149	173	205	216
60–64	157	103	108	130	153	173	197	231
65–69	158	95	102	129	156	190	211	228
70+	153	99	111	131	151	175	195	212

*All values have been converted from plasma to serum (Plasma Value $\times$ 1.03 = Serum Value).

From The Lipid Research Clinics population studies data book, Vol 1: The prevalence study. NIH Publication No. 80-1527. U.S. Department of Health and Human Services, Public Health Service, July 1980.

18 / *The Scope of Practice for Diabetes Educators and the Standards of Practice for Diabetes Educators*

Developed under the algis of a multidisciplinary task force of the American Association of Diabetes Educators.

The American Association of Diabetes Educators is a professional organization dedicated to enhancing the competence of health professionals who teach people with diabetes, advancing the specialty practice of diabetes education, and improving the quality of diabetes education and care. In keeping with this mission, a multidisciplinary task force of health professionals has developed a Scope of Practice for Diabetes Educators and a Standards of Practice for Diabetes Educators. These guidelines will not only foster high professional standards for those who teach people with diabetes, but will also provide a consistent point of reference for developing evaluation tools, quality assurance programs, orientation procedures, and professional appraisal systems.

The American Association of Diabetes Educators (AADE) was established in 1974 as a multidisciplinary organization of health professionals who teach people with diabetes. Since then the Association has achieved many milestones in the professional specialty, including the development of a Certification Program for Diabetes Educators, a Core Curriculum for Diabetes Education, and accreditation as a provider and approver of continuing education in nursing.

MISSION OF THE ASSOCIATION

As a professional organization, AADE has a responsibility to foster high professional standards of diabetes education and practice, and to identify for the consumer competencies and excellence in practice. The Association's purpose is embodied in the following mission statement adopted by the AADE Board of Directors:

The American Association of Diabetes Educators is dedicated to enhancing the competence of health professionals who teach people with diabetes, advancing the specialty practice of diabetes education, and improving the quality of diabetes education and care for all those affected by diabetes.

---

*Developed under the aegis of a multidisciplinary task force of the American Association of Diabetes Educators. Reprinted with permission from the American Association of Diabetes Educators, 400 North Michigan Avenue, Suite 1240, Chicago, IL 60611.

In keeping with this mission, the AADE has developed the Scope of Practice for Diabetes Educators and the Standards of Practice for Diabetes Educators to provide guidelines for achieving excellence and improving the quality of diabetes patient education and care.

These documents represent the combined expertise and experience of a multidisciplinary task force of health professionals involved in diabetes education and an extensive review process embracing a broad spectrum of practice areas. Together the Scope of Practice and the Standards of Practice provide a framework for health professionals who teach people with diabetes.

By also providing a consistent point of reference, the Standards of Practice may be used as the basis for the development of evaluation tools, quality assurance programs, orientation procedures, and performance appraisal systems. Additionally they support the specialty by

- Stimulating the process of peer review
- Promoting documentation of the benefits and outcomes of the diabetes education experience
- Encouraging research to validate practice and lead toward improved quality of patient education

The Scope of Practice for Diabetes Educators and the Standards of Practice for Diabetes Educators are designed to complement the National Standards and Recognition for Diabetes Patient Education Programs, the Core Curriculum for Diabetes Patient Education, and the Certification Program for Diabetes Educators. Thus these documents will further enhance and promote quality diabetes education for people with diabetes.

DEVELOPMENT OF THE DOCUMENTS

The Scope of Practice for Diabetes Educators and the Standards of Practice for Diabetes Educators were developed by a specially appointed multidisciplinary task force of the American Association of Diabetes Educators. The following members were selected for their expertise, professional discipline, and geographical location to gain a broad representation of perspectives and practices.

Chairs:	Darlene Paduano, MSN, RN, CDE (Standards)
	Elizabeth Walker, RN, DNSc, CDE (Scope)
Members:	Karmeen Kulkarni, MS, RD, CDE
	Eileen Otsuji, PharmD, CDE
	Sue Thom, RD, LD, CDE
Executive liaison:	Jean Betschart, MN, RN, CDE

Special thanks and acknowledgement are owed to the following individuals who also provided input and review:

Robert Anderson, EdD
Rosanna Baicich, MS, RD, CDE
Betty Brackenridge, MS, RD, CDE
Marjorie Cypress, RN, C-ANP, CDE
Judy Davis, RN, CDE

Liz DeShetler, RD, CDE
Kathryn Godley, RN, MS, CDE
Linda Haas, MN, RN, CDE
Marilyn Hergert, RN, MSN, CDE
Deborah Hinnen, RN, MN, CDE
Sharon Johnson, RN, MS, CDE
Phyllis Jones, RN, PhD
Sandra Knott, RN-C, MA, CDE
Theresa Lovett, RN, CDE
Jan Luckenbill, RN, CDE
Jane Morton, RD, CDE
Robert Ratner, MD, CDE
Rita Schluneger, RN, CDE
Rita Saltiel, RN, MPH, CDE
Sue Thom, RD, LD, CDE
Hope Warshaw, MMSc, RD, CDE
Review and comments were also provided by AADE Boards of Directors from 1988 through 1991.

SCOPE OF PRACTICE FOR DIABETES EDUCATORS

Purpose

The American Association of Diabetes Educators developed this Scope of Practice to delineate: (1) selected beliefs and definitions related to the practice of diabetes education, and (2) the dimensions of this practice in relation to other components of care for persons with diabetes, their families, and appropriate support systems. This Scope of Practice describes the present practice of diabetes education of multidisciplinary health care professionals.

Beliefs and Definitions

Living well with diabetes requires a positive psychosocial adaptation to, and the effective self-management of, the disease. To achieve effective self-management of diabetes mellitus, a patient must learn the body of knowledge, attitudes, and self-management skills related to the control of this chronic disease. *Diabetes education* is defined as the teaching and the learning of this body of knowledge and skills, with the ultimate goal being to promote the behavior changes necessary for optimal health outcomes, psychosocial adaptation, and quality of life. This planned educational experience is most effectively provided by qualified diabetes educators. Diabetes education is considered a therapeutic modality, and it is integral to the care of these patients.

A *diabetes educator* is defined as a health care professional who has mastered the core of knowledge and skill in the biological and social sciences, communication and counseling, and education, and who has experience in the care of patients with diabetes. The role of the diabetes educator can be assumed by various health care professionals, including but not limited to: registered dietitians, registered nurses, physicians, pharmacists, social workers, podiatrists, and exercise physiologists. A goal for all diabetes educators should be to meet the academic, professional, and experiential requirements to become a certified diabetes educator (CDE).

Dimensions of Practice

The role of the diabetes educator is multidimensional, with boundaries for accountability that interface with other members of the health care team. This role involves the education of patients, their families, and appropriate support systems, as well as other health care professionals who do not specialize in diabetes management, and the public. While a multidisciplinary team approach is the preferred delivery system for diabetes education, this specialty practice can occur successfully in a wide variety of settings and formats.

The primary area of responsibility for diabetes educators is the education of patients, their families, and appropriate support systems about diabetes self-management and related issues. The content of this educational experience should include, but not be limited to, the following topics:

- Pathophysiology of diabetes mellitus
- Nutrition management and diet
- Pharmacologic interventions
- Exercise and activity
- Self-monitoring for glycemic control
- Prevention and management of acute and chronic complications
- Psychosocial adjustment
- Problem-solving skills
- Stress management
- Use of the health care delivery system

The diabetes educator should present the necessary information, using established principles of teaching-learning theory and life-style counseling. The instruction is individualized for persons of all ages, incorporating their cultural preferences, health beliefs, and preferred learning styles, when feasible. The diabetes educator should perform the following:

- Assessment of educational needs
- Planning of the teaching-learning process
- Implementation of the educational plan
- Documentation of the process
- Evaluation based on outcome criteria

The Scope of Practice of a diabetes educator *should intersect* with the practice of other members of the health care team. The diabetes educator should appreciate the impact of acute or chronic problems on patients' health behaviors and on the teaching-learning process. Such appreciation is essential for the development of a comprehensive plan for continuing education and cost-effective, managed care.

Members of the various health care professions who practice diabetes education bring their particular focus to the educational process. This phenomenon widens or narrows the Scope of Practice for the individual educators, as is appropriate within the boundaries of each health profession, which may be regulated by national or state agencies or accrediting bodies. Other roles for the diabetes educator may involve consultation with other health care providers or agencies and research in diabetes management and education.

Diabetes education occurs in a variety of settings, depending on the needs of the patient, the practice of the educator, and the local environment. Inpatient and outpatient settings, as well as home settings, are used effectively for both individual and group education. Diabetes education should be a planned, individualized, and evaluated activity wherever it occurs.

Summary

This Scope of Practice incorporates definitions of *diabetes educator* and *diabetes education,* while providing statements of beliefs regarding the educational process inherent in this practice. The scope of practice of a diabetes educator has changing dimensions because of the multidisciplinary nature of the health care professionals who provide it. The primary role of a diabetes educator is to provide an educational experience for patients, their families, and appropriate support systems to learn the effective management of diabetes. Thus Scope of Practice delineates the multifaceted role and responsibilities of the health care professional who engages in this teaching-learning process. This Scope of Practice does not constitute an exhaustive description of diabetes education as a specialty practice because there are various interpretations of the role of the diabetes educator in a health care team.

STANDARDS OF PRACTICE FOR DIABETES EDUCATORS

Purpose

This document has been developed by the American Association of Diabetes Educators to: (1) provide standards for a nationally acceptable level of practice for diabetes educators; and (2) assure quality in the professional practice of diabetes education. The individual diabetes educator is responsible for adhering to these Standards.

The Standards of Practice will provide:

1. Diabetes educators with
   - direction to assess and improve the quality of diabetes education services provided
   - a framework within which to practice
2. Patients with
   - a means of assessing the quality of diabetes education services provided
   - a basis for forming expectations of the diabetes education experience
3. Health care professionals who do not specialize in diabetes management with a means of
   - understanding the role of the diabetes educator
   - assessing the quality of diabetes education services provided
   - understanding diabetes education as an integral component of diabetes patient care

4. Insurers, government agencies, industry, and the general public with
   - a description of the specialized educational services provided by a diabetes educator
   - information about the benefits of diabetes education in developing self-management skills
   - an awareness of the importance of diabetes education in improving the quality of life for persons with diabetes

Standards of Education

Standard I. Assessment

The diabetes educator should conduct a thorough, individualized needs assessment with the participation of the patient, family, or support systems, when appropriate, prior to the development of the education plan and intervention.

Practice Guidelines

The needs assessment should include information from the patient on the following:

1. Health history
2. Medical history
3. Previous use of medication
4. Diet history
5. Current mental health status
6. Use of health care delivery systems
7. Life-style practices such as occupation, vocation, education, financial status, social, cultural, and religious practices
8. Physical and psychological factors including age, mobility, visual acuity, hearing, manual dexterity, alertness, attention span, and ability to concentrate
9. Barriers to learning such as education, literacy levels, perceived learning needs, motivation to learn, and attitudes
10. Family and social supports
11. Previous diabetes education, actual knowledge, and skills

Standard II. Use of Resources

The diabetes educator should strive to create an educational setting conducive to learning, with adequate resources to facilitate the learning process.

Practice Guidelines

Appropriate resources for effective teaching should include:

1. A teaching environment that
   a. provides privacy, safety, and accessibility
   b. includes ample teaching and storage space, adequate furniture, lighting, and ventilation
2. A variety of teaching materials and audiovisual teaching aids to meet the individual patient's needs
3. Adequate staffing for the needs of the patient population

Standard III. Planning

The written educational plan should be developed from information obtained from the needs assessment and based on the components of the educational process: assessment, planning, implementation, and evaluation. The plan is coordinated among diabetes health team members, including the patient with diabetes, family, and support system.

Practice Guidelines

The written educational plan should include the following:

1. Goals of the educational intervention
2. Measurable, behaviorally stated learner objectives
3. Content outline
4. Instructional methods, including discussion, demonstration, role playing, simulations
5. Learner outcomes based on the evaluation process

Standard IV. Implementation

The diabetes educator should provide individualized education based on a progression from basic survival skills to advanced information for daily self-management.

Practice Guidelines

Considerations in developing the individualized education plan should include:

1. The need for diabetes education to be lifelong because of the chronicity of the condition
2. The need for a dynamic education plan that will reflect the inevitable changes in life-style
3. Survival skills that include safe practices of medication administration, meal planning, self-monitoring for glycemic control, and recognition of when to access professional assistance for emergencies
4. Advanced information for daily self-management practices that may include prevention and management of chronic complications, problem-solving skills, exercise, psychosocial adjustment, stress management, and travel situations

Standard V. Documentation

The diabetes educator should completely and accurately document the educational experience.

Practice Guidelines

Accurate documentation:

1. Establishes a record to substantiate the provision of education
2. Contributes information for retrospective, concurrent, and prospective reviews
3. Provides data for scientific and economic analysis
4. Serves as a resource for continuity of care
5. Aids in planning subsequent education

Standard VI. Evaluation and Outcome

The diabetes educator should participate in at least an annual review of the quality and outcome of the education process.

Practice Guidelines

Evaluation of the diabetes education process should:

1. Occur periodically and as part of a comprehensive quality assurance program
2. Be consistent with the National Standards for Diabetes Patient Education Programs as established by the National Diabetes Advisory Board

3. Determine the impact of education on patients, institutions, and the community
4. Use outcome measures such as:
    a. cost effectiveness
    b. changes in use of health care delivery systems, e.g., emergency room visits, hospital length of stay
    c. changes in knowledge and attitudes
    d. changes in physiological measures, e.g., glycosylated hemoglobin values, weight

Standards of Professional Practice

Standard VII. Multidisciplinary Collaboration

The diabetes educator should collaborate with the multidisciplinary team of health care professionals and integrate their knowledge and skills to provide a comprehensive educational experience.

Practice Guidelines

The multidisciplinary education team should:
1. Include, but not be limited to, the registered nurse, registered dietitian, physician, pharmacist, social worker, psychologist, exercise physiologist, and podiatrist
2. Observe professional practice boundaries in light of each member's discipline
3. Have a responsibility to:
    a. share with team members information from individual patient assessments
    b. prioritize learning needs
    c. make education relevant to medical management
    d. promote delivery of consistent information from various team members to patients
    e. hold patient management conferences on a regular basis
    f. provide referrals for appropriate follow-up

Standard VIII. Professional Development

The diabetes educator should assume responsibility for professional development and pursue continuing education to acquire current knowledge and skills.

Practice Guidelines

The diabetes educator should:
1. Incorporate into practice the generally accepted new techniques and knowledge acquired through continuing education
2. Deliver education based on a continuous process of review and evaluation of scientific theory, clinical and educational research
3. Pursue professional education based on progression from basic through advanced curriculum
4. Strive to meet the academic, professional, and experiential requirement to become a certified diabetes educator (CDE)

Standard IX. Professional Accountability

The diabetes educator should accept responsibility for self-assessment of performance and peer review to assure the delivery of high quality diabetes education.

Practice Guidelines

The diabetes educator should:

1. Participate in an annual systematic review and evaluation of practice
2. Incorporate into practice the appropriate changes based on the results of self-evaluation, peer review, and patients' evaluations

Standard X. Ethics

The diabetes educator should respect and uphold the basic human rights of all persons.

Practice Guidelines

The diabetes educator should:

1. Maintain confidentiality of appropriate information, and allow freedom of expression, decision making, and action
2. Demonstrate concern for personal dignity
3. Consider that a person with diabetes balances many daily tasks for management which may require a gradual incorporation into life-style
4. Appreciate the impact of diabetes management on daily living so that reasonable expectations are established with the patient
5. Display honesty, warmth, and openness to reinforce positive behavior change

Bibliography

American Diabetes Association. Standards of medical care for patients with diabetes mellitus. Diabetes Care 1991;14(suppl 2):10–13.

American Nurses' Association and Association of Rehabilitation Nurses. Standards of rehabilitative nursing practice. Kansas City, MO: American Nurses' Association, 1986.

Bartlett E. At last a definition of patient education [Editorial]. Patient Educ Couns 1985;7:323-324.

Beebe CA. Self-monitoring of blood glucose: an adjunct to dietary and insulin management of the patient with diabetes. J Am Diet Assoc 1987;87:61–65.

Brookfield SD. Understanding and facilitating adult learning. San Francisco: Jossey-Bass, 1986.

Dunst C, Trivette C, Deal A. Enabling and empowering families: principles and guidelines for practice. Cambridge, MA: Brookline Books, 1988.

Green LW, Kreuter MW. Health promotion planning: an educational and environmental approach. 2d ed. Mountain View, CA: Mayfield Publishing Co, 1991.

Guthrie DW, ed. Diabetes education: a core curriculum for health professionals. Chicago: American Association of Diabetes Educators, 1988.

National Coalition for Recognition of Diabetes Patient Education Programs. Self-study and application handbook. Rockville, MD: NACOR, 1986.

Powers, MA, ed. Nutrition guide for professionals: diabetes education and meal planning. Alexandria, VA/Chicago: American Diabetes Association/American Dietetic Association, 1987.

Redman BK. The process of patient education. 6th ed. St. Louis: CV Mosby, 1988.

Van Hoozer HL. The teaching process: theory and practice in nursing. East Norwalk, CT: Appleton & Lange, 1987.

19 / *Position Papers of The American Dietetic Association*

The following is a listing of position papers of The American Dietetic Association current at the time of publication of this manual.

- The position of the ADA on a national nutrition policy. JADA 1980;76:596–597. (Reaffirmed)
- Promotion of breast feeding. JADA 1993;93:467–469. (Expires in 1996)
- Issues in feeding the terminally ill adult. JADA 1992;92:996. (Expires in 1996 with update of cases in 1994)
- Child nutrition services. JADA 1993;93:334–336. (Expires in 1996)
- Nutrition, aging, and the continuum of health care. JADA 1993;93:80–82. (Expires in 1996).
- Nutrition standards in day care programs for children. JADA 1987;87:503–506. (Reaffirmed)
- Nutrition—essential component of medical education. JADA 1987;87:642–643. (Reaffirmed)
- Nutrition for physical fitness and athletic performance for adults. JADA 1993; 93:691–696. (Reaffirmed; expires 1998)
- Nutrition services in health maintenance organizations and other forms of managed care. JADA 1993;93:1171–1172. (Expires 1997)
- Use of nutritive and non-nutritive sweeteners. JADA 1993;93:816–821.
- Nutrition intervention in the treatment of anorexia nervosa and bulimia. JADA 1988;88:68. (Reaffirmed)
- Health implications of dietary fiber. JADA 1993;93:1446–1447. (Expires in 1997)
- Vegetarian diets. JADA 1993;93:1317–1319. (Expires 1997)
- Identifying food and nutrition misinformation. JADA 1988;88;1589-1591. (Reaffirmed)
- Nutrition management of adolescent pregnancy. JADA 1989;89:104. (Reaffirmed)
- Nutritional monitoring of the home parenteral and enteral patient. JADA 1989;89:263–265. (Reaffirmed)
- Nutritional intervention in the treatment of human immunodeficiency virus infections. JADA 1989;89:839–841. (Reaffirmed)
- The impact of fluoride on dental health. JADA 1989;89:971–974. (Expires in 1994)
- Nutrition services for children with special health care needs. JADA 1989;89:1133–1137. (Expires in 1994)

- Optimal weight as a health promotion strategy. JADA 1989;89:1814–1817. (Expires in 1994)
- Nutrition education for the public. JADA 1990;90:107–110. (Expires in 1994)
- Nutrition and health information on food labels. J Am Diet Assoc. 1990;90:583–585. (Expires in 1995)
- Very-low-calorie weight loss diets. JADA 1990;90:722–726. (Expires in 1994)
- Nutrition intervention in the treatment and recovery from chemical dependency. JADA 1990;90:1274–1277. (Expires in 1995)
- Domestic hunger and inadequate access to food. JADA 1990;90:1437–1441. (Expires in 1995)
- Nutrition in food service establishments. JADA 1991;91:480–482. (Expires 1996)
- Nutrition education of health professionals. JADA 1991;91:611–613. (Expires in 1995)
- Competitive foods in schools. JADA 1991;91:1123–1125. (Expires in 1996)
- Fat replacements. JADA. 1991;91:1285–1288. (Expires in 1996)
- The role of the registered dietitian in enteral and parenteral nutrition support. JADA 1991;91:1440–1441. (Expires in 1996)
- Affordable and accessible health care services. JADA 1992;92:746. (Expires in 1996)
- Nutrition in comprehensive program planning for persons with developmental disabilities. JADA 1992;92:613. (Expires in 1996)
- Management of health care food and nutrition services. 1993;93:914–915. (Expires in 1997)
- Biotechnology and the future of food. JADA 1993;93:189–194. (Expires in 1997)
- Environmental issues. JADA 1993;93:589–591. (Expires in 1996)
- Appropriate use of nutritive and non-nutritive sweeteners. JADA 1993;93:816–821. (Expires in 1997)

Currently, ADA has 36 position papers. For more information about ADA position papers, call (800) 877-1600, ext 4896.

20 / *Multiple Vitamin Preparations*

					Vitamins					
	A (IU)	D (IU)	E (IU)	K (µg)	C (mg)	FA (µg)	B$_1$ (mg)	B$_2$ (mg)	B$_6$ (mg)	Niacin (mg)
Adult MVI-12 Injection (10 ml, Armour)	3,300	200	10	—	100	400	3	3.6	4	40
Peds IV MV's (5 ml, Armour)	2,300	400	7	200	80	140	1.2	1.4	1.0	17
Centrum Liquid (15 ml, Lederle)	2,500	400	30	—	60	—	1.5	1.7	2	20
Theragran Liquid (5 ml, Squibb)	10,000	400	—	—	200	—	10	10	4.1	100
Vi-Daylin Liquid (5 ml, Ross)	2,500	400	15	—	60	—	1.05	1.2	1.05	13.5
Tri-Vi-Sol Drops (1 ml, Mead Johnson Nutritional)	1,500	400	—	—	35	—	—	—	—	—
Poly-Vi-Sol Drops 1 ml, Mead Johnson Nutritional)	1,500	400	5	—	35	—	0.5	0.6	0.4	8
Poly-Vi-Sol + Fe Drops (1 ml, Mead Johnson Nutritional)	1,500	400	5	—	35	—	0.5	0.6	0.4	8
Vi-Daylin Drops (1 ml, Ross)	1,500	400	4.1	—	35	—	0.5	0.6	0.4	8
Vi-Daylin + Fe Drops (1 ml, Ross)	1,500	400	4.1	—	35	—	0.5	0.6	0.4	8
Flintstones (Chewable, Miles)	2,500	400	15	—	60	300	1.05	1.2	1.05	13.5
Flintstones + Iron (Chewable, Miles)	2,500	400	15	—	60	300	1.05	1.2	1.05	13.5
Poly-Vi-Sol (Chewable, Mead Johnson Nutritional)	2,500	400	15	—	60	300	1.05	1.2	1.05	13.5
Poly-Vi-Sol + Iron (Chewable, Mead Johnson Nutritional)	2,500	400	15	—	60	300	1.05	1.2	1.05	13.5

| Vitamins | | | Minerals | | | | | | | | |
B$_{12}$ (μg)	PA (mg)	Biotin (μg)	Fe (mg)	I (μg)	Zn (mg)	Cu (mg)	Mn (mg)	Cr (μg)	Se (μg)	Mo (μg)	Other
5	15	60									
1	5	20									
6	10	300	9	150	3	—	2.5	25	—	25	
5	21.4	—	—	—	—	—	—	—	—	—	
4.5	—	—	—	—	—	—	—	—	—	—	
—	—	—	10								
2	—	—									
—	—	—	10								
1.5	—	—									
—	—	—	10								
4.5	—	—									
4.5	—	—	15								
4.5	—	—									
4.5	—	—	12								

Continued.

	Vitamins									
	A (IU)	D (IU)	E (IU)	K (μg)	C (mg)	FA (μg)	B$_1$ (mg)	B$_2$ (mg)	B$_6$ (mg)	Niacin (mg)
Theragran-M (Tablet, Squibb)	5,000	400	30	—	90	400	3.0	3.4	3.0	20
Centrum (Tablet, Lederle)	5,000	400	30	2.5	60	400	1.5	1.7	2.0	20
One-A-Day Essential (Tablet, Miles)	5,000	400	30	—	60	400	1.5	1.7	2.0	20
Theragran (Tablet, Squibb)	5,000	400	30	—	90	400	3	3.4	3	30
Nephro Vite (Tablet, R and D Laboratories)	—	—	—	—	60	800	10	1.7	10	20
Materna (Tablet, Lederle)	5,000	400	30	—	100	1,000	3	3.4	10	20

Vitamins			Minerals								Other
B_{12} (µg)	PA (mg)	Biotin (µg)	Fe (mg)	I (µg)	Zn (mg)	Cu (mg)	Mn (mg)	Cr (µg)	Se (µg)	Mo (µg)	
9.0	10	35	27	150	15	2.0	5.0	15	10	15	400 mg Ca 31 mg P 100 mg Mg 7.5 mg Cl 7.5 mg K
6.0	10	30	18	150	15	2.0	2.5	25	20	25	162 mg Ca 109 mg P 100 mg Mg 40 mg K 36 mg Cl 5 µg Ni 10 µg Tn 20 mg Si 10 µg V 150 µg B
6.0	10	—									—
9	10	35									1,250 IU beta carotene
6	10	300	—	—	—	—	—	—	—	—	—
12	10	30	60	150	25	2.0	5.0	25	—	25	250 mg Ca 25 mg Mg

Vitamin Sources, Functions, Deficiency, and Toxic Effects

Fat-Soluble Vitamins	U.S. RDA for Adults and Children ≥ 4 Yr	Significant Sources	Major Functions	Deficiency Conditions	Toxicity Symptoms
Vitamin A	5,000 IU	Liver, whole milk or fortified dairy products, eggs, carrots, dark leafy vegetables, dark yellow squashes, sweet potato, pumpkin	Essential for vision, growth, reproduction Assists formation and maintenance of skin mucous membranes; thus increases resistance to infection	Mild: night blindness, hyperkeratosis Severe: xerophthalmia, keratomalacia	Level: Children: >20,000 IU daily Adults: >50,000 IU daily Mild: headache, prolonged vomiting, diplopia, liver damage, hair loss, dermal Severe: spontaneous abortions, birth defects
Vitamin D	400 IU	Fortified dairy products, egg yolk; synthesized by skin with sunlight exposure	Proper formation of skeleton, teeth; mineral homeostasis; increases intestinal absorption of calcium	Rickets in children, osteomalacia in adults	Level: Children: 1,800 IU daily Adults: unknown Mild: nausea, weight loss, irritability Severe: hypercalcemia, hypercalcuria, irreversible renal & cardiovascular damage secondary to calcification

Vitamin	USRDA	Sources	Functions	Deficiency	Toxic Effects
Vitamin E	30 IU	Vegetable oil, margarine, wheat germ, nuts, green leafy vegetables	An antioxidant that protects unsaturated fatty acids from destruction; helps prevent cell membrane damage	Patients with long-standing fat malabsorption through the digestive process	Level: Adults: 150–1,200 IU daily tolerated without signs of toxicity Possible effects: headaches, nausea, diarrhea, rapid pulse, extreme fatigue, fatty liver, elevated lipid profile, increase bleeding time when on anticoagulants
Vitamin K	Not established	Green leafy vegetables, milk, dairy products, meats, eggs, cereals, fruits. Also produced by bacterial flora in the gut	Essential for formation of prothrombin and other proteins necessary in regulation of blood clotting Also required for biosynthesis of some proteins in plasma, bone, kidney	Long-term hyperalimentation or broad spectrum antibiotics, chronic biliary obstruction, lipid malabsorption syndromes	Toxic range unknown. Be cautious when taking anticoagulants

USRDA = U.S. Recommended Dietary Allowances; GI = gastrointestinal.

Water Soluble Vitamins	U.S. RDA for Adults and Children ≥ 4 Yr	Significant Sources	Major Functions	Deficiency Conditions	Toxicity Symptoms
Vitamin C	60 mg	Green & red peppers, collard greens, broccoli, spinach, tomatoes, potatoes, strawberries, and citrus fruit	An antioxidant necessary in formation of collagen; thus strengthens blood vessels, hastens healing process, increases resistance to infection Aids in absorption of iron	Mild: bleeding gums, easily bruised Severe: scurvy	Level: Adults: ≤2000 mg daily tolerated without signs of toxicity Signs of toxicity: nausea, diarrhea, kidney stones When megadoses are discontinued, deficiency symptoms may occur until the body adapts
Thiamin (B₁)	1.5 mg	Unrefined cereals, brewer's yeast, organ meats, pork, legumes, seeds, nuts	Functions as part of a coenzyme in carbohydrate metabolism & production of ribose for DNA & RNA formation Promotes normal function of nervous system	Mild: impaired growth, mental confusion, muscle wasting, edema Severe: beriberi	Toxic range unknown
Riboflavin (B₂)	1.7 mg	Animal protein, dairy products, enriched fortified grains, cereals, bakery products	Functions as part of coenzymes that release energy within the cell Essential for maintenance of skin, mucous membranes, cornea, nervous system	Cornea lesions, cracks in corners of mouth	Toxic range unknown

		Functions	Deficiency	Toxic/Excess
Niacin (nico-tinamide, nicotinic acid)	20 mg	Animal protein, synthesized from tryptophan (60 mg tryptophan = 1 mg niacin) Dairy products are high in tryptophan	Functions as part of a coenzyme involved in fat & carbohydrate metabolism, tissue respiration. Essential for growth and hormone production Promotes healthy skin production	Mild: skin & GI lesions, anorexia, weakness, irritability, vertigo Severe: pellagra	Toxic: >1000 mg nicotinic acid may cause vascular dilation, flushing, decreased lipids, increased blood sugars, decreased mobilization of fatty acids from adipose tissue during exercise, hepatoxicity, cardiac arrhythmias
Vitamin B$_6$ (pyridoxine, pyridoxal)	2.0 mg	Chicken, fish, pork, kidney, liver	Functions as part of a coenzyme involved in protein & lipid metabolism, assists in the conversion of tryptophan to niacin, red blood cell formation	Epileptiform convulsions, dermatitis, hypochromic anemia, irritability, insomnia	Toxic: >200 mg daily: ataxia and severe sensory neuropathy
Folacin (folic acid)	0.4 mg	Liver, yeast, legumes, green leafy vegetables	Functions as part of a coenzyme for amino acid metabolism & nucleic acid formation Promotes red & white blood cell formation	Diarrhea, sore tongue, anemia, severe weight loss	Level: >15 mg daily May disguise existence of pernicious anemia

Continued.

Water Soluble Vitamins	U.S. RDA for Adults and Children ≥ 4 Yr	Significant Sources	Major Functions	Deficiency Conditions	Toxicity Symptoms
Vitamin B$_{12}$ (cobalamin)	6.0 μg	Animal & dairy products	Functions as part of a coenzyme involved in nucleic acid formation & biologic methylation	Pernicious anemia, neurological disorders	Toxic: >100 mg daily: polycythemia, parenteral administration—optic nerve atrophy in patients with Leber's disease, acneiform rash
			Assists development of red blood cells, maintenance of nerve tissue		
Biotin	0.3 mg	Kidney, liver, milk, egg yolk, fresh vegetables	Functions as part of a coenzyme involved in fat synthesis, amino acid metabolism, & glycogen formation	Anorexia, nausea, vomiting, dermatitis, depression	No known toxicity
			Assists in maintenance of nerve tissue, skin, hair, blood cells, sex organs		
Pantothenic acid	10 mg	Animal products, whole-grain cereals, legumes	Functions as a coenzyme involved in gluconeogenesis, synthesis, & degradation of fatty acids & synthesis of some hormones	Rare since it is found in most foods, but when induced, fatigue, nausea, & sleep disturbances occur	Minimal toxicity, but diarrhea and water retention associated with >10 g daily

References:
National Research Council. Recommended Dietary Allowances, 10th Edition. Washington, DC: National Academy Press, 1989.
Blair KA. Vitamin supplementation and megadoses. Nurse Pract 1986:11(7):19–36.

22 / *Fat Substitutes*

Extensive data are available that associate excess dietary fat with an increased risk for heart disease, certain types of cancer, and obesity. In turn, obesity is associated with an increased risk of hypertension, hyperlipidemia, and adult onset diabetes. This information has caused government agencies and national health organizations to recommend a reduction in dietary fat to 30% or less of total calories consumed. Studies show that the dropout rate is high for those who attempt to reduce the amount of fat in their diet. Because of this, the National Institute of Health Consensus Development Conference and Surgeon General's report have encouraged food manufacturers to develop foods that will make it easier for individuals to adhere to a low fat diet.[1,2,3]

Industry is responding by developing several low calorie and calorie-free fat substitutes. Some of these are currently being used by food processors, others are being reviewed by the Food and Drug Administration (FDA), and still others are in developmental or testing stages. These new ingredients are formulated to provide the flavor, mouth feel, viscosity, and other organoleptic properties of fat but with fewer calories. These substitutes for fat can be classified into three major categories: carbohydrate-based, protein-based, and fat-based.[1,4] Following are descriptions of these fat substitutes.

The American Dietetic Association states in its position statement on fat replacements that it "recognizes the innovative development and use of traditional food ingredients and processing methods to reduce or replace fat in foods. Such foods should be used within the context of a diet consistent with the Dietary Guidelines for Americans."[5]

Extensive programs are needed to assure the safety and effectiveness of some of these fat substitutes. No fat substitute is a panacea against heart disease, cancer, or obesity, but when combined with a prudent diet and healthy lifestyle, products made with fat substitutes may make reducing the fat content of the diet easier and more enjoyable.

No fat substitute can replace the benefits of a diet rich in whole grains and fresh fruits and vegetables. Therefore, nutrition education continues to be an important component in the goal to reduce dietary fat intake to 30% or less of total calories while maintaining a balanced and healthy diet.[6]

References

1. Anon. Fat substitute update. Food Technology 1990; March: 92–97.
2. Drewnowski A. The new fat replacements: a strategy for reducing fat consumption. Postgrad Med 1990;87(6):111–121.
3. Anon. Summary of Olestra safety research. Procter & Gamble: rev Feb 1991.
4. Dziezak J. Fats, oils, and fat substitutes. Food Technology 1989; July; 66–74.
5. American Dietetic Association. Position of the American Dietetic Association: fat replacements. JADA 1991;91(10):1285–1288.
6. Anon. Simplesse all natural fat substitute: a scientific overview. Deerfield, IL: The NutraSweet Co., 1989:1–2.

Fat Substitutes—Carbohydrate-Based*

Some carbohydrates and carbohydrate-based compounds have been used to partially or totally replace fats or oils in food products since the late 1970s. These provide 1–4 kcal/g and are categorized as generally recognized as safe (GRAS). These substitutes include gums, corn starch maltodextrin (Maltrin™ MO40), tapioca dextrins (N-Oil™), potato starch maltodextrin (Paselli SA2), modified potato starch (Sta-Slim™ 143), modified food starch/maltodextrin (N-LITE series), acid modified cornstarch (STELLAR), and oat fiber amylodextrin (Oatrim). Polydextrose, an approved food additive, is also included in this category. These are used in a variety of products, including salad dressings, margarine-like products, mayonnaise-like products, imitation sour cream, dips, imitation cream cheese, frozen dairy products, dry mixes, puddings, bakery products, frostings, confections, chewing gum, cereals, snacks, meats, cheese sauces and soups.[1-6]

Fat Substitute	Derivation	Description	Use
Gums	Long-chain, high molecular weight polymers	Increase viscosity, leading to emulsion stability; give a thickening and sometimes gelling effect; used as formulation tools and do not serve as direct substitutes for fats or oils	Used since the early 1980s to produce reduced calorie, fat-free salad dressings and to reduce the fat content of a wide variety of formulated foods
Maltrin™ MO40 (Grain Processing Corp.)	Cornstarch maltodextrin, spray-dried, nonsweet saccharide polymer produced by a limited hydrolysis of cornstarch	Completely soluble in hot water and forms thermoreversible gels when cooled. The gels have a bland flavor, smooth mouth feel, and texture similar to that of hydrogenated oils. Typical M040 reduced calorie table spreads contain about 4.5 kcal/g; low fat salad dressings about 1.5 kcal/g	Used as a partial or total replacement for fats and oils in margarine-type products, imitation sour cream, salad dressings, frozen desserts, extruded high-fiber cereals and snacks
N-Oil™, Instant N-Oil™, Instant N-Oil™ II (National Starch and Chemical Corp.)	Tapioca dextrin	The dextrin products are usually used as a 20–35% aqueous solution. Generally, one part of a 25% solution is considered the equivalent of one part of oil, providing 1 kcal/g. The maltodextrin product is used as a 30–40% solution. One part of a 30% solution is equivalent to one part oil, providing 1.2 kcal/g. N-Oil can with-	Used to produce no-fat frozen desserts and reduce the fat or oil content of salad dressings, puddings, margarine type products, imitation sour cream, cheese sauces

Continued.

*This is not a complete listing of all carbohydrate-based substitutes.

Fat Substitutes—Carbohydrate-Based—cont'd

Fat Substitute	Derivation	Description	Use
N-Oil™, Instant N-Oil™, Instant N-Oil™ II (National Starch and Chemical Corp.) —cont'd		stand processing under high temperatures, high shear, and acidic conditions. The instant form is designed for use in processes requiring little or no heat. It can also be used for applications requiring high temperatures for a short period of time	
Paselli SA2 (Avebe American Inc.)	Potato starch maltodextrin	Thermostable gels that present a smooth, fat-like texture and bland flavor. One part Paselli SA2 is usually used to replace 4 parts oil or fat, contributing 3.8 kcal/g	Used to replace fats or oils in bakery products, dips, salad dressings, frostings, frozen desserts, mayonnaise and margarine-like products, meat products, confections, dessert toppings
Sta-Slim™ 143 (A.E. Staley Mfg. Co.)	Modified potato starch	Provides the mouth feel and texture of fats and oils. Contributes 4 kcal/g but is used at reduced levels compared to the fats or oils it replaces, further reducing caloric contribution	Used to partially replace fats and oils in salad dressings, cheesecakes, imitation cream cheese, soups, dips, frozen desserts, baked products, frostings, meats
N-LITE series: N-LITE L	Modified food starch	Disperses readily in water, has stability to gelling, and is resistant to acid, heat, and shear	Used in spoonable salad dressings, soups, microwavable cheese sauces
N-LITE LP	Modified food starch	Has viscosity stability in liquid systems and is stable to heat, acid, and shear	Used in pourable salad dressings, dry mix soups, microwavable cheese sauces

Product (Company)	Composition	Description	Uses
N-LITE F	Modified food starch, nonfat dried milk, emulsifiers, and guar gum	Has a unique ability to entrap air and create light and rich textures	Used in icings and fillings
N-LITE B	Food grade maltodextrin	Free-flowing powder that solubilizes into a smooth, shortening-like creme	Used in bakery products; can replace 100% of the shortening in laminated products
N-LITE D (National Starch and Chemical Co.)	Food grade maltodextrin	Resistant to heat and sets to a gel	Used in frozen desserts, yogurts, imitation cheeses, sour cream
STELLAR (A.E. Staley Co.)	Acid modified corn starch	An insoluble crystallite. When processed in an aqueous system, it develops a firm plastic fat-like creme with properties similar to shortening	Used to replace fats and oils in salad dressings, margarines, baked goods, dairy products, meats
Oatrim (Developed by U.S. Dept. of Agriculture)	Beta-glucan amylodextrin derived from oat fiber	Designed as a fat substitute that would provide the additional cholesterol-lowering benefits of beta-glucan fiber in oats	Can be incorporated into dips, dressings, ice cream, bakery products
Polydextrose (Pfizer Inc.)	Polymer of dextrose with small amounts of sorbitol and citric acid	Water-soluble, stable, functions as a humectant, marketed primarily as a bulking agent, but may be used as a partial substitute for fat. Caloric value is 1 kcal/g	Used in candy, chewing gum, frozen dairy products, dry mixes, frostings

Fat Substitutes—Protein-Based*

These substitutes are derived from proteins found in eggs and milk. The first of these to receive approval from the FDA was Simplesse™. The NutraSweet Company received GRAS approval for this product in February 1990. The egg white and milk in Simplesse™ produces allergic reactions in those allergic to eggs or milk. Because protein is not an effective conductor of heat, Simplesse™ Simplesse™ can be used in a wide variety of foods. However, it can be used in high heat processes such as pasteurization and canning.[1-4, 7-12] cannot be used in frying.

Fat Substitute	Derivation	Description	Use
Simplesse™ (NutraSweet Co.)	Milk and/or egg protein substance, obtained by microparticulation, a heating and shearing process that shapes the protein into small, round particles that are perceived by the tongue as fluid	Has richness and creaminess associated with fat; provides 1–2 kcal/g, depending on development process; current forms of Simplesse™ are not effective in frying but can be used in high heat processes	Currently approved for use in frozen desserts, hard cheese, cheese spreads, sour cream, pizza, cheesecake; approval expected for use in yogurt, salad dressings, mayonnaise- and margarine-like products, dips, puddings, baked goods

*This is not a complete listing of all protein-based substitutes.

Fat Substitutes—Fat-Based*

These are substances that use traditional fatty acids to provide organoleptic properties similar to conventional fat, but are resistant to hydrolysis by digestive enzymes. Currently only the manufacturer of one product has filed a food additive petition (FAP) with the FDA. This product, developed by Procter & Gamble, is Olestra™. Olestra™ is composed of sucrose with six to eight fatty acids. Its large size prevents it from being digested and absorbed.[1,2,4,12-14]

In the FAP, submitted in 1987, Procter & Gamble submitted the results of over 100 animal studies and more than 25 clinical investigations. At this time, there is controversy over interpretation of the results of these studies. Procter & Gamble is requesting approval to use Olestra™ as 100% replacement of oil in the preparation of fried snack foods. Olestra™ has the potential to be used in frozen desserts, margarine-like products, salad dressings, and cheese also. Approval for these uses has not yet been requested.[1-4,13,14]

Other compounds that are resistant to enzymatic hydrolysis or that are minimally digested include EPG, TATCA, and DDM. These are similar to Olestra™ in that they have good stability for baking and frying and have potential in any formulation in which vegetable oils are used.[1,3]

Caprenin is a reduced-calorie triglyceride also developed by Procter & Gamble. A petition for GRAS approval has been filed with the FDA. It has been developed to replace some of the cocoa butter in soft candy and confectionery coatings.[4]

Fat Substitute	Derivation	Description	Use
Olestra™, formerly called sucrose polyester (Procter & Gamble Co.)	A mixture of hexa-, hepta-, and octa-esters of sucrose with long-chain fatty acids from traditional fats	Has appearance, flavor, texture, mouth feel, heat stability, flash point, and shelf-life similar to conventional fats; contributes no calories since it is not digested or absorbed	Has the potential to be used wherever fats are used
EPG—esterified propoxylated glycerols (ARCO Chemical Co./Best Foods)	Modified fats/oils. Glycerine is reacted with propylene oxide to form a polyether polyol, which is esterified with a fatty acid or acids	A non- or low caloric triglyceride with properites similar to natural fats and oils; has good stability for frying and baking; is resistant to enzymatic hydrolysis	Has the potential to be substituted for fats and oils in items such as margarine-like products, fried snacks, frozen desserts, salad dressings, and bakery products. Petition for FDA approval expected to be filed in the mid-1990s

Continued.

*This is not a complete list of fat-based substitutes.

Fat Substitutes—Fat-Based—cont'd

Fat Substitute	Derivation	Description	Use
DDM—dialkyl dihexa-decylmalonate (Frito-Lay Inc.)	A fatty alcohol ester of malonic and alkyl-malonic acids	Suitable for high temperature applications; blends with other oils are being tested; DDM-soybean oil blend results in 33% reduction in calories and 60% reduction in fats; DDM is minimally digested and absorbed	A DDM-oil blend has been used to produce potato and tortilla chips. No FAP has been filed for any DDM-based fat substitutes
TATCA—trialkoxytricar-ballyate (Best Foods)	Tricarballylic acid ester-ified with fatty alco-hols	Has conventional fat properties but is resistant to hydrolysis by diges-tive enzymes	Being evaluated as an oil substitute in margarine- and mayonnaise-like products; may have potential applications wherever vegetable oils are used. No FAP has been filed
Caprenin (Procter & Gamble Co.)	A triglyceride formed by the esterification of glycerol with three naturally occurring fatty acids: caprylic, capric, and behenic acids	Caprenin is digested, absorbed, and metabolized by the same pathways as other triglycerides; because behenic acid is only partially absorbed, caprenin supplies 5 kcal/g. Caprenin has functional properties similar to cocoa butter	Can replace some cocoa butter in soft candy and confectionery coatings

References

1. Anon. Fat substitute update. Food Technology 1990; March:92–97.
2. Drewnowski A. The new fat replacements: a strategy for reducing fat consumption. Postgrad Med 1990;87(6):111–121.
3. Dziezak J. Fats, oils, and fat substitutes. Food Technology 1989; July :66–74.
4. American Dietetic Association. Position of the American Dietetic Association: fat replacements. JADA 1991;91(10):1285–1288.
5. Manufacturer's data. Bridgewater, NJ: National Starch & Chemical Co., 1992.
6. Anon. The ingredient for the future: STELLAR, a new dimension in fat replacement. Decatur, IL: A.E. Staley Manufacturing Co., 1992.
7. Anon. Simplesse all natural fat substitute: a scientific overview. Deerfield, IL: The NutraSweet Co., 1989:1–12.
8. Anon. Simplesse all natural fat substitute: a nutrition overview. Deerfield, IL: The Nutrasweet Co., 1992:1–4.
9. Young UR, Fukagawa NK, Pellett PL. Nutritional implications of microparticulated protein. J Am Coll Nutr 1990;9 (4):418–426.
10. Sampson HA, Cooke SK. Food allergy and the potential allergenicity-antigenicity of microparticulated egg and cows' milk proteins. J Am Coll Nutr 1990;9(4):410–417.
11. Harrigan KA, Breene WM. Fat substitutes: sucrose esters and Simplesse. Cereal Food World 1990;34(3):261–266.
12. Segal M. Fat substitutes, a taste of the future? FDA Consumer 1990;24(10):25–27.
13. Jandacek R, Ramirez MM, Crouse JR III. Effects of partial replacement of dietary fat by Olestra on dietary cholesterol absorption in man. Metabolism 1990;39(8):848–852.
14. Anon. Summary of Olestra safety research. Procter & Gamble Co., 1991.

23 / *Caffeine*

Caffeine Content of Beverages and Foods

	mg/Serving
COFFEE, 6-OZ CUP	
Brewed, drip method	103
Brewed, percolator method	75
Instant, 1 rounded tsp	57
Decaffeinated	2
Flavored, regular and sugar-free	25–75
TEA	
3-minute brew, 6 oz cup	36
Instant, 1 rounded tsp in 8 oz of water	25–35
Decaffeinated, 5-min brew, 6 oz cup	1
COLA BEVERAGES, 12 OZ	
Regular or diet	35–50
Decaffeinated	Trace
CHERRY COLAS, DR. PEPPER™, MR. PIBB™, 12 OZ	
Regular or diet	35–50
Decaffeinated	Trace
MELLOW YELLOW™, 12 OZ	
Regular or diet	52
MOUNTAIN DEW™, 12 OZ	
Regular or diet	54
COCOA AND CHOCOLATE	
Cocoa beverage, 6 oz cup	4
Chocolate milk, 8 oz	8
Chocolate, sweet, semisweet, dark, milk, 1 oz	8–20
Chocolate, baking, unsweetened, 1 oz	58
Chocolate flavored syrup, 1 oz	5
Chocolate pudding, ½ cup	4–8

Adapted from Pennington JAT: Bowes and Church's food values of portions commonly used, 16th ed. Philadelphia: JB Lippincott, 1994.

Caffeine Content of Common Medications

	mg/Serving
STAY-AWAKE TABLETS	
No Doz	100
Vivarin	200
PAIN RELIEVERS	
Anacin	32
Excedrin	65
Excedrin PM	0
Vanquish	33
Aspirin, any brand	0

Physicians' Desk Reference (PDR) for Nonprescription Drugs, 14th edition. Montvale, NJ: Medical Economics Company, 1993.

Beverages without Caffeine*

A & W Root Beer, regular and sugar-free
Bigelow Herbal Teas
Caffeine-Free Coke, Caffeine-Free Diet Coke
Caffeine-Free Dr. Pepper, Caffeine and Sugar-Free Dr. Pepper
Caffeine-Free Tab
Caffeine-free tea
Cafix
Carob chocolate substitute
Celestial Seasonings Herbal Teas
Club soda
Crush drinks
Crystal Pepsi, Diet Crystal Pepsi
Dad's Root Beer, regular and sugar-free
Diet Rite (all flavors)
Fresca
Fruit drinks
Fruit juices
Gatorade
Ginger ale
Grape soda
Hires Root Beer, regular and sugar-free
Lemon-lime soda
Lemonade
Lipton Herbal Teas
Mineral water
Caffeine free Mountain Dew, Caffeine and Sugar free Mountain Dew
Orange soda
Pepsi-Free, Diet Pepsi-Free
Pero or Postum coffee-flavored beverage
Diet RC, caffeine free
Root beer
Seltzer
Seven-Up, Diet Seven-Up, Cherry and Diet Cherry Seven-Up
Shasta beverages (except colas and cherry colas)
Slice, Diet Slice, Orange Slice, Lemon-Lime Slice
Sparkling water
Sprite, Diet Sprite
Squirt, Diet Squirt
Sunkist, Diet Sunkist
Tonic water

*Per confirmation by manufacturer.

24 / *Phosphorus Content of Common Foods*[1]

Milk Group	Milligrams of Phosphorus
⅓ cup custard, homemade	103
½ cup half and half	112
¾ cup ice cream, vanilla	100
½ cup milk, whole	114
½ cup pudding (vanilla, homemade)	116
½ cup yogurt (plain, whole milk)	108

Meat and Meat Substitutes	
⅓ cup beans, cooked, great northern	98
1 oz beef	65
1 oz cheese, cheddar	145
¼ cup cheese, cottage, creamed	70
1 oz cheese, processed American	211
1 oz cheese, Swiss	171
1 oz chicken (average)	55
1 egg	90
1 oz fish, haddock, cooked by dry heat	68
⅓ cup lentils, cooked	119
1 oz liver	105
2 Tbsp peanut butter, creamy/smooth	120
1 oz pork, lean, roasted	70
1 oz turkey (average)	60

Starch	
½ cup cereal (100% Bran)	344
⅓ cup cereal (All Bran, Bran Buds, granola-type)	246
½ cup cereal (Bran Flakes)	108
1 waffle (frozen)	130
2 4-in pancakes, prepared with mix	251
1 biscuit, from mix	128
⅓ cup brown rice	47
1 Tbsp wheat germ	81
½ cup oatmeal, cooked	89
1 slice whole-wheat bread	65
⅓ cup lima beans, boiled	69
1/12 cake, white (from mix)	170

Vegetables	Milligrams of Phosphorus
½ cup green peas, boiled	94
½ cup mushrooms, raw pieces	36
½ cup mushrooms, boiled	68

Fruit	
1 oz coconut, dried	59

Fats and Oils	
1 oz peanuts, dry-roasted	100
1 oz sunflower seeds, dry roasted	328

Carbohydrate Supplements	
8 oz carbonated colas	35
1 oz caramels	35
1 oz chocolate, semi-sweet	43
1 Tbsp cocoa powder	35
1 Tbsp molasses, blackstrap	17
12 fl oz beer	44

Reference

1. Pennington JAT, Church HN. Bowes and Churchs' food values of portions commonly used. 16th ed. Philadelphia: JB Lippincott, 1994.

B. PEDIATRIC APPENDICES

25 / *Infant Formulas and Feedings*

Note: Formula compositions change over time. The information in this appendix is accurate at the time of publication. The reader is encouraged to check with the product manufacturers for the most current information.

References

1. Pennington JAT. Food values of portions commonly used. 16th ed. Philadelphia: JB Lippincott, 1994.
2. Manufacturer's information.
3. Committee on nutrition, American Academy of Pediatrics: Pediatric nutrition handbook. 2nd ed. American Academy of Pediatrics, 1985:363–368.

Infant and Pediatric Formulas and Feedings[1-3]

Name	Company	Classification	Food Source	Use	Form Available	Composition per 1,000 ml Normal Dilution					
						Normal Dilution (kcal/oz)	Protein (g/% kcals)	Fat (g/% kcals)	Carbohydrate (g/% kcals)	Calcium (mg)	Phosphorus (mg)
Advance™	Ross	Infant formula	Nonfat cows' milk, soy protein isolate; lactose, corn syrup; soy and coconut oils	Transitional beverage between infant formula and cows' milk for the older infant	Ready-to-feed; concentrate	16	20/15	27/45	55/40	510	390
Alimentum™	Ross	Infant formula	Hydrolyzed casein; free amino acids; sucrose; modified tapioca starch; coconut, soy, and safflower oil, MCT oil	For infants with sensitivity to intact proteins, multiple food allergies, pancreatic insufficiency, chronic diarrhea	Ready-to-feed	20	19/11	37/48	69/41	710	510
Carnation Good Start™	Carnation	Infant formula	Hydrolyzed whey, palm, soy, coconut, and safflower oil; maltodextrin; lactose	Infant feeding	Ready-to-feed; concentrate; powder	20	16/9.6	34/46	74/44	433	243
Carnation Follow Up™	Carnation	Infant formula	Nonfat milk; corn syrup; palm and corn oil	Feeding 6–12-mo-olds who are eating solid foods	Ready-to-feed; concentrate; powder	20	18/10	28/37	89/53	913	609
Enfamil™ with or without iron	Mead Johnson	Infant formula	Reduced mineral whey; nonfat milk; lactose, mono- and diglycerides; soy and coconut oils	Infant feeding	Ready-to-feed; concentrate; powder	20	15/9	38/50	70/41	530	360

| | Composition per 1,000 ml Normal Dilution | | | | | | | | | | | Osmotic Characteristics | |
Name	Iron* (w/wo) (mg)	Sodium (mEq)	Potassium (mEq)	Vitamin A (IU)	Vitamin D (IU)	Thiamin (mg)	Riboflavin (mg)	Niacin (mg)	Ascorbic Acid (mg)	Other	Miscellaneous Information	Renal Solute Load (mOsm)	Osmolality (mOsm/kg H₂O)
Advance™	10	8	20	1,620	320	0.7	0.9	7	50	Other vitamins and minerals		122	200
Alimentum™	12	13	20	2,030	410	0.4	0.6	10	60	Other vitamins and minerals	Lactose-free, corn-free 50% of fat as MCT	123	370
Carnation Good Start™	10	7	17	2,029	406	0.4	0.9	5	54	Other vitamins and minerals	Protein is 100% whey	122	265
Carnation Follow Up™	13	12	23	1,691	440	0.5	0.6	8.6	54	Other vitamins and minerals		99	326
Enfamil™ with or without iron	13/3	8	19	2,100	430	0.5	1.0	8	55	Other vitamins and minerals	60:40 whey: casein ratio. Powder contains corn oil instead of soy oil. Also available as 13 and 24 kcal/oz formula with appropriate adjustments in all nutrients	134	300

*With or without iron.

Continued.

Infant and Pediatric Formulas and Feedings[1-3]—cont'd

Name	Company	Classification	Food Source	Use	Form Available	Composition per 1,000 ml Normal Dilution					
						Normal Dilution (kcal/oz)	Protein (g/% kcals)	Fat (g/% kcals)	Carbohydrate (g/% kcals)	Calcium (mg)	Phosphorus (mg)
Enfamil Premature Formula™ with or without iron	Mead Johnson	Premature infant formula	Nonfat milk, whey protein concentrate; corn syrup solids, lactose; MCT, soy, and coconut oils	For growing, healthy, low-birth-weight infants (<2,000 g)	Ready-to-feed	24	24/12	41/44	90/44	1,340	670
Gerber Baby Formula™ with or without iron	Gerber	Infant formula	Nonfat milk, lactose, soy and coconut oil, palm, sunflower oil	Infant feeding	Ready-to-feed; concentrate; powder	20	15/9	37/48	73/43	510	390
Gerber Soy Formula™	Gerber	Infant formula	Soy protein isolate; corn syrup; sucrose; soy, coconut, and sunflower oil	Same as Isomil	Ready-to-feed, concentrate powder	20	20/12	36/48	68/40	640	500
Isomil™	Ross	Infant formula	Soy-protein isolate, sucrose, corn syrup; soy and coconut oils	For infants allergic or sensitive to cows' milk protein or lactose; galactosemia; temporary feeding following diarrhea until lactase regenerates	Ready-to-feed; concentrate; powder	20	17/11	37/49	70/40	710	510

				Composition per 1,000 ml Normal Dilution									Osmotic Characteristics	
Name	Iron* (w/wo) (mg)	Sodium (mEq)	Potas- sium (mEq)	Vita- min A (IU)	Vita- min D (IU)	Thia- min (mg)	Ribo- flavin (mg)	Niacin (mg)	Ascorbic Acid (mg)	Other	Miscellaneous Information	Renal Solute Load (mOsm)	Osmolality (mOsm/kg H₂O)
Enfamil Premature Formula™ with or without iron	2/15	14	21	10,100	2,200	1.6	2.4	32	162	Other vitamins and miner- als in amounts to meet esti- mated needs of prema- ture infants except for iron and possibly vita- min E	60:40 whey: casein ra- tio. Also available as 20 kcal/oz formula	210	310
Gerber Baby Formula™ with or without iron	12/1	9	18	1,997	395	0.66	1.0	7	60	Other vitamins and miner- als	82:18 casein: whey ratio; powder contains corn oil in- stead of soy oil	138	240
Gerber Soy™ Formula	12	14	20	2,000	410	.4	.6	9.2	61	Other vitamins and miner- als		162	230
Isomil™	12	13	19	2,030	410	0.4	0.6	9	60	Other vitamins and miner- als		115	240

*With or without iron.

Continued.

767

Infant and Pediatric Formulas and Feedings[1-3]—cont'd

Name	Company	Classification	Food Source	Use	Form Available	Composition per 1,000 ml Normal Dilution					
						Normal Dilution (kcal/oz)	Protein (g/% kcals)	Fat (g/% kcals)	Carbohydrate (g/% kcals)	Calcium (mg)	Phosphorus (mg)
MSUD Diet Powder™	Mead Johnson	Modified infant formula	Amino acids (except leucine, isoleucine, and valine); corn syrup solids, modified tapioca starch; corn oil	For infants and children with maple syrup urine disease or other disorders in branched-chain amino acid metabolism	Powder	20	14/8	28/38	89/54	686	374
Nursoy™	Wyeth	Infant formula	Soy protein isolate; sucrose; oleo, oleic, coconut, soy oils	For infants allergic or sensitive to cows' milk protein or lactose; galactosemia	Ready-to-feed; concentrate; powder	20	18/13	36/48	69/41	600	420
Nutramigen™	Mead Johnson	Modified infant formula	Hydrolyzed casein; sucrose; modified tapioca starch; corn oil	For infants with sensitivity to intact proteins or severe food allergies; diarrhea, colic, or other gastrointestinal disturbances	Powder; ready-to-feed (for hospital use only)	20	19/11	27/35	91/54	640	430
PediaSure™	Ross	Pediatric formula	Hydrolyzed cornstarch, sucrose, sodium caseinate, soy, coconut, and whey protein concentrate, safflower oil, mono- and diglycerides, soy lecithin	Enteral feeding or oral supplement for 1–10-year-olds	Ready-to-feed liquid	30 (1 cal/ml)	30/12	50/44	110/44	970	800

		Composition per 1,000 ml Normal Dilution										Osmotic Characteristics	
Name	Iron† (w/wo) (mg)	Sodium (mEq)	Potassium (mEq)	Vitamin A (IU)	Vitamin D (IU)	Thiamin (mg)	Riboflavin (mg)	Niacin (mg)	Ascorbic Acid (mg)	Other	Miscellaneous Information	Renal Solute Load (mOsm)	Osmolality (mOsm/kg H$_2$O)
MSUD Diet Powder™	12	11	18	2,080	416	0.5	0.6	8	54	Other vitamins and minerals	Needs to be supplemented with appropriate amounts of leucine, isoleucine, and valine according to patient tolerance	138	300
Nursoy™	12	8.7	18	2,000	400	0.67	1.0	5	55	Other vitamins and minerals	Lower in sodium than other soy formulas. Nursoy powder contains corn syrup solids and sucrose	154	296
Nutramigen™	13	14	19	2,100	430	0.5	0.6	8	55	Other vitamins and minerals		172	320
PediaSure™	14	16	34	2,570	510	2.7	2.1	17	100	Other vitamins and minerals	1,000 ml meets RDA for protein, vitamins, and minerals for 1–6-yr-olds. Essentially lactose-free and gluten-free. Protein: 82% casein, 18% whey. Kosher	198	310

*With or without iron.

Continued.

Infant and Pediatric Formulas and Feedings[1-3]—cont'd

Name	Company	Classification	Food Source	Use	Form Available	Composition per 1,000 ml Normal Dilution					
						Normal Dilution (kcal/oz)	Protein (g/% kcals)	Fat (g/% kcals)	Carbohydrate (g/% kcals)	Calcium (mg)	Phosphorus (mg)
PediaSure with Fiber™	Ross	Pediatric formula	Same as Pediasure	Same as Pediasure			30/12	50/44	114/44	970	800
Phenyl-Free™	Mead Johnson	Phenylalanine-free food	Amino acids (no phenylalanine); sucrose, corn syrup solids, modified tapioca starch; corn and coconut oils	For children with phenylketonuria	Powder	25	42/20	14/15	140/64	1040	1,040
Portagen™	Mead Johnson	Modified infant formula	Sodium caseinate; corn syrup solids, sucrose; MCT, corn oil	For infants, children, or adults with fat malabsorption such as steatorrhea, pancreatic insufficiency, lymphatic anomalies, chylothorax	Powder	20	24/14	33/40	78/46	640	480

Name	Iron* (w/wo) (mg)	Sodium (mEq)	Potassium (mEq)	Vitamin A (IU)	Vitamin D (IU)	Thiamin (mg)	Riboflavin (mg)	Niacin (mg)	Ascorbic Acid (mg)	Other	Miscellaneous Information	Renal Solute Load (mOsm)	Osmolality (mOsm/kg H$_2$O)
PediaSure with Fiber™	14	16	34	2,570	510	2.7	2.1	17	100	Other vitamins and minerals	Same as Pediasure Contains 5 g dietary fiber per liter.	198	310
Phenyl-Free™	25	36	72	2,496	312	1.2	2.1	17	108	Other vitamins and minerals	Not an infant formula. Designed to complement remainder of diet of children ≥2 yr. Not intended as sole source of nutrition	450	790
Portagen™	13	16	22	5,300	530	1.0	1.3	14	55	Other vitamins and minerals	Fat content approximately 85% MCT and 15% corn oil (to supply essential fatty acids)	200	230

*With or without iron.

Continued.

Infant and Pediatric Formulas and Feedings[1-3]—cont'd

Name	Company	Classification	Food Source	Use	Form Available	Composition per 1,000 ml Normal Dilution					
						Normal Dilution (kcal/oz)	Protein (g/% kcals)	Fat (g/% kcals)	Carbohydrate (g/% kcals)	Calcium (mg)	Phosphorus (mg)
Pregestimil™	Mead Johnson	Modified infant formula	Hydrolyzed casein; corn syrup solids, modified tapioca starch; corn oil and MCT and sunflower oil	For infants with malabsorption disorders, intractable diarrhea, severe allergies or sensitivity to intact protein, cystic fibrosis, intestinal resections, steatorrhea, lactase or sucrase deficiency	Powder	20	19/11	38/48	69/41	640	430
ProSobee™	Mead Johnson	Infant formula	Soy protein isolate; corn syrup solids; palm, coconut and sunflower oils	For infants allergic or sensitive to cows' milk or lactase; galactosemia; temporary feeding following diarrhea until lactase regenerates; sucrose intolerance	Ready-to-feed; concentrate; powder	20	20/12	36/48	68/40	640	500

Composition per 1,000 ml Normal Dilution

Name	Iron* (w/wo) (mg)	Sodium (mEq)	Potas-sium (mEq)	Vita-min A (IU)	Vita-min D (IU)	Thia-min (mg)	Ribo-flavin (mg)	Niacin (mg)	Ascorbic Acid (mg)	Other	Miscellaneous Information	Renal Solute Load (mOsm)	Osmolality (mOsm/kg H₂O)
												Osmotic Characteristics	
Pregestimil™	13	12	19	2,600	510	0.5	0.6	8	80	Other vitamins and miner-als	Fat content is 60% MCT, 20% corn oil, and 20% high oleic saf-flower oil	169	320
ProSobee™	13	10	21	2,100	430	0.5	0.6	8	55	Other vitamins and miner-als	Powder con-tains corn oil instead of soy oil	178	200

*With or without iron.

Continued.

Infant and Pediatric Formulas and Feedings[1-3]—cont'd

Name	Company	Classification	Food Source	Use	Form Available	Normal Dilution (kcal/oz)	Composition per 1,000 ml Normal Dilution				
							Protein (g/% kcals)	Fat (g/% kcals)	Carbohydrate (g/% kcals)	Calcium (mg)	Phosphorus (mg)
Protein Free Diet Powder™ (Product 80056)	Mead Johnson	Formula base	Corn syrup solids, modified tapioca starch, corn oil	Protein-free formula base for infants who require specific mixtures of amino acids such as with hyperlysinemia, isovaleric acidemia, propionic aciduria, urea cycle disorders, B₁₂ independent methylmalonic aciduria, argininemia, gyrate atrophy, histidinemia	Powder		§	26	83	624	343
Ross Carbohydrate-Free (RCF) Low-Iron Soy Protein Formula Base	Ross	Formula Base	Soy protein isolate; soy and coconut oils	For infants intolerant to all types of carbohydrate; intractable diarrhea	Concentrate	12*	20	36	—*	700	500

Composition per 1,000 ml Normal Dilution

Name	Iron† (w/wo) (mg)	Sodium (mEq)	Potassium (mEq)	Vitamin A (IU)	Vitamin D (IU)	Thiamin (mg)	Riboflavin (mg)	Niacin (mg)	Ascorbic Acid (mg)	Other	Miscellaneous Information	Renal Solute Load (mOsm)	Osmotic Characteristics Osmolality (mOsm/kg H_2O)
Protein Free Diet Powder™ (Product 80056)	12	8	18	2,080	416	0.5	0.6	8	54	Other vitamins and minerals	Adequate sodium, potassium, and chloride must be added		200‡
Ross Carbohydrate-Free™ (RCF) Low-Iron Soy Protein Formula Base	1.5	13	20	2,030	410	0.4	0.6	9	55	Other vitamins and minerals	Carbohydrates added according to tolerance. A carbohydrate concentration of at least 2% is needed to prevent hypoglycemia and ketosis. IV glucose should be used as a supplement until then. Use only under medical supervision	124	74 (no carbohydrate added)

*Normal dilution without carbohydrate.

†With or without iron.

§Appropriate amino acids (or other protein source) must be added.

Continued.

Infant and Pediatric Formulas and Feedings[1-3]—cont'd

Name	Company	Classification	Food Source	Use	Form Available	Composition per 1,000 ml Normal Dilution					
						Normal Dilution (kcal/oz)	Protein (g/% kcals)	Fat (g/% kcals)	Carbohydrate (g/% kcals)	Calcium (mg)	Phosphorus (mg)
SMA™ with or without iron	Wyeth	Infant formula	Nonfat cows' milk and demineralized whey; lactose; coconut, oleic, oleo, and soybean oils	Infant feeding; use for infants with cardiac or renal problems who could benefit from reduced sodium or renal solute load	Ready-to-feed; concentrate; powder	20	15/9	36/48	72/43	420	280
SMA "Premie"™	Wyeth	Premature infant formula	Nonfat cows' milk, partially demineralized whey; lactose, glucose polymers; MCT, oleo, oleic, coconut, and soy oils	For growing, healthy low-birth-weight infants (<2,000 g) Infant feeding	Ready-to-feed (hospital use only)	24	20/10	44/47	86/42	750	400
Similac with or without iron	Ross	Infant formula	Nonfat cows' milk; lactose; coconut and soy oils		Ready-to-feed; concentrate; powder	20	14.5/9	36/48	72/43	490	380

				Composition per 1,000 ml Normal Dilution								Osmotic Characteristics	
Name	Iron* (w/wo) (mg)	Sodium (mEq)	Potassium (mEq)	Vitamin A (IU)	Vitamin D (IU)	Thiamin (mg)	Riboflavin (mg)	Niacin (mg)	Ascorbic Acid (mg)	Other	Miscellaneous Information	Renal Solute Load (mOsm)	Osmolality (mOsm/kg H₂O)
SMA™ with or without iron	12/1.5	6.5	14	2,000	400	0.67	1.0	5	55	Other vitamins and minerals	60:40 whey: casein ratio. For hospital use only: 24 kcal/oz with proportional adjustments in all nutrients	91	300
SMA "Premie"™	3	14	19	2,400	480	0.8	1.3	6	70	Other vitamins and minerals. Needs to be supplemented with vitamins and minerals when used for infants <2,000 g	60:40 whey: casein ratio	128	280
Similac with or without iron	12/1.5	8	18	2,030	410	0.7	1.0	7	60	Other vitamins and minerals	For hospital use only; available as 13, 24, and 27 kcal/oz with proportional adjustments in all nutrients. Powder contains corn oil instead of soy oil	100	300

*With or without iron.

Continued.

Infant and Pediatric Formulas and Feedings[1-3]—cont'd

Name	Company	Classification	Food Source	Use	Form Available	Composition per 1,000 ml Normal Dilution					
						Normal Dilution (kcal/oz)	Protein (g/% kcals)	Fat (g/% kcals)	Carbohydrate (g/% kcals)	Calcium (mg)	Phosphorus (mg)
Similac Natural Care	Ross	Human milk supplement	Nonfat cows' milk, whey protein concentrate; hydrolyzed corn starch, lactose; MCT, soy and coconut oils	To fortify human milk for premature infants	Ready-to-feed (hospital use only)	24	22/11	44/47	86/42	1705	853
Similac PM 60/40	Ross	Infant formula	Demineralized whey solids, sodium caseinate; lactose; corn and coconut oils	For infants whose renal or cardiovascular system might be taxed by a sodium or solute load greater than that of human milk or who have hyperphosphatemia	Ready-to-feed (for hospital use only); powder	20	15/9	38/50	69/41	379	189

Composition per 1,000 ml Normal Dilution

Name	Iron* (w/wo) (mg)	Sodium (mEq)	Potassium (mEq)	Vitamin A (IU)	Vitamin D (IU)	Thiamin (mg)	Riboflavin (mg)	Niacin (mg)	Ascorbic Acid (mg)	Other	Miscellaneous Information	Renal Solute Load (mOsm)	Osmotic Characteristics — Osmolality (mOsm/kg H_2O)
Similac Natural Care™	3.0	15	27	5,520	1,220	2.0	5.0	41	300	Other vitamins and minerals	Mix 50:50 with human milk; or feed alternately with human milk; 60:40 whey:casein ratio. May require supplementation with some nutrients to meet estimated needs of premature infants	148	300
Similac PM 60/40™	1.5	7	15	2,030	406	0.7	1.0	7	60	Other vitamins and minerals	60:40 whey:casein ratio. May be necessary to supplement with electrolytes or minerals for premature infants or with abnormally high losses. Ready-to-feed formula contains corn instead of soy oil	96	280

*With or without iron.

Continued.

Infant and Pediatric Formulas and Feedings[1-3]—cont'd

Name	Company	Classification	Food Source	Use	Form Available	Composition per 1,000 ml Normal Dilution						
						Normal Dilution (kcal/oz)	Protein (g/% kcals)	Fat (g/% kcals)	Carbohydrate (g/% kcals)	Calcium (mg)	Phosphorus (mg)
Similac Special Care™ with or without iron	Ross	Premature infant formula	Nonfat cows' milk, whey protein concentrate; corn syrup solids, lactose; MCT, soy and coconut oils	For growing healthy low-birth-weight (<2,000 g) infants	Ready-to-feed; (hospital use only)	24	22/11	44/47	86/42	1,460	730
Soyalac™	Loma Linda	Infant formula	Soy protein solids, corn syrup solids, carbohydrates from soybean, sucrose; soy oil	For infants allergic or sensitive to cows' milk protein or lactose; galactosemia	Ready-to-feed; concentrate; powder	20	20/12	37/49	66/39	634	528
I-Soyalac™	Loma Linda	Infant formula	Soy protein isolate; sucrose, tapioca, dextrin starch; soy oil	For infants allergic or sensitive to cows' milk protein or lactose; galactosemia	Ready-to-feed; concentrate	20	20/12	37/49	66/39	690	480

| Name | Composition per 1,000 ml Normal Dilution | | | | | | | | | | | Osmotic Characteristics | |
	Iron* (w/wo) (mg)	Sodium (mEq)	Potassium (mEq)	Vitamin A (IU)	Vitamin D (IU)	Thiamin (mg)	Riboflavin (mg)	Niacin (mg)	Ascorbic Acid (mg)	Other	Miscellaneous Information	Renal Solute Load (mOsm)	Osmolality (mOsm/kg H₂O)
Similac Special Care with or without iron	15/3	15	27	5,520	1,220	2.0	5.0	40	300	Other vitamins and minerals in amounts to meet estimated needs of premature infants, except for iron and possibly vitamins D and E	60:40 whey:casein ratio. Also available in 20 kcal/oz with proportional adjustments in all nutrients	148	300
Soyalac	10	15	24	2,114	423	0.5	0.6	8.5	63	Other vitamins and minerals		129	210
I-Soyalac	13	12	20	2,114	423	0.5	0.6	8.5	63	Other vitamins and minerals	Corn free	134	280

*With or without iron.

Feeding Supplements and Modules[2]

Name	Company	Food Source	Use	Composition per 100 g		
				Form Available	Kilo-calories	Protein (g)
Ketonex-1™	Ross	Hydrolyzed corn starch, palm, coconut and soy oil, amino acids	For infants and toddlers with maple syrup urine disease or other disorders in branched-chain amino acid metabolism	Powder	480	15
I-Valex-1™	Ross	Hydrolyzed cornstarch, palm & coconut, soy oils, amino acids	For infants and toddlers with disorders of leucine metabolism	Powder	480	15
Glutarex-1™	Ross	Hydrolyzed corn starch, palm, coconut & soy oils, amino acids	For infants and toddlers with glutaric aciduria type 1	Powder	480	15

							Composition per 100 g	
Fat (g)	Carbo-hydrate (g)	Calcium (mg)	Phos-phorus (g)	Iron (mg)	Sodium (mEq)	Potas-sium (mEq)	Other	Miscellaneous Information
23.9	46.3	575	400	9	8	17	Isoleucine-, leucine-, and valine-free	Formula dilution will vary as prescribed by physician. Diet must be supplemented with prescribed amounts of standard infant formula to provide adequate nutrients and amino acids
23.9	46.3	575	400	9	8	17	Leucine-free	Formula dilution will vary as prescribed by physician. Diet must be supplemented with prescribed amounts of standard infant formula to provide adequate nutrients and amino acids
23.9	46.3	575	400	9	8	17	Lysine- and tryptophan- free	Formula dilution will vary as prescribed by physician. Diet must be supplemented with prescribed amounts of standard infant formula to provide adequate nutrients and amino acids

Continued.

Feeding Supplements and Modules[2]—cont'd

Name	Company	Food Source	Use	Form Available	Kilo-calories	Protein (g)
			Composition per 100 g			
Hominex I™	Ross	Hydrolyzed corn-starch, palm, co-conut, soy oils, amino acids	For infants and tod-dlers with B_6 non-responsive homo-cystinuria or hypermethio-ninemia	Powder	480	15
Propimex I™	Ross	Hydrolyzed corn-starch, palm, co-conut, soy oils, amino acids	For infants and tod-dlers with methyl-malonic or propi-onic acidemia	Powder	480	15
Phenex-I™	Ross	Hydrolyzed corn-starch, palm, co-conut, soy oils, amino acids	For infants and tod-dlers with phenylketonuria	Powder	480	15

							Composition per 100 g	
Fat (g)	**Carbo-hydrate (g)**	**Calcium (mg)**	**Phos-phorus (g)**	**Iron (mg)**	**Sodium (mEq)**	**Potas-sium (mEq)**	**Other**	**Miscellaneous Information**
23.9	46.3	575	400	9	8	17	Methionine-free	Formula dilution will vary as prescribed by physician. Diet must be supplemented with prescribed amounts of standard infant formula to provide adequate nutrients and amino acids
23.9	46.3	575	400	9	8	17	Methionine- and valine-free; low isoleucine and threonine	Formula dilution will vary as prescribed by physician. Diet must be supplemented with prescribed amounts of standard infant formula to provide adequate nutrients and amino acids
23.9	46.3	575	400	9	8	17	Phenylalanine-free	Formula dilution will vary as prescribed by physician. Diet must be supplemented with prescribed amounts of standard infant formula to provide adequate nutrients and amino acids

Continued.

Feeding Supplements and Modules[2]—cont'd

Name	Company	Food Source	Use	Form Available	Kilo-calories	Protein (g)
Tyromex-1™	Ross	Hydrolyzed cornstarch, palm, coconut, soy oils, amino acids	For infants and toddlers with tyrosinemia type I	Powder	480	15
Calcilo XD™	Ross	Lactose, whey protein concentrate, corn and coconut oil	For infants with hypercalcemia requiring a low calcium vitamin D-free formula	Powder	513	11.4
Casec™	Mead Johnson	Calcium caseinate	Protein supplement; to increase protein for low sodium and low fat diets	Powder	370	88
Enfamil Human Milk Fortifier™	Mead Johnson	Whey protein concentrate, casein, corn syrup solids, lactose	To fortify human milk for premature infants	Powder	14†	0.7†

†Per 4 packets (3.8 g), which should be mixed with 100 ml of human milk

	Composition per 100 g							
Fat (g)	Carbo-hydrate (g)	Calcium (mg)	Phos-phorus (g)	Iron (mg)	Sodium (mEq)	Potas-sium (mEq)	Other	Miscellaneous Information
23.9	46.3	575	400	9	8	17	Phenylalanine- and tyrosine-free	Formula dilution will vary as pre-scribed by physi-cian. Diet must be supple-mented with prescribed amounts of stan-dard infant for-mula to provide adequate nutri-ents and amino acids
28.7	52.3	<50	128	1.1	5	11		Additional iron needed. Calcium and vitamin D requirements should be deter-mined by appro-priate laboratory tests
2	—	1,600	800	—	5.2	0.25	10 mg chloride per 100 g	
0.05†	2.7†	90†	45†	—	0.3†	0.4†	Other vitamins and minerals in amounts to nearly meet es-timated needs of premature infants except for iron and possibly vita-min E	Mix 1 packet with 25 ml human milk

Continued.

Feeding Supplements and Modules[2]—cont'd

Name	Company	Food Source	Use	Composition per 100 g		
				Form Available	Kilo-calories	Protein (g)
MCT* oil	Mead Johnson	Lipid fraction of co-conut oil	Supplement for people who cannot digest and absorb long-chain fats	Liquid	830	—
Microlipid™	Sherwood Medical	Safflower oil emulsion	Calorie supplementation from fat	Liquid	450	—
Moducal™	Mead Johnson	Glucose polymers from hydrolyzed corn starch	Carbohydrate supplement	Powder	380	—
Polycose™	Ross	Glucose polymers from hydrolyzed corn starch	Carbohydrate supplement	Powder	380	—
				Liquid	200	—
Pro Mod™	Ross	D-whey protein concentrate; soy lecithin	Protein supplement	Powder	423	76
ProViMin™	Ross	Casein	Protein base for preparing formula for infants and children with chronic diarrhea and other malabsorptive disorders requiring fat and carbohydrate restriction	Powder	313	73

*MCT = medium-chain triglycerides

							Composition per 100 g	
Fat (g)	**Carbo-hydrate (g)**	**Calcium (mg)**	**Phos-phorus (g)**	**Iron (mg)**	**Sodium (mEq)**	**Potas-sium (mEq)**	**Other**	**Miscellaneous Information**
100	—	—	—	—	—	—		
50	—	—	—	—	—	—		5.5 g linoleic acid per 15 ml
—	95	—	—	—	3	<0.26	4.2 mEq chloride	Osmolality is approximately $\frac{1}{6}$ of a glucose solution
—	94	≤30	≤5	—	≤4.8	≤0.3	≤ 6.3 mEq chloride	Osmolality is approximately $\frac{1}{6}$ of a glucose solution
—	50	20	3	—	3	0.15	3.9 mEq chloride	Osmolality of liquid polycose is 835 mOsm/kg H_2O
9	10	665	498	—	9.8	25		1 scoop = 6.6 g and contains 5 g protein
1.4	2	2,400	1,700	40	52	84		Carbohydrate and fat need to be added per individual tolerance; adequate vitamin D needs to be added

Exchange Values for Commercial Baby Foods[1]

The following exchange values were determined from Gerber Products Company and Heinz, U.S.A., 1992 nutrient data. These manufacturers use similar size jars, but different names to designate the texture or consistency of the baby foods. The names and jar sizes are listed below. The abbreviated name in parenthesis will be used throughout the exchange list.

HEINZ (H)

Beginner Foods	2½ oz	(Beginner)
Strained Foods	4 oz	(Strained)
Junior Foods	6 oz	(Junior)

GERBER (G)

First Foods	2½ oz	(First)
Second Foods	4 oz	(Second)
Third Foods	6 oz	(Third)
Tropical Foods	4 oz	(Tropical)
Graduates	6 oz	(Graduates)
Chunky Main Dishes	6 oz	(Chunky)

CONVERSIONS*

2 Tbsp = 1 oz
8 Tbsp = 4 oz = ½ cup
9 Tbsp = 4½ oz jar
12 Tbsp = 8 oz = ¾ cup

---

*The above conversions do not apply to dry cereals because the weights of dry cereals vary so do not directly convert to a volume measure.

OTHER NOTES

Desserts, including fruit with tapioca and yogurt desserts, are generally not acceptable because of their higher sugar content.

Foods that should only be used occasionally, because their sugar content is higher than other foods listed, are noted with an asterisk(*). Occasional use is considered to be 2 to 3 times per week or at the discretion of the dietitian who is able to assess the infant's individual needs.

These exchange values are calculated for use with calorie control or diabetic diets and are *not* specific enough for protein and/or mineral restricted diets.

Note that mixed dinners contain less protein (1 to 7 g of protein per 8 Tbsp or ½ cup) when compared with plain meats (15 to 18 g of protein per 8 Tbsp or ½ cup). To ensure adequate intake of high biological value protein, it is recommended that the care giver mix meat and vegetables together rather than use the mixed dinners.

This appendix is a partial listing and does not imply an endorsement of any product or manufacturer. For further information on baby food composition, contact the following:

1. Gerber Products Company
   445 State Street
   Fremont, MI 49413-0001
   1 (800) 443-7237 or (616) 928-2000
2. Growing Healthy, Inc.
   7615 Golden Triangle Drive
   Eden Prairie, MN 55344
   1 (800) 755-4999
3. Heinz, U.S.A.
   Communications Department
   PO Box 57
   Pittsburgh, PA 15230-0057
   1 (800) USA-BABY
4. Beechnut Nutrition Corporation
   Office of Consumer Affairs
   Checkerboard Square
   St. Louis, MO 63164
   1 (800) 523-6633

Reference

1. Adapted and revised from: Holzmeister LA. Baby food exchanges and meal planning for the infant with diabetes. Diabetes Educator 1992;18 (Sept/Oct):375–385.

Milk Exchange per 8 oz

Milk Exchange based on one serving of whole milk that contains approximately 12 g of carbohydrates, 8 g of protein, and 8 g of fat.

Formula/Milk	Calories	Carbohydrate (g)	Protein (g)	Fat (g)
Breast milk[a]	160	17.3	2.5	9.6
Carnation Follow-Up[b]	160	21.1	4.8	6.2
Enfamil[c]	160	16.5	3.5	9.0
Gerber[d]	160	17.3	3.6	8.8
Good Start[e]	160	17.6	3.8	8.2
Isomil[f]	160	16.7	4.3	8.7
Prosobee[c]	160	16.0	4.8	8.5
Similac[f]	160	17.1	3.6	8.6
SMA[g]	160	17.3	3.6	8.6

[a]Committee on Nutrition, American Academy of Pediatrics. Pediatric nutrition handbook, 2nd ed. Elk Grove, IL: AAP, 1985;363–368.

[b]Carnation follow-up. Product monograph, 1988.

[c]Pediatric product's handbook. Mead Johnson Nutritionals, 1990.

[d]Gerber product monograph, 1989.

[e]Carnation Good Start. H.A. product monograph, 1988.

[f]Ross Laboratories product handbook, 1990.

[g]SMA infant formula comparison chart, Wyeth Laboratories, July 1991.

Starch/Bread Exchange

Each starch/bread exchange contains approximately 15 g of carbohydrate, 3 g of protein, and 80 cal.

Item	Amount	Brand
CEREALS	**(TBSP)**	
Dry Infant cereal, First/Second/Tropical (Barley, Rice, Mixed, Corn)	5	G
Dry Infant cereal, First (Oatmeal)	4	G
Dry Infant cereal, Beginner (Mixed, Oatmeal)	9	H
Dry Infant cereal, Beginner (Barley, Rice)	8	H
Rice cereal w/mango, Tropical*	5	G
Dry Infant cereal w/banana, Second (Oatmeal)*	6	G
Dry Infant cereal w/banana, Second (Mixed, Rice*)	5	G
Dry Infant cereal, Beginner (High protein)	15	H
Dry Infant cereal, Second (High protein)	10	G
Infant cereal w/fruit in jars, Second/Third (Mixed, Oatmeal, Rice)	6	G
Infant cereal w/fruit in jars, strained (Rice)	6	H
Infant cereal w/fruit in jars, strained (Mixed,* Oatmeal)	7	H
FINGER FOODS	**(EACH)**	
Animal Crackers (cinnamon), Graduates	6	G
Arrowroot Cookies, Graduates	4	G
Biter Biscuits, Chunky*	2	G
Animal-shaped Cookies, Chunky*	3	G
Pretzels, Graduates	3	G
Zwieback Toast, Chunky*	2	G
STARCHY VEGETABLES	**(TBSP)**	
Corn, creamed; Second/Strained	8	G, H
Corn, creamed; Junior	7	H
Peas, Beginner	11	H
Peas, First/Second	14	G
Peas, Third	13	G
Peas, creamed; Strained	14	H
Squash, First/Second/Third	15	G
Squash, Beginner	14	H
Squash, Strained	16	H
Sweet Potatoes, First/Second/Third/Beginner/Strained/Junior	7	G, H

*Use occasionally (see introduction).

Meat Exchange

Each meat exchange contains approximately 7 g of protein, 3 g of fat, and 55 cal.

Item	Amount (TBSP)	Brand
Beef, Second/Third	4	G
Chicken, Second/Third	4	G
Ham, Second/Third	4	G
Lamb, Second/Third	4	G
Turkey, Second/Third	4	G
Veal, Second/Third	4	G
Egg yolks, Second	5	G
Beef and broth, Strained/Junior	3	H
Chicken and broth, Strained/Junior	4	H
Lamb and broth, Strained/Junior	3	H
Turkey and broth, Strained/Junior	3	H
Veal and broth, Strained/Junior	3	H
Liver and liver broth, Strained/Junior	3	H
Chicken sticks, Graduates	5 sticks	G
Meat sticks, Graduates	5 sticks	G
Turkey sticks, Graduates	5 sticks	G

Fruit Exchange

Each fruit exchange contains approximately 15 g of carbohydrate and 60 cal.

	Amount	Brand
FRUIT	**(TBSP)**	
Apples/blueberry, Second/Third	9	G
Applesauce, Beginner	6	H
Applesauce, First/Strained/Junior	8	G, H
Applesauce, Second/Third	9	G
Applesauce apricot, Second	8	G
Apples and apricots, Strained/Junior	8	H
Apples and pears, Strained/Junior	8	H
Bananas, First/Beginner	4	G, H
Peaches, First	11	G
Peaches, Beginner	6	H
Peaches, Second/Third/Strained/Junior*	7	G, H
Pears, First/Second/Third	8	G
Pears, Beginner	6	H
Pears, Strained/Junior	7	H
Pears/pineapple, Second/Third	8	G
Pears/pineapple, Strained	8	H
Prunes, First	4	G
FRUIT JUICES	**(OZ)**	
Apple, First/Strained	4	G, H
Apple apricot, Strained	4	H
Apple/banana, Second/Strained	4	G, H
Apple/cherry, Second/Strained	4	G, H
Apple/cranberry, Strained	4	H
Apple/grape, Second/Strained	4	G, H
Apple/peach, Second	4	G
Apple/peach, Strained	5	H
Apple/pineapple, Strained	4	H
Apple/plum, Second	4	G
Apple/prune, Second/Strained	4	G, H
Guava/mixed fruit, Tropical	3	G
Mango/mixed fruit, Tropical	3	G
Papaya/mixed fruit, Tropical	3	G
Mixed fruit, Second/Strained	4	G, H
Orange, Strained	4	H
Orange, Second	5	G
Orange/apple, Strained	4	H
Orange/apple/banana, Strained	4	H
Pear, First/Strained	4	G, H
Pear/grape, Strained	5	H
Apple/carrot, Third	5	G

*Use occasionally (see introduction).

Fruit Exchange—cont'd

	Amount	Brand
FRUIT JUICES—cont'd	(OZ)	
Apple/sweet potato, Third	4	G
Orange/carrot, Third	5	G
Pineapple/carrot, Third	5	G
Red grape, First	3	G
White grape, First/Strained	3	G, H

Vegetable Exchange

Each vegetable exchange contains approximately 5 g of carbohydrate, 2 g of protein, and 25 cal.

Item	Amount	Brand
	(TBSP)	
Beets, Second/Strained	4	G, H
Broccoli/carrots/cheese, Third	5	G
Carrots, First	5	G
Carrots, Second/Third/Beginner	6	G, H
Carrots, Strained/Junior	7	H
Corn, creamed; Junior	2	H
Corn, creamed; Second/Strained	3	G, H
Garden vegetables, Second	5	G
Green beans, First/Second/Beginner	6	G, H
Green beans, Strained	7	H
Green beans, creamed; Third	4	G
Green beans, creamed; Junior	5	H
Mixed vegetables, Second/Third/Strained	4	G, H
Peas, First/Second	5	G
Peas, Beginner/Third	4	G, H
Peas, creamed; Strained	5	H
Spinach, creamed; Second	5	G
Squash, First/Second/Third/Beginner/Strained	5	G, H
Sweet potatoes, First/Second/Third/Beginner/Strained/Junior	2	G, H

Combination Foods

Combination foods vary in their nutrient composition.

Item	Amount	Exchange	Brand
DINNERS	**(CUPS)**		
Beef/egg noodle, Second	½	½ starch, ½ meat	G
Beef/egg noodle, Strained	½	½ starch, ½ vegetable	H
Beef/egg noodle, Third	¾	½ starch, ½ fat	G
Beef/egg noodle, Junior	¾	1 vegetable, ½ starch, ½ fat	H
Carrots/beef, Second (Simple Recipes)	½	1 vegetable, ½ meat	G
Broccoli/chicken, Second (Simple Recipes)	½	1 vegetable, ½ meat	G
Chicken noodle, Second	½	½ starch, ½ meat	G
Chicken noodle, Strained	½	½ vegetable, ½ starch, ½ fat	H
Chicken noodle, Third	¾	½ meat, 1 starch	G
Chicken noodle, Junior	¾	1 vegetable, ½ starch, ½ fat	H
Apples/chicken, Second (Simple Recipes)	½	1 fruit	G
Apples/ham, Second (Simple Recipes)	½	1 fruit, ½ meat	G
Apples/turkey, Second (Simple Recipes)	½	1 fruit, ½ meat	G
Green beans/turkey, Second (Simple recipes)	½	1 vegetable, ½ meat	G
Macaroni/cheese, Second	½	½ starch, ½ meat	G
Macaroni/tomato/beef, Second	½	1 starch	G
Macaroni/tomato/beef, Strained	½	½ vegetable, ½ starch	H
Macaroni/tomato/beef, Third	¾	½ meat, 1 starch	G
Macaroni/tomato/beef, Junior	¾	1 vegetable, ½ starch, ½ fat	H
Spaghetti tomato sauce/beef, Third	¾	1 starch, ½ meat	G
Spaghetti tomato sauce/beef, Junior	¾	½ vegetable, 1 starch, ½ fat	H
Turkey rice, Second	½	½ starch, ½ meat	G
Turkey rice, Third	¾	½ meat, 1 starch	G
Turkey rice dinner/vegetables, Strained	½	½ vegetable, ½ starch	H
Turkey rice dinner/vegetables, Junior	¾	1 vegetable, ½ starch	H
Vegetable Turkey, Second	½	½ starch	G
Vegetable Turkey, Third	¾	½ meat, 1 starch	G
Vegetable bacon, Second	½	1 starch, 1 fat	G
Vegetable bacon, Strained	½	½ vegetable, ½ starch, ½ fat	H
Vegetable bacon, Third	¾	½ meat, 1 starch, 1 fat	G
Vegetable bacon, Junior	¾	1 vegetable, ½ starch, ½ fat	H
Vegetable beef, Second	½	½ starch	G

Combination Foods—cont'd

Item	Amount	Exchange	Brand
DINNERS—cont'd	**(CUPS)**		
Vegetable beef, Strained	½	½ vegetable, ½ starch, ½ fat	H
Vegetable beef, Third	¾	½ meat, 1 starch	G
Vegetable beef, Junior	¾	1 vegetable, ½ starch, ½ fat	H
Vegetable chicken, Second	½	1 starch	G
Vegetable chicken, Third	¾	½ meat, 1 starch	G
Vegetable ham, Second	½	½ starch	G
Vegetable ham, Strained	½	½ vegetable, ½ starch	H
Vegetable ham, Third	¾	½ meat, 1 starch	G
Vegetable ham, Junior	¾	½ vegetable, ½ starch, ½ fat	H
Vegetable lamb, Strained	½	½ vegetable, ½ starch	H
Vegetable turkey, Second	½	½ starch	G
Vegetable turkey, Third	¾	½ meat, 1 starch	G
Vegetables, egg noodles/chicken, Strained	½	½ vegetable, ½ starch	H
Vegetables, egg noodles/chicken, Junior	¾	1 vegetable, ½ starch, ½ fat	H
Vegetables, egg noodles/turkey, Strained	½	½ vegetable, ½ starch	H
Vegetables, egg noodles/turkey, Junior	¾	1 vegetable, ½ starch, ½ fat	H
Vegetables, dumplings/beef, Strained	½	½ vegetable, ½ starch	H
Vegetables, dumplings/beef, Junior	¾	1 vegetable, ½ starch, ½ fat	H
TODDLER FOODS			
Chunky Products			
Homestyle noodles/beef	¾	1 starch, ½ meat, ½ fat	G
Macaroni alphabets/beef/tomato sauce	¾	1 starch, ½ meat, 1 vegetable	G
Noodles/chicken/carrots/peas	¾	1 starch, ½ meat,	G
Rice/beef/tomato sauce	¾	1 starch, 1 vegetable, ½ meat	G
Saucy rice/chicken	¾	1 starch, 1 vegetable	G
Spaghetti/tomato sauce/beef	¾	1 starch, 1 vegetable, ½ meat	G
Vegetables/beef	¾	1 starch, ½ meat	G
Vegetables/chicken	¾	1 starch, ½ meat	G
Vegetables/ham	¾	1 starch, ½ meat	G
Vegetables/turkey	¾	1 starch, ½ meat	G
Graduates			
Macaroni/beef in sauce	¾	1 starch, 1 meat	G
Tomato sauce w/beef ravioli	¾	2 starch, 1 meat	G
Tomato sauce w/cheese ravioli	¾	2 starch, 1 meat	G

Continued.

Combination Foods—cont'd

Item	Amount	Exchange	Brand
TODDLER FOODS—cont'd	(CUPS)		
Graduates—cont'd			
Turkey stew w/rice	¾	1 starch, 1 meat	G
Chicken stew/noodles	¾	1 starch, 1 meat	G
Spaghetti/mini-meatballs/sauce	¾	1½ starch, 1 meat	G
Vegetable stew/beef	¾	1 starch, 1 meat	G
Soups			
Chicken, Strained	½	½ vegetable, ½ starch	H
Cream of Broccoli, Third	¾	1 vegetable	G
Cream of Potato, Third	½	½ starch	G
Cream of Tomato, Third	¾	1 starch	G
Cream of Vegetable, Third	¾	½ starch	G

27 / Common Carbohydrates in Foods (per 100 g Edible Portion)

| Food | Monosaccharides | | Reducing Sugars* | Disaccharides | | | Polysaccharides | | | | | |
	Fructose (g)	Glucose (g)	(g)	Lactose (g)	Maltose (g)	Sucrose (g)	Cellulose (g)	Dextrins (g)	Hemicellulose (g)	Pectin (g)	Pentosans (g)	Starch (g)
FRUITS												
Agave juice	17.0		19.0	†								
Apple	5.0	1.7	8.3			3.1	0.4		0.7	0.6		0.6
Apple juice			8.0			4.2	0.8		1.2	1.0		
Apricots	0.4	1.9				5.5						
Banana												
Yellow green			5.0			5.1						8.8
Yellow			8.4			8.9						1.9
Flecked	3.5	4.5				11.9						1.2
Powder			32.6			33.2						7.8
Blackberries	2.9	3.2				0.2						
Blueberry juice, commercial			9.6			0.2						
Boysenberries			5.3			1.1				0.3		
Breadfruit												
Hawaiian			1.8			7.7		9.6				
Samoan			4.9			9.7						
Cherries												
Eating	7.2	4.7	12.5			0.1				0.3		
Cooking	6.1	5.5	11.6			0.1						
Cranberries	0.7	2.7				0.1						
Currants												
Black	3.7	2.4				0.6						
Red	1.9	2.3				0.2						
White	2.6	3.0										
Dates												
Invert sugar, seedling type	23.9	24.9				0.3						

Deglet Noor			16.2	45.4		3.0
Egyptian			35.8	48.5		
Figs, Kadota						
Fresh	8.2	9.6		0.9		0.1
Dried	30.9	42.0		0.1		0.3
Gooseberries	4.1	4.4		0.7		
Grapes						
Black	7.3	8.2				
Concord	4.3	4.8	9.5	0.2		
Malaga			22.2	0.2		
White	8.0	8.1				
Grapefruit	1.2	2.0		2.9		
Guava			4.4	1.9	1.3	
Lemon						
Edible portion			1.3	0.2	0.7	
Whole	1.4	1.4		0.4	3.0	
Juice	0.9	0.5		0.1		
Peel			3.4	0.1		
Loganberries	1.3	1.9		0.2		
Loquat						
Champagne	12.0			0.8		
Thales	9.0			0.9		
Mango			3.4	11.6		
Melon						
Cantaloupe	0.9	1.2	2.3	4.4	0.3	0.3
Cassaba						
Vine						
ripened			2.8	6.2		
Picked						
green			3.2	3.9		

*Mainly monosaccharides plus the disaccharides maltose and lactose.

†Blanks indicate lack of acceptable data.

‡Also known as Alaska pea, field pea, and common pea.

§Trace = less than 0.05 g.

From: Hardinge MG, Swarner JB, Crooks H. Carbohydrate in foods. Copyright The American Dietetic Association. Reprinted by permission from Journal of the American Dietetic Association 1965;46:197.

Continued.

| Food | Mono-Saccharides | | Reducing Sugars* | Disaccharides | | | Polysaccharides | | | | | |
	Fructose (g)	Glucose (g)		Lactose (g)	Maltose (g)	Sucrose (g)	Cellulose (g)	Dextrins (g)	Hemicellulose (g)	Pectin (g)	Pentosans (g)	Starch (g)
FRUITS—cont'd												
Honeydew												
Vine ripened			3.3			7.4						
Picked green			3.6			3.3						
Yellow	1.5	2.1				1.4						
Mulberries	3.6	4.4										
Orange												
Valencia (Calif)	2.3	2.4	4.7			4.2						
Composite values	1.8	2.5	5.0			4.6	0.3		0.3	1.3	0.3	
Juice												
Fresh	2.4	2.4	5.1			4.7						
Frozen, reconstituted			4.6			3.2						
Palmyra palm, tender kernal	1.5	3.2				0.4						
Papaw (Asimina triloba) (North America)			5.9			2.7						
Papaya (Carica papaya) (Tropics)			9.0			0.5						
Passion fruit juice	3.6	3.6				3.8		0.7				
Peaches	1.6	1.5	3.1			6.6				0.7		1.8

Food											
Pears											
Anjou	5.0		7.6		1.9				0.7		
Bartlett	6.5	2.5	8.0		1.5				0.6		
Bosc		2.6			1.7				0.6		
Persimmon			17.7								
Pineapple											
Ripened on plant	1.4	2.3	4.2		7.9						
Picked green			1.3		2.4						
Plums											
Damson	3.4	5.2	8.4		1.0						
Green gage	4.0	5.5			2.9						
Italian prunes			4.6		5.4				0.9		
Sweet	2.9	4.5	7.4		4.4		0.5		1.0	0.1	
Sour	1.3	3.5			1.5				1.0		
Pomegranate			12.0		0.6						
Prunes, uncooked	15.0	30.0	47.0		2.0	2.8		10.7	0.9	2.0	0.7
Raisins, Thompson seedless			70.0								
Raspberries	2.4	2.3			1.0				1.0		
Sapote	3.8	4.2	5.0	0.7					0.8		
Strawberries											
Ripe	2.3	2.6			1.4						
Medium ripe			3.8		0.3						
Tangerine	4.8	1.6			9.0				0.3		
Tomatoes	1.2		3.4								
Canned			3.0		0.3	0.2		0.3			
Seedless pulp			6.5		0.4	0.4		0.5			

Continued.

Food	Monosaccharides		Reducing Sugars*	Disaccharides			Polysaccharides					
	Fructose (g)	Glucose (g)		Lactose (g)	Maltose (g)	Sucrose (g)	Cellulose (g)	Dextrins (g)	Hemicellulose (g)	Pectin (g)	Pentosans (g)	Starch (g)
FRUITS—cont'd												
Watermelon												
Flesh red and firm, ripe	3.8					4.0				0.1		
Red, mealy, overripe	3.0					4.9				0.1		
VEGETABLES												
Asparagus, raw			1.2						0.3			
Bamboo shoots			0.5			0.2	1.2					
Beans												
Lima												
Canned						1.4						
Fresh						1.4						
Snap, fresh			1.7			0.5	0.5	0.3	1.0	0.5	1.2	2.0
Beets, sugar						12.9	0.9		0.8			
Broccoli							0.9		0.9		0.9	1.3
Brussels sprouts							1.1		1.5			
Cabbage, raw			3.4			0.3	0.8		1.0			
Carrots, raw		2.8	5.8			1.7	1.0		1.7	0.9		
Cauliflower						0.3	0.7		0.6			
Celery												
Fresh			0.3			0.3						
Hearts			1.7			0.2						
Corn												
Fresh		0.5				0.3	0.6	0.1	0.9		1.3	14.5
Bran									77.1		4.0	
Cucumber			2.5			0.1						
Eggplant			2.1			0.6			0.5			
Lettuce			1.4			0.2	0.4		0.6			
Licorice root		1.4				3.2						22.0

Food									
Mushrooms, fresh		0.1							2.5
Onions, raw		5.4		2.9	0.9		0.7	0.6	7.0
Parsnips, fresh				3.5			0.3		4.1
Peas, green				5.5	1.1				17.0
Potatoes, white	0.1	0.8		0.1	0.4		2.2		0.1
Pumpkin		2.2		0.6			0.3		
Radishes		3.1		0.3			0.5	0.4	
Rutabagas	5.0			1.3	0.4		0.3		
Spinach		0.2						0.8	
Squash									
Butternut	0.1			0.4	0.7				2.6
Blue hubbard	1.1			0.4					4.8
Golden crook-neck		2.8		1.0					
Sweet potato									
Raw	0.4	0.8		4.1			0.8		16.5
Baked		14.5	1.6	7.2	0.6		1.4		4.0
MATURE DRY LEGUMES									
Beans									
Mung				1.6					
Black gram									
Green gram				1.8					
Navy		1.6		7.2	3.1	3.7	6.4	8.2	35.2
Soy					2.6	1.4	6.6	4.0	1.9
Cow pea				1.5	5.4		4.8		
Garbanzo (chick peas)				2.4					

Continued.

Food	Monosaccharides		Reducing Sugars* (g)	Disaccharides			Polysaccharides					
	Fructose (g)	Glucose (g)		Lactose (g)	Maltose (g)	Sucrose (g)	Cellulose (g)	Dextrins (g)	Hemicellulose (g)	Pectin (g)	Pentosans (g)	Starch (g)
MATURE DRY LEGUMES—cont'd												
Garden pea (Pisum sativum)‡						6.7	5.0		5.1			38.0
Horse gram (Dolichos biplorus)					2.7							
Lentils					2.1							28.5
Pigeon pea (red gram)					1.6							
Soybean Flour					6.8							
Meal					6.8							
MILK AND MILK PRODUCTS												
Buttermilk Dry				39.9								
Fluid, genuine and cultured				5.0								
Casein		0.1		4.9								
Ice cream (14.5% cream)				3.6		16.6						
Milk												
Ass				6.0								
Cow				4.9								
Dried												
Skim				52.0								
Whole				38.1								

Food								
Fluid								
Skim			5.0					
Whole			4.9					
Sweetened, condensed			14.1				43.5	
Ewe			4.9					
Goat			4.7					
Human								
Colostrum			5.3					
Mature			6.9					
Whey			4.9					
Yogurt			3.8					
NUTS AND NUT PRODUCTS								
Almonds, blanched		0.2		2.3			2.1	
Chestnuts		2.2		3.6			1.2	18.0
Virginia		1.2		8.1			2.8	18.6
French		3.3		3.6		0.3	2.5	33.1
Coconut, milk ripe				2.6				
Copra meal, dried	1.2			14.3	15.6			
Macadamia nut		0.3		5.5		0.6	2.2	0.9
Peanuts		0.2		4.5	2.4	2.5		
Peanut butter		0.9				3.8		4.0
Pecans				1.1			0.2	5.9
SPICES AND CONDIMENTS								
Allspice (pimenta)		18.0		3.0				
Cassia		23.3						
Cinnamon		19.3						
Cloves		9.0						2.7
Nutmeg		17.2						14.6
Pepper, black		38.6						34.2

Continued.

‡See footnote on p. 809

Food	Monosaccharides		Reducing Sugars* (g)	Disaccharides			Polysaccharides					
	Fructose (g)	Glucose (g)		Lactose (g)	Maltose (g)	Sucrose (g)	Cellulose (g)	Dextrins (g)	Hemicellulose (g)	Pectin (g)	Pentosans (g)	Starch (g)
CEREALS AND CEREAL PRODUCTS												
Barley												
Grain, hulled							2.6		6.0		8.5	62.0
Flour						3.1					1.2	69.0
Corn, yellow							4.5		4.9		6.2	62.0
Flaxseed							1.8		5.2			56.0
Millet grain											6.5	56.0
Oats, hulled									0.9		6.4	56.4
Rice												
Bran			1.4			10.6	11.4		7.0		7.4	69.7
Brown, raw		2.0	0.1			0.8		2.1			2.1	72.9
Polished, raw			trace§			0.4	0.3	0.9			1.8	
Polish			0.7								3.8	
Rye												
Grain							3.8		5.6		6.8	57.0
Flour											4.1	71.4
Sorghum grain											2.5	70.2
Soya-wheat (cereal)											3.3	46.4
Wheat												
Germ, de-fatted						8.3					6.2	
Grain			2.0			1.5	2.0	2.5	5.8		6.6	59.0
Flour, patent			2.0		0.1	0.2		5.5			2.1	68.8

SYRUPS AND OTHER SWEETS

Corn syrup		21.2			26.4		34.7			
High conversion		33.0			23.0		19.0			
Medium conversion		26.0			21.0		23.0			
Corn sugar		87.5			3.5		0.5			
Chocolate, sweet dry						56.4				
Golden syrup	40.5		37.5			31.0				
Honey		34.2				1.9	1.5			
Invert sugar			74.0			6.0				
Jellies, pectin	11.3	9.8				40–65				
Royal jelly						0.9				
Jellies, starch						25–60				
Maple syrup			1.5			62.9				
Milk chocolate				8.1		43.0				
Molasses	8.0	8.8	26.9			53.6				
Blackstrap	6.8	6.8	27.0			36.9				
Sorghum syrup						36.0				

MISCELLANEOUS

Beer			1.5				2.8			7–12
Cacao beans, raw, Arriba	0.6	0.5	1.1		1.9					
Carob bean										
Pod			11.2		23.2			1.4		
Pod and seeds			11.1		19.4					
Soy Sauce	0.9								0.3	

§See footnote on p. 809.

28 / *National Center for Health Statistics (NCHS) Growth Graphs*

Boys: Birth to 36 Months; Physical Growth; NCHS Percentiles

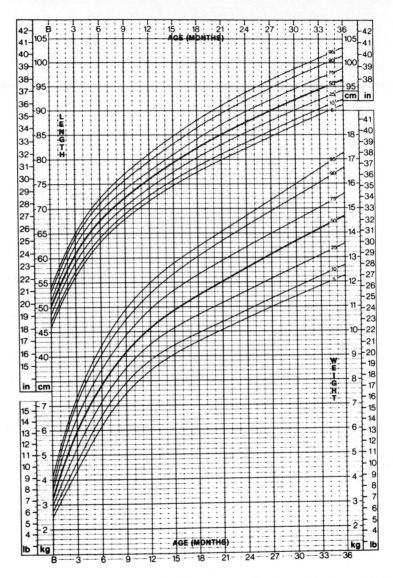

With permission from Hamill PVV, Drizd TA, Johnson CL, Reed RB, Roche AF, Moore WM. Physical growth: National Center for Health Statistics percentiles. Am J Clin Nutr 1979; 32:607–629. Data from the Fels Longitudinal Study, Wright State University School of Medicine, Yellow Springs, Ohio.

Boys: Birth to 36 Months; Physical Growth; NCHS Percentiles

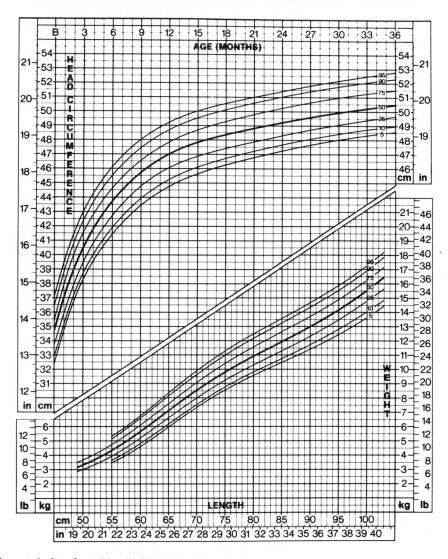

With permission from Hamill PVV, Drizd TA, Johnson CL, Reed RB, Roche AF, Moore WM. Physical growth: National Center for Health Statistics percentiles. Am J Clin Nutr 1979; 32:607–629. Data from the Fels Longitudinal Study, Wright State University School of Medicine, Yellow Springs, Ohio.

Girls: Birth to 36 months; Physical Growth; NCHS Percentiles

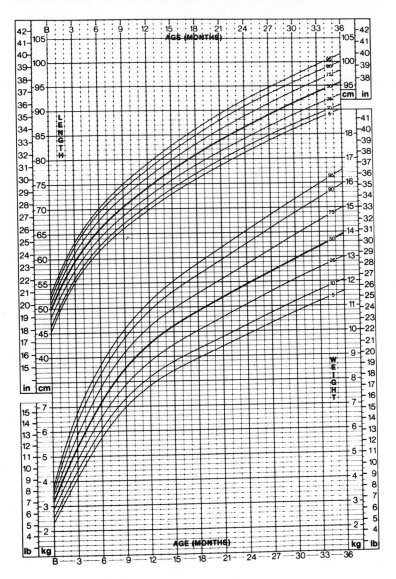

With permission from Hamill PVV, Drizd TA, Johnson CL, Reed RB, Roche AF, Moore WM. Physical growth: National Center for Health Statistics percentiles. Am J Clin Nutr 1979; 32:607–629. Data from the Fels Longitudinal Study, Wright State University School of Medicine, Yellow Springs, Ohio.

Girls: Birth to 36 Months; Physical Growth; NCHS Percentiles

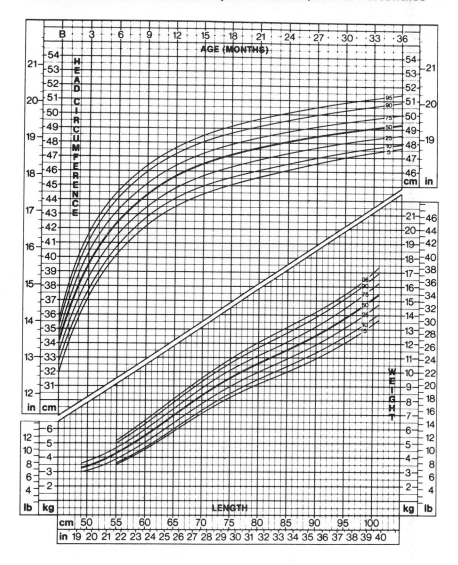

With permission from Hamill PVV, Drizd TA, Johnson CL, Reed RB, Roche AF, Moore WM. Physical growth: National Center for Health Statistics percentiles. Am J Clin Nutr 1979; 32:607–629. Data from the Fels Longitudinal Study, Wright State University School of Medicine, Yellow Springs, Ohio.

Boys: 2 to 18 Years; Physical Growth; NCHS Percentiles

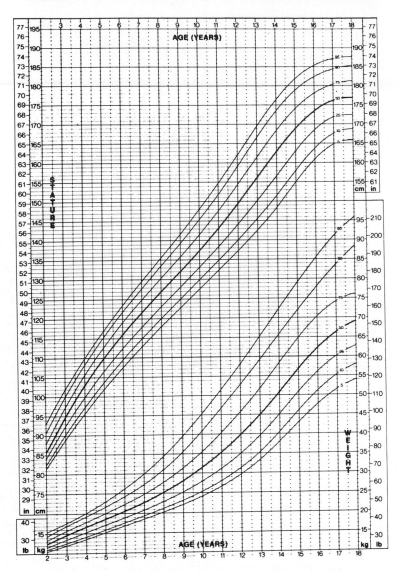

With permission from Hamill PVV, Drizd TA, Johnson CL, Reed RB, Roche AF, Moore WM. Physical growth: National Center for Health Statistics percentiles. Am J Clin Nutr 1979; 32:607–629. Data from the Fels Longitudinal Study, Wright State University School of Medicine, Yellow Springs, Ohio.

Boys: Prepubescent Physical Growth; NCHS Percentiles

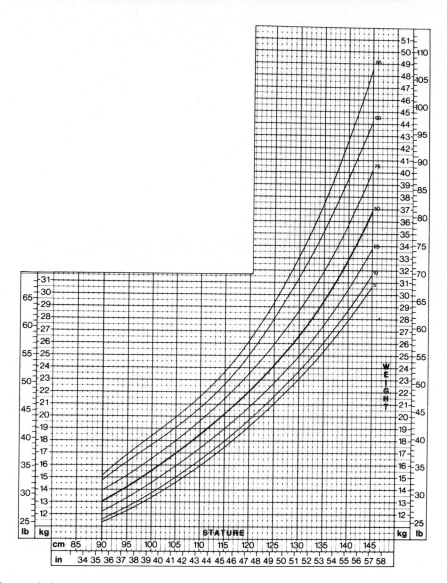

With permission from Hamill PVV, Drizd TA, Johnson CL, Reed RB, Roche AF, Moore WM. Physical growth: National Center for Health Statistics percentiles. Am J Clin Nutr 1979; 32:607–629. Data from the Fels Longitudinal Study, Wright State University School of Medicine, Yellow Springs, Ohio.

Girls: 2 to 18 Years; Physical Growth; NCHS Percentiles

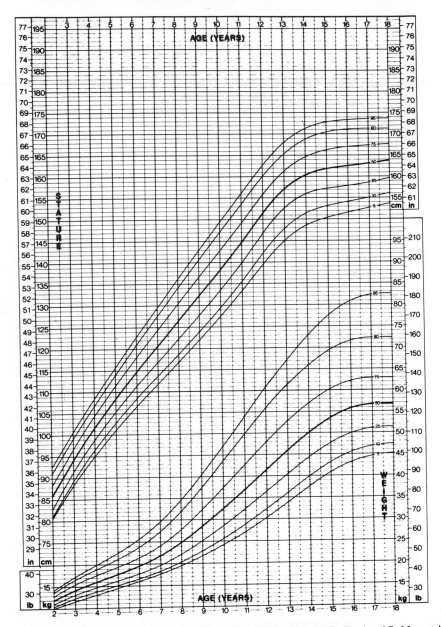

With permission from Hamill PVV, Drizd TA, Johnson CL, Reed RB, Roche AF, Moore WM. Physical growth: National Center for Health Statistics percentiles. Am J Clin Nutr 1979; 32:607–629. Data from the Fels Longitudinal Study, Wright State University School of Medicine, Yellow Springs, Ohio.

Girls: Prepubescent Physical Growth; NCHS Percentiles

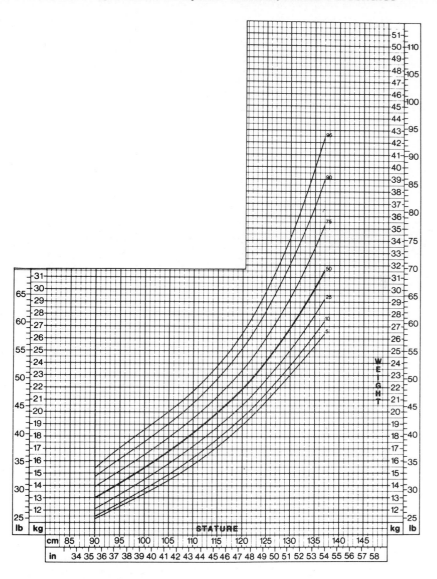

With permission from Hamill PVV, Drizd TA, Johnson CL, Reed RB, Roche AF, Moore WM. Physical growth: National Center for Health Statistics percentiles. Am J Clin Nutr 1979; 32:607–629. Data from the Fels Longitudinal Study, Wright State University School of Medicine, Yellow Springs, Ohio.

29 / *Baldwin-Wood Tables*

Weight-for-Height in Older Children

Height (cm)	\ Age (yr) 8	9	10	11	12	13	14	15	16	17	18	19
						MALES						
140	*31.6	31.6	32.2	32.2	32.4	32.4	*32.5					
141	*32.1	32.3	32.9	32.8	32.9	33.2	*33.1					
142	*32.6	33.1	33.7	33.5	33.4	34.0	*33.7					
143		*33.6	34.1	34.2	34.1	34.7	34.5	*35.3				
144		*34.1	34.4	35.0	34.7	35.2	35.5	*35.8				
145		*35.6	34.9	35.7	35.4	35.8	36.3	*36.3				
146		*36.3	35.7	36.2	36.2	36.5	36.9	*37.0				
147		*34.0	36.5	36.7	36.9	37.1	37.4	*37.7				
148			37.0	37.2	37.6	37.8	38.0	38.2				
149			37.5	37.8	38.2	38.4	38.6	38.7				
150			38.1	38.5	39.0	39.1	39.3	39.3	39.2			
151			*38.7	39.2	39.5	39.7	40.0	40.3	40.3			
152			*39.4	39.9	40.0	40.3	40.7	41.3	41.5			
153				40.5	40.6	41.1	41.6	42.1	42.6			
154				41.0	41.4	41.9	42.5	42.8	43.7			
155				41.5	42.1	42.7	43.4	43.5	44.8	*46.3		
156				*42.3	42.9	43.4	44.0	44.2	45.5	*47.2		
157				*43.2	43.8	44.1	44.7	44.9	46.3	48.1		
158				*44.0	44.6	44.9	45.5	45.8	47.3	49.2	*51.3	
159				*44.9	45.4	45.8	46.4	46.9	48.6	50.3	*52.6	
160				*45.8	46.2	46.7	47.4	48.0	49.8	51.5	53.9	*55.4
161					47.4	47.3	48.1	48.8	50.2	52.0	54.4	*55.9
162					48.7	48.0	48.8	49.6	50.6	52.5	54.9	*56.4

Figures with asterisks represent values based on theoretical computations rather than on exact ages. Age is taken at the nearest birthday, height at the nearest centimeter, and weight at the nearest tenth of a kilogram.

With permission from Jellifee DB. The assessment of the nutritional status of the community. Monograph No. 53. Geneva: World Health Organization, 1966.

Continued.

Weight-for-Height in Older Children—cont'd

Height (cm)	8	9	10	11	12	13	14	15	16	17	18	19
						MALES—cont'd						
163					49.4	48.8	49.6	50.5	51.2	53.2	55.5	*57.0
164					*49.6	49.9	50.5	51.4	52.1	54.1	56.3	*57.7
165					*49.7	50.9	51.4	52.3	53.1	55.1	57.1	58.3
166						51.4	52.1	53.2	54.1	56.1	57.9	59.3
167						51.8	52.9	54.0	55.1	57.0	58.7	60.3
168						52.3	53.7	54.8	56.1	57.8	59.4	61.0
169						*53.1	54.7	55.7	57.1	58.5	60.0	61.4
170						*53.9	55.6	56.5	58.1	59.1	60.5	61.7
171							56.7	57.3	58.8	59.9	61.2	62.5
172							57.8	58.0	59.5	60.9	62.0	63.4
173							58.7	58.7	60.2	61.8	62.8	64.2
174							59.2	59.6	61.1	62.7	63.8	65.1
175							59.7	60.4	61.9	63.5	64.7	65.9
176							60.5	61.2	62.5	64.0	65.3	66.5
177							61.4	62.0	62.9	64.3	65.7	67.2
178							62.4	62.8	63.4	64.7	66.1	67.8
179							*63.3	63.9	64.5	65.4	66.6	68.4
180							*64.2	65.1	65.7	66.1	67.1	68.8
181								65.8	66.4	66.7	67.7	69.6
182								66.3	67.0	67.3	68.3	70.4
183								66.9	67.6	68.0	69.0	71.2
184								*67.5	68.6	69.1	70.1	71.8
185								*68.2	69.5	70.3	71.3	72.5
186								*68.8	70.3	71.3	72.2	73.2
187								*69.3	71.0	72.3	73.1	73.8
188								*69.8	71.7	73.3	73.9	74.4
						FEMALES						
138	*30.9	31.6	31.6	31.9	32.0	32.8						
139	*31.4	32.3	32.3	32.5	32.6	33.4						
140		32.9	32.9	33.1	33.2	34.1	*34.8					
141		33.3	33.6	33.7	34.0	34.9	*35.6					
142		33.6	34.4	34.3	34.8	35.8	*36.5					
143		*34.2	35.1	35.0	35.5	36.3	*37.4					
144		*34.9	35.9	35.6	36.0	36.7	*38.4					
145			36.6	36.4	36.6	37.2	39.3	*41.1				
146			36.8	37.3	37.3	38.0	40.3	*42.0				
147			37.1	38.2	37.9	38.8	41.4	*42.8				
148			37.6	38.9	38.6	39.5	42.0	*43.5	*45.1			
149			38.2	39.5	39.2	40.3	42.5	*44.0	*45.5			
150			38.8	40.2	39.9	41.1	43.0	44.6	*45.9	*46.4		
151			*39.5	41.0	40.8	41.9	43.8	45.5	*46.8	47.3		
152			*40.2	41.8	41.7	42.7	44.6	46.4	*47.7	48.1		

Weight-for-Height in Older Children—cont'd

Height (cm)	Age (yr)											
	8	9	10	11	12	13	14	15	16	17	18	19
					FEMALES—cont'd							
153				42.6	42.7	43.5	45.4	47.1	48.6	*48.9	*49.9	
154				43.4	43.8	44.2	46.2	47.6	49.4	49.7	*50.7	
155				44.0	44.8	45.0	47.0	48.1	50.2	50.4	51.4	
156				*44.1	45.5	45.7	47.5	48.9	50.7	51.1	51.7	
157				*44.2	46.2	46.5	48.1	49.8	51.1	51.8	52.0	
158					47.0	47.4	48.7	50.5	51.4	52.2	52.4	
159					47.9	48.3	49.2	51.0	51.7	52.5	52.7	
160					48.9	49.2	49.8	51.5	51.9	52.8	53.1	
161					*49.6	49.9	50.7	52.1	52.6	53.3	53.6	
162					*50.3	50.6	51.5	52.7	53.2	53.7	54.0	
163					*51.0	51.4	52.3	53.3	53.8	54.2	54.6	
164					*51.7	52.2	53.2	53.7	54.3	54.8	55.3	
165					*52.4	53.1	54.0	54.2	54.8	55.4	55.9	
166						54.0	54.5	54.6	55.7	56.1	56.6	
167						54.9	54.9	55.0	56.6	56.9	57.4	
168						*55.6	55.5	55.7	57.4	57.6	58.2	
169						*56.2	56.6	56.9	58.2	58.2	59.2	
170						*56.8	57.6	58.0	58.9	58.9	60.1	
171						*57.2	58.2	58.8	59.5	59.7	60.7	
172						*57.8	58.7	59.5	60.0	60.7	61.1	
173							59.1	60.1	60.5	61.4	61.6	
174							*59.6	*60.5	*60.9	*61.8	*62.3	
175							*60.0	*60.8	*61.2	*62.1	*62.9	
176							*60.2	*61.0	*61.6	*62.5	*63.4	
177							*60.4	*61.2	*62.0	*62.8	*63.7	
178							*60.6	*61.5	*62.4	*63.2	*64.0	
179							*60.9	*61.8	*62.7	*63.5	*64.2	
180							*61.3	*62.2	*63.0	*63.9	*64.4	

Girls with Down's syndrome: Physical Growth, 1 to 36 Months

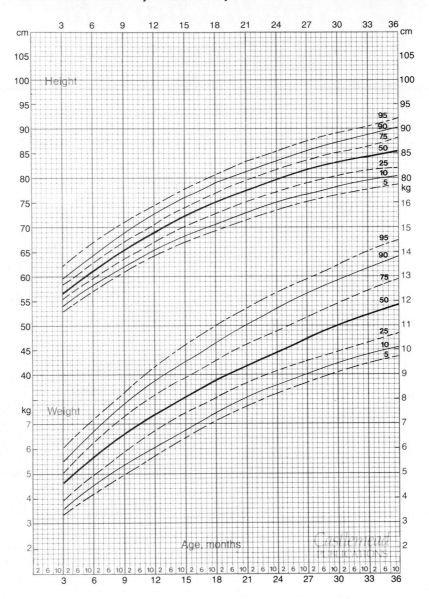

This chart provides reference percentiles for girls with Down's syndrome from birth to 36 months of age. It is based on mixed longitudinal data on approximately 300 girls with Down's syndrome born between 1960 and 1986 and reared at home. Children with congenital heart disease are included in the sample. The percentile rank for a given child indicates the relative position she would hold in a series of 100 girls with Down's syndrome. For example, a girl at the 10th percentile is larger than 10% and smaller than 90% of girls her age with Down's syndrome. The 50th percentile is the midposition, equivalent to "average" height or weight for a girl with Down's syndrome.

These charts correct for both the smaller size and the slower growth rate of girls with Down's syndrome, and a girl with Down's syndrome would be expected to conform better to the percentile channels on this chart than to those on the NCHS charts. However, because deficiencies in growth velocity occur at varying times and are of widely different magnitudes, a child may not remain in a single growth channel on this chart. Downward percentile shifts are common between 6 and 36 months of age.

Children with moderate or severe heart disease show greater growth deficiencies than those without or with only mild heart disease during the first 3 years of life. On the average, girls with significant cardiac disease are 1.5 cm smaller than those without or with only mild disease beginning in the first 6 months of life. As with normal children with heart disease, catch-up growth may occur following surgical repair or spontaneous closure of the lesion.

Weight gain for children with Down's syndrome is more rapid than height growth. This often results in overweight by 36 months of age. The cause of this problem is not well understood but may relate to decreased activity level and/or appetite disorder. Because the present chart reflects this tendency to overweight, it should always be used in conjunction with charts for normal children when assessing body weight.

Growth Record

Date	Age	Height	Weight	Date	Age	Height	Weight

With permission: Castlemead Publications, 12 Little Mundells, Welwyn Garden City, Herts. England AL7 1EW; and based on data from the Developmental Evaluation Clinic of the Children's Hospital, Boston; The Child Development Center of Rhode Island Hospital; and the Clinical Genetics Service of the Children's Hospital of Philadelphia; supported by March of Dimes grant 6-449; Cronk CE, Crocker AC, Pueschel SM, Zachai E.

Girls with Down's syndrome: Physical Growth, 2 to 18 Years

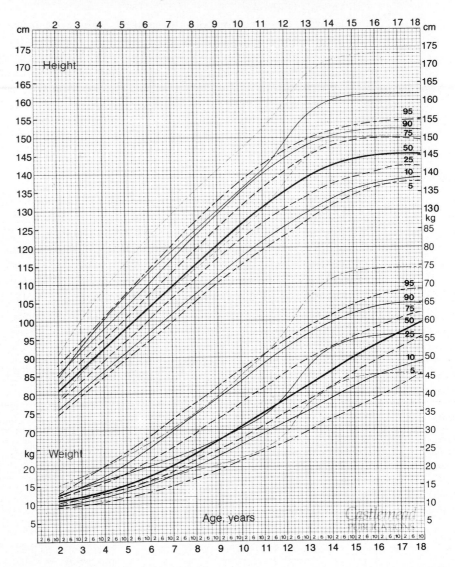

This chart provides reference percentiles for girls with Down's syndrome from 2 to 18 years of age. It is based on mixed longitudinal data on approximately 300 girls with Down's syndrome born between 1960 and 1984 and reared at home. Children with congenital heart disease are included in the sample. The percentile rank for a given child indicates the relative position she would hold in a series of 100 girls with

Down's syndrome. For example, a girl at the 10th percentile is larger than 10% and smaller than 90% of girls her age with Down's syndrome. The 50th percentile is the midposition, equivalent to "average" height or weight for a girl with Down's syndrome.

These charts correct for both the smaller size and the slower growth rate of girls with Down's syndrome, and a girl with Down's syndrome would be expected to conform better to the percentile channels on this chart than those on the NCHS charts. During the childhood years, girls with Down's syndrome grow very similarly to normal girls. However at adolescence, their growth spurts tend to occur slightly later than normal and are not as dramatic as those seen in normal girls. Some girls with Down's syndrome do not exhibit an adolescent growth spurt.

Children with moderate or severe heart disease show greater growth deficiencies than those without or with only mild heart disease. On the average, girls with significant cardiac disease are 1.5 cm smaller than those without or with only mild disease beginning in the first 6 months of life and continuing up through the adolescent period. As with normal children with heart disease, catch-up growth may occur following surgical repair or spontaneous closure of the lesion.

Weight gain for children with Down's syndrome is more rapid than height growth. This often results in overweight by 36 months of age, which is often enhanced during adolescence. The cause of this problem is not well understood but may relate to decreased activity level and/or appetite disorder. Because the present chart reflects this tendency to overweight, particularly in values for the 90th and 95th percentiles, it should always be used in conjunction with charts for normal children when assessing body weight.

Growth Record

Date	Age	Height	Weight	Date	Age	Height	Weight

With permission: Castlemead Publications, 12 Little Mundells, Welwyn Garden City, Herts. England AL7 1EW and based on data from the Developmental Evaluation Clinic of the Children's Hospital, Boston; The Child Development Center of Rhode Island Hospital; and the Clinical Genetics Service of the Children's Hospital of Philadelphia; supported by March of Dimes grant 6-449; Cronk CE, Crocker AC, Pueschel SM, Zachai E.

Boys with Down's syndrome: Physical Growth, 1 to 36 months

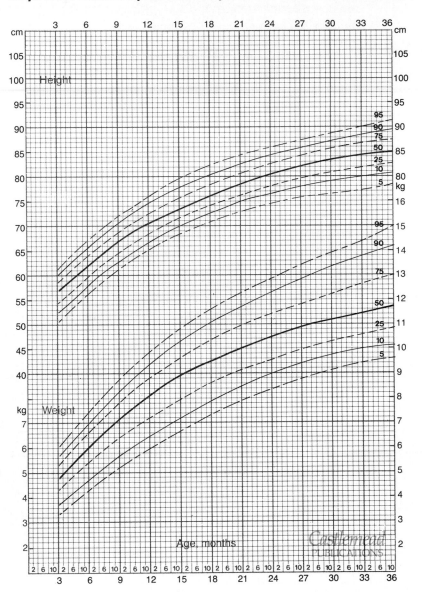

This chart provides reference percentiles for boys with Down's syndrome from birth to 36 months of age. It is based on mixed longitudinal data for approximately 400 boys with Down's syndrome born between 1960 and 1986 and reared at home. Children with congenital heart disease are included in the sample. The percentile rank for a given child indicates the relative position he would hold in a series of 100 boys with Down's syndrome. For example, a boy at the 10th percentile is larger than 10% and smaller than 90% of boys his age with Down's syndrome. The 50th percentile is the midposition, equivalent to "average" height or weight for a boy with Down's syndrome.

These charts correct for both the smaller size and the slower growth rate of boys with Down's syndrome, and a boy with Down's syndrome would be expected to conform better to the percentile channels on this chart than those on the NCHS charts. However, because deficiencies in growth velocity occur at varying times and are of widely different magnitudes, a child may not remain in a single growth channel on this chart. Downward percentile shifts are common between 6 and 36 months of age.

Children with moderate or severe heart disease show greater growth deficiencies than those without or with only mild heart disease during the first 3 years of life. On the average, boys with significant cardiac disease are 2 cm smaller than those without or with only mild disease beginning in the first 6 months of life. As with normal children with heart disease, catch-up growth may occur following surgical repair or spontaneous closure of the lesion.

Weight gain for children with Down's syndrome is more rapid than height growth. This often results in overweight by 36 months of age. The cause of this problem is not well understood but may relate to decreased activity level and/or appetite disorder. Because the present chart reflects this tendency to overweight, it should always be used in conjunction with charts for normal children when assessing body weight.

Growth Record

Date	Age	Height	Weight	Date	Age	Height	Weight

With permission: Castlemead Publications, 12 Little Mundells, Welwyn Garden City, Herts. England AL7 1EW and based on data from the Developmental Evaluation Clinic of the Children's Hospital, Boston; The Child Development Center of Rhode Island Hospital; and the Clinical Genetics Service of the Children's Hospital of Philadelphia; supported by March of Dimes grant 6-449; Cronk CE, Crocker AC, Pueschel SM, Zachai E.

Boys with Down's syndrome: Physical Growth, 2 to 18 years

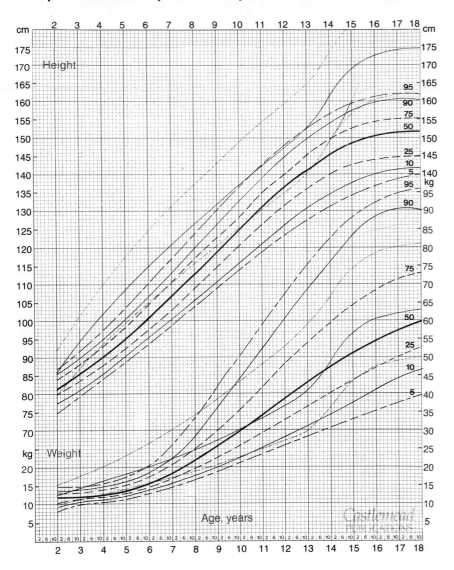

This chart provides reference percentiles for boys with Down's syndrome from 2 to 18 years of age. It is based on mixed longitudinal data for approximately 400 boys with Down's syndrome born between 1960 and 1984 and reared at home. Children with congenital heart disease are included in the sample. The percentile rank for a given child indicates the relative position he would hold in a series of 100 boys with Down's syndrome. For example, a boy at the 10th percentile is larger than 10% and smaller than 90% of boys his age with Down's syndrome. The 50th percentile is the midposition, equivalent to "average" height or weight for a boy with Down's syndrome.

These charts correct for both the smaller size and the slower growth rate of boys with Down's syndrome, and a boy with Down's syndrome would be expected to conform better to the percentile channels on this chart than to those on the NCHS charts. During the childhood years, boys with Down's syndrome grow very similarly to normal boys. However, at adolescence, their growth spurts tend to occur slightly later than normal and are not as dramatic as those seen in normal boys. A small percentage of boys with Down's syndrome do not have an adolescent growth spurt.

Children with moderate or severe heart disease show greater growth deficiencies than those without or with only mild heart disease during the first 3 years of life. On the average, boys with significant cardiac disease are 2 cm smaller than those without or with only mild disease beginning in the first 6 months of life and continuing up through the adolescent period. As with normal children with heart disease, catch-up growth may occur following surgical repair or spontaneous closure of the lesion.

Weight gain for children with Down's syndrome is more rapid than height growth. This often results in overweight by 36 months of age, which is often enhanced during adolescence. The cause of this problem is not well understood but may relate to decreased activity level and/or appetite disorder. Because the present chart reflects this tendency to overweight, particularly in values for the 90th and 95th percentiles, it should always be used in conjunction with charts for normal children when assessing body weight.

Growth Record

Date	Age	Height	Weight	Date	Age	Height	Weight

With permission: Castlemead Publications, 12 Little Mundells, Welwyn Garden City, Herts. England AL7 1EW and based on data from the Developmental Evaluation Clinic of the Children's Hospital, Boston; The Child Development Center of Rhode Island Hospital; and the Clinical Genetics Service of the Children's Hospital of Philadelphia; supported by March of Dimes grant 6-449; Cronk CE, Crocker AC, Pueschel SM, Zachai E.

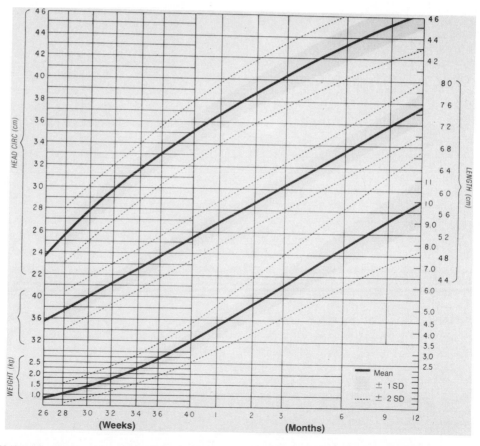

Birth to 1 year, sexes combined. (Adapted with permission from Babson SG, Benda GI. Growth graphs for the clinical assessment of infants of varying gestational age. J Pediatr 1976; 89:814–820.)

Triceps Skinfold Percentiles (mm²)

Age Group	n	5	10	25	50	75	90	95	n	5	10	25	50	75	90	95
				MALES									**FEMALES**			
1–1.9	228	6	7	8	10	12	14	16	204	6	7	8	10	12	14	16
2–2.9	223	6	7	8	10	12	14	15	208	6	8	9	10	12	15	16
3–3.9	220	6	7	8	10	11	14	15	208	7	8	9	11	12	14	15
4–4.9	230	6	6	8	9	11	12	14	208	7	8	8	10	12	14	16
5–5.9	214	6	6	8	9	11	14	15	219	6	7	8	10	12	15	18
6–6.9	117	5	6	7	8	10	13	16	118	6	6	8	10	12	14	16
7–7.9	122	5	6	7	9	12	15	17	126	6	7	9	11	13	16	18
8–8.9	117	5	6	7	8	10	13	16	118	6	8	9	12	15	18	24
9–9.9	121	6	6	7	10	13	17	18	125	8	8	10	13	16	20	22
10–10.9	146	6	6	8	10	14	18	21	152	7	8	10	12	17	23	27
11–11.9	122	6	6	8	11	16	20	24	117	7	8	10	13	18	24	28
12–12.9	153	6	6	8	11	14	22	28	129	8	9	11	14	18	23	27
13–13.9	134	5	5	7	10	14	22	26	151	8	8	12	15	21	26	30
14–14.9	131	4	5	7	9	14	21	24	141	9	10	13	16	21	26	28
15–15.9	128	4	5	6	8	11	18	24	117	8	10	12	17	21	25	32
16–16.9	131	4	5	6	8	12	16	22	142	10	12	15	18	22	26	31
17–17.9	133	5	5	6	8	12	16	19	114	10	12	13	19	24	30	37

*For whites ages 1 through 18, based on U.S. Health and Nutrition Examination Survey I of 1971–1974.

With permission from Frisancho AR. New norms of upper limb fat and muscle areas for assessment of nutritional status. Am J Clin Nutr 1981;34:2540–2545.

Nomogram for Anthropometry for Children

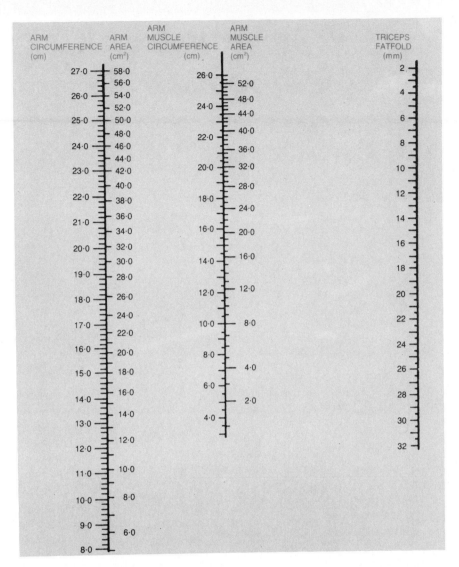

To obtain muscle circumference: (1) lay ruler between values of arm circumference and fatfold; (2) read off muscle circumference on middle line. To obtain tissue areas: (1) the arm areas and muscle areas are alongside their respective circumferences. (2) fat area = arm area − muscle area.

With permission from Gurney JM, Jelliffe DM. Arm anthropometry in nutritional assessment: nomogram for rapid calculation of muscle circumference and cross-sectional muscle and fat areas. Am J Clin Nutr 1973;26:912–915.

*Arm and Arm Muscle Circumference Percentiles**

*Percentiles of upper arm circumference (mm) and estimated upper arm muscle circumference (mm) for whites ages 1 through 18, based on U.S. Health and Nutrition Examination Survey I of 1971–1974

Age Group	Arm Circumference (mm)							Arm Muscle Circumference (mm)						
	5	10	25	50	75	90	95	5	10	25	50	75	90	95
MALES														
1–1.9	142	146	150	159	170	176	183	110	113	119	127	135	144	147
2–2.9	141	145	153	162	170	178	185	111	114	122	130	140	146	150
3–3.9	150	153	160	167	175	184	190	117	123	131	137	143	148	153
4–4.9	149	154	162	171	180	186	192	123	126	133	141	148	156	159
5–5.9	153	160	167	175	185	195	204	128	133	140	147	154	162	169
6–6.9	155	159	167	179	188	209	228	131	135	142	151	161	170	177
7–7.9	162	167	177	187	201	223	230	137	139	151	160	168	177	190
8–8.9	162	170	177	190	202	220	245	140	145	154	162	170	182	187
9–9.9	175	178	187	200	217	249	257	151	154	161	170	183	196	202
10–10.9	181	184	196	210	231	262	274	156	160	166	180	191	209	221
11–11.9	186	190	202	223	244	261	280	159	165	173	183	195	205	230
12–12.9	193	200	214	232	254	282	303	167	171	182	195	210	223	241
13–13.9	194	211	228	247	263	286	301	172	179	196	211	226	238	245
14–14.9	220	226	237	253	283	303	322	189	199	212	223	240	260	264
15–15.9	222	229	244	264	284	311	320	199	204	218	237	254	266	272
16–16.9	244	248	262	278	303	324	343	213	225	234	249	269	287	296
17–17.9	246	253	267	285	308	336	347	224	231	245	258	273	294	312
FEMALES														
1–1.9	138	142	148	156	164	172	177	105	111	117	124	132	139	143
2–2.9	142	145	152	160	167	176	184	111	114	119	126	133	142	147
3–3.9	143	150	158	167	175	183	189	113	119	124	132	140	146	152
4–4.9	149	154	160	169	177	184	191	115	121	128	136	144	152	157
5–5.9	153	157	165	175	185	203	211	125	128	134	142	151	159	165
6–6.9	156	162	170	176	187	204	211	130	133	138	145	154	166	171
7–7.9	164	167	174	183	199	216	231	129	135	142	151	160	171	176
8–8.9	168	172	183	195	214	247	261	138	140	151	160	171	183	194
9–9.9	178	182	194	211	224	251	260	147	150	159	167	180	194	198
10–10.9	174	182	193	210	228	251	265	148	150	159	170	180	190	197
11–11.9	185	194	208	224	248	276	303	150	158	171	181	196	217	223
12–12.9	194	203	216	237	256	282	294	162	166	180	191	201	214	220
13–13.9	202	211	223	243	271	301	338	169	175	183	198	211	226	240
14–14.9	214	223	237	252	272	304	322	174	179	190	201	216	232	247
15–15.9	208	221	239	254	279	300	322	175	178	189	202	215	228	244
16–16.9	218	224	241	258	283	318	334	170	180	190	202	216	234	249
17–17.9	220	227	241	264	295	324	350	175	183	194	205	221	239	257

With permission from Frisancho AR. New norms of upper limb fat and muscle areas for assessment of nutritional status. Am J Clin Nutr 1981;34:2540–2545.

*Percentiles for estimates of upper arm fat (mm²) and upper arm muscle fat (mm²) for whites ages 1 through 18, based on U.S. Health and Nutrition Examination Survey I of 1971 to 1974

Age Group	Arm Muscle Area Percentiles (mm²)							Arm Fat Area Percentiles (mm²)						
	5	10	25	50	75	90	95	5	10	25	50	75	90	95
MALES														
1–1.9	956	1,014	1,133	1,278	1,447	1,644	1,720	452	486	590	741	895	1,036	1,176
2–2.9	973	1,040	1,190	1,345	1,557	1,690	1,787	434	504	578	737	871	1,044	1,148
3–3.9	1,095	1,201	1,357	1,484	1,618	1,750	1,853	464	519	590	736	868	1,071	1,151
4–4.9	1,207	1,264	1,408	1,579	1,747	1,926	2,008	428	494	598	722	859	989	1,085
5–5.9	1,298	1,411	1,550	1,720	1,884	2,089	2,285	446	488	582	713	914	1,176	1,299
6–6.9	1,360	1,447	1,605	1,815	2,056	2,297	2,493	371	446	539	678	896	1,115	1,519
7–7.9	1,497	1,548	1,808	2,027	2,246	2,494	2,886	423	473	574	758	1,011	1,393	1,511
8–8.9	1,550	1,664	1,895	2,089	2,296	2,628	2,788	410	460	588	725	1,003	1,248	1,558
9–9.9	1,811	1,884	2,067	2,288	2,657	3,053	3,257	485	527	635	859	1,252	1,864	2,081
10–10.9	1,930	2,027	2,182	2,575	2,903	3,486	3,882	523	543	738	982	1,376	1,906	2,609
11–11.9	2,016	2,156	2,382	2,670	3,022	3,359	4,226	536	595	754	1,148	1,710	2,348	2,574
12–12.9	2,216	2,339	2,649	3,022	3,496	3,968	4,640	554	650	874	1,172	1,558	2,536	3,580
13–13.9	2,363	2,546	3,044	3,553	4,081	4,502	4,794	475	570	812	1,096	1,702	2,744	3,322
14–14.9	2,803	3,147	3,586	3,963	4,575	5,368	5,530	453	536	786	1,082	1,608	2,746	3,508
15–15.9	3,138	3,317	3,788	4,481	5,134	5,631	5,900	521	595	690	931	1,423	2,434	3,100
16–16.9	3,625	4,044	4,352	4,951	5,753	6,576	6,980	542	593	844	1,078	1,746	2,280	3,041
17–17.9	3,998	4,252	4,777	5,286	5,950	6,886	7,726	598	698	827	1,096	1,636	2,407	2,888
FEMALES														
1–1.9	885	973	1,084	1,221	1,378	1,535	1,621	401	466	578	706	847	1,022	1,140
2–2.9	973	1,029	1,119	1,269	1,405	1,595	1,727	469	526	642	474	894	1,061	1,173
3–3.9	1,014	1,133	1,227	1,396	1,563	1,690	1,846	473	529	656	822	967	1,106	1,158
4–4.9	1,058	1,171	1,313	1,475	1,644	1,832	1,958	490	541	654	766	907	1,109	1,236
5–5.9	1,238	1,301	1,423	1,598	1,825	2,012	2,159	470	529	647	812	991	1,330	1,536
6–6.9	1,354	1,414	1,513	1,683	1,877	2,182	2,323	464	508	638	827	1,009	1,263	1,436
7–7.9	1,330	1,441	1,602	1,815	2,045	2,332	2,469	491	560	706	920	1,135	1,407	1,644
8–8.9	1,513	1,566	1,808	2,034	2,327	2,657	2,996	527	634	769	1,042	1,383	1,872	2,482
9–9.9	1,723	1,788	1,976	2,227	2,571	2,987	3,112	642	690	933	1,219	1,584	2,171	2,524
10–10.9	1,740	1,784	2,019	2,296	2,583	2,872	3,093	616	702	842	1,141	1,608	2,500	3,005
11–11.9	1,784	1,987	2,316	2,612	3,071	3,739	3,953	707	802	1,015	1,301	1,942	2,730	3,690
12–12.9	2,092	2,182	2,579	2,904	3,225	3,655	3,847	782	854	1,090	1,511	2,056	2,666	3,369
13–13.9	2,269	2,426	2,657	3,130	3,529	4,081	4,568	726	838	1,219	1,625	2,374	3,272	4,150
14–14.9	2,418	2,562	2,874	3,220	3,704	4,294	4,850	981	1,043	1,423	1,818	2,403	3,250	3,765
15–15.9	2,426	2,518	2,847	3,248	3,689	4,123	4,756	839	1,126	1,396	1,886	2,544	3,093	4,195
16–16.9	2,308	2,567	2,865	3,248	3,718	4,353	4,946	1,126	1,351	1,663	2,006	2,598	3,374	4,236
17–17.9	2,442	2,674	2,996	3,336	3,883	4,552	5,251	1,042	1,267	1,463	2,104	2,977	3,864	5,159

With permission from Frisancho AR. New norms of upper limb fat and muscle areas for assessment of nutritional status. Am J Clin Nutr 1981;34:2540–2545.

36 / *Selected References for Pediatric Laboratory Values*

Normal ranges for laboratory tests in pediatric patients are in the process of being developed at the Mayo Clinic. The following are four sources of published pediatric normal laboratory values.

1. Rowe PC. The Harriet Lane handbook: a manual for pediatric house officers, 12th ed. Chicago: Year Book Medical Publishers, 1991:378–385.
2. Nelson WE, Behrman RE, Vaughan VC III. Nelson textbook of pediatrics, 13th ed. Philadelphia: WB Saunders, 1987:1535–1558.
3. Oski FA, DeAngelis CD, Feigin RD, Warshaw JB. Principles and practice of pediatrics. Philadelphia: JB Lippincott, 1987:1973–1980.
4. Burritt MF, Slockbower JM, Forsman RW, Offord KP, Bergstrath EJ, Smithson WA. Pediatric reference intervals for 19 biologic variables in healthy children. Mayo Clin Proc 1990;65:329–336.

Tanner Height for Age and Height Velocity Graphs— Girls and Boys, Birth through 19 Years

Girls: Birth through 19 Years, Height-for-Age Graphs

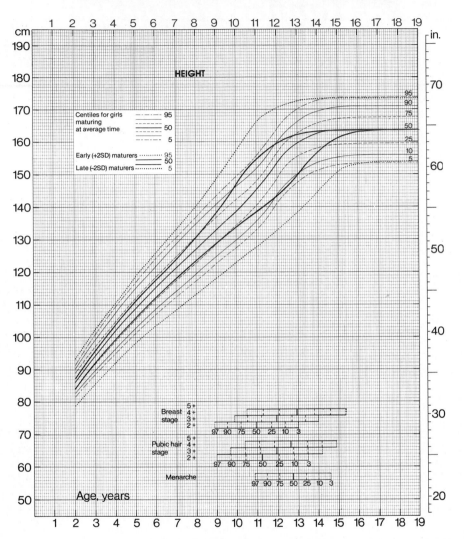

With permission from Castlemead Publications, 12 Little Mundells, Welwyn Garden City, Herts. England AL7 1EW and Tanner JM, Davies PSW. J Pediatr 1985; 107.

Girls: Birth through 19 Years, Height-Velocity Graph

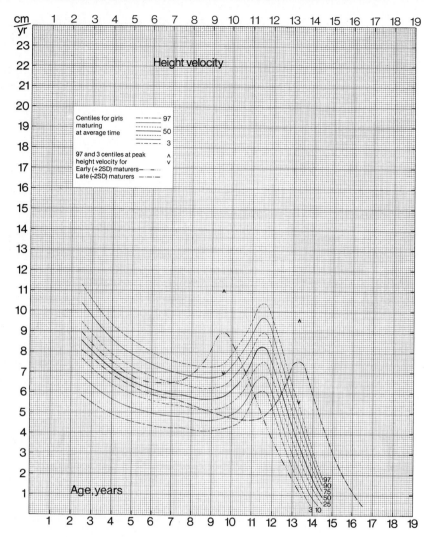

With permission from Castlemead Publications, 12 Little Mundells, Welwyn Garden City, Herts. England AL7 1EW and Tanner JM, Davies PSW. J Pediatr 1985; 107.

Boys: Birth through 19 Years, Height-for-Age Graph

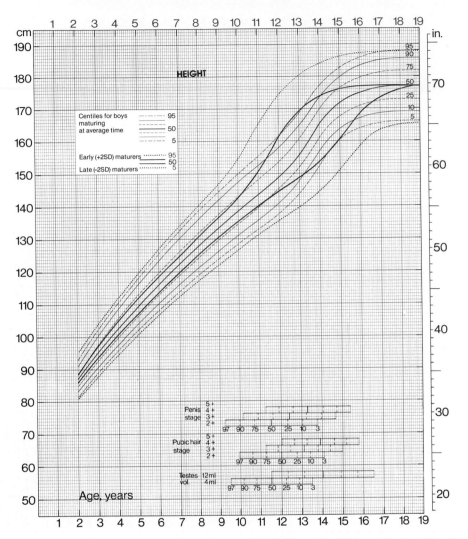

With permission from Castlemead Publications, 12 Little Mundells, Welwyn Garden City, Herts. England AL7 1EW and Tanner JM, Davies PSW. J Pediatr 1985; 107.

Boys: Birth through 19 Years, Height-Velocity Graph

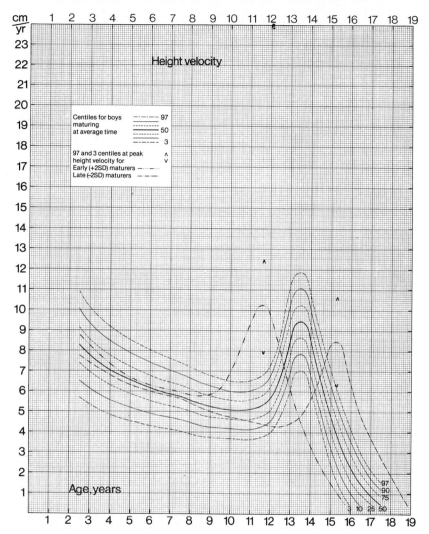

With permission from Castlemead Publications, 12 Little Mundells, Welwyn Garden City, Herts. England AL7 1EW and Tanner JM, Davies PSW. J Pediatr 1985; 107.

38 / *Oral Rehydration Solutions*[1]

Solution (Manufacturer)	Sodium (mEq/L)	Potassium (mEq/L)	Chloride (mEq/L)	Citrate (mEq/L)	Glucose (g/L)	Rice Syrup Solids (g/L)	Osmolality (mOsm)
Rehydralyte (Ross)	75	20	65	30	25	—	305
World Health Organization Formula*	90	20	80	30	20	—	310
Pedialyte (Ross)	45	20	35	30	25	—	250
Ricelyte (Mead Johnson)	50	25	45	34	—	30	200
Resol (Wyeth)	50	20	50	34	20	—	270

*World Health Organization formula[2]:

    3.5 g table salt (NaCl)
    2.5 g baking soda (NaHCO$_3$)
    1.5 g potassium chloride (KCl)
  20.0 g glucose
 960   g water

To improve palatability, noncaloric flavoring can be added (e.g., commercial enteral formula flavor packets, unsweetened or artificially sweetened beverage mixes).

References

1. Manufacturers' data.
2. MacMahon RA. The use of the World Health Organization's oral rehydration solution in patients on home parenteral nutrition. JPEN 1984;8:720–721.

Index

A

Abbreviations, 709-714
Abdominal discomfort, 215, 216
Abdominal gas and flatulence
  in cancer, 298
  dietary recommendations, 215-216
  factors contributing to, 214
  indications and rationale, 213-215
  in irritable bowel syndrome, 262
  nutritional inadequacy and, 213
  treatment, 213
Abdominal radiation, 296-297
Absorption blockers, 25
Acesulfame K, 162
Acetate, in parenteral nutrition, 400
Acetylsalicylic acid intolerance, 121
Acid-ash diet, 346-347
Acidemia, 502
Acidic foods, peptic ulcer disease
  and, 269
Acidosis, metabolic, 319
Aciduria, 502, 503
Acquired immune deficiency syndrome, patients targeted for fraud,
  27-28
Activity (*see* Exercise)
Acute renal failure
  dietary management goals, 316-317
  dietary recommendations, 316, 317
  diet order, 317
  indications and rationale, 315-316
  nutritional inadequacy and, 315
  nutritional problems, 316
Additives, 111-121
  cancer risk and, 17
Adenoidectomy, diet progression, 89
Adolescents
  athletes, 442-446

Adolescents—cont'd
  cystic fibrosis, 584
  eating habits, 439-440
  nutritional implications of substance
    abuse, 440
  nutritional requirements, 438-439
  obesity, 540, 543-544
  pregnancy, 44-46
  recommended food intake, 437
  sick, 469-473
  Tanner rating stages of maturity,
    543
Adults, nutritional support
  enteral, 385-399
  parenteral, 399-409
Aerobic activity (*see* Exercise)
Aerophagia, 214-215
Aging, 58 (*see also* Geriatric nutrition)
  laboratory values affected by, 62-63
  osteoporosis and, 205
AIDS, patients targeted for fraud, 27-
  28
AIDS Nutrition Network, address and
  phone number, 26
Air embolism, in parenteral nutrition,
  404-405
Albumin
  hypoalbuminemia, 33, 255
  nephrotic syndrome and, 333
  pediatric protein status and, 425
Alcohol
  ACS/NCI guidelines for cancer risk
    reduction, 17
  adolescent abuse, 440
  diabetes and, 162-163
  hyperlipidemia and, 140
  hypertension and, 125, 131
  hypertriglyceridemia and, 142

Alcohol—cont'd
  kidney transplantation and, 370
  lactation and, 49
  osteoporosis and, 207
  pancreas transplantation and, 373
  peptic ulcer disease and, 269
  peritoneal dialysis and, 328
  in pregnancy, normal, 43
  USDA/USDHHS guidelines, 6
Alcoholic beverages and mixes, nutritive values, 645-646
Alkaline-ash diet, 346-347
Allergies (*see* Food allergies)
American Academy of Allergy and
  Immunology, address and phone
  number, 99
American Cancer Society dietary
  guidelines, 15-17
American Celiac Society, address and
  phone number, 249
American Diabetes Association,
  address, 168
American Dietetic Association
  address and phone number, 26
  Exchange Lists for Meal Planning,
    169
  position papers, 733-734
American Heart Association
  address, 132
  dietary guidelines, 8
    pediatric, 490
Amino acids
  athletes and, 56
  branched-chain
    in enteral formulas, 388
    ketoaciduria (*see* Maple syrup
      urine disease)
    in liver disease, 277, 278, 280
  deficiency, in liver disease, 275

Amino acids—cont'd
  in enteral formulas, 388, 389
  hereditary metabolic disorders and,
    502-503, 506
  for maple syrup urine disease, 521-
    522
  in parenteral nutrition, 399, 400, 401
    pediatric, 606
  in Parkinson's disease, 287, 288
  vegetarian diet and, 71-72, 74
Ammonia, hepatic encephalopathy
    and, 277, 278
Amphetamines, 25
Amygdalin, 26-27
Anabolic steroids, for muscle build-
    ing, 24-25, 56
Anafranil, 313
Analog MSUD, 521
Analog XP, 525, 526
Analog X-Phen, 530
Anaphylaxis, 97
Anemia
  dumping syndrome and, 273
  in elderly, 62
  in inflammatory bowel disease, 255
  iron deficiency, pediatric screen-
    ing, 424-425
Animal sources of foods, 478
Anorexia in cancer, 294
  pediatric, 575-576
Anorexia nervosa
  dietary management goals, 306
  dietary recommendations, 303
    diet history, 306-307
    diet plan design, 307-308
    diet plan for weight mainte-
      nance, 309
    diet progression, 308-309
    kilocalories content of ideal diet,
      307
    weight gain expectations, 309
  indications and rationale, 303-305
  nutritional inadequacy and, 303
  treatment, 304-305
Antabuse, 162
Anthropometrics, 31-32, 453-454
  nomogram for children, 848
Anticonvulsants, developmental dis-
    ability and, 458
Appetite loss
  in cancer, 298
  hemodialysis and, 325-326
Argininosuccinic aciduria, 503
Arm and arm muscle circumference
    percentiles, 850
Arm fat area and arm muscle area
    percentiles, 852
Arthritis, in elderly, nutrition misin-
    formation and, 24
Arthritis Foundation, address and
    phone number, 26

Artificial sweeteners (*see also*
    Aspartame)
  cancer risk and, 17
  in diabetes, pediatric, 496
  ketogenic diet and, 569
  phenylketonuria and, 529
  in pregnancy, normal, 43-44
Ascorbic acid (*see* Vitamin C)
Aspartame
  diabetes and, 161
  intolerance, 111-112
  phenylketonuria and, 529
  in pregnancy, normal, 43-44, 161
Aspirin intolerance, 121
Assessment (*see* Nutritional screening
    and assessment)
Association for Glycogen Storage
    Disease, address, 518
Asthma, 121
Asthma and Allergy Foundation of
    America, address and phone num-
    ber, 99
Atherosclerosis
  cholesterol and, 488
  diabetes and, 159
    pediatric, 497
  hyperlipidemia and, 134
Athletes
  nutritional needs, 51
    carbohydrate, 53-54
    drugs and special dietary supple-
      ments, 55-57
    fat, 54-55
    fluid and electrolyte replacement,
      51-53
    kilocalories, 53
    precompetition meal, 57
    protein, 54
    vitamins and minerals, 55
  targeted for fraud, 24-25
  young, 442
    achieving competing weight,
      445-446
    energy needs, 443-444
    fluid and electrolyte replace-
      ment, 442-443
    pregame and postgame meal,
      445
    protein requirements, 444
    vitamins and minerals for, 444-
      445
Atropine sulfate, diphenoxylate with,
    224
Azathioprine, 365
Azotemia, 612

B

Baby foods, commercial, exchange
    values, 797-807

Bacteria, diet low in, for transplanta-
    tion, 367-368, 373, 376, 378, 382
Baked goods, for infants, phenylala-
    nine content, 531
Baldwin-Wood tables, 454, 829-831
Bariatric surgery
  dietary management goals, 196
  dietary recommendations, 197-200
  diet order, 204
  follow-up, 201-204
  indications and rationale, 196
  pancreaticobiliary bypass, 200-201,
    203
  patient and family education after,
    201
  types, 195
  vertical banded gastroplasty and
    gastric bypass, 196-200, 202
Basal energy expenditure, 34
Basal metabolic rate, formulas, 471
Basic Four Food Guide, 6-7
  vegetarian diet modifications, 73-74
BEE (basal energy expenditure), 34
Behavioral patterns in obesity, 189,
    193
Belching, excessive, 214, 215
Benzoic acid intolerance, 112-113
Beverages
  alcoholic, nutritive values, 645-646
  carbohydrate-containing, 51-52,
    443
  copper in, 284
  decaffeinated, peptic ulcer disease
    and, 269
  food exchanges for protein, sodi-
    um, and potassium control, 355-
    356
  gluten in, 147
  glycogen storage disease and, type
    I, 515
  oxalate in, 341
  potassium in, low content, 358
  sodium in, 129, 130
  sugar-containing, carbohydrate
    content, 163
  tyramine in, 312
Bezoars, 219
BHA intolerance, 113
BHT intolerance, 113
Bile acids, fat malabsorption and, 230
Binge eating, in bulimia nervosa, 305,
    310
Biochemical assessment, 32-33
Biotin
  in parenteral nutrition, pediatric,
    608
  safe and adequate daily dietary
    intake, 20
Bismuth subsalicylate, 224
Bleeding, esophageal variceal, scle-
    rotherapy for, 286

Blenderized foods, for intermaxillary
fixation diet, 90-91
Bloating, 215, 216
in cancer, 298
Blood pressure, high (*see* Hypertension)
BMR (basal metabolic rate), formulas,
471
Body composition, fat distribution
and, 189
Bodyfuel 450, 52
Body mass index, 186
nomogram, 657-658
Body parts, contribution of each to
total body weight, 32
Body weight (*see* Weight)
Bolus feeding, in enteral nutrition,
391
Bone loss (*see* Osteoporosis)
Bone marrow transplantation, 380-381
dietary management of gastrointestinal GVHD, 383
immediate post-transplant management, 381-383
long-term post-transplant management, 381-383
nutritional care guidelines, 382
pretransplant management, 381
Bone mineralization, in infants, 428
low-birth-weight, 465, 467
Borborygmus, from high fiber diet,
236
Bowels
fistulas, restricted fiber diet for, 240
inflamed (*see* Inflammatory bowel
disease)
irritable (*see* Irritable bowel syndrome)
preparation for surgery, restricted
fiber diet for, 240
regulation, high fiber diet for, 235
Branched-chain amino acids
in enteral formulas, 388
ketoaciduria (*see* Maple syrup urine
disease)
in liver disease, 277, 278, 280
BRAT diet, for pediatric diarrhea,
554
Breads
exchanges in ketogenic diet
with MCT oil, 573
without MCT oil, 570
in lacto-ovo diet, pediatric, 450
number of daily servings, 7
oxalate in, 342
recommended intake for children
and teens, 437
in vegan diet, pediatric, 451
Breast cancer, 235, 296, 300
Breast milk, 428-430, 431
Breath hydrogen analysis test, diet
for, 411-412

Brewer's yeast, in vegan diet, pediatric,
451
Bulimia nervosa
dietary management goals, 306
dietary recommendations, 303,
309-310
indications and rationale, 305-306
treatment, 305-306
Burns, pediatric, 472
Butylated hydroxyanisole (BHA)
intolerance, 113
Butylated hydroxytoluene (BHT)
intolerance, 113

C

Cachectin, cancer and, 294
Cachexia
cancer, 293-294
cardiac, 148, 149, 377
Caffeine
in athlete's diet, 55-56
in beverages and foods, 757
beverages without, 759
cancer risk and, 17
hyperlipidemia and, 140
lactation and, 49
in medications, 758
myocardial infarction and, 150, 151
osteoporosis and, 207
peptic ulcer disease and, 269
in pregnancy, normal, 43
thoracic organ transplantation and,
378
Calcium
adolescent needs, 439
in athlete's diet, 55
bone marrow transplantation and,
382
chronic renal failure and, 317, 318,
320
pediatric, 586, 588
control, 336-339
deficiency, in short bowel syndrome, 258
food sources, 208-209
hemodialysis and, 323, 325
pediatric, 591, 592
hypercalciuria, 336-338, 339
infant RDA and content in milk
sources, 431
kidney transplantation and, 370,
371
lactation and, 48
in liver disease, 279
liver transplantation and, 376
for low-birth-weight infants, 464,
465
osteoporosis and, 206, 207-210
oxalate absorption and, 340

Calcium—cont'd
pancreas transplantation and, 373
pancreaticobiliary bypass and, 201
in parenteral nutrition, 400, 407
pediatric, 607, 612
peritoneal dialysis and, 328, 330-
331
pediatric, 593, 594
in pregnancy
in adolescents, 45-46
normal, 41, 42
recommended dietary allowances,
19, 206
thoracic organ transplantation and,
378
in vegetarian diet, 72
pediatric, 448, 449
Calcium carbonate, 209, 210
Calcium citrate, 209, 210
Calcium gluconate, 210
Calcium lactate, 209, 210
Calcium supplements, 209-210, 264
Calories
adolescent needs, 438-439
from alcohol, 162
anorexia nervosa and, 307, 308-309
athletic needs, 53, 55
bone marrow transplantation and,
382
bulimia nervosa and, 309-310
cancer and, 297
chronic renal failure and, 318, 319
pediatric, 586, 587
congestive heart failure and, 149
cystic fibrosis and, supplementation, 580
developmental disabilities and, 457
diabetes and, 158
pediatric, 496
in pregnancy, 167-168
enteral nutrition and, 386
estimating needs, 34-35
failure to thrive and, 461
hemodialysis and, 323, 324
pediatric, 590, 591
infant RDA and content in milk
sources, 431
infant requirements, 427
in ketogenic diet
with MCT oil, 568
without MCT oil, 563-565
kidney transplantation and, 369-
370
lactation and, 47-48
liver disease and, 276, 280
liver transplantation and, 374, 375,
376
for low-birth-weight infants, 464,
467
maple syrup urine disease and, 522
nephrotic syndrome and, 333-334

Calories—cont'd
nomogram for estimating requirements, 655-656
obesity and, 168, 191-192
pediatric, 541, 542-543, 544
in one serving from each food
exchange group, 348
pancreas transplantation and, 372,
373
peritoneal dialysis and, 328, 329
pediatric, 592-594
phenylketonuria and, 529
in pregnancy
adolescents, 44-45
diabetes and, 46-47
normal, 40-41
for preschool and school age children, 436
requirements for ICU, ward, and
obese patient, 33
thoracic organ transplantation and,
378, 379
for young athletes, 443-444
Canadian Diabetes Association,
address, 169
Cancer, 293-302
dietary management goals, 297
dietary recommendations, 297-300
high fiber diet and, 235-236
indications and rationale, 293
nutritional effects, 293-294
nutritional problems and
approaches, 298-299
patients targeted for fraud, 26-27
pediatric, 575
malnutrition causes, 575-576
nutritional assessment, 576
nutritional intervention, 576-578
protective role of nutrition, 300
protein-calorie malnutrition from,
293
risk, diet and, 15-17
Cancer therapies, nutritional effects,
294-295
chemotherapy, 295-296
radiation therapy, 296-297
surgery, 295
CAPD (continuous ambulatory peritoneal dialysis), 328-329, 330-331
Carbamylphosphate synthetase
defect, 503
Carbidopa, 287, 288, 289
Carbohydrate(s)
in athlete's diet, 53-54
in beverages, 51-52, 443
bone marrow transplantation and,
382
competition and, 445
diabetes and, 159-160, 163, 164
pediatric, 496, 498, 499, 500
flatulence and, 215, 262

Carbohydrates—cont'd
food exchanges for protein, sodium, and potassium control, 355
from food groups, 163
glycemic effects, 160
hereditary metabolic disorders,
504-505
hypertriglyceridemia and, 144
hypoglycemia and, 184-185
infant requirements, 427
in ketogenic diet
with MCT oil, 568
without MCT oil, 563-565
kidney transplantation and, 370
liver transplantation and, 376
loading, 54
for low-birth-weight infants, 465
malabsorption, 504
metabolism, diet before testing,
412-413
in milk sources for infants, 431
in one serving from each food
exchange group, 348
pancreas transplantation and, 372,
373
peritoneal dialysis and, 328
pediatric, 593, 594
in specific foods, 809-820
in sugar-containing foods and beverages, 163
thoracic organ transplantation and,
378
Carbohydrate-Free formula, 554
Carbon dioxide, as bowel gas, 213-
214, 215
Cardiac cachexia, 148, 149, 377
Cardiac surgery
dietary management goals, 147
dietary recommendations, 147-148
dietary restrictions, 146
diet order, 148
indications and rationale, 146-147
nutritional inadequacy and, 146
pediatric, 491-492
Cardiovascular diseases, 123-151
pediatric, 483-492
Carnitine, in vegetarian diet, pediatric, 449
Carotid artery puncture, in parenteral nutrition, 404
Casein, 104-105
Catheter-related problems, in parenteral nutrition, 404, 405
CCPD (continuous cyclic peritoneal
dialysis), 329, 330-331
Celiac disease, 245
pediatric, 555-556
Celiac sprue, 108-109, 245-246
Celiac Sprue Association, address and
phone number, 249
Cellulose, food sources, 234

Central nervous system stimulants,
458
Cereals
exchanges in ketogenic diet, with
MCT oil, 573
for infants, phenylalanine content,
531
in lacto-ovo diet, pediatric, 450
recommended intake for children
and teens, 437
in vegan diet, pediatric, 451
Cerebral palsy, calorie requirements,
457
CHD (see Coronary disease)
Chemotherapy
before bone marrow transplant,
side effects, 381
nutritional effects, 295-296
pediatric, 576
Chest pain, in gastroplasty, 197
Chewing difficulties, in cancer, 298
Children (see Pediatric nutrition)
Chloride
for low-birth-weight infants, 464
minimum requirements, 21
in parenteral nutrition, 400
Chlorine, in pediatric parenteral
nutrition, 607
Chlorpropamide, 162-163
Cholecystectomy, 195
Cholestasis, from parenteral nutrition
in children, 612
Cholesterol (blood or serum)
atherosclerosis and, 488
diets for lowering, 489
elevated levels (see
Hypercholesterolemia)
fiber and, 139, 235
guidelines by age and sex, 137
high density lipoprotein (see HDL
cholesterol)
levels in United States, 717-718
low density lipoprotein (see LDL
cholesterol)
pediatric levels, 488-489
peritoneal dialysis and, 331
total, ratio to HLD cholesterol, 135
Cholesterol (dietary)
cardiovascular disease and, pediatric,
488, 489
diabetes and, 159
hemodialysis and, pediatric, 592
in infant formulas, 430
intake reduction, 141
kidney transplantation and, 370
myocardial infarction and, 150, 151
pancreas transplantation and, 373
peritoneal dialysis and, 328, 331
pediatric, 593, 594
thoracic organ transplantation and,
378

Cholesterol (dietary)—cont'd
USDA/USDHHS guidelines, 5-6
Cholestyramine, 557
for inflammatory bowel disease,
251
for short bowel syndrome, 259
Chromium
in parenteral nutrition, pediatric,
608
safe and adequate daily dietary
intake, 20
Chronic renal failure
calcium and phosphorus and, 318,
320
diabetes and, 166-167, 321
dietary management goals, 320
dietary recommendations, 318, 321
diet order, 321
indications and rationale, 318-320
kilocalories and, 318, 319
nutritional inadequacy and, 317
pediatric
dietary management, 585, 586,
587-588
indications and rationale, 585-586
nutritional inadequacy and, 585
potassium and, 318, 320
protein and, 318-319
sodium and, 318, 319-320
Chylomicrons, 144, 230
Cigarette smoking, 138, 270
Cirrhosis, 231, 276
Citrullinemia, 503
Clear liquid diet, 79-80
Colitis, ulcerative, 250, 251 (*see also*
Inflammatory bowel disease)
pediatric, 557
Colon cancer, high fiber diet and,
235
Colon surgery, 295
Colostomy, 255-256, 257
Compazine (prochlorperazine), 297
Competition, meal before, 57
Condiments
peptic ulcer disease and, 269
sodium content, 129, 130
Congenital heart defect surgery, 147
Congestive heart failure, 148-150
Constipation
in cancer, 298
gastroplasty and, 197
high fiber diet for, 235
Parkinson's disease and, 289-290
from tube feeding, 393
pediatric, 604
Constipation and encopresis, 547
causes, 548
definitions, 547-548
dietary recommendations, 548-550
indications and rationale, 547-548
water requirements by age, 549

Continuous ambulatory peritoneal
dialysis, 328-329, 330-331
Continuous cyclic peritoneal dialysis,
329, 330-331
Continuous infusion, in enteral nutrition, 391
Conversions
metric measures, 707-708
milligrams to milliequivalents, 705
Copper
content of foods, 283-284
liver disease and, 279
for low-birth-weight infants, 465, 466
metabolism, in Wilson's disease,
282-285
in parenteral nutrition, pediatric,
608, 609
in pregnancy, normal, 42
safe and adequate daily dietary
intake, 20
Corn, terms indicating presence of,
101
Corn allergy, 101-102
Cornstarch, for glycogen storage disease
type I, 511-512
type III and type VI, 517
Coronary artery bypass grafting, 147
Coronary disease
childhood risk, dietary recommendations, 488-490
in elderly, 61
HDL cholesterol and, 10, 13-14
LDL cholesterol and, 11, 13-14
Corticosteroids (*see* Steroids)
Counseling, dietary, for Crohn's disease, 254
Cow's milk, in infant nutrition, 429,
430-432
Crackers, exchanges in ketogenic
diet, with MCT oil, 573
Cranial nerves, swallowing and, 92
Crohn's disease, 250, 251, 258 (*see
also* Inflammatory bowel disease)
pediatric, 557, 558
treatment, 253-255
Cronk's growth graphs, 454
Cyclosporine, 365, 371, 380
Cystic fibrosis
dietary assessment, 584
dietary management goals, 581-582
dietary recommendations, 579,
582-584
energy requirements, 582
indications and rationale, 580-581
nutritional inadequacy and, 579-
580
treatment, 579, 581
vitamin supplementation, 579-580
Cystinuria, 344
Cytokines, cancer and, 294

D

Daily Reference Values, 23
Dairy products
food exchanges for protein,
sodium, and potassium control,
349-350
in lacto-ovo diet, pediatric, 450
penicillin in, 118
potassium in
high, 361
low, 358
moderate, 359
in pregnancy, number of food servings, 45
Debrancher enzyme defect, 505
Decaffeinated beverages, 269, 759
Dehydration
diarrhea and, pediatric, 551-553
in parenteral nutrition, 406
in peritoneal dialysis, 331
Delayed gastric emptying
dietary management goals, 220
dietary recommendations, 220-221
gastric motility dysfunction, 218-
220, 220-221
indications and rationale, 217-220
mechanical obstruction, 217-218, 220
nutritional inadequacy and, 217
treatment, 217
Demerol, 313
Dermatitis, from nickel, 116
Dermatitis herpetiformis, 246
Desserts
copper in, 284
gluten in, 148
for infants, phenylalanine content,
533
recommended intake for children
and teens, 437
sodium content, 129, 130
Determine Your Nutritional Health,
64-68
Developmental abilities, infant nutrition and, 433-434
Developmental disability, 422, 453
(*see also* Growth entries)
dietary recommendations, 457-459
failure to thrive, 459-462
nutritional assessment
anthropometrics, 453-454
diet, 454-455
feeding, 455-456
syndromes associated with growth
retardation, 454
Dexpanthenol, 608
Dextrose, in parenteral nutrition,
400, 401
pediatric, 606
Diabetes educators, scope of practice
and standards of practice, 723-732

Diabetes mellitus, 153-183
  alcohol and, 162-163
  carbohydrates and, 159-160, 163, 164
  chronic renal failure and, 166-167, 321
  community support programs, 168-169
  dietary management goals, 155-156
  dietary modifications
    chronic renal failure, 166-167
    exercise and, 165, 166
    after gastroplasty for weight reduction, 168
    hypoglycemia, 164-165
    in illness, 163-164
    liberalized diabetic diet, 165-166, 167
    pregnancy, 167-168
    tube feeding, 168
  dietary recommendations, 156-161
  dietetic foods and, 162
  diet order, 168
  feeding limitations, 33
  fiber and, 160-161, 235
  food exchange lists, 169
    fat, 180
    foods containing sugar, 170
    "free" foods, 170-171
    fruit, 179
    meat, 171-173
    milk, 174
    nutrients in one serving from each exchange list, 169
    starch, 175-177
    vegetable, 178
  gestational, 155, 167
  impaired glucose tolerance and, 155
  indications and rationale, 153-155
  insulin-dependent, 154, 156
  kilocalories and, 158-159
  meal timing and composition, 158
  non–insulin-dependent, 154-155, 157
  nutritional inadequacy and, 153
  pediatric, 495-500
    changing preferences and needs, 497
    dietary management goals, 496-500
    diet during illness, 498-500
    eating for extra activity, 498, 499
    energy and protein needs, 496-497
    fat and sodium needs, 497
    fiber and, 497
    indications and rationale, 495-496
    management, 495
    school lunch, 497-498
  pregnancy and, 46-47

Diabetes mellitus—cont'd
  secondary, 155
  sweeteners and, 159, 161-162
  very low calorie diets, 158
  weight and, 156, 158
Diabinese (chlorpropamide), 162-163
Diagnostic testing, preparatory diets
  carbohydrate metabolism, 412-413
  fat absorption, 413-415
  5-HIAA, 415
Dialysis (see Hemodialysis; Peritoneal dialysis)
Diarrhea, 222
  acute, 222-223
  cancer and, 298
  causes, 222-223
  chronic, 223, 224
  dietary management goals, 225
  dietary recommendations, 225
  diet order, 225
  gastroplasty and, 197
  indications and rationale, 222-224
  large bowel inflammation and, 253
  medications for, 224
  nutritional inadequacy and, 222
  short bowel syndrome and, 259
  treatment, 223-224
  from tube feeding, 393, 394
Diarrhea in children, 550-551
  chronic, 551, 554
  from enteral nutrition, 604
  fluid and electrolyte therapy, 553
  indications and rationale, 551
  nutritional inadequacy and, 551
  nutritional therapy, 553-554
  oral rehydration solutions, 551-553
  treatment chart, 552
Diet (see Food entries and Nutritional entries)
Dietary counseling, for Crohn's disease, 254
Dietary guidelines
  American Heart Association, 8
  cancer risk and, 15-17
  USDA/USDHHS Dietary Guidelines for Americans, 5-6
Dietary misinformation (see Fraud in food claims)
Dietetic foods, diabetes and, 162
Diet pills, 25
Digestion, in infants, 433
Dinners for infants, phenylalanine content, 532
Diphenoxylate with atropine sulfate, 224
Disulfiram, 162
Diverticulitis, 240
Diverticulosis, 235
Dopamine, 288, 290
Down's syndrome, 422, 454
  calorie requirements, 457

Down's syndrome—cont'd
  growth charts, 834-841
  obesity and, 458-459
D-penicillamine, 282, 285
Drugs (see also Medications)
  adolescent abuse, 440
  athletes and, 55-57
  effect on nutrition, 625-643
  lactation and, 49
DRVs (Daily Reference Values), 23
Dry mouth, in cancer, 298
Dumping symptoms, in gastroplasty, 197
Dumping syndrome, postgastrectomy
  dietary management goals, 270, 272
  dietary recommendations, 272-273
  indications and rationale, 271-272
  nutritional inadequacy and, 271
  phases and symptoms, 271-272
Duodenal ulcers, 268, 269
Dyes, 111
Dyslipidemia, 134
Dysphagia, 61, 92
Dysphagia diet
  description, 91
  feeding guidelines, 93-94
  food thickeners and, 93
  goals, 92
  indications and rationale, 91
  nutritional inadequacy, 91
  recommendations, 92-93

E

Eating disorders, 303-313
  dietary management goals, 306
  dietary recommendations, 303, 306-310
  indications and rationale, 303-306
  nutritional inadequacy and, 303
Eating habits
  adolescents, 439-440
  infants, 436
  preschool and school age children, 438
Edema, 149, 304
Education
  bariatric surgery, 201
  developmental disability nutrition, 458-459
  failure to thrive, 462
  tube feeding, 395
Egg allergy, 102-103
Eggs
  in lacto-ovo diet, pediatric, 450
  terms indicating presence of, 103
Elderly (see also Geriatric nutrition)
  drug use, 60-61
  targeted for fraud, 24
Electrical muscle stimulators, 25

Electrolytes (*see also* Fluids and electrolytes), in parenteral nutrition, 400, 401
  pediatric, 608
Elimination diet, for food allergy, 98
Embolism, in parenteral nutrition, 404-405
Encephalopathy, hepatic, in liver disease, 276-280
Encopresis (*see* Constipation and encopresis)
Endocrine diseases and disorders, 153-212
  pediatric, 495-545
End-stage renal disease (*see* Hemodialysis)
Energy balance, obesity and, 168-169
Energy intake, in normal pregnancy, 40-41
Energy needs
  athletic, 53
  bone marrow transplantation, 381-382
  cancer, 297
  congestive heart failure, 149
  diabetes, 158-159
  estimating, 34-35
  lactation, 47-48
  liver disease, 276, 280
  in pregnancy
    adolescents, 44-45
    diabetes and, 46-47
  thoracic organ transplantation, 377-378, 379
Energy needs of children
  adolescents, 438
  cardiac surgery, 492
  chronic renal failure, 587
  cystic fibrosis, 582-583
  developmental disability, 457
  diabetes, 496-497
  hemodialysis, 590, 591
  infants, 427
  maple syrup urine disease, 521, 522
  nephrotic syndrome, 596
  peritoneal dialysis, 592-594
  preschool and school age children, 436
  sick infants, children, and adolescents, 470-471
  on vegetarian diet, 447
  young athletes, 443-444
Enteral nutrition for children, 599
  administration, 600, 603
  cancer and, 577
  inititiating tube feeding, 603
  low-birth-weight infants, 468
  monitoring, 603-604
  physician's order sheet, 601
  recommendations, 602
  selecting tube feeding formulas, 599-600

Enteral nutrition for children—cont'd
  sick infants, children, adolescents, 473
  vomiting, diarrhea, and constipation from, 604
  water requirements, 604
Enteral nutrition formulas, 666-683
Enteral nutrition support of adults, 385-399
  access routes, 390
  administration, 390-392
  complications and their prevention
    gastrointestinal, 393-394
    mechanical, 392-393
    metabolic, 394-395
  Crohn's disease, 254
  determination of nutrient needs, 386-387
  formulations, 387
    intestinal fuels, 389
    modular products, 388
    polymeric formulas, 387
    predigested formulas, 387-388
    selection, 389
    special disease-specific formulas, 388-389
  general description, 385
  at home, 395
  indications and rationale, 385-386
  order for, 396, 686-688
  patient education, 395
Enteritis, radiation, 240
Enterostomies, tube, 390 (*see also* Tube feeding)
Enzymes, in inborn errors of metabolism, 501, 506
Epilepsy, ketogenic diet, 561-574
Equal (*see* Aspartame)
Erythropoietin, in end-stage renal disease, 326
Esophageal cancer, 296
Esophageal reflux, 226
  dietary recommendations, 228
  indications and rationale, 226-227
  pharmaceutical management, 227
Esophageal variceal bleeding, sclerotherapy for, 286
European guidelines for hyperlipidemia, 138
Exceed Fluid Replacement, 52
Exercise (*see also* Athletes)
  diabetes and, 165, 166
    pediatric, 498, 499
  fluid and electrolyte replacement, 51-53
  for hypertriglyceridemia, 142
  for obesity, 139, 192-193
    pediatric, 544
  osteoporosis and, 211
  transplantation and, 366
Extrapancreatic tumors, hypoglycemia and, 183, 184

F

Facial nerve, swallowing and, 92
Faddism (*see* Fraud in food claims)
Failure to thrive
  causes and symptoms, 460
  definition, 459-460
  dietary recommendations
    catch-up growth, 461-462
    feeding trial, 460-461
    nutrition assessment, 460
    patient education and follow-up, 462
Fat (body)
  distribution, body composition and, 189
  pediatric measurement, 423
  percent of body weight as, 139
  in young athletes, 445-446
Fat (dietary)
  ACS/NCI guidelines for cancer risk reduction, 17
  in athlete's diet, 54-55
  bone marrow transplantation and, 382
  cardiovascular disease and, pediatric, 488, 489
  copper in, 283
  in cow's milk, infants and, 432
  cystic fibrosis and, 583
  diabetes and, 159
    pediatric, 497
  exchanges, 180
    for glycogen storage disease, type I, 514-515
    in ketogenic diet, without MCT oil, 571
  fat absorption test diet, pediatric, 559-560
  fiber content, 239
  food, exchanges for protein, sodium, and potassium control, 354
  gluten in, 147
  hemodialysis and, 325
  infant requirements, 427-428
  intake reduction, 141
  intolerance, pediatric, 555, 556
  in ketogenic diet, 571
    with MCT oil, 568
    without MCT oil, 563-565
  kidney transplantation and, 370, 371
  liver disease and, 278
  liver transplantation and, 376
  for low-birth-weight infants, 464
  malabsorption
    dietary recommendations, 229, 232
    indications and rationale, 229-230
    medium-chain triglycerides and, 230-232

Fat (dietary)—cont'd
  malabsorption—cont'd
    nutritional inadequacy and, 229
  maldigestion, 229-230
  maple syrup urine disease and, 522
  meal plans for 100-g daily intake,
    414
  in milk sources for infants, 431
  myocardial infarction and, 150, 151
  in one serving from each food
    exchange group, 348
  oxalate in, 342
  pancreas transplantation and, 372-
    373
  peritoneal dialysis and, 328
    pediatric, 593
  in predigested formulas, 388
  recommended intake for children
    and teens, 437
  requirements for ICU, ward, and
    obese patient, 33
  in restricted fiber diet, 241
  short bowel syndrome and, 259
  sodium content, 129, 130
  substitutes, 747-755
  thoracic organ transplantation and,
    378
  transport defects, 230
  USDA/USDHHS guidelines, 5-6
  utilization defects, 230
Fat emulsions, in parenteral nutrition, 400, 402
  pediatric, 606-607
Fat test diet, 413-414
  meal planning suggestion, 414-415
  order for, 414
Fatty acids
  in enteral nutrition, 389
  in parenteral nutrition, 407
FDA-HFY40, address and phone number, 26
Feeding (*see also* Enteral nutrition
  and Parenteral nutrition entries)
  in developmetal disability, 455-456,
    458
  for low-birth-weight infants, 466-
    468
  skills and attitudes assessment, 424
  trial, in failure to thrive, 460-461
Ferritin, 425
Fetal alcohol syndrome, 43
Fiber
  ACS/NCI guidelines for cancer risk
    reduction, 16
  bone marrow transplantation and,
    382
  cholesterol and, 139
  components, food sources, 234
  constipation and encopresis and,
    548, 549-550
  content in selected foods, 237-239

Fiber—cont'd
  developmental disabilities and, 458
  diabetes and, 160-161
    pediatric, 497
  geriatric needs, 64
  high fiber diet, 233
    for bowel regulation, 235
    for cancer prevention, 235-236
    for diabetes, 235
    dietary management goals, 236
    dietary recommendations, 236
    for hyperlipidemia, 235
    indications and rationale, 233-236
    for irritable bowel syndrome, 263
    nutritional inadequacy and, 233
    undesirable effects, 236
  hypercalciuria and, 338
  inflammatory bowel disease and,
    253, 255
  irritable bowel syndrome and, 263
  kidney transplantation and, 370
  low residue diet, 242-243
  osteoporosis and, 207
  pancreas transplantation and, 373
  physiological effects, 234
  restricted fiber diet, 240
    dietary recommendations, 242
    food groups and, 241
    indications and rationale, 241
    for specific diseases, 240
  short bowel syndrome and, 259
  terminology, 233-234
Fiber and residue modifications, 233-
  244
Fiber-containing enteral formulas,
  389
Fiber supplements, 236
Fish allergy, 103-104
Fish oils, 139, 253
FK 506 (tacrolimus), 365
Flatulence, 213-216
  carbohydrate and, 215, 262
  from high fiber diet, 236
Fluids
  bariatric surgery and, 198-199
  in chronic renal failure, pediatric,
    586, 587
  in congestive heart failure, 148, 149
  in constipation and encopresis,
    549, 550
  in developmental disabilities, 457
  in dumping syndrome, 272
  in enteral nutrition, 386
  geriatric needs, 64
  hemodialysis and, 323, 324-325
    pediatric, 591, 592
  infant requirements, 427-428
  lactation and, 49
  for low-birth-weight infants, 466
  in parenteral nutrition, pediatric,
    605-606

Fluids—cont'd
  peritoneal dialysis and, 328, 330
    pediatric, 593, 594
  urolithiasis and, 336
Fluids and electrolytes
  in acute renal failure, 316
  athletic needs, 51-53
  bone marrow transplantation and,
    382
  diarrhea and, 223, 225
    pediatric, 551-553
  kidney transplantation and, 370,
    371
  in liver disease, 278-279, 280, 281
  liver transplantation and, 376
  pancreas transplantation and, 373
  in short bowel syndrome, 259
  thoracic organ transplantation and,
    378
  in young athletes, 442-443
Fluoride
  bones and, 210
  infant requirements, 428, 429
  lactation and, 48
  safe and adequate daily dietary
    intake, 20
Folacin, infant RDA and content in
  milk sources, 431
Folate
  deficiency, in megaloblastic ane-
    mia, 62
  in pregnancy, normal, 42
  recommended dietary allowances, 19
Folic acid
  chronic renal failure and, 317
    pediatric, 588
  in hemodialysis, pediatric, 592
  liver disease and, 275-276
  for low-birth-weight infants, 465
  in parenteral nutrition, pediatric,
    608
  in peritoneal dialysis, pediatric, 594
  in pregnancy, normal, 41-42
Food additives, 111-121
  cancer risk and, 17
Food allergies, 97-111 (*see also* Food
  intolerance)
  associations and organizations, 99-
    100
  corn, 101-102
  cross-reactivity, 100
  diagnosis, 97-98
  diet modification, 100
  eggs, 102-103
  fish or shellfish, 103-104
  food challenge, 98
  heat and processing effects, 100
  milk, 104-106
  peanut and soy, 107-108
  reactions, 97, 100
  treatment overview, 99

Food allergies—cont'd
wheat, 108-110
Food allergies in children, 477-481
classification of foods into families,
478-479
dietary recommendations, 477, 480
diet order, 480
indications and rationale, 477, 479-
480
Food Allergy Network, address and
phone number, 100
Food and Drug Administration, food
labeling standards, 21-23
Food classification into families, 478-
479
Food dyes, 111
Food exchange lists, 169-180
average nutrient content in one
serving from each exchange
group, 348
commercial baby foods, 797-806
for glycogen storage disease, type I,
513, 514-516
for ketogenic diet, 568-569
with MCT oil, 572-573
without MCT oil, 565, 569-572
for protein, sodium, and potassium
control, 348-356
Food groups, 6-8
available carbohydrate from, 163
in hospital diets, 78, 80, 82, 83, 85,
87
in restricted fiber diet, 241
in vegetarian diet, 73-74
Food guide pyramid, 6-8
Food intolerance, 97-100, 111-122 (*see
also* Food allergies)
aspartame, 111-112
associations and organizations, 99-100
benzoates and parabens, 112-113
BHA and BHT, 113
diagnosis, 98
after gastroplasty or gastric bypass,
199-200
in irritable bowel syndrome, 262-
263
mold, 114-115
monosodium glutamate (MSG),
115-116
nickel, 116-117
nitrates and nitrites, 117-118
penicillin, 118-119
reactions, 97, 110-111
sulfites, 119-120
tartrazine and acetylsalicylic acid,
121
Food labeling, 21-23
additives, 111
gluten, 248-249
sodium, 131
specific labels, 659-660

Food misinformation (*see* Fraud in
food claims)
Food preparation methods, cancer
risk and, 17
Food preservatives, 111
Food servings
definitions, 8
number required daily, 7
in pregnancy and lactation, 45
Food thickeners, 93
Food variety
ACS/NCI guidelines for cancer risk
reduction, 16
USDA/USDHHS guidelines, 5
Forbes disease, 505
Formulas
for enteral nutrition, 666-683
administration, 390-392
types, 387-389
for infant nutrition, 429, 430, 431,
763-795
for low-birth-weight infants, 467
for maple syrup urine disease, 521
phenylalanine and, 526-527, 530
for tube feeding in children, selection, 599-600
Four Food Groups, 6-7
vegetarian diet modifications, 73-74
Fraud in food claims, 23-28
combatting, 28
resources, 26
target groups, 24-28
where to report, 27
Fredrickson classification of hyperlipoproteinemia, 138
Friedewald Formula, 12, 134-135, 489
Fructose
flatulence and, 215
hereditary intolerance, 504
Fruits
ACS/NCI guidelines for cancer risk
reduction, 16
cholesterol and fat from, 141
copper in, 284
diabetes and, pediatric, 500
exchanges, 179
in ketogenic diet, without MCT
oil, 571-572
for protein, sodium, and potassium control, 353-354
fiber in, 237
restricted fiber diet, 241
gluten in, 147
for infants
dietary guidelines, 435
phenylalanine content, 533-534
in lacto-ovo diet, pediatric, 450
in low residue diet, 243
number of daily servings, 7
in pregnancy, 45
oxalate in, 341-342

Fruits—cont'd
potassium in
high, 360
low, 358
moderate, 359
very high, 361
recommended intake for children
and teens, 437
sodium in, 128, 130
USDA/USDHHS guidelines, 6
in vegan diet, pediatric, 451
FTT (*see* Failure to thrive)
Full liquid diet, 81-82

G

Galactokinase deficiency, hereditary,
504
Galactosemia, 504
Gas, 213-216, 262
Gastrectomy, 200, 270-273
Gastric acid secretion, in peptic ulcer
disease, 268, 269
Gastric bypass
complications and dietary modifications, 197
dietary recommendations, 197-200
follow-up, 202
food intolerances and, 199-200
nutritional inadequacy and, 196-
197
Gastric emptying, delayed (*see*
Delayed gastric emptying)
Gastric motility dysfunction, 218-220
associated conditions, 218
dietary recommendations, 220-221
Gastric obstruction, 217-218, 220
Gastric reflux, 226-228
Gastric ulcers, 268, 269
Gastrointestinal complications of
tube feeding, 393-394
Gastrointestinal diseases and disorders, 213-274
in children, 547-560
Gastroparesis, 218-221, 240
Gastroplasty
food intolerances and, 199-200
for weight reduction, 195
complications and dietary modifications, 197
diabetes and, 168
vertical banded, 197-200
Gatorade, 52
Geriatric nutrition, 58-68
aging process, 58
anemias and, 62
in chronic disease, 60-61
community-based long-term care,
65
diet modifications, 61-62

Geriatric nutrition—cont'd
  drug use and, 60-61
  hypercholesterolemia and, 61-62
  indicators of nutritional status, 66-
    68
  laboratory values and, 62-63
  metabolic, physiological, and bio-
    chemical factors, 58-59
  osteoporosis and, 62
  requirements, 63-64
  socioeconomic and psychological
    factors, 59-60
Gestational diabetes, 46
Glandular products, 24-25
Gliadin, 108
Glomerular filtration, in nephrotic
  syndrome, 333
Glossopharyngeal nerve, swallowing
  and, 92
Glucose
  altered levels (see Hyperglycemia;
    Hypoglycemia)
  in diabetes and pregnancy, 46-47,
    167, 168
  exercise and, 165, 166
  impaired tolerance, 155
  lactose intolerance test and, 265-
    266
  in parenteral nutrition, pediatric,
    606
  production, in glycogen storage
    disease, type I, 510, 511
  short bowel syndrome and, 259
  tube feeding and, 168
Glucose-galactose malabsorption, 504
Glucose-6-P defect, 505
Glucose polymers, in glycogen storage disease, type I, 511
Glucose tolerance test, diet for, 412-
  413
Glutamic acid (glutamate), in MSG,
  115
Glutamine, in enteral nutrition, 389
Gluten, sources of, 247-248
Gluten-Intolerance Group, address
  and phone number, 249
Gluten-sensitive enteropathy in children, 555-556
Gluten sensitivity, 108-109, 244-250
  celiac sprue, 245-246
  dermatitis herpetiformis, 246
  dietary recommendations, 246, 248
  diet order, 248
  food labeling and, 248-249
  indications and rationale, 245-246
  nutritional inadequacy and, 245
  patient support groups, 249
  wheat flour substitutions, 249
Glycemic effects of carbohydrates, 160
Glycogen diseases, substrate restriction treatment, 505

Glycogen packing, 54
Glycogen storage diseases, 508
  diet order, 518
  nutritional therapy, 509
  support group, 518
  type I, 508
    cornstarch therapy, 511-512
    dietary management goals, 510
    dietary recommendations, 510-
      513
    food exchanges, 513, 514-516
    foods restricted in intake, 516
    indications and rationale, 509-
      510
    nocturnal tube feedings, 511
    nutritional inadequacy and, 509
    oral feedings, 512-513
  type III and type VI, 513, 516
    dietary recommendations, 517
    indications and rationale, 517
    nutritional inadequacy and, 516
  type IV, 517-518
Glycogen synthetase deficiency, 505
Gout, 344, 345
Graft atherosclerosis, in thoracic
  organ transplantation, 379
Graft versus host disease (GVHD),
  381, 382, 383
Grains
  cholesterol and fat from, 141
  dietary guidelines for infants, 435
  exchanges in ketogenic diet, with
    MCT oil, 573
  gluten in, 147
  in lacto-ovo diet, pediatric, 450
  in low residue diet, 243
  recommended intake for children
    and teens, 437
  USDA/USDHHS guidelines, 6
  in vegan diet, pediatric, 451
Growth (see also Developmental disability), anthropometrics, 31-32,
  453-454, 848
Growth charts
  Down's syndrome, 834-841
  premature infants, 843
Growth graphs, 422, 454
  from National Center for Health
    Statistics, 820-827
  Tanner height for age and height
    velocity graphs, 856-859
Growth hormone, athletes and, 56
Growth quotient, 462
Growth retardation
  in chronic renal failure, 585-586
  failure to thrive, 459-462
  from inflammatory bowel disease,
    557-558
  syndromes associated with, 454
GSD (see Glycogen storage diseases)
Gums, food sources, 234

GVHD (graft versus host disease),
  381, 382, 383

H

Harris-Benedict equations, 34, 471
HDL cholesterol
  coronary heart disease and, 10, 13-
    14
  levels, 135
    causes of reduced serum levels,
      135
    in United States, 719-720
  NCEP guidelines, 10, 11, 13-14
  ratio to LDL cholesterol, 135
  ratio to total cholesterol, 135
Head and neck surgery, malnutrition
  from, 295
Head circumference measurements,
  421-422
Heart disease, 123-151 (see also
  Coronary disease)
Heart surgery, 146-148
Heart transplantation, 377-380
Height
  in nutritional screening and assess-
    ment, 31
  pediatric development and, 421,
    422
  Tanner height for age and height
    velocity graphs, 856-859
Hematocrit, pediatric iron deficiency
  anemia and, 424
Hemicellulose, food sources, 234
Hemodialysis
  calcium and phosphorus and, 323,
    325
  dietary management goals, 326
  dietary recommendations, 322, 327
  diet order, 327
  erythropoitein and, 326
  fluid and, 323, 324-325
  indications and rationale, 322-325
  kilocalories and, 323, 324
  nutritional inadequacy and, 322
  nutritional problems, 325-326
  pediatric
    dietary management, 588, 590-
      592
    diet order, 594
    indications and rationale, 590
    nutritional inadequacy and, 589-
      590
  potassium and, 323, 324
  protein and, 323-324
  sodium and, 323, 324
Hemoglobin, pediatric iron deficiency anemia and, 424
Hepatic encephalopathy, in liver disease, 276-280

Hepatic phosphorylase deficiency glycogenosis, 505
Hepatobiliary diseases, 275-286
    copper metabolism and, 282-285
    dietary management goals, 279
    dietary recommendations, 280
    diet order, 281
    energy needs, 276
    fat and, 278
    fluids and electrolytes and, 278-279, 280, 281
    general description, 275
    indications and rationale, 276-279
    malnutrition causes, 276
    nutritional inadequacy and, 275-276
    protein and, 275, 276-278, 280
    sclerotherapy, 286
    staging of hepatic encephalopathy, 277
    vitamins and minerals and, 279
Hepatolenticular degeneration (Wilson's disease), 279, 282, 285
Hereditary metabolic disorders (see Inborn errors of metabolism)
5-HIAA test, diet for, 415
High blood pressure (see Hypertension)
High density lipoprotein cholesterol (see HDL cholesterol)
High fiber diet, 233-240
Histidine requirements, 506
History (medical) review, 29-30
Home tube feeding, 395
Homocystinuria, 503
Hospital diet, general, 77-78
Hospital diet progressions, 77-94
    clear liquid diet, 79-80
    consistency and texture modifications, 77-78
    for dysphagia, 91-94
    full liquid diet, 81-82
    for intermaxillary fixation, 89-91
    mechanical soft diet, 84-86
    pureed diet, 82-84
    soft diet, 86-88
    for tonsillectomy and adenoidectomy, 89
    transitional feeding, 88-89
Hydrogen, as bowel gas, 213-214
Hydrogen breath analysis, diet for, 411-412
5-Hydroxyindoleacetic acid test, diet for, 415
Hypercalciuria
    dietary recommendations, 338, 339
    indications and rationale, 336-338
    nutritional inadequacy and, 336
Hypercholesterolemia, 134
    classification and typing, 136-139
    dietary guidelines, 141

Hypercholesterolemia—cont'd
    dietary modifications, 143, 144
    in elderly, 61-62
    in hemodialysis, 325
    NCEP treatment guidelines, 8-12
    pediatric, 489
    in thoracic organ transplantation, 379
Hyperchylomicronemia, 230
Hyperglycemia
    from parenteral nutrition, 406
        pediatric, 612
    stress, feeding limitations, 33
Hyperkalemia
    in parenteral nutrition, 406-407
    postassium control in, 356-357
Hyperlipidemia, 133-146
    assessment, 143
    cardiac surgery and, 146
    cardiovascular risk factors, 138-139
    cholesterol and, 134
    diagnosis, 134
    dietary factors, 139-140
    dietary management goals, 140
    dietary recommendations, 140-144
    HDL cholesterol and, 135
    high fiber diet and, 235
    indications and rationale, 134-140
    LDL cholesterol and, 134-135
    nephrotic syndrome and, 334, 597
    nutritional inadequacy and, 123
    pediatric
        dietary management goals, 488
        dietary recommendations, 488-490
        diet order, 490
        indications and rationale, 488
        management, 487
        nephrotic syndrome and, 597
        nutritional inadequacy and, 487-488
    peritoneal dialysis and, 331
    thoracic organ transplantation and, 379
    treatment, 133, 140
    triglycerides and, 135-136
Hyperlipoproteinemia, 134
    fat utilization and, 138
    type I, 230
Hyperoxaluria, enteric, 340, 343
Hypertension
    alcohol and, 125, 131
    associations and organizations, 132
    as cardiovascular risk factor, 138
    classification, 124
    definition and causes, 123
    dietary management goals, 126
    dietary recommendations, 127-131
    diet order, 131-132
    epidemiology, 124
    indications and rationale, 123-126
    nutritional inadequacy and, 123

Hypertension—cont'd
    pediatric
        algorithm for identification, 485
        classification by age group, 484
        definitions, 484
        dietary management goals, 486
        dietary recommendations, 486-487
        indications and rationale, 483, 485-486
        management, 483
    portal, 286
    postural, in Parkinson's disease, 290
    sodium and, 125, 127, 130-131
    treatment, 124, 125-126
    weight and, 124-125, 127
Hypertriglyceridemia, 136
    causes, 136
    dietary guidelines, 142
    dietary modifications, 143-144
    in hemodialysis, 325
    NCEP guidelines, 12-13
Hyperuricemia, 344, 345
Hypervalinemia, 502
Hypoalbuminemia, 33, 255
Hypocalcemia, in parenteral nutrition, 407
Hypoglossal nerve, swallowing and, 92
Hypoglycemia, 183-185
    in diabetes, 164-165
    dietary management goals, 184-185
    dietary recommendations, 183, 185
    in glycogen storage disease
        type I, 510, 511, 513
        type III and type VI, 517
    indications and rationale, 183-184
    in parenteral nutrition, 406
    pediatric, 498, 499
    reactive, 183-184, 185
    types and causes, 183-184
Hypokalemia, postassium management in, 356-357
Hypomagnesemia, in parenteral nutrition, 407
Hypophosphatemia, in parenteral nutrition, 407
Hypoproteinemia, pancreaticobiliary bypass and, 201

I

IBD (see Inflammatory bowel disease)
IBS (see Irritable bowel syndrome)
Idiopathic calcium urolithiasis, 336, 337
Ileal pouch/anal anastomosis, 256, 258
Ileal resection, 258

Ileostomy, 256, 257
Immunological testing, for food allergy, 98
Immunosuppressive therapy, 364, 365
Imodium (loperamide), 224
Imuran (azathioprine), 365
Inborn errors of metabolism, 501, 506
　amino acid requirements, 506
　defects, 501
　dietary management goals, 506
　dietary recommendations, 506-507
　information sources for parents and
　　health professionals, 507-508
　substrate restriction treatment, 502-
　　505
Infants
　cystic fibrosis and, 583
　formulas and feedings, 763-795
　low-birth-weight (*see* Low-birth-
　　weight infants)
　nutritional requirements
　　developmental abilities and, 433-
　　　434
　　dietary guidelines, 435
　　digestion and, 433
　　energy, 440
　　feeding guidelines, 434
　　fluid, 428
　　food introduction by age, 435
　　human milk, cow's milk, and for-
　　　mulas, 429-432
　　protein, carbohydrates, and fat,
　　　427-428
　　solid foods, 432-436
　　vitamins and minerals, 428-429
　premature, 422
　　growth chart, 843
　sick, 469-473
　tube feeding formula selection,
　　599-600
Infection in transplantation, low bac-
　teria diet and, 368
Inflammatory bowel disease, 250-259
　dietary management goals, 251
　dietary recommendations, 251
　　colostomy, 255-256, 257
　　ileal pouch/anal anastomosis,
　　　256, 258
　　ileostomy, 256, 257
　　large bowel inflammation, 253
　　short bowel syndrome, 258-259
　　small bowel inflammation, 253-255
　indications and rationale, 250-251
　management, 251
　nutritional inadequacy and, 250
　pediatric
　　dietary management goals, 558
　　dietary recommendations, 558-559
　　indications and rationale, 557-558
　　management, 557
　　nutritional inadequacy and, 557

Inflammatory bowel disease—cont'd
　restricted fiber diet, 240
　signs and symptoms, 251
　site and extent of disease process,
　　nutrient absorption and, 252
　types, 250
Insulin, diabetes and, 46-47, 154-155
　pediatric, 496, 498, 499
Intensive care unit, assessing nutri-
　tional needs in, 33
Interleukin-1, cancer and, 294
Intermaxillary fixation, diet progres-
　sion, 89-91
Intermittent infusion, in enteral
　nutrition, 391
Interview with patient, 31
Intestinal feedings, 390 (*see also* Tube
　feeding)
Intestinal resection, 295
Intolerance (*see* Food intolerance)
Intradialytic parenteral nutrition, 326
Intubation, nasal, 390 (*see also* Tube
　feeding)
Iodine
　infant RDA and content in milk
　　sources, 431
　recommended dietary allowances, 19
Iron
　adolescent needs, 439
　in athlete's diet, 55
　infant RDA and content in milk
　　sources, 431
　infant requirements, 428, 429
　lactation and, 48
　in liver disease, 279
　for low-birth-weight infants, 465,
　　466
　in parenteral nutrition, pediatric,
　　608, 609
　in pregnancy
　　adolescents, 45-46
　　normal, 41, 42
　recommended dietary allowances, 19
　in vegetarian diet, 72
　　pediatric, 448, 449
　for young athletes, 444-445
Iron deficiency
　in hypoproliferative anemia, 62
　in infants, cow's milk and, 432
　in parenteral nutrition, 407
　in young athletes, 444-445
Iron deficiency anemia, pediatric
　screening, 424-425
Irradiation
　before bone marrow transplant,
　　side effects, 381
　nutritional effects, 296-297
　pediatric, 576
Irritable bowel syndrome
　dietary recommendations, 261, 263
　high fiber diet and, 235, 236

Irritable bowel syndrome—cont'd
　indications and rationale, 261-263
　nutritional inadequacy and, 261
　symptoms and causes, 261-262
Islet cell tumors, hypoglycemia and,
　183, 184
Isocarboxazid, 312
Isoleucine
　in maple syrup urine disease, 521-
　　522
　requirements, 506
Isovaleric acidemia, 502

J

Jejunoileal bypass, 195
Jejunostomy, 390
Jewish dietary practices, 75-76
Juices
　for infants, phenylalanine content,
　　534
　oxalate in, 341-342
Juvenile Diabetes Foundation,
　address, 169

K

Kaolin-containing products, 224
Ketoacidosis, medium-chain triglyc-
　erides and, 231
Ketoaciduria, branched-chain (*see*
　Maple syrup urine disease)
Ketogenic diet, 561-574
　artificial sweeteners and, 569
　calculation
　　with MCT oil, 567, 568
　　without MCT oil, 563-566
　carbohydrate-containing foods to
　　avoid, 568
　description, 561
　dietary management goals, 562
　dietary recommendations, 562-563
　diet order, 567
　food exchange list, 565, 568-569
　　with MCT oil, 572-573
　　without MCT oil, 569-572
　indications and rationale, 561-562
　K:AK ratio calculation table, 567
　nutritional inadequacy and, 561
　sample meal plan, 566
Kidney diseases and disorders, 315-362
　in children, 585-597
Kidney transplantation, 369
　immediate and long-term post-
　　transplant management, 369-371
　nutritional care guidelines, 370
　pretransplant management, 369
Kilocalories (*see* Calories)
Kosher foods, 75-76

L

Labeling of foods, 21-23
  additives, 111
  gluten, 248-249
  sodium, 131
  specific labels, 659-660
Laboratory monitoring of parenteral
  nutrition, 403
Laboratory nutritional assessment,
  32-33
  pediatric, 420, 424-425
Laboratory test values
  aging and, 62-63
  normal, 651-654
  pediatric, selected references, 853
Lactase deficiency, 265
Lactase enzyme products, 267
Lactation, 45, 47-49
Lacto-ovovegetarian diet, 70, 71, 72
  food guide for children, 450
Lactose, content of foods, 266
Lactose intolerance, 209, 264
  breath hydrogen analysis test, 411
  dietary recommendations, 267
  gastroplasty and, 197
  indications and rationale, 265-266
  inflammatory bowel disease and,
    253, 254-255
  mechanism and diagnosis, 265-266
  nutritional inadequacy and, 264-265
  pediatric, 555, 556
Lactose malabsorption, 504
Lactovegetarian diet, 70, 72
Laetrile, 26-27
Large bowel inflammation, 253
LDL cholesterol
  calculation, 488-489
  coronary heart disease and, NCEP
    guidelines, 11, 13-14
  elevated (see Hyperlipidemia)
  Friedewald equation, 12
  levels
    calculation and, 134-135
    pediatric, 488-489
    in United States, 722-723
  ratio to HDL cholesterol, 135
L-dopa, for Parkinson's disease, 287-
  288, 289
Legumes
  allergy, 107-108
  breath hydrogen concentration
    and, 412
Length, pediatric development and,
  421, 422
Leucine
  in maple syrup urine disease, 521, 522
  requirements, 506
Leucinosis, 502
Levodopa, for Parkinson's disease,
  287-288, 289

Lignin, food sources, 234
Limit dextrinosis, 505
Lipids, elevated levels (see
  Hyperlipidemia)
Lipoproteins, 134, 138, 230
  levels in United States, 721-723
Liquid diet
  clear, 79-80
  full, 81-82
Liquids (see Fluids)
Liver disease (see Hepatobiliary diseases)
Liver transplantation, 374
  candidates, 374, 375
  immediate post-transplant manage-
    ment, 375
  long-term post-transplant manage-
    ment, 376
  nutritional care guidelines, 376
  pretransplant management, 374
Lofenalac, 525, 526-527
  composition, 530
  diet calculation for infants with,
    535
  diet calculation for toddlers with,
    536
Lomotil (diphenoxylate with atropine
  sulfate), 224
Lonox (diphenoxylate with atropine
  sulfate), 224
Loperamide, 224
Low bacteria diet, for transplantation,
  367-368, 373, 376, 378, 382
Low-birth-weight infants, 463
  dietary assessment, 463-466
  feedings
    formulas, 467
    human milk, 466-467
    techniques, 467-468
  fluids for, 466
Low density lipoprotein cholesterol
  (see LDL cholesterol)
Lower esophageal sphincter, reflux
  and, 226-227, 228
Low residue diet, 242-243
L-tryptophan, 288
Lung transplantation, 377-380
Lysine intolerance with ammonia
  intoxication, 503
Lysine requirements, 506

M

Macrobiotic diet, in chronic illness,
  26
Magnesium
  deficiency, in short bowel syndrome,
    258
  infant RDA and content in milk
    sources, 431

Magnesium—cont'd
  in liver disease, 279
  for low-birth-weight infants, 464
  in parenteral nutrition, 400, 407
    pediatric, 607
  recommended dietary allowances, 19
Malabsorption
  in celiac sprue, 245
  fat, 229-232
  pancreaticobiliary bypass and, 200
Malnutrition
  in cancer, 293-294
    pediatric, 575-576
    from treatment, 294-295
  in celiac disease, pediatric, 555
  in liver disease, causes, 276
  pathophysiological mechanisms,
    29-30
  in sick infants, children, and ado-
    lescents, 470
  in transplantation, 363, 364, 377
Manganese
  in parenteral nutrition, pediatric,
    608, 609
  safe and adequate daily dietary
    intake, 20
MAO inhibitors, tyramine controlled
  diet and, 311-312, 313
Maple syrup urine disease
  branched-chain amino acids and, 519
  classification by branched-chain
    ketoacid decarboxylase activity,
    520
  defective pathway and treatment,
    502
  dietary management goals, 520-521
  dietary recommendations, 521-523
  diet order, 523
  family resources, 524
  indications and rationale, 519-520
  nutritional inadequacy and, 519
  variants, 520
Marijuana abuse, adolescent, 440
Marplan (isocarboxazid), 312
Maxamaid, 525, 527, 530
Maxamum XP, 525, 526, 530
McArdle-Schmidt-Pearson disease, 505
MCTs (see Medium-chain triglycerides)
Meal plans, hospital
  clear liquid diet, 80
  full liquid diet, 81
  general, 78
  mechanical soft diet, 85
  pureed diet, 83
  soft diet, 87
Meals
  planning guidelines, 5-28
  precompetition, 57
  pregame and postgame, 445
Mean corpuscular volume, pediatric
  iron deficiency anemia and, 424

Measurements, pediatric, 419, 420, 421-423
Meat
　alternatives, 173
　cholesterol and fat from, 141
　copper in, 283
　exchanges, 171-172
　　for glycogen storage disease, type I, 514
　　in ketogenic diet, without MCT oil, 570
　　for protein, sodium, and potassium control, 349
　gluten in, 147
　for infants
　　dietary guidelines, 435
　　phenylalanine content of products, 531
　in low residue diet, 243
　number of daily servings, 7
　　in pregnancy, 45
　oxalate in, 341
　penicillin in, 118
　recommended intake for children and teens, 437
　in restricted fiber diet, 241
　sodium in, 128, 130
　tyramine in, 312
Mechanical soft diet, 84-86
Medical history review, 29-30
Medications
　breast feeding and, 429-430
　in developmental disability, 458
　effect on nutrition of specific drugs, 625-643
　geriatric nutrition and, 60-61, 68
　lactation and, 49
　obesity and, 190
　with parenteral nutrition, 402, 408
　sodium content, 131
　for transplantation, 365
Medium-chain triglycerides, 230-232
　MCT oil in ketogenic diet, 563
　　diet calculation, 567, 568
　　food exchange list, 572-573
　　in predigested formulas, 388
Menopause, osteoporosis and, 205, 208
Mental retardation, from phenylketonuria, 525, 535
Metabolic acidosis, 319
Metabolic diseases and disorders, 153-212
　pediatric, 495-545
Metabolic rate, basal, formulas, 471
Metabolism
　in bulimia nervosa, 305
　changes in elderly, 58
　complications of parenteral nutrition, 394-395, 406-407
　　pediatric, 612
　inborn errors, 501-508

Methane, as bowel gas, 213-214
Methionine
　requirements, 506
　restriction, 344
Methotrexate, 365
Methylmalonic aciduria, 502
Metric measures, conversions, 707-708
Mexican-American children, growth graphs and, 422
Milk
　allergy, 104-106
　cholesterol and fat from, 141
　copper in, 283
　diabetes and, pediatric, 498, 500
　dumping syndrome and, 272
　exchanges, 174
　　for protein, sodium, and potassium control, 349-350
　gluten in, 147
　human, 47-49
　　for low-birth-weight infants, 466-467
　in infant nutrition
　　breast milk, 428-430, 431
　　cow's milk, 429, 430-432
　　dietary guidelines, 435
　　formulas, 429, 430, 431
　intolerance (see Lactose intolerance)
　in lacto-ovo diet, pediatric, 450
　in low residue diet, 243
　number of daily servings, 7
　nutrients in, alternative food sources, 105
　oxalate in, 341
　penicillin in, 118
　peptic ulcer disease and, 269
　peritoneal dialysis and, 330
　recommended intake for children and teens, 437
　in restricted fiber diet, 241
　skim, in school lunch, 498
　sodium content, 128, 130
　soy, in vegan diet, pediatric, 451
　terms indicating presence of, 106
Milliequivalents, conversion from milligrams, 705
Milligrams, conversion to milliequivalents, 705
Minerals
　in athlete's diet, 54-55
　deficiencies in elderly, 64
　enteral nutrition and, 386
　estimating needs, 35
　fraudulent claims, 23
　infant requirements, 428
　kidney transplantation and, 371
　in liver disease, 279
　for low-birth-weight infants, 464, 465
　in parenteral nutrition, 400, 401
　　pediatric, 607
　for preschool and school age children, 436

Minerals—cont'd
　recommended dietary allowances, 19
　in vegetarian diet, pediatric, 449
　for young athletes, 444-445
Mineral supplements, in normal pregnancy, 42
MIV-Pediatric, 608
Molasses, in vegan diet, pediatric, 451
Mold intolerance, 114-115
Molybdenum, safe and adequate daily dietary intake, 20
Monoamine oxidase inhibitors, tyramine controlled diet and, 311-312, 313
Monosodium glutamate intolerance, 115-116
Motility dysfunction
　gastric, 218-220
　　associated conditions, 218
　　dietary recommendations, 220-221
　intestinal, in irritable bowel syndrome, 262
Mouth, dry, in cancer, 298
MSG intolerance, 115-116
MSUD (see Maple syrup urine disease)
MSUD diet powder, 521
Mucositis, from chemotherapy, 295
Multiple vitamin preparations, 738-741
Muscle, of athletes, 53, 54, 446
Muscle building, 24-25, 56
Muscle stimulators, electrical, 25
Myelomeningocele, 457
Myocardial infarction, 150-151
Myophosphorylase deficiency, 505

N

Nardil (phenelzine), 312
Nasal intubation, 390
Natabec Rx, 276
National Academy of Sciences, recommended dietary allowances, 18-21
National Cancer Institute
　address and phone number, 26
　dietary guidelines, 15-17
National Center for Education in Maternal and Child Health, address and phone number, 507
National Center for Health Statistics, growth graphs, 820-827
National Cholesterol Education Program guidelines
　HDL cholesterol, 13-14
　hypercholesterolemia, 8-12
　hypertriglyceridemia, 12-13
　pediatric diet, 489
National Council Against Health Fraud, address and phone number, 26

National Diabetes Information Clearinghouse, address, 169

National Health and Nutrition Examination Survey, calcium and, 206

National Heart, Lung, and Blood Institute, address and phone number, 132

National Institute of Allergy and Infectious Diseases, address and phone number, 100

Nausea
cancer and, 295, 297, 298
from dopamine, 288-289
gastroplasty and, 197
ketogenic diet and, 562
pediatric diabetes and, 499-500

Nephrotic syndrome, 333
dietary management goals, 334-335
dietary recommendations, 334, 335
indications and rationale, 333-334
nutritional problems, 334
pediatric
dietary management, 595, 596-597
hyperlipidemia in, 597
indications and rationale, 595-596
nutritional inadequacy and, 595

Nerves, swallowing and, 92

Neurologic disease
ketogenic diet for children, 561-574
Parkinson's disease, 287-291

NHANES II, calcium and, 206

Niacin
infant RDA and content in milk sources, 431
in parenteral nutrition, pediatric, 608
recommended dietary allowances, 19

Nickel intolerance, 116-117

Nickel restricted diet, 117

Nicotine (smoking), 138, 270

Nitrates intolerance, 117-118

Nitrite-preserved foods, ACS/NCI guidelines for cancer risk reduction, 17

Nitrites intolerance, 117-118

Nitrogen
as bowel gas, 213
in parenteral nutrition, 400
stool, fat test diet and, 414

Nomograms
anthropometry for children, 848
body mass index, 657-658
estimating caloric requirements, 655-656

Normal nutrition, 39-76
pediatric, 427-452

Nutramigen, 554

NutraSweet (*see* Aspartame)

Nutra-Thik, 93

Nutrient requirements
in elderly, 63-64

Nutrient requirements—cont'd
estimating, 33-35
new proposals, 23
Recommended Dietary Allowances, 18-21

Nutritional care
definition, 3
plan, 36

Nutritional monitoring
enteral nutrition for children, 603-604
parenteral nutrition for adults, 408
parenteral nutrition for children, 609

Nutritional screening and assessment, 29-37
anthropometrics, 31-32
biochemical assessment, 32-33
care plan, 36
estimation of nutrient requirements, 33
guidelines for ICU, ward, and obese patient, 33-35
malnutrition mechanisms, 29-30
patient interview, 31
pediatric assessment, 419-426
anthropometric evaluation, 419, 420, 421-423
biochemical data, 424-425
diet, 423-424
technique selection guidelines, 420
review of medical history, 29-30

Nutritional support (*see* Enteral nutrition and Parenteral nutrition entries)

Nutrition Screening Initiative (NSI), 64

Nutrition support dietitians, standards of practice, 617-624

Nuts
in lacto-ovo diet, pediatric, 450
low in potassium, 358
in vegan diet, pediatric, 451

O

Obesity, 185-195
bariatric surgery, 195-196
body composition and fat distribution, 189
cancer and, 300
as cardiovascular risk factor, 139
complications and associated conditions, 189-190
definitions, 186-187
determination of desirable weight, 190
developmental patterns, 187
in diabetes, 156, 158
pediatric, 497
dietary management goals, 190
dietary recommendations, 191-192

Obesity—cont'd
diet order, 193
energy balance and, 188-189
exercise for, 192-193
family history, 187-188
fraud and, 25
hypertension and, 124-125, 127
indications and rationale, 186-190
nutritional inadequacy and, 185-186
nutritional needs assessment, 33
pediatric (see Weight control, pediatric)
personal and demographic data, 187
pregnancy and, 46
psychological and behavioral factors, 189, 193
treatment, 185, 190-193

Obstruction
gastric, 217-218, 220
small bowel, restricted fiber diet for, 240

Octreotide, 259

Oils
cholesterol and fat from, 141
copper in, 283
fiber content, 239
food exchanges for protein, sodium, and potassium control, 354
gluten in, 147
oxalate in, 342
recommended intake for children and teens, 437
in restricted fiber diet, 241

OKT3, 365

Omega-3 fatty acids, heart disease and, 139

Oncologic diseases (*see* Cancer)

Opium, tincture of, 224

Oral rehydration solutions, 863
in pediatric diarrhea, 551-553

Organ transplantation (*see* Transplantation)

Ornithine transcarbamylase deficiency, 503

Osteomalacia, in dumping syndrome, 273

Osteoporosis, 204-211
calcium and, 206, 207-210
dietary recommendations, 207-211
diet order, 211
in elderly, 62
epidemiology, 205
exercise and, 211
indications and rationale, 205-207
lifestyle habits and, 207
liver transplantation and, 376
nutritional inadequacy and, 205
risk factors, 205
types, 205-206

Overweight, obesity vs., 186 (*see also* Obesity)
Oxalate content of selected foods, 341-342
Oxalate restriction
    dietary recommendations, 339, 340
    indications and rationale, 340, 343
Oxygen, as bowel gas, 213

P

Pancreas (and pancreas-renal) transplantation, 372-373
Pancreatic cancer surgery, 295
Pancreatic lipase, 229-230
Pancreaticobiliary bypass
    dietary recommendations, 201
    effect of procedure, 200
    follow-up, 203
    nutritional inadequacy and, 200-201
    partial, 195
    patient selection, 200
Pantothenic acid, safe and adequate daily dietary intake, 20
Parabens intolerance, 113
Parenteral nutrition for children, 605
    in cancer, 577
    complications, 609, 612
    components, 605-609
    indications and rationale, 605
    low-birth-weight infants, 468
    monitoring, 609
    nutrient recommendations, 607-608
    ordering, 610-611, 612
    sick infants, children, and adolescents, 473
Parenteral nutrition solutions, 690-698
Parenteral nutrition support of adults, 399-409
    central, 399, 400, 408
    complications, 408
        metabolic, 406-407
        septic, 405
        technical, 404-405
    component products, 399-402
    in Crohn's disease, 254
    general description, 399
    indications and rationale, 399
    intradialytic, 326
    laboratory monitoring guidelines, 403
    medications provided with, 402, 408
    ordering, 408-409, 700-703
    patient monitoring, 408
    peripheral, 399, 400, 408
    in short bowel syndrome, 259
    total, 402
Pareve, 106

Parkinson's disease
    dietary recommendations, 290
    diet order, 290
    indications and rationale, 288-290
    management, 287
    nutritional inadequacy and, 287-288
Parnate (tranylcypromine), 312
Patient interview, 31
Peanut, terms indicating presence of, 108
Peanut allergy, 107-108
Pectin, 224, 234
Pedialyte, 552
PediaSure, 600
Pediatric nutrition
    developmental disability, 453-459
    enteral, 599-604
    failure to thrive, 459-462
    laboratory values, selected references, 853
    low-birth-weight infants, 463-468
    normal, 427-452
        adolescents, 438-440
        infants, 427-436
        preschool and school age children, 436-438
        young athletes, 442-446
    parenteral, 605-612
    sick infants, children, and adolescents, 469-473
    vegetarian diet, 447-452
    weight control, 539-545
Pediatric nutritional assessment, 419-426
    anthropometric evaluation, 419, 420, 421-423
    biochemical data, 424-425
    dietary assessment, 423-424
    technique selection guidelines, 420
Pelvic radiation, 296-297
D-penicillamine, 282, 285
Penicillin intolerance, 118-119
Peptic ulcer disease
    dietary management goals, 270
    dietary recommendations, 270
    indications and rationale, 268-270
Pepto Bismol (bismuth subsalicylate), 224
Peritoneal dialysis, 327
    calcium and, 328, 330-331
    calories and, 328, 329
    continuous ambulatory, 328-329, 330-331
        pediatric, 589-590, 592-594, 595
    continuous cyclic, 329, 330-331
    dietary management goals, 332
    dietary recommendations, 328, 332
    diet order, 332
    fluid and, 328, 330
    indications and rationale, 328-331

Peritoneal dialysis—cont'd
    nutritional inadequacy and, 328
    nutritional problems, 331-332
    pediatric
        dietary management, 588, 592-594
        diet order, 595
        indications and rationale, 590
        nutritional inadequacy and, 589-590
    phosphorus and, 328, 330
    potassium and, 328, 330
    protein and, 328, 329
    sodium and, 328, 330
Phenelzine, 312
Phenylalanine
    content of infant foods, 531-534
    in phenylketonuria, 524, 525 (*see also* Phenylketonuria)
    requirements, 506
Phenyl Free, 525, 527, 530
Phenylketonuria
    artificial sweeteners and, 529
    aspartame and, 161
    calculation of diet, 529-530, 534-537
    dietary management goals, 526
    dietary recommendations, 524, 526-529
    maternal and paternal, 536-537
    nutritional inadequacy and, 524-525
    parent resources, 537-538
    phenylalanine-controlled diet meal plan, 528
Phenytoin, 393
Phosphate restriction, 343
Phosphorus
    chronic renal failure and, 318, 320
        pediatric, 586, 588
    content in common foods, 761-762
    estimating needs, 35
    hemodialysis and, 323, 325
        pediatric, 591, 592
    infant RDA and content in milk sources, 431
    kidney transplantation and, 371
    for low-birth-weight infants, 464, 465
    in one serving from each food exchange group, 348
    osteoporosis and, 207
    in parenteral nutrition, 400
        pediatric, 607, 612
    peritoneal dialysis and, 328, 330
        pediatric, 593, 594
    recommended dietary allowances, 19
Physical examination, for food allergy, 98
Physical performance (*see* Athletes)
Physiological changes in elderly, 58-59

Physiological values, normal, 651-654
· Pickled foods, ACS/NCI guidelines
  for cancer risk reduction, 17
PKU (*see* Phenylketonuria)
PKU-1, 525, 526, 530
PKU-2, 525, 526, 530
PKU Children's Network, address
  and phone number, 537
Plant sources of foods, 478-479
Pneumothorax, in parenteral nutri-
  tion, 404
Polymeric formulas, 387
Portal hypertension, 286
Postgastrectomy dumping syndrome,
  270-273
Postural hypertension, in Parkinson's
  disease, 290
Potassium
  altered levels (*see* Hyprkalemia;
    Hypokalemia)
  chronic renal failure and, 318, 320
    pediatric, 586, 587-588
  control, 356-357
    food exchange lists, 348-356
  estimating needs, 35
  food sources, 357-358
    high potassium, 360-361
    low potassium, 358
    moderate potassium, 359
    very high potassium, 361
  hemodialysis and, 323, 324
    pediatric, 591, 592
  infant RDA and content in milk
    sources, 431
  kidney transplantation and, 370, 371
  in liver disease, 279
  lost during exercise, 52-53
  for low-birth-weight infants, 464
  minimum requirements, 21
  in one serving from each food
    exchange group, 348
  pancreas transplantation and, 373
  in parenteral nutrition, 400
    pediatric, 607
  peritoneal dialysis and, 328, 330
    pediatric, 593
  for young athletes, 444
Potassium chloride supplements, 356-
  357
Prader-Willi syndrome, 422, 457
Predigested formulas, 387-388
Prednisone, 365, 379-380
Prefixes, 715
Pregestimil, 554
Pregnancy
  adolescent, 44-46
  diabetes and, 46-47, 167-168
  diet order, 49
  normal
    energy intake, 40-41
    nutritional needs, 41-44

Pregnancy—cont'd
  normal—cont'd
    weight gain, 40, 41
    number of daily food servings by
      group, 45
    nutritional inadequacy and, 39
    nutritional indications and ratio-
      nale, 39
    nutritional risk factors, 40
    obesity and, 46
Premature infants, 422 (*see also* Low-
  birth-weight infants)
  growth chart, 845
Preschool children, nutritional
  needs, 436-438
Preservatives, 111
President's Council on Physical
  Fitness and Sports, address and
  phone number, 26
Prochlorperazine, 297
Prograf (tacrolimus), 365
Prosthetic valve replacement, 147
Protein(s) (*see also* Amino acids)
  acute renal failure and, 316
  for adolescents, 438-439
  in athlete's diet, 54
  bone marrow transplantation and,
    381-382
  chronic renal failure and, 318-319
    pediatric, 586, 587
  control, food exchange lists, 348-356
  in cow's milk, infants and, 430, 432
  Crohn's disease and, 254
  cystic fibrosis and, 583
  developmental disabilities and, 457
  diabetes and, 158-159
    pediatric, 496-497
  dumping syndrome and, 273
  enteral nutrition and, 386
  estimating needs, 35
  failure to thrive and, 461
  fat test and, 414
  geriatric needs, 63
  glycogen storage disease and, type
    III and type VI, 517
  hemodialysis and, 323-324
    pediatric, 590, 591
  hypoglycemia and, 184
  infant RDA and content in milk
    sources, 431
  infant requirements, 427
  in ketogenic diet
    with MCT oil, 568
    without MCT oil, 563-565
  kidney transplantation and, 370
  lactation and, 48
  liver disease and, 275, 276-278, 280
  liver transplantation and, 374, 375,
    376
  for low-birth-weight infants, 464,
    467

Protein(s)—cont'd
  in maple syrup urine disease, 522
  in milk, 104-105
  nephrotic syndrome and, 333, 334
    pediatric, 596-597
  in one serving from each food
    exchange group, 348
  osteoporosis and, 207
  pancreas transplantation and, 372,
    373
  pancreaticobiliary bypass and, 201
  in parenteral nutrition, pediatric,
    606, 607
  Parkinson's disease and, 287, 288,
    289
  pediatric assessment, 423, 425
  peritoneal dialysis and, 328, 329
    pediatric, 593, 594
  phenylketonuria and, 529
  in predigested formulas, 388
  in pregnancy
    adolescents, 45
    normal, 41
  for preschool and school age chil-
    dren, 436
  products low in, 354
  requirements for ICU, ward, and
    obese patient, 33
  for sick infants, children, and ado-
    lescents, 471-472
  thoracic organ transplantation and,
    378, 379
  in vegetarian diet, 71-72
    pediatric, 447-448, 450, 451
Protein-calorie malnutrition, in cancer, 293
Protein catabolic rate (PCR), 323
Psychological factors
  in cancer, 294
  in geriatric nutrition, 59-60
  in irritable bowel syndrome, 262
  in obesity, 189, 193
Pulmonary aspiration, from tube
  feeding, 393-394
Pulmonary disease in children (*see*
  Cystic fibrosis)
Pureed diet, 82-84
Purging, in bulimia nervosa, 305, 309
Purine restriction, 344-346
Pyridoxine (*see also* Vitamin B_6), in
  parenteral nutrition, pediatric, 608

R

Radiation enteritis, restricted fiber
  diet for, 240
Radiation therapy
  before bone marrow transplant,
    side effects, 381
  nutritional effects, 296-297

Radiation therapy—cont'd
  pediatric, 576
RDAs (*see* Recommended Dietary
  Allowances)
RDIs (Reference Daily Intakes), 23
Recharge, 52
Recommended Dietary Allowances,
  18-21
  for calcium, 206
  for elderly, 63, 64
  safe and adequate intakes, 20
  sodium, chloride, and potassium
    minimum requirements, 21
  for specific vitamins and minerals, 19
REE (resting energy expenditure),
  34, 188
Reference Daily Intakes, 23
Reflux, esophageal, 226-228
Rehydration solutions, 223, 861
Renal diseases and disorders, 315-
  362, 369
  in children, 585-597
Renal failure (*see* Acute renal failure;
  Chronic renal failure)
Renal transplantation, pancreas transplantation with, 372-374
Respiratory quotient, 34-35
Resting energy expenditure, 34, 188
Restricted fiber diet, 240-242
Riboflavin
  adolescent needs, 439
  infant RDA and content in milk
    sources, 431
  in parenteral nutrition, pediatric, 608
  recommended dietary allowances, 19
  in vegetarian diet, 72
    pediatric, 448, 449
Ricelyte, 552
Rickets, 612
RQ (respiratory quotient), 34-35

S

Saccharin, 161
Salivary glands, radiation and, 296
Salt (*see* Sodium)
Salt-cured foods, ACS/NCI guidelines
  for cancer risk reduction, 17
Salt substitutes, potassium chloride,
  356-357
Satiety, early, 298, 332
Saturated fat, peritoneal dialysis and,
  328
Sauces, in glycogen storage disease,
  type I, 515
School age children, nutritional
  needs, 436-438
School lunch, in pediatric diabetes,
  497-498
Sclerotherapy, 286

Screening (*see* Nutritional screening
  and assessment)
Seashore formula for basal metabolic
  rate, 471
Seasonings
  in glycogen storage disease, type I, 515
  sodium content, 129, 130
*See*ds
  in lacto-ovo diet, pediatric, 450
  in vegan diet, pediatric, 451
Seizures, ketogenic diet and, 561-574
Selenium
  in parenteral nutrition, pediatric, 609
  recommended dietary allowances, 19
Sepsis
  in parenteral nutrition, 405, 609
  pediatric, 470, 472, 609
Serotonin, 5-HIAA test and, 415
Sexual maturation, Tanner rating
  stages, 543
Shellfish allergy, 103-104
Short bowel syndrome
  dietary recommendations, 258-259
  fat malabsorption in, 230
Short-chain fatty acids, in enteral
  nutrition, 389
Shoulder pain, in gastroplasty, 197
Sick infants, children, and adolescents, 469-470
  nutritional considerations, 470-472
  nutritional support, 472-473
Sinemet, 287, 289
Small bowel inflammation, dietary
  recommendations, 253-255
Small bowel obstruction or stricture,
  restricted fiber diet, 240
Smell, cancer and, 298
Smoked foods, ACS/NCI guidelines
  for cancer risk reduction, 17
Smoking, 138, 270
Socioeconomic factors in geriatric
  nutrition, 59
Sodium
  bone marrow transplantation and,
    382
  cardiac surgery and, 146
    pediatric, 491, 492
  chronic renal failure and, 318, 319-
    320
    pediatric, 586, 587
  congestive heart failure and, 148, 149
  content in selected foods, 128-129
  control, food exchange lists, 348-356
  cystic fibrosis and, 583
  diabetes and, pediatric, 497
  food categorization for, 130
  hemodialysis and, 323, 324
    pediatric, 591-592
  hypercalciuria and, 338
  hypertension and, 125, 127, 130-131
    pediatric, 486-487

Sodium—cont'd
  infant RDA and content in milk
    sources, 431
  kidney transplantation and, 370
  liver disease and, 278-279, 280, 281
  liver transplantation and, 376
  lost during exercise, 52-53
  for low-birth-weight infants, 464
  minimum requirements, 21
  myocardial infarction and, 150, 151
  nephrotic syndrome and, 334
    pediatric, 597
  in one serving from each food
    exchange group, 348
  pancreas transplantation and, 373
  parenteral nutrition and, 400
    pediatric, 607
  peritoneal dialysis and, 328, 330
    pediatric, 593
  in pregnancy, normal, 43
  thoracic organ transplantation and,
    378
  USDA/USDHHS guidelines, 6
  for young athletes, 444
Sodium benzoate intolerance, 112-113
Soft diet, 86-88
  mechanical, 84-86
Soups
  gluten in, 147
  in glycogen storage disease, type I,
    515
  tyramine in, 312
Southeast Asian children, growth
  graphs and, 422
Soy, terms indicating presence of, 108
Soy allergy, 107-108
Soy formulas, for infant nutrition, 430
Soy milk, in vegan diet, pediatric, 451
Spices, peptic ulcer disease and, 269
Spinal cord injury, hypercalciuria
  and, 338, 339
Sports (*see* Athletes)
Sports drinks, 51-52
Sprue, celiac, 108-109, 245-246
Sqwincher, 52
Starches
  copper in, 283
  diabetes and, pediatric, 500
  exchanges, 175-177
    for glycogen storage disease, type
      I, 514
    in ketogenic diet, without MCT
      oil, 570
    for protein, sodium, and potassi-
      um control, 350-352
  fiber content, 238-239
  glycogen storage disease and, 510-
    513
  number of food servings in preg-
    nancy, 45
  oxalate in, 342

Starches—cont'd
in restricted fiber diet, 241
sodium content, 128, 130
Starchy vegetables, exchanges in ketogenic diet, with MCT oil, 573
Starvation, in anorexia nervosa, 303, 304
Steatorrhea
in Crohn's disease, 255
in cystic fibrosis, 581
in dumping syndrome, 273
pediatric, 558, 559
in short bowel syndrome, 258
test diet for, 413-415
Steroids, 557
developmetal disability and, 458
for inflammatory bowel disease, 251
for muscle building, 24-25, 56
for nephrotic syndrome, pediatric,
596
Stress
cancer and, 294
hyperglycemia and, feeding limitations, 33
irritable bowel syndrome and, 262
Subclavian artery puncture, 404
Substance abuse, adolescent, 440
Sucrase-isomaltase deficiency, 505
Sucrose-isomaltose malabsorption, 504
Suffixes, 716
Sugar
copper in, 284
dumping syndrome and, 272
foods and beverages containing,
carbohydrate content, 163
foods high in, 170
hypertriglyceridemia and, 142
hypoglycemia, 183-185
osteoporosis and, 207
USDA/USDHHS guidelines, 6
Sulfasalazine, 251, 557
Sulfites
additives and, 120
foods containing, 120
intolerance, 119-120
Sunette (acesulfame K), 162
Supplements (see also Vitamin supplements), mineral, in pregnancy, 42
Surgery
bariatric, 196-204
cancer, nutritional effects, 295
cardiac, 146-148
pediatric, 491-492
for inflammatory bowel disease, 251
postgastrectomy dumping syndrome, 270-273
postoperative diet, 88-89
preoperative diet, 88
Swallowing difficulties (see also
Dysphagia), in cancer, 298
Sweeteners
artificial (see Artificial sweeteners)

Sweeteners—cont'd
diabetes and, 159, 161-162
flatulence and, 215
non-nutritive, 161-162
characteristics, 662-664
nutritive, 161
characteristics, 662-664
Sweet One (acesulfame K), 162
Sweets
copper in, 284
gluten in, 148
recommended intake for children
and teens, 437

T

Tacrolimus, 365
Tanner height for age and height
velocity graphs, 856-859
Tanner rating stages of maturity, 543
Tartrazine intolerance, 121
Taste
cancer and, 294, 298
radiation and, 296, 298
Teenagers (see Adolescents)
Testing (see also Laboratory entries),
diagnostic, preparatory diets, 411-
415
Thiamine
infant RDA and content in milk
sources, 431
for maple syrup urine disease, 520
in parenteral nutrition, pediatric, 608
recommended dietary allowances, 19
Thick-It, 93
Thick 'N Easy, 93
Thirst, exercise and, 51
Thoracic organ transplantation, 377
immediate post-transplant management, 379
long-term post-transplant management, 379-380
nutritional care guidelines, 378
pretransplant management, 377-379
Threonine requirements, 506
Thrombosis, in parenteral nutrition,
405
Tincture of opium, 224
Tolbutamide response testing, diet
for, 412
Tolerex, 511
Tonsillectomy, diet progression, 89
Total parenteral nutrition, 402 (see
also Parenteral nutrition entries)
Trace elements
enteral nutrition and, 386
estimating needs, 35
for low-birth-weight infants, 465-466
in parenteral nutrition, 401-402
pediatric, 608-609

Trace elements—cont'd
safe and adequate daily dietary
intake, 20
Transferrin, 425
Transplantation, 363-384
bone marrow, 380-383
diet order, 368
drug therapy side effects, 365
kidney, 369-371
liver, 374-376
low bacteria diet, 367-368
malnutrition mechanisms, 364
nutrition assessment and management
immediate post-transplantation,
364
long-term post-transplantation,
364, 366
pretransplantation, 363-364
pancreas and pancreas-renal, 372-373
thoracic organ, 377-380
Tranylcypromine, 311-312
Trauma, pediatric, 470, 471, 472
Triceps skinfold percentiles, 845
Trientine, 285
Trigeminal nerve, swallowing and, 92
Triglycerides, 135-136
elevated levels (see
Hypertriglyceridemia)
guidelines by age and sex, 137
hemodialysis and, pediatric, 592
levels in United States, 718-719
medium-chain (see Medium-chain
triglycerides)
peritoneal dialysis and, 331
pediatric, 594
Tryptophan, 288, 506
Tube feeding, 385 (see also Enteral
nutrition)
access routes, 390
administration, 390-392
complications and their prevention, 392-395
diabetes and, 168
at home, 395
indications, 386
patient education, 395
Tumor necrosis factor, cancer and,
294
Tumors, metabolic changes and, 294
Turner syndrome, 422, 454
Tyramine, food sources, 312
Tyramine controlled diet, 311-312
Tyrosinosis, 503

U

Ulcerative colitis, 250, 251 (see also
Inflammatory bowel disease)
pediatric, 557

Ulcers, 268-270
United States Department of
    Agriculture
    Dietary Guidelines for Americans,
        5-6
    food labeling standards, 21-23
    school lunch pattern, 498
United States Department of Health
    and Human Services, Dietary
    Guidelines for Americans, 5-6
Urea cycle, 503
Urea kinetic modeling, 323
    pediatric, 590
Uric acid, 344
    ketogenic diet and, 562-563
Urine, acid-ash and alkaline-ash diets,
    346-347
Urolithiasis, 335-336, 337
Urticaria, 121
USDA Dietary Guidelines for
    Americans, 5-6
USDA food labeling standards, 21-23
USDA school lunch pattern, 498
USDHHS Dietary Guidelines for
    Americans, 5-6

V

Vagus nerve, swallowing and, 92
Valine
    in maple syrup urine disease, 521-522
    requirements, 506
Van Creveld/Von Gierke's disease, 505
Vegan diet, food guide for children, 450
Vegetables
    ACS/NCI guidelines for cancer risk
        reduction, 16
    cholesterol and fat from, 141
    copper in, 284
    exchanges, 178
        in ketogenic diet, 570-571, 573
        for protein, sodium, and potassi-
            um control, 353
    fiber content, 237-238
    gluten in, 147
    glycogen storage disease and, type
        I, 515
    for infants
        dietary guidelines, 435
        phenylalanine content, 532-533
    in lacto-ovo diet, pediatric, 450
    in low residue diet, 243
    number of daily servings, 7
        in pregnancy, 45
    oxalate in, 341
    potassium in
        high, 360
        low, 358
        moderate, 359
        very high, 361

Vegetables—cont'd
    recommended intake for children
        and teens, 437
    in restricted fiber diet, 241
    sodium content, 128, 130
    tyramine in, 312
    USDA/USDHHS guidelines, 6
    in vegan diet, pediatric, 451
Vegetarian diet
    for children, 447
        dietary management goals, 449,
            452
        guide for lacto-ovo diets, 450
        guide for vegan diet, 451
        nutritional inadequacy and, 447-
            449
    classification, 71
    description, 70-71
    dietary recommendations, 71-72
    goals, 71
    nutritional inadequacy, 71
    planning and evaluating, 72-74
    sources of clinical nutrients, 448
Vertical banded gastroplasty
    complications and dietary modifi-
        cations, 197
    dietary recommendations, 197-200
    follow-up, 202
    nutritional inadequacy and, 196-197
Very low calorie diets, 158, 192
Vitamin A
    adolescent needs, 439
    cystic fibrosis and, 580
    infant RDA and content in milk
        sources, 431
    in parenteral nutrition, pediatric, 608
    recommended dietary allowances, 19
Vitamin B_1 (*see* Thiamine)
Vitamin B_2 (*see* Riboflavin)
Vitamin B_6
    deficiency, D-penicillamine and, 282
    infant RDA and content in milk
        sources, 431
Vitamin B_{12}
    deficiency, in megaloblastic anemia,
        62
    infant RDA and content in milk
        sources, 431
    lactation and, 48
    in parenteral nutrition, pediatric, 608
    in pregnancy, normal, 42
    recommended dietary allowances, 19
    in vegetarian diet, 72
        pediatric, 448-449
Vitamin B_{17}, 26-27
Vitamin C (ascorbic acid)
    infant RDA and content in milk
        sources, 431
    for low-birth-weight infants, 465
    oxalate and, 343
    in parenteral nutrition, pediatric, 608

Vitamin C—cont'd
    in pregnancy, normal, 42
    recommended dietary allowances, 19
Vitamin D
    bones and, 210
    cystic fibrosis and, 580
    hemodialysis and, 325
    infant RDA and content in milk
        sources, 431
    infant requirements, 428, 429
    lactation and, 48
    for low-birth-weight infants, 465
    osteoporosis and, 206
    in parenteral nutrition, pediatric,
        608
    in pregnancy, normal, 42
    recommended dietary allowances, 19
    in vegetarian diet, 72
        pediatric, 449
Vitamin D supplements, in lactose
    intolerance, 265
Vitamin E
    cystic fibrosis and, 580
    fraudulent claims, 24
    infant RDA and content in milk
        sources, 431
    for low-birth-weight infants, 465, 466
    in parenteral nutrition, pediatric, 608
    recommended dietary allowances, 19
Vitamin K
    cystic fibrosis and, 580
    deficiency, in parenteral nutrition,
        407
    recommended dietary allowances, 19
Vitamin K_1, in parenteral nutrition,
    pediatric, 608
Vitamins
    in athlete's diet, 54-55
    deficiencies in elderly, 64
    enteral nutrition and, 386
    estimating needs, 35
    fraudulent claims, 23, 26
    in hemodialysis, pediatric, 591, 592
    infant requirements, 428
    liver disease and, 279
    for low-birth-weight infants, 465-466
    multiple vitamin preparations, 736-
        739
    in parenteral nutrition, 400, 401
        pediatric, 608
    in peritoneal dialysis, pediatric,
        593, 594
    for preschool and school age chil-
        dren, 436
    recommended dietary allowances, 19
    sources, functions, deficiency, and
        toxic effects, 742-744
    in vegetarian diet, pediatric, 448-449
    for young athletes, 444-445
Vitamin supplements
    chronic illness and, 26

Vitamin supplements—cont'd
  chronic renal failure and, pediatric, 588
  cystic fibrosis and, 579-580
  diarrhea and, 22
  in pregnancy, normal, 42
VLCDs (very low calorie diets), 158, 192
Vomiting
  cancer and, 295, 298
  diabetes and, pediatric, 499-500
  gastroplasty and, 197
  ketogenic diet and, 562
  from tube feeding, 393
    pediatric, 604

W

Water (*see also* Fluids)
  constipation and encopresis and, 549, 550
  enteral nutrition and, 386
    pediatric requirements, 604
  in milk sources for infants, 431
  sodium content, 131
Weight
  ACS/NCI guidelines for cancer risk reduction, 16
  in anorexia nervosa treatment, 309
  of athletes, 53
    competing weight for young athletes, 445-446
  in bulimia nervosa treatment, 310
  cardiovascular risk and, 139
  change in, 32
  desirable, determination, 186, 190
  diabetes and, 156, 158
    pediatric, 497
  excessive (*see* Obesity)
  failure to thrive and, 459, 461
  hypertension and, 124-125, 127
    pediatric, 483, 486
  low at birth, 463-469

Weight—cont'd
  nutritional misinformation and, 25
  in nutritional screening and assessment, 31-32
  pediatric development and, 421, 422
  standards, 186
  USDA/USDHHS guidelines, 5
Weight control, pediatric, 539
  assessment, 541
  blood pressure and, 483
  caloric allowances, 541
  caloric needs by activity level, 542, 543
  dietary management goals, 541
  dietary recommendations, 541-544
  indications and rationale, 540
  long-term weight-control guidelines, 544-545
  nutritional inadequacy and, 540
Weight for height tables
  for adults, 647-650
  for older children, 829-831
Weight gain
  breast cancer and, 296, 300
  cancer and, 300
  gastroplasty and, 197
  peritoneal dialysis and, 331
  in pregnancy
    normal, 40, 41
    obese patients, 46
  transplantation and, 366
Weight loss
  in anorexia nervosa, 303, 304
  bariatric surgery for, 195-196
  chronic renal failure and, 319
  diets, 185, 192
  gastroplasty for, diabetes and, 168
  hemodialysis and, 324
  pancreatic cancer and, 295
  Parkinson's disease and, 289
Wheat
  foods containing, breath hydrogen concentration and, 412
  terms indicating presence of, 109

Wheat allergy, 108-110
Wheat flour substitutes, 110, 249
Whey proteins, 104, 105
Whipping cream exchange in ketogenic diet, 571
Wilson's disease, 279
  dietary recommendations, 285
  indications and rationale, 282, 285
  management, 282
  nutritional inadequacy and, 282
World Health Organization, Program for Control of Diarrheal Diseases, 553-554

Y

Yogurt, lactose intolerance and, 267
Yogurt juices for infants, phenylalanine content, 534

Z

Zinc
  infant RDA and content in milk sources, 431
  liver disease and, 279
  for low-birth-weight infants, 465, 466
  parenteral nutrition and deficiency, 407
    pediatric, 608
  in pregnancy, normal, 42
  recommended dietary allowances, 19
  in vegetarian diet, 72
    pediatric, 448, 449

HELP US BUILD BETTER BOOKS

Mayo Clinic Diet Manual, 7th Edition, (23782)

ABOUT YOURSELF:

Name:

Title:

Business Address:

ABOUT THIS BOOK:

How/When do you use this book?

What did you like best?

Least?

How can we Improve?

Has your institution adopted this manual for its use?   ❑ **YES**   ❑ **NO**

   If yes, what is the institution:

Thank you. Your comments are very important to us!

Please send this form to:
Mosby
Medical Editorial
11830 Westline Industrial Drive
St. Louis, MO 63146